CURRENT CLINICAL UROLOGY

ERIC A. KLEIN, MD, SERIES EDITOR

For other titles published in the series, go to
www.springer.com/series/7635

Bladder Cancer

Diagnosis, Therapeutics, and Management

Edited by
Cheryl T. Lee, M.D.
and
David P. Wood, M.D.

Humana Press

Editors:
Cheryl T. Lee, MD
Department of Urology
University of Michigan
Ann Arbor, MI
USA

David P. Wood, MD
Department of Urology
University of Michigan
Ann Arbor, MI
USA

Series Editor
Eric A. Klein, MD
Professor of Surgery
Cleveland Clinic Lerner College of Medicine
Head, Section of Urologic Oncology
Glickman Urological and Kidney Institute
Cleveland, OH

ISBN: 978-1-58829-988-8 e-ISBN: 978-1-59745-417-9
DOI 10.1007/978-1-59745-417-9

Library of Congress Control Number: 2009921444

Printed on acid-free paper

springer.com

This book is dedicated to William Joseph Amato, an individual who has contributed greatly to my personal and professional development. He is my friend, my confidant, and my husband.

We also dedicate this book to the memory of Dr. Saroja Adusumilli.

Preface

Bladder cancer continues to be a major disease affecting the healthcare system in the United States, consuming almost $3 billion annually. Patients at low risk for disease-related death require long-term surveillance because of high recurrence rates. Treatment of intermediate- and high-risk disease requires complex management that is often misapplied due to difficulties in tumor staging and uncertainty about the natural history of non–muscle-invasive cancers. Radical surgery for muscle-invasive disease is underutilized because of concerns about complications, surgical technique, altered quality of life, and diminished reimbursement. Neoadjuvant chemotherapy is rarely incorporated in the management of locally advanced tumors, despite mounting evidence that it offers a modest, but real, survival advantage. Metastatic disease remains a deadly condition, as systemic therapies are largely palliative and not curative. Taken together, there are many challenging hurdles for clinicians when managing patients with this disease. Unfortunately, real progress in improving life expectancy from the disease has been slow.

A fundamental lack of clinical research in the field, coupled with disproportionately low funding from federal and foundation sources, has limited advances in multidisciplinary bladder cancer care. As a result, our practice patterns in 2008 are surprisingly similar to those in 1988. In consideration of the major challenges facing patients and providers, we developed this text focused on clinical management. Within *Bladder Cancer: Diagnosis, Therapeutics, and Management*, a group of accomplished authors examine emerging techniques and strategies developed to address common clinical scenarios. Authors provide insight into obstacles to improved survival, discuss methods to advance the field, and review the related supporting evidence. Our intended goal in creating this text is not to create a summary of bladder cancer, but to spur innovative thoughts and approaches to common problems in the management of early and advanced stage of the disease.

The book consists of four parts addressing diagnostics, surgical technique, and multidisciplinary care. Part I is dedicated to bladder cancer staging, which continues to plague clinicians who unknowingly understage 40–60% of patients. Inaccurate staging greatly undermines therapeutic efficacy and often leaves the patient undertreated. This section particularly focuses on understaging of invasive bladder cancer as well as improved pelvic staging with updated imaging. Part II addresses optimization of treatment for localized disease. Novel approaches to intravesical therapy are discussed, as are specific surgical techniques used to ensure cancer control but also provide improved organ preservation and quality of life. Part III briefly reviews applications of existing systemic therapies in the treatment of locally advanced tumors and metastatic disease. Consideration is given to new types of systemic therapies used in combination with standard drugs to provide a synergistic effect. Finally, Part IV is devoted to a discussion of infrastructure needed to support the translational research efforts that will propel this field forward. Contributors in this and earlier sections represent a mix of seasoned veterans and junior scientists representing the next generation to embrace novel technologies and innovative practice strategies.

Ann Arbor, MI, USA — Cheryl T. Lee
Ann Arbor, MI, USA — David P. Wood

Contents

Contributors

Saroja Adusumilli
Department of Radiology, University of Michigan, Ann Arbor, MI, USA

Tara Allen
Department of Urology, University of Arkansas, Little Rock, AK, USA

David Berger
Section of Urological Surgery, Kansas University, Kansas City, KS, USA

Bernard H. Bochner
Division of Urology, Memorial Sloan Kettering Cancer Center, New York, NY, USA

Stephen Boorjian
Department of Urology, Cornell University, New York, NY, USA

Deborah Bradley
Division of Hematology-Oncology, University of Michigan, Ann Arbor, MI, USA

Marta Sanchez-Carbayo
Tumor Markers Group, Spanish National Cancer Center, Madrid, Spain

Carlos Cordon-Cardo
Department of Pathology, Division of Molecular Pathology, Columbia University, New York, NY, USA

Sam S. Chang
Department of Urologic Surgery, Vanderbilt University, Nashville, TN, USA

Karen Giselle Chee
Division of Hematology-Oncology, University of California, Davis Cancer Center, Sacramento, CA, USA

Richard H. Cohan
Department of Radiology, University of Michigan, Ann Arbor, MI, USA

Jonathon Coleman
Division of Urology, Memorial Sloan-Kettering Cancer Center, New York, NY, USA

Michael S. Cookson
Department of Urologic Surgery, Vanderbilt University, Nashville, TN, USA

Matthew R. Cooperberg
Department of Urology, University of California San Francisco, San Francisco, CA, USA

Guido Dalbagni
Department of Urology, Memorial Sloan Kettering Cancer Center, New York, NY, USA

Thomas A. Gardiner
Department of Urology, Indiana University, Bloomington, IN, USA

Scott M. Gilbert
Department of Urology, University of Michigan, Ann Arbor, MI, USA

Timothy Gilligan
Department of Solid Tumor Oncology, Cleveland Clinic Clinic Taussig Cancer, Cleveland, OH, USA

Mark. L. Gonzalgo
Department of Urology, Johns Hopkins University School of Medicine, Baltimore, MD, USA

Graham Greene
Department of Urology, University of Arkansas for Medical Sciences, Little Rock, AK, USA

H. Barton Grossman
Department of Urology, The University of Texas, MD Anderson Cancer Center, Houston, TX, USA

Jeffrey M. Holzbeierlein
Section of Urological Surgery, Kansas University, Kansas City, KS, USA

Hero Hussain
Department of Radiology, University of Michigan, Ann Arbor, MI, USA

Maha Hussain
Division of Hematology-Oncology, University of Michigan Medical Center, Ann Arbor, MI, USA

Niels-Erik B. Jacobsen
Department of Urology, Indiana University School of Medicine, Bloomington, IN, USA

Shida Jin
Clinical Research Informations Systems, University of Texas, MD Anderson Cancer Center, Houston, TX, USA

J. Stephen Jones
Glickman Urological Institute, Cleveland Clinic Foundation, Cleveland, OH, USA

Nicholas Karanikolas
State University of New York, Downstate, Brooklyn, NY, USA

Badrinath R. Konety
Department of Urology, University of California San Francisco, San Francisco, CA, USA

Primo N. Lara
Division of Hematology-Oncology, University of California, Davis Cancer Center, Sacramento, CA, USA

Jerilyn M. Latini
Department of Urology, University of Michigan, Ann Arbor, MI, USA

Cheryl T. Lee
Department of Urology, University of Michigan, Ann Arbor, MI, USA

Ralph Madeb
Department of Urology, University of Rochester, Rochester, NY, USA

James M. McKiernan
Department of Urology, Columbia University Medical Center, New York, NY, USA

Edward Messing
Department of Urology, University of Rochester, Rochester, NY, USA

Randall E. Milikan
Department of Genitourinary Medical Oncology, University of Texas, MD Anderson Cancer Center, Houston, TX, USA

Lambda Msezane
Section of Urology, University of Chicago, Chicago, IL, USA

Matthew E. Nielsen
Department of Urology, Johns Hopkins University School of Medicine, Baltimore, MD, USA

Phillip M. Pierorazio
Department of Urology, Columbia University Medical Center, New York, NY, USA

Morand Piert
Department of Radiology, Division of Nuclear Medicine, University of Michigan, Ann Arbor, MI, USA

Marcus L. Quek
Department of Urology, Loyola University Stritch School of Medicine, Maywood, IL, USA

Ganesh V. Raj
Division of Urology, Memorial Sloan Kettering Cancer Center, New York, NY, USA

Edward M. Schaeffer
Department of Urology, Johns Hopkins University School of Medicine, Baltimore, MD, USA

Douglas S. Scherr
Department of Urology, New York Presbyterian Hospital-Weill Cornell University, New York, NY, USA

Mark P. Schoenberg
Department of Urology, Johns Hopkins University School of Medicine, Baltimore, MD, USA

Timothy Schuster
Department of Urology, University of Michigan, Ann Arbor, MI, USA

Stephen Smith
Department of Solid Tumor Oncology, Cleveland Clinic Foundation, Cleveland, OH, USA

Philippe E. Spiess
Department of Urology, MD Anderson Cancer Center, Houston, TX, USA

Andrew A. Stec
Department of Urologic Surgery, Vanderbilt University, Nashville, TN, USA

Gary D. Steinberg
Section of Urology, University of Chicago, Chicago, IL, USA

Daniel Theodorescu
Department of Medicine, University of Virginia, Charlottesville, VA, USA

Christopher Y. Thomas
Division of Hematology-Oncology, University of Virginia, Charlottesville, VA, USA

Alon Z. Weizer
Department of Urology, University of Michigan, Ann Arbor, MI, USA

Jon M. Willatt
Department of Radiology, University of Michigan, Ann Arbor, MI, USA

David P. Wood Jr.
Department of Urology, University of Michigan, Ann Arbor, MI, USA

Michael E. Woods
Department of Urology, Loyola University Stritch School of Medicine, Maywood, IL, USA

Stuart O. Zimmerman
Clinical Research Informations Systems, University of Texas, MD Anderson Cancer Center, Houston, TX, USA

Part I
Improving Bladder Cancer Staging

Section 1
CIS

1
Approaches to Carcinoma In Situ (CIS)

J. Stephen Jones

Contents

Abstract Despite its traditional categorization as "superficial," Carcinoma in situ (CIS) is a high grade, flat, noninvasive bladder cancer confined to the urothelium. Bladder biopsy is required to establish a diagnosis. Cytology to examine voided or bladder wash urine can allow identification of malignant cells, but failure to recognize such cells does not rule out CIS. Options to improve cystoscopic recognition of malignant areas such as fluorescence cystoscopy and narrow band imaging are promising developments. A number of tumor markers have been developed. Most have high sensitivity, but these tests have varying specificity. The urologist must understand the implications of a negative or positive test in order to successfully integrate these tests into clinical practice.

Keywords Carcinoma in situ, Cytology, Cystoscopy, Intravesical therapy, Surveillance

1. Introduction

Malignant urothelial tumors confined to the bladder mucosa are accurately termed nonmuscle invasive instead of being given the traditional "superficial" label (1, 2). The traditional term suggested that all such tumors shared the relatively benign course of low grade papillary tumors. In contrast, patients with highly malignant lesions, including carcinoma in situ (CIS), actually have a serious prognosis if not recognized and treated successfully. CIS is often

From: *Current Clinical Urology: Bladder Cancer*, Edited by: C.T. Lee and D.P. Wood,
DOI: 10.1007/978-1-59745-417-9_1,

mischaracterized as "premalignant" (3), but by definition it is actually a flat, noninvasive high grade urothelial carcinoma (UC) (Figs. 1 and 2). CIS is regarded as a precursor lesion for the development of invasive high-grade cancer that has simply been identified prior to invasion of the lamina propria. These lesions comprise 10% of bladder cancer (4).

The presence of CIS is usually suspected by hematuria or irritative voiding symptoms. Patients with macroscopic (gross) hematuria have reported rates of bladder cancer of 13–34.5% (5, 6). Bladder cancer is identified in 0.5–10.5% of patients with microscopic hematuria (7–10). The presence of irritative voiding symptoms doubled the risk in one study (5 vs. 10.5%) (10). The Mayo Clinic reported that 80% of patients with CIS presented with irritative symptoms (11). In a large review of patients diagnosed with interstitial cystitis, 1% had a missed diagnosis of CIS or UC. Two-thirds of these patients did not have hematuria (12). The presence of irritative voiding symptoms has been associated with diffuse disease, invasion, and a compromised prognosis, but there is no consensus on this finding in the literature (1, 3). Thus, cystoscopy and upper tract imaging are indicated in patients with hematuria and/or unexplained irritative symptoms (13).

2. Pathology

The bladder has three histological layers: (1) urothelium, (2) suburothelial loose connective tissue (lamina propria), and (3) detrusor or muscularis propria. CIS is a flat, high-grade lesion confined to the lamina propria. The TNM staging system for nonmuscle invasive tumors is shown in Fig. 1.1.

CIS lesions are comprised of severely dysplastic urothelium, and in older series were often categorized as "severe dysplasia." Disorderly histology with nuclear atypia characteristic of high-grade malignancy is microscopically diagnostic. Denudement of some or all of the mucosa due to loss of cellular cohesion is often identified. Most pathologists consider mild versions of dysplasia or atypia to be benign. However, lesions interpreted as severe dysplasia or severe atypia are now regarded as being the same entity as CIS (2). Precise communication between pathologist and urologist can minimize the risk for misinterpretation.

Between 40 and 83% of patients with CIS will develop muscle invasion if untreated, especially if associated with papillary tumors (14). Among patients believed to have CIS alone, as many as 20% who are treated with cystectomy are found to contain invasive

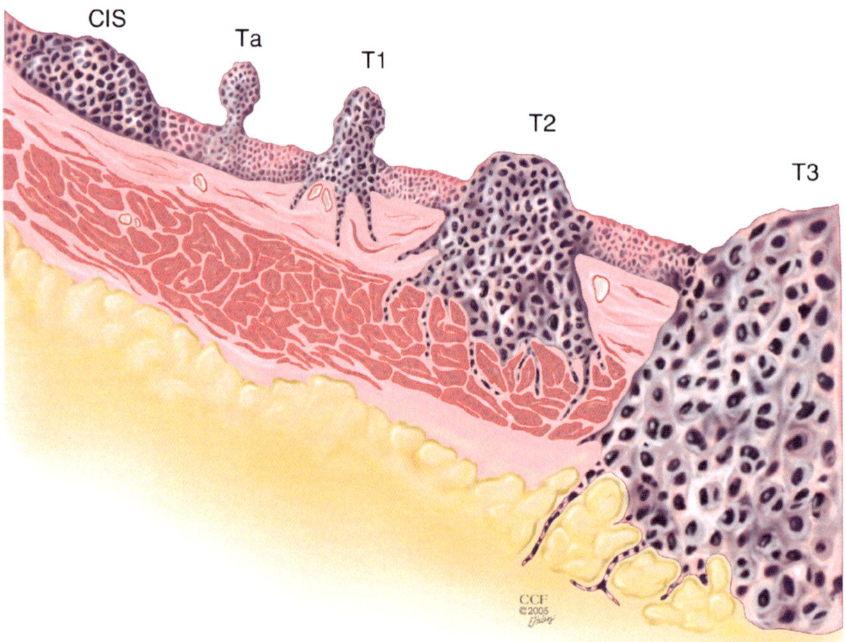

Fig. 1.1. CIS is a high-grade, flat malignancy confined to the urothelium.

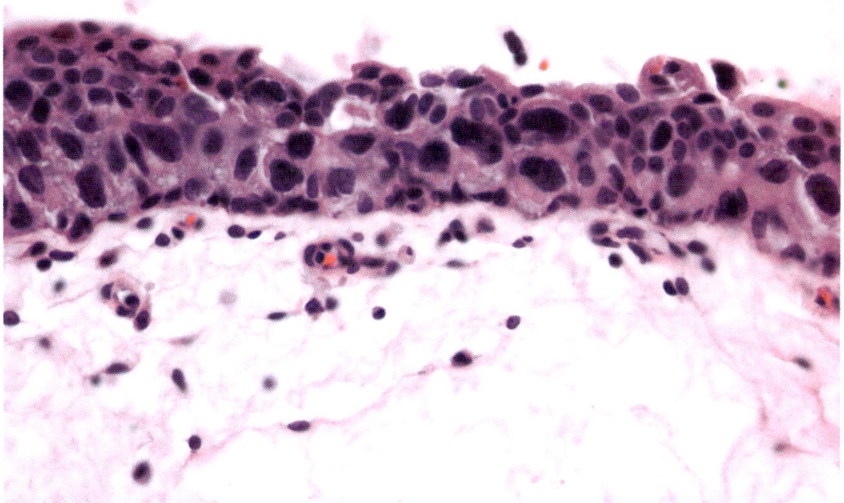

FIG. 1.2. CIS exhibits severe irregularity of cellular structure and nuclear pleomorphism

solid tumors on final pathology (15). The presence of CIS in cystectomy specimens performed for presumed T1 tumors was associated with upstaging in over half of the patients, compared to 6% upstaging in patients without CIS, in a recent series (16). Multicentricity of CIS is especially prone to progression (17). In a large series, presence of CIS was the second most important prognostic factor after grade (18).

There is a substantial risk of underestimation of the probability of progression in some patients with presumed "superficial" disease, and the risk of underestimation of the disease status based on sampling errors as shown in Tables 1.1 and 1.2.

3. Endoscopic Diagnosis

The goal of endoscopic biopsy is to provide specimens for pathological examination, and to remove all visibly abnormal tissue. Due to its tendency for multifocality, complete endoscopic eradication is often not feasible. Excessive use of electrocautery causes cellular reorientation and creates difficulty in the interpretation the pathology, so "cold cup" biopsies are the mainstay of diagnosis. Sampling of erythematous or otherwise suspicious mucosa is occasionally the source of tissue diagnostics for CIS, but normal-appearing tissue in patients with positive or suspicious cytology is often the actual site of CIS as described below.

A number of "tumor markers" have been developed to assist in the management of these patients. Several are approved in the United States for surveillance in patients with known bladder cancer, but most are not approved for initial diagnosis or screening, so are considered below along with conventional urinary cytology in the section labeled "Surveillance Strategies."

4. "Random" Biopsies

CIS can exist in normal-appearing urothelium, so some random biopsies are often performed to identify CIS in patients undergoing surgery for visible tumors, in patients with positive cytology, or in those following intravesical or surgical therapy. However, the value of doing so is largely unproved. Random biopsies in high-risk patients were positive in 12.4% in one report, and altered treatment in 7%, including 14 of 1,033 patients in whom the only positive tissue was in the random biopsy – not in the area appearing abnormal (19). However, even when velvety red patches were biopsied in one report, only 11.9% of samples were positive (20). Fujimoto et al. prospectively evaluated the role of random biopsies of normal-appearing

TABLE 1.1. Estimates of disease progression in nonmuscle-invasive bladder cancer WHO/International society of Urological Pathology Consensus Classification (*source*: [102]).

Tumor type	% Relative frequency	% Progression	% Deaths
Noninvasive			
Papilloma	10	0–1	0
PUNLMP	20	3	0–1
Papillary cancer low grade (TaG1)	20	5–10	1–5
Papillary cancer high grade (TaG3)	30	15–40	10–25
Invasive			
Papillary cancer (T1G3)	20	30–50	33
CIS			
Primary	10	>50	–
Secondary	90		

TABLE 1.2. Risk of understaging when cystectomy is performed for presumed nonmuscle-invasive disease (*source*: [103]).

Author	Institution	Year	Risk (%) of understaging
Ghoneim et al.	Urology and Nephrology Center Mansoura, Egypt	1997	62
Stein et al.	USC	2000	39
Dutta et al.	Vanderbilt	2001	40
Bianco et al.	Wayne State University	2004	27
Bayraktar	Vakif Gureba Hospital Urology Department Aksaray-Istanbul, Turkey	2004	50
Huguet et al.	Servicio de Urologia, Fundacion Puigvert Barcelona	2005	27
Ficarra et al.	University of Verona, Italy	2005	43

urothelium and found cancer in only 8 of 100 biopsies, five of which were CIS. They concluded that random biopsies are indicated only in the setting of multiple tumors or positive cytology (21). An EORTC retrospective review concluded that random biopsies were not warranted because only 10% were positive (3.5% CIS) (22). As a result, current consensus is that random biopsies are not indicated in low-risk patients, i.e., those with low-grade papillary tumors and negative cytology, but may be of value in high risk patients such as those with high grade or multiple tumors, especially in patients with a history of CIS. Random biopsies are always indicated in the setting of a positive urinary cytology in the absence of abnormal cystoscopic findings.

Prostatic urethral biopsy using the cutting loop will occasionally identify urethral CIS, but bleeding may be more common (23). The theoretical risk that random biopsies provide an exposed bed for tumor implantation must be weighed against the additional value of the information obtained (24–26).

5. Diagnostic Strategies Following Intravesical Therapy

American urologists use BCG by a 2:1 margin compared to intravesical chemotherapy, whereas European urologists favor chemotherapy. The initial tumor-free response rate is as high as 80% (27–30). Approximately 50% of the patients experience a durable response for a median period of 4 years. Over a 10-year period, approximately 30% of the patients remain free of tumor progression or recurrence, so diligent surveillance is mandatory. The majority of these occur within the first 5 years (31). Herr reported progression in 19% of initial responders at 5 years, but 95% in nonresponders – findings confirmed by other investigators (32, 33).

The necessity of biopsy to determine a BCG response is unclear, although it should be strongly considered in high risk patients to determine disease status at this key point in time. Urine cytology can be useful in this setting, as a positive result is in essence a positive biopsy of the shed urothelium. Dalbagni reported minimal utility in routine biopsy following BCG if cystoscopy and urinary cytology were both negative. Whereas 5/11 patients with erythematous bladder mucosa and positive cytology had positive bladder biopsies, none of 37 with erythematous lesions and negative cytology was positive, and only 1/13 patients with a normal mucosa had positive biopsies (34). Other studies have suggested that the value of routine post-BCG biopsy is limited (35). UroVysion FISH (Abbott Molecular, Chicago IL. See below) conversion from positive to negative has been shown to correlate with BCG response in a single-center study (36).

Declaring failure may take up to 6 months, as the response rate for patients with high grade bladder cancer treated with BCG rose from 57 to 80% between 3 and 6 months after therapy. Tumoricidal activity clearly continues for some period after cessation of therapy. This has obvious implications not only for declaring BCG failure and the need for subsequent therapy, but also for the interpretation of success rates of salvage protocols if administered soon after therapy (37).

6. Fluorescence Cystoscopy

Endoscopically, urologists suspect CIS on the basis of the presence of visible changes such as mucosal edema, denudement or "red spots." However, CIS often creates no visible abnormalities, and it appears likely that the classic visible changes may be due solely to an inflammatory reaction and not to the actual CIS. A multicenter study found that 37% of the biopsies performed on the basis of suspicious endoscopic findings resulted in false negative biopsy (38). The failure of cystoscopy to identify all tumor for removal potentially explains the high rate of cancer recurrence soon after complete removal of all visible tumors (tumor cell implantation also contributing as described above). The most complete consideration of such issues has been in studies of fluorescence cystoscopy as described in the following chapter.

7. Molecular Aspects of CIS

Like most malignancies, CIS is a genetic disease. Chromosomal alterations caused by oxidative DNA damage create genetic abnormalities in tissues of the affected organ. There appear to be two separate genetic pathways leading to the development of urothelial carcinoma (39, 40). One leads to noninvasive, papillary tumors that tend to recur frequently, but rarely progress. These cancers usually follow an indolent course unless they convert to the second pathway, which occurs in less than 5% of cases (41). The second pathway leads to the development of CIS and ultimately to its natural outcome of invasive high-grade cancer.

Such genetic alterations can be evaluated using karyotyping, microsatellite analysis for allelic imbalance (42), comparative genomic hybridization (43), DNA ploidy analysis by flow cytometry (44), or fluorescence in situ hybridization (FISH) of probes or labels to site-specific chromosomal abnormalities (45). These technologies have allowed for the discovery that noninvasive papillary tumors tend to demonstrate relatively few chromosomal abnormalities, primarily involving loss of all or part of chromosome 9 and its p16 tumor suppressor gene at the 9p21 locus. In contrast, high-grade tumors (whether CIS, T1, or invasive) tend to have numerous and greatly variable chromosomal gains and losses. In addition to their relatively predictable aneuploidy, high-grade tumors also often have loss of all or part of chromosome 9 as the initial step in malignant degeneration (46). Although almost any chromosome can be affected, aneuploidy of chromosomes 7, 9, and 17 appear to be indicative of especially aggressive tumors (47–49).

Most solid tumors exhibit a marked degree of chromosomal instability, such that different cells of the tumor exhibit significant karyotypic variation. In combination with aneuploidy, this is virtually pathognomonic of the malignancy (50). Moreover, the degree of aneuploidy is related to the likelihood of progression to invasive disease (51–53).

Currently there is no known molecular marker to accurately predict progression from CIS to invasive disease. However, p53, pRb, or other molecular markers have been proposed as potential predictors of prognosis. Patients with p53-negative lesions progress 25% of the time, compared to the 75% progression rate for p53 positive lesions. Ten-year survival is 60% in patients with p53-positive lesions, and 88% in patients with p53-negative lesions (54). Nuclear p53 overexpression before BCG therapy has not been shown to predict response to therapy, but posttherapy p53 overexpression suggests a high likelihood of the disease progression (55, 56).

Other studies have failed to find a clear role for p53 status, so the role of p53 for the prediction of tumor behavior and response to therapy remains unclear, but the subject of intense investigation (57).

Multiple investigators are pursuing molecular markers to predict progression as well as markers to provide therapeutic targets.

8. Surveillance Strategies

According to the Agency for Health Care Policy and Research, annual expenditures are $2.2 billion for bladder cancer vs. $1.4 billion for prostate cancer (Donat 2003, 58 (102)). A significant portion of this cost is due to the potential need for lifelong surveillance, especially in high risk patients such as those with CIS (58).

Despite these financial resources, in an era of high-technology medical diagnostics, UC surveillance remains dominated by subjective modalities that rely on phenotypic alterations significant enough for the interpreter to differentiate the malignant from the normal structure (cystoscopy) or histology (conventional urinary cytology). Most protocols include this combination every 3 months for 18–24 months after the initial diagnosis, then every 6 months for the following 2 years, and then annually, resetting the clock with each newly identified tumor (59). Their traditional presumed status as the "gold standard" has been widely accepted despite evidence that both suffer from accuracy limitations (60). In addition, only 40% of patients fully comply with a standard surveillance protocol (61).

General guidelines for bladder cancer surveillance are shown in Table 1.3.

9. Cystoscopic Surveillance

Cystoscopy is a rapid, relatively painless method to visualize the urothelium in the office setting. The endoscopic appearance of CIS is classically described as a velvety red mucosal patch, although this finding has been shown to be unreliable as discussed above. The role of cystoscopy as a "gold standard" in cancer detection has come under scrutiny with the emergence of tumor markers and the development of newer endoscopic technology, including fluorescence cystoscopy (62).

Most lesions believed to be malignant are proven so pathologically, although the classic description of CIS is often absent (63, 64). Flexible fiberoptic cystoscopes are almost as sensitive, and are markedly more comfortable for men compared to rigid rod lens systems (65, 66), although there is no clear advantage to their use in women due to the short, relatively straight female urethra. Phase II studies reportedly show that flexible office-based fluorescence cystoscopy can improve the detection of CIS (67, 68). Moreover, the use of Narrow Band Imaging or NBI (Olympus Surgical, USA) in order to define differences in tissue vascularization has allowed identification of CIS in areas that appear normal by white light cystoscopy (unpublished data). This technology is under consideration for approval by the U.S. Food and Drug Administration (FDA) based on previous and ongoing investigations at our institution.

The vast majority of both men and women tolerate office-based cystoscopy with minimal discomfort.

TABLE 1.3. Surveillance strategies (*source*: Jones (45)).

Risk	Tumor status	Cystoscopy schedule	Upper tract imaging
Low	Solitary TaG1	3 months following initial resection Annually beginning 9 months after initial surveillance if no recurrence Consider cessation at 5 or more years Consider cytology or tumor markers	Not necessary unless hematuria present
Intermediate	Multiple TaG1 Large tumor Recurrence at 3 months	Q 3 months for 1–2 years Semiannual or annual after 2 years Consider cytology or tumor markers Restart clock with each recurrence	Consider imaging, especially for recurrence Imaging for hematuria
High	Any High Grade (inc. CIS)	Q 3 months for 2 years Semiannual for 2 years Annually for lifetime Cytology at same schedule Consider tumor markers Restart clock with each recurrence	Imaging annually for 2 years, then consider lengthening interval

Most studies have failed to identify benefit to intraurethral lidocaine injection (69, 70), and recent studies actually found that the experience of pain was higher with the use of local anesthetics than in patients cystoscoped using aqueous lubricant alone (71–73). Use of a video monitor allows the patient to see and understand the findings, theoretically distracting them from discomfort. Men who are unable to do so experience almost twice as much pain (14.1 vs. 22.9 $p < 0.01$) as those who can see their findings on the monitor. This has not been found to be of significant benefit in women for unclear reasons (74).

10. Urine Cytology

Urinary cytology is not a laboratory test. Rather, it is a pathologist's interpretation of the morphological features of dislodged urothelial cells. Poor cellular cohesion in CIS enhances the yield of cytology (Figs. 1.3 and 1.4). Its very high specificity is the strongest feature of cytology, because a positive reading even in the absence of cystoscopic or radiographic findings suggests the existence of malignancy in the vast majority of patients. Patients with a negative workup (cystoscopy and upper tract imaging) and a persistently positive cytology are found to have genitourinary cancer within 24 months (mean 5.6 months) in 40% of the cases (75).

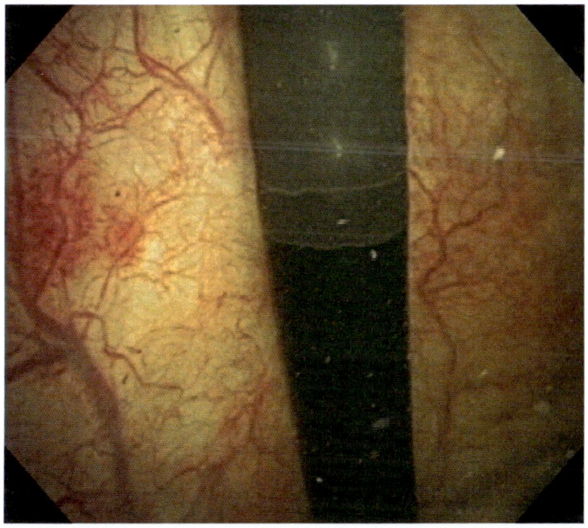

FIG. 1.3. Narrow band imaging allows enhanced visualization of tissue characteristics based on differences in vascularization. The classic appearance of CIS is a "red velvety patch." If vascularity is only slightly increased, this may not be obvious

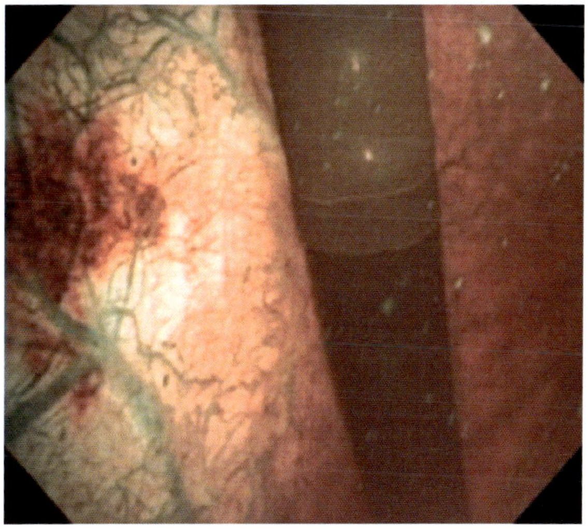

FIG. 1.4. Subtle changes in Fig. 3 become obvious when visualized with NBI technology in Fig. 4

Bladder irrigation (or barbotage) dislodges cells with poor cellular cohesion, which is common in CIS. This increases the cellularity available for evaluation compared to voided urine. Nevertheless, Murphy et al. showed that urine collected cystoscopically prior to obtaining a bladder wash provided additional diagnostic information. Bladder washings had a higher yield in their study of 313 patients, but 13.1% of cancers would have been missed in bladder washings alone. Moreover, mechanical trauma has the potential to create cellular alterations that might interfere with the interpretation (76). Radiographic contrast has also been implicated in creating fragmentation, nuclear pyknosis, cellular shrinkage, and cytoplasmic vacuolization that might lead to a false positive reading, especially when injected for retrograde pyelography (77). This appears to be less likely with low osmolar ionic as well as nonionic contrast media (78).

Recent studies fail to support the traditional reputation of cytology as being highly accurate for high grade lesions such as CIS. The Mayo Clinic recently observed that only 58% of bladder tumors were identified using cytology. Its sensitivity was not limited to low-grade tumors, as only 71% of high-grade cancers were identified. They reviewed the literature and found that series published after 1990 reported that cytology only identified 11% of grade 1, 31% of grade 2, and 60% of grade 3 tumors (79). These recent findings were well below those reported prior to 1990, when their review found that the sensitivity of cytology was 94% for grade 3 tumors in published reports. The authors identified no explanation for this deterioration. A change in the stringency of cytological criteria for determining a case as positive was ruled out, as the very high specificity for studies before and after 1990 was not significantly different and was consistent with specificity in their own laboratory. These findings are consistent with numerous other studies, most strikingly by a recent multicenter study involving several institutions noted for bladder cancer expertise that found cytology had an overall sensitivity of 15.8% (80).

Thus, cytology has very high specificity, but low sensitivity for both high-grade and low-grade tumors, including CIS, in recently published reports (Fig. 1.5).

11. Tumor Markers

Based on the limitations of cytology, several biomarkers have been developed for diagnosis or surveillance. Most have adequate sensitivity but poor specificity and costs usually exceeding that for cytology. The most significant issue limiting widespread adoption of tumor markers is the lack of prospective data to support their impact on prognosis or disease management (81). Moreover, incomplete understanding of the significance of positive or negative marker results based on unclear levels of positive predictive value and negative predictive value create a scenario where clinicians often receive test results that do not / clarify whether the patient is likely or unlikely to have bladder cancer. The economic impact of a false-positive cancer test in a screening population was calculated to be $1,024 for women and $1,171 for men, so tests with low specificity can lead to significant negative consequence even in the absence of malignancy (82). Despite continuing advances including those described herein, the above issues will limit the role of tumor markers in the foreseeable future.

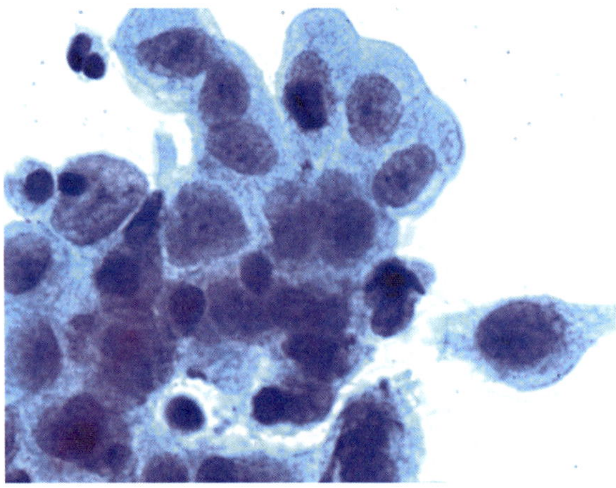

FIG. 1.5. CIS (40×) exhibits severe irregularity of cellular structure and nuclear pleomorphism. The lamina propria is uninvolved

Tumor markers can either be point-of-care tests (performed in the office) or laboratory based. These tests identify factors at different levels of cancer cell evolution, including tumor-associated antigens, blood group antigens, growth factors, cell cycle/apoptosis, and extracellular matrix proteins.

The qualitative point-of-care test, BTA stat® (Polymedco, Inc., Cortlandt Manor, NY, USA), and the quantitative BTA TRAK® (Polymedco) assays detect the human complement factor H-related protein. The sensitivity of these tests ranges from 50 to 80%, with a specificity of 50–75%. These tests are more sensitive than cytology, but can be falsely positive in patients with inflammation, infection, caffeine, nicotine, acetaminophen, acetyl salicylic acid or hematuria (83, 84). They are approved by the FDA for UC surveillance.

ImmunoCyt™ (DiagnoCure, Inc., Saint Foy, Canada) is a hybrid of cytology and an immunofluorescence assay. Three fluorescent-labeled monoclonal antibodies are targeted at a UC variant of CEA and two bladder mucins. Sensitivity and specificity are reported to be 86 and 79%, respectively. It has not been shown to be significantly affected by benign conditions, but adoption has been limited because interpretation is complex and requires a highly trained laboratory technician at this time (85, 86). This test is approved for UC surveillance.

The NMP22® BladderChek Test® (Matritech, Inc., Newton, MA, USA) is based on the detection of nuclear matrix protein 22, part of the mitotic apparatus released from urothelial nuclei upon cellular apoptosis. The protein is elevated in bladder cancer, but it is also released from the dead and dying urothelial cells. Benign conditions tract such as stones, infection, inflammation, hematuria, and cystoscopy can cause a false positive reading. Both a laboratory-based, quantitative immunoassay and a qualitative point-of-care test are available. The sensitivities and specificities range from 68.5 to 88.5% for sensitivity and from 65.2 to 91.3% for specificity (84). A multi-institutional trial involving 1,331 patients showed that the NMP22 was more sensitive but less specific than cytology. Overall sensitivity was 55.7%. Overall specificity was higher for cytology at 99.2% compared with NMP22 at 85.7%. Combining NMP22 with cystoscopy increased sensitivity from 88.6 to 93.7% (79).

UroVysion® (Abbott Molecular, Chicago IL) is not truly a tumor marker, but is rather a cytology-based test that uses fluorescent in situ hybridization (FISH) of DNA probes or "labels" specific to certain chromosomal foci. Probes to identify centromeres to chromosomes 3, 7, and 17 are combined with a probe to the 9p21 locus. FISH probes can be developed to identify essentially any locus, but this combination has been shown to have the best combination of sensitivity and specificity (78). Cumulative data from comparative studies show sensitivity of 19 vs. 58% for grade 1, 50 vs. 77% for grade 2, and 71 vs. 96% for grade 3 for cytology compared to FISH. Similar findings occurred by stage where the sensitivity for cytology compared to FISH was 35 vs. 64% for Ta, 66 vs. 83% for T1, and 76 vs. 94% for muscle invasive carcinoma (74).

Notably, cytology detected only 67% of the cases with CIS vs. 100% detection by FISH in a review of all comparative studies published as of 2005. UroVysion has a specificity approaching that of cytology (74), but it will sometimes detect chromosomal changes before the development of phenotypic expression of malignancy, so leads to an "anticipatory positive" reading in some patients. Such readings will lead to identification of clinical tumors within 3–15 months in the majority of cases (37). This may allow identification of patients at risk of recurrence vs. those unlikely to recur in order to individualize surveillance protocols.

UroVysion has also been shown to clarify equivocal findings in patients with atypical or negative cytology (87). It is not affected by hematuria, inflammation, or other factors that can cause false positive readings with some tumor markers, so appears to be useful as a marker of CIS response to BCG (35).

Determining the utility of tumor markers and the choice of which one to use is not clear at this point in time. For example, if indication for biopsy in the operating room is the desired, then high specificity is preferred to limit the number of anesthetics and negative biopsies. Conversely, if increasing the interval of cystoscopic surveillance is the endpoint, then high sensitivity, particularly for high-grade tumors, is desired. Defining that a patient has a low likelihood of recurrence within the following year can allow individualism of surveillance protocols (Table 1.4, Fig. 1.6).

12. Investigational Markers

The Accu-Dx® (Intracel Corp, Rockville, Maryland, USA) point-of-care immunoassay is based on the higher level of VEGF that increases the permeability of the blood vessels to serum proteins, including plasminogen, fibrinogen, and the members of the clotting cascade in bladder cancer patients. This test detects fibrin and its degradation products. Its sensitivity and specificity is 68 and 86%, respectively, but it can also be falsely positive in patients with hematuria (88, 89). The test is currently not commercially available, but has been approved by the FDA.

The telomerase assay has shown high specificity but suboptimal sensitivity. Telomerase is a protein/RNA complex involved in extension of telomeres during cell cycle DNA replication, so is elevated in malignant cells. The stability of telomerase RNA is variable, yielding reports with unpredictable reproducibility (90, 91).

Hyaluronic acid is a nonsulphated glycosaminoglycan in the basement membrane that is degraded by

TABLE 1.4. Commercially available markers (adapted from Liou (84)).

Commercially available markers	Sensitivity		Specificity	
	Mean%	Range%	Mean%	Range%
Cytology	48	16–89	96	81–100
Hematuria dipstick	68	40–93	68	51–97
NMP22®	75	32–92	75	51–94
NMP22 BladderChek®	55.7		85.7	
BTA stat®	68	53–89	74	54–93
BTA TRAK®	61	17–78	71	51–89
ImmunoCyt™	74	39–100	80	73–84
UroVysion®	77	73–81	98	96–100

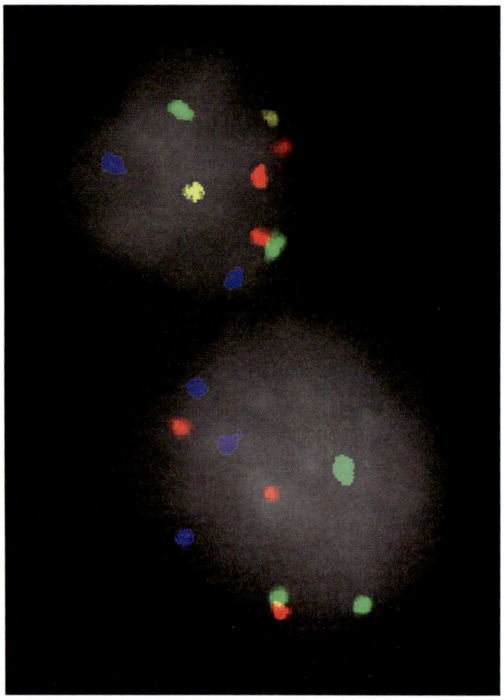

FIG. 1.6. An abnormal enlarged cell (*lower right*) demonstrates three copies of chromosome 3 (*red*), chromosome 7 (*green*), and chromosome 17 (*aqua*) using Fluorescence in situ hybridization (FISH). Homozygous deletion of band 9p21 locus (*yellow*) is also present. (Courtesy of Raymond Tubbs, MD; Department of Laboratory Pathology, Cleveland Clinic Foundation)

hyaluronidase. The sensitivity and specificity for this test is between 80 and 85%, respectively. Cytokeratins 18, 19, and 20 are highly expressed in bladder cancer. However, all 3 are also induced with infections. The test for cytokeratin 8 and 18 is the UBC™ II ELISA (84).

Miscellaneous proteins with promise are BLCA4, a nuclear matrix bladder cancer protein; mucin 7, a glycoprotein that is mainly found in invasive and CIS bladder cancer; survivin, an antiapoptotic protein; Lewis X, found mainly in low-grade cancer; and CD44, a metastatic/invasive protein marker (84).

13. Management of Tumor Marker Results

Because most of the above tumor markers have low positive predictive value, a positive test is often associated with a benign condition. As long as the clinician recognizes this fact, simple diligence in assuring that malignancy is ruled out may be sufficient to address this situation. All tumor markers have a higher sensitivity than cytology, so are often positive in the presence of visible tumor despite a negative cytology. This is offset in many clinical scenarios by the disadvantage of excessive false positives in patients without malignancy. In addition, UroVysion is uniquely associated with the potential for "anticipatory positive" results due to the detection of chromosomal changes prior to phenotypic expression of those findings. Close surveillance and a low threshold to biopsy the bladder and image the extravesical urothelium is in order.

The negative predictive value of these tests is greatly variable. The highest NPV appears to occur with Urovysion. Our experience is that patients with a negative cystoscopy and negative UroVysion have a 5% chance of tumor recurrence within 2 years, compared to 62% with negative cystoscopy and positive UroVysion (92). Tests with a high negative predictive value may be useful for individualizing surveillance protocols in patients with low grade cancer, but this approach should be used with caution in patients with CIS.

Although conventional cytology is associated with a woefully low negative predictive value (NPV), its positive predictive value (PPV) is very high. Therefore, cytology can serve as a useful adjunct to tumor markers and their low PPV. For example, a screening tumor marker such as BTA stat or NMP-22 might be positive in the setting of a negative cystoscopy. A positive cytology at that point in time would automatically warrant biopsy. Conversely, the high NPV of UroVysion might preclude automatic biopsy in the same setting if it and cytology were negative.

14. Extravesical Surveillance

The likelihood of patients developing upper tract CIS or invasive UC after the diagnosis and treatment of nonmuscle-invasive disease has been reported as 0.002–2.4% over surveillance intervals of 5–13 years (93–96), although the risk increases substantially over time to as high as 18% in very high risk populations (97). Most reviews have concluded that patients with CIS should undergo upper tract imaging.

In a review of 591 patients with a median follow-up of 86 months, upper tract recurrence was 2.2% in patients at intermediate risk (recurrent or multifocal disease), and 9.8% in high-risk patients, including intravesical chemotherapy failures (98).

Excretory urography is the traditional choice for upper tract imaging, but gives limited information about renal parenchyma and can miss small tumors. Retrograde pyelography requires instrumentation. CT urography is a promising technology for the evaluation of hematuria, but its role in the evaluation of patients with CIS has not been reported (99).

The synchronous or metachrynous appearance of upper tract disease is associated with mortality rates of 40–70%. Patients with high-risk disease treated with BCG experience upper tract recurrence risk of 13–18% (97, 100). The risk for recurrence appears greatest over the first 5 years after treatment, yet persists for at least 15 years.

Selective cytology of the upper tract may increase the yield, but, in the presence of a bladder tumor, selective upper tract cytology may be falsely positive and is not recommended for most patients (96, 101). Bilateral ureteroscopy is often employed, but data on its yield are lacking. Nevertheless, patients with positive cytologies and a negative cystoscopic and radiographic evaluation may warrant bilateral flexible ureteroscopy. Although selective collection of tumor markers is logical, there is no evidence to date to support this practice.

15. Conclusion

Despite its traditional categorization as "superficial," CIS is a high grade, flat, noninvasive bladder cancer confined to the urothelium. Bladder biopsy is required to establish a diagnosis. Cytology to examine voided or bladder wash urine can allow identification of malignant cells, but failure to recognize such cells does not rule out CIS. Options to improve cystoscopic recognition of malignant areas such as fluorescence cystoscopy and narrow band imaging are promising developments that have not received FDA approval in the United States at the time of this writing. A number of tumor markers have been developed. Most have high sensitivity, but these tests have varying specificity. The urologist must understand the implications of a negative or positive test in order to successfully integrate these tests into clinical practice.

References

1. Smith JA Jr. Labasky RF, Cockett AT, Fracchia JA, Montie JE, Rowland RG. Bladder cancer clinicial guidelines panel summary report on the management of nonmuscle invasive bladder cancer (stages Ta, T1 and TIS). The American Urological Association. J Urol 1999 Nov;162(5):1697–701.
2. Epstein JI, Amin MB, Reuter VR, Mostofi FK. The World Health Organization/International Society of Urological Pathology consensus classification of urothelial (transitional cell) neoplasms of the urinary bladder. Bladder Consensus Conference Committee. Am J Surg Pathol 1998 Dec;22(12):1435–48.
3. Sylvester RJ, van der Meijden A, Witjes JA, Jakse G, Nonomura N, Cheng C, Torres A, Watson R, Kurth KH. High-grade Ta urothelial carcinoma and carcinoma in situ of the bladder. Urology 2005 Dec;66(6 Suppl 1):90–107.
4. Ro JY, Staerkel GA, Ayala AG. Cytologic and histologic features of superficial bladder cancer. Urol Clin North Am 1992;19:435–453.
5. Lee LW, and Davis E Jr. Gross urinary hemorrhage: a symptom, not a disease. JAMA 1953;153:782–784.
6. Varkarakis MJ, Gaeta J, Moore RH, et al. Superficial bladder tumor. Aspects of clinical progression. Urology 1974;4:414–420.
7. Sultana SR, Goodman CM, Byrne DJ, et al. Microscopic hematuria: urological investigation using a standard protocol. Br J Urol 1996;78:691–698.
8. Khadra MH, Pickard RS, Charlton M, et al. A prospective analysis of 1,930 patients with hematuria to evaluate current diagnostic practice. J Urol 2000;163:524–527.
9. Golin AL and Howard RS. Asymptomatic microscopic hematuria. J Urol 1980;124:389–391.
10. Mohr DN, Offord KP, Owen RA, et al. Asymptomatic microhematuria and urologic disease. A population-based study. JAMA 1986;256:224–229.
11. Zincke H, Utz DC, Farrow GM: Review of Mayo Clinic experience with carcinoma in situ. Urology 1985;26:39–46.
12. Tissot WD, Diokno AC, Peters KM. A referral center's experience with transitional cell carcinoma misdiagnosed as interstitial cystitis. J Urol 2004;172:478–480.
13. Grossfeld GD, Wolf JS Jr, Litwan MS, et al. Asymptomatic microscopic hematuria in adults: summary of the AUA best practice policy recommendations. Am Fam Physician 2001;63:1145–1154.
14. Althausen AF, Prout GR Jr, Daly JJ. Non-invasive papillary carcinoma of the bladder associated with carcinoma in situ. J Urol 1976;116:575–580.
15. Farrow GM, Utz DC, Rife CC. Morphological and clinical observations of patients with early bladder cancer treated with total cystectomy. Cancer Res 1976;36:2495–2501.
16. Masood S, Sriprasad S, Palmer JH. T1G3 bladder cancer–indications for early cystectomy. Int Urol Nephrol 2004; 36:41–44.
17. Koch MO and Smith JA Jr. Natural history and surgical management of superficial bladder cancer (stages Ta/T1/Tis). In Vogelzang N, Miles BJ. (eds.) Comprehensive Textbook of Genitourinary Oncology. 1996; Chapter 26:405–15.
18. Millan-Rodriguez F, Chechile-Toniolo G, Salvador-Bayarri J, Palou J, and Vicente-Rodriquez J. Multivariate analysis of the prognostic factors of primary superficial bladder cancer. J Urol 2000;163:73–78.

19. May F, Treiber V, Hartung R, Schwaibald H. Significance of random bladder biopsies in superficial bladder cancer. Eur Urol 2003;44:47–50.
20. Swinn MJ, Walker MM, Harbin LJ, Adshead JM, O'N Witherow R, Vale JA, Patel A. Biopsy of the red patch at cystoscopy: is it worthwhile?: Eur Urol 2004;45:471–474.
21. Fujimoto N, Haradas S, Terado M, Sato H, et al. Multiple biopsies of normal looking urothelium in patients with superficial bladder cancer: are they necessary?: Int J Urol 2003;10:631–635.
22. van der Meijden A, Oosterlinck W, Brausi M, Kurth KH, Sylvester R, de Balincourt C. Significance of bladder biopsies in Ta,T1 bladder tumors: a report from the EORTC Genito-Urinary Tract Cancer Cooperative Group. EORTC-GU Group Superficial Bladder Committee. Eur Urol 1999 Apr;35(4):267–271.
23. Holzbeierlein JM, Smith JA Jr. Surgical management of noninvasive bladder cancer (stages Ta/T1/CIS). Urol Clin North Am 2000 Feb;27(1):15–24; vii-viii.
24. Mufti GR, Singh M. Value of random mucosal biopsies in the management of superficial bladder cancer. Eur Urol 1992;22:288–293.
25. Kiemeney LA, Witjes JA, Hiejbroek RP, et al. Should random urothelial biopsies be taken from patients with primary superficial bladder cancer? A decision analysis. Br J Urol 1994;73:164–171.
26. Yamada Y, Hayashi Y, Kohri K, et al. Random biopsy and recurrence risk in patients with bladder cancer. Jpn J Urol 1996;87:61–66.
27. Lamm DL. Carcinoma in situ. Urol Clin North Am 1992a;19:499–508.
28. Lamm DL: Complications of bacillus Calmette-Guérin immunotherapy. Urol Clin North Am 1992b;19:565–572.
29. Hudson MA, Herr HW. Carcinoma in situ of the bladder. J Urol 1995;153:564–572.
30. Brosman SA. Experience with bacillus Calmette-Guerin in patients with superficial bladder carcinoma. J Urol 1982 Jul;128(1):27–30.
31. Herr HW, Wartinger DD, Fair WR, et al. Bacillus Calmette-Guérin therapy for superficial bladder cancer: A 10-year follow-up. J Urol 1992;147:1020–1023.
32. Coplen DE, Marcus MD, Myers JA, et al. Long-term follow-up of patients treated with 1 or 2, 6-week courses of intravesical bacillus Calmette-Guérin: Analysis of possible predictors of response free of tumor. J Urol 1990;144:652–657.
33. Harland SJ, Charig CR, Highman W, et al. Outcome in carcinoma in situ of bladder treatment with intravesical bacille Calmette-Guérin. Br J Urol 1992;70:271.
34. Dalbagni G, Rechtschaffen T, Herr HW. Is transurethral biopsy of the bladder necessary after 3 months to evaluate response to bacillus Calmette-Guérin therapy? J Urol 1999;162:708–709.
35. Highsaw RA, Tanaka ST, Evans CP, deVere White RW. Is bladder biopsy necessary at three or six months post BCG therapy? Urol Oncol 2003 May–June;21(3):207–209.
36. Kipp BR, Karnes RJ, Brankley SM, et al. Monitoring intravesical therapy for superficial bladder cancer using fluorescence in situ hybridization. J Urol 2005;173:401–404.
37. Herr HW, Dalbagni G. Defining bacillus Calmette-Guerin refractory superficial bladder tumors. J Urol 2003;169:1706–1708.
38. Sarosdy AF, Schellhammer P, Bokinsky G, et al. Clinical evaluation of a multi-target fluorescent in situ hybridization assay for detection of bladder cancer. J Urol 2002;168: 1950–1954.
39. Richter J, Jiang F, Gorog JP, et al. Marked genetic differences between stage pTa and stage pT1 papillary bladder cancer detected by comparative genomic hybridization. Cancer Res 1997;57:2860–2864.
40. Spruck CH 3rd, Ohneseit PF, Gonzalez-Zulueta M, et al. Two molecular pathways to transitional cell carcinoma of the bladder. Cancer Res 1994;54:784–748.
41. Kiemeney LA, Witjes JA, Verbeek AL, et al. The clinical epidemiology of superficial bladder cancer. Dutch South-East Cooperative Urological Group. Br J Cancer 1993;67:806–812.
42. Mao L, Schoenberg MP, Scicchitano M, et al. Molecular detection of primary bladder cancer by microsatellite analysis. Science 1996;271:659–662.
43. Kallioniemi A, Kallioniemi OP, Citro G, et al. Identification of gains and losses of DNA sequences in primary bladder cancer by comparative genomic hybridization. Genes Chromosomes Cancer 1995;12:213–219.
44. Bittard H, Lamy B, and Billery C. Clinical evaluation of cell deoxyribonucleic acid content measured by flow cytometry in bladder cancer. J Urol 1996;155:1887–1891.
45. Jones JS. DNA-based molecular cytology for bladder cancer surveillance. Urology 2006 Mar;67(3 Suppl 1):35–45; discussion 45–47.
46. Richter J, Jiang F, Gorog JP, et al. Marked genetic differences between stage pTa and stage pT1 papillary bladder cancer detected by comparative genomic hybridization. Cancer Res 1997;57:2860–2864.
47. Sauter G, and Mihatsch MJ. Pussycats and baby tigers: non-invasive (pTa) and minimally invasive (pT1) bladder carcinomas are not the same! J Pathol 1998;185:339–341.
48. Waldman FM, Carroll PR, Kerschmann R, et al. Centromeric copy number of chromosome 7 is strongly correlated with tumor grade and labeling index in human bladder cancer. Cancer Res 1991;51:3807–3813.
49. Olumi AF, Tsai YC, Nichols PW, et al. Allelic loss of chromosome 17p distinguishes high grade from low grade transitional cell carcinomas of the bladder. Cancer Res 1990;50:7081–7083.
50. Degtyar P, Neulander E, Zirkin H, et al. Fluorescence in situ hybridization performed on exfoliated urothelial cells in patients with transitional cell carcinoma of the bladder. Urology 2004;63:398–401.
51. Halling KC. Vysis UroVysion for the detection of urothelial carcinoma. Expert Rev Mol Diagn 2003;3:507–519; Erratum in: Expert Rev Mol Diagn 2004;4:266.
52. Pycha A, Mian C, Haitel A, et al. Fluorescence in situ hybridization identifies more aggressive types of primarily noninvasive (stage pTa) bladder cancer. J Urol 1997;157:2116–2119.
53. Troxler H, Neuheiser F, Kleinert P, et al. Detection of a novel variant human hemoglobin by electrospray ionization mass spectrometry. Biochem Biophys Res Commun 2002;292:1044–1047.
54. Sarkis AS, Zhang ZF, Cordon-Cardo C, et al. p53 nuclear overexpression and disease progression in Ta bladder carcinoma. Int J Oncol 1993;3:355.

55. Lacome L, Dalbagni G, Zuo-Feng Z, et al. Overexpression of p53 protein in a high risk population of patients with superficial bladder cancer before and after bacillus Calmette-Guérin: Correlation to clinical outcome. J Clin Oncol 1996;14:2646–2652.
56. Lebret T, Becette V, Burbagelatta M, et al. Correlation between p53 overexpression and response to bacillus Calmette-Guérin therapy in a high risk select population of patients with T1G3 bladder cancer. J Urol 1998;159: 788–791.
57. Peyromaure M, Weibing S, Sebe P, Verpillat P, Toublanc M, Dauge MC, Boccon-Gibod L, Ravery V. Prognostic value of p53 overexpression in T1G3 bladder tumors treated with bacillus Calmette-Guerin therapy. Urology 2002 Mar;59(3): 409–413.
58. Hedelin H, Holmang S, Wiman L. The cost of bladder tumour treatment and follow-up. Scand J Urol Nephrol 2002;36(5):344–347.
59. Fitzpatrick JM, West AB, Butler MR, et al. Superficial bladder tumors (stage pTa, grades 1 and 2): The importance of recurrence pattern following initial resection. J Urol 1986;135:920–922.
60. Brown FM. Urine cytology. It is still the gold standard for screening? Urol Clin North Am 2000 Feb;27(1):25–37.
61. Schrag D, Hsieh LJ, Rabbani F, Bach PB, Herr H, Begg CB. Adherence to surveillance among patients with superficial bladder cancer. J Natl Cancer Inst 2003 Apr;95(8): 588–597.
62. Kriegmair M, Zaak D, Stepp H, et al. Transurethral resection and surveillance of bladder cancer supported by 5-aminolevulinic acid-induced fluorescence endoscopy. Eur Urol 1999;36:386–392.
63. Cina SJ, Epstein JI, Endrizzi JM, Harmon WJ, Seay TM, Schoenberg MP. Correlation of cystoscopic impression with histologic diagnosis of biopsy specimens of the bladder. Hum Pathol 2001 Jun;32(6):630–637.
64. Mitropoulos D, Kiroudi-Voulgari A, Nikolopoulos P, Manousakas T, Zervas A. Accuracy of cystoscopy in predicting histologic features of bladder lesions. J Endourol 2005 Sep;19(7):861–864.
65. Walker L, Liston TG and Lloyd-Davies RW. Does flexible cystoscopy miss more tumors than rod-lens examination? Br J Urol 1993;72(4):449.
66. Meyoff HH, Andersen JT, Klarskov P, Steven K. Flexible fiberoptic versus conventional cystourethroscopy in bladder tumor patients. A prospective study. Scand J Urol Nephrol Suppl 1988;110:237–240.
67. Witjes JA. Bladder carcinoma in situ in 2003: state of the art. Eur Urol 2004;45:142–146.
68. Loidl W, Schmidbauer J, Susani M, Marberger M. Flexible cystoscopy assisted by hexaminolevulinate induced fluorescence: a new approach for bladder cancer detection and surveillance? Eur Urol 2005 Mar;47(3):323–326.
69. Rodriguez-Rubio F, Sanz G, Garrido S, Sanchez C, Estudillo F. Patient tolerance during outpatient flexible cystoscopy–a prospective, randomized, double-blind study comparing plain lubrication and lidocaine gel. Scand J Urol Nephrol 2004;38(6):477–480.
70. Palit V, Ashurst HN, Biyani CS, Elmasray Y, Puri R, Shah T. Is using lignocaine gel prior to flexible cystoscopy justified? A randomized prospective study. Urol Int 2003;71(4):389–392.
71. Ho KJ, Thompson TJ, O'Brien A, Young MR, McCleane G. Lignocaine gel: does it cause urethral pain rather than prevent it? Eur Urol. 2003 Feb;43(2):194–196.
72. Chen YT, Hsiao PJ, Wong WY, Wang CC, Yang SS, Hsieh CH. Randomized double-blind comparison of lidocaine gel and plain lubricating gel in relieving pain during flexible cystoscopy. J Endourol 2005 Mar;19(2):163–166.
73. Chen YT, Hsiao PJ, Wong WY, Wang CC, Yang SS, Hsieh CH. Randomized double-blind comparison of lidocaine gel and plain lubricating gel in relieving pain during flexible cystoscopy. J Endourol 2005 Mar;19(2):163–166.
74. Jones JS, Patel A, Angie M, Kitay R, Sanders S. Office cystoscopy more tolerated with patient visualized real-time video monitoring. Abstract#: 94765, presented AUA Annual Meeting, Atlanta, GA, May 20, 2006.
75. Nabi G, Greene D, O'Donnell MO. Suspicious urinary cytology with negative evaluation for malignancy in the diagnostic investigation of hematuria: how to follow up?. J Clin Pathol 2004 Jun;57(6):672.
76. Murphy WM, Crabtree WN, Jukkola AF, Soloway MS. The diagnostic value of urine versus bladder washing in patients with bladder cancer. J Urol 1981 Sep;126(3):320–322.
77. McClennan BL, Oertel YC, Malmgren RA, Mendoza M. The effect of water soluble contrast material on urine cytology. Acta Cytol 1978 Jul–Aug;22(4):230–233.
78. Andriole GL, McClennan BL, Becich MJ, Picus DD. Effect of low osmolar, ionic and nonionic, contrast media on the cytologic features of exfoliated urothelial cells. Urol Radiol 1989;11(3):133–135.
79. Halling K, King W, Sokolova I, et al. A comparison of cytology and fluorescence in situ hybridization for the detection of urothelial carcinoma. J Urol 2000;164:1768–1175.
80. Grossman HB, Messing E, Soloway M, et al. Detection of bladder cancer using a point-of-care proteomic assay. JAMA 2005;293:810–816.
81. Lokeshwar VB, Habuchi T, Grossman HB, Murphy WM, Hautmann SH, Hemstreet GP 3rd, Bono AV, Getzenberg RH, Goebell P, Schmitz-Drager BJ, Schalken JA, Fradet Y, Marberger M, Messing E, Droller MJ. Bladder tumor markers beyond cytology: International Consensus Panel on bladder tumor markers. Urology 2005 Dec;66(6 Suppl 1):35–63.
82. Lafata JE, Simpkins J, Lamerato L, et al. The economic impact of false-positive cancer screens. Cancer Epidemiol Biomarkers Prev 2004;13:2126–2132.
83. Irani J, Desgrandcamps F, Millet C, et al. BTA stat and BTA TRAK: A comparative evaluation of urine testing for the diagnosis of transitional cell carcinoma of the bladder. Eur Urol 1999;35:89–92.
84. Liou LS. Urothelial cancer biomarkers for detection and surveillance. Urology 2006 Mar;67(3 Suppl 1):25–33; discussion 33–34.
85. Tetu B, Tiguert R, Harel F, et al. ImmunoCyt/uCyt +improves the sensitivity of urine cytology in patients followed for urothelial carcinoma. Mod Pathol 2005;18:83–89.
86. Toma MI, Friedrich MG, Hautmann SH, et al. Comparison of the ImmunoCyt test and urinary cytology with other urine tests in the detection and surveillance of bladder cancer. World J Urol 2004;22:145–149.
87. Skacel M, Fahmy M, Brainard JA, Pettay JD, Biscotti CV, Liou LS, Procop GW, Jones JS, Ulchaker J, Zippe CD, Tubbs RR. Multitarget fluorescence in situ gybridization

assay detects transitional cell carcinoma in the majority of patients with bladder cancer and atypical or negative urine cytology. J Urol 2003 Jun;169(6):2101–2105.
88. Ewing R, Tate GM and Hetherington JW. Urinary fibrin/fibrinogen degradation products in transitional cell carcinoma of the bladder. Br J Urol 1987;59:53–58.
89. Lokeshwar VB and Soloway MS. Current bladder tumor tests: does their projected utility fulfill clinical necessity? J Urol 2001;165:1067–1077.
90. de Kok JB, van Balkan MR, Ruers TJ, et al. Detection of telomerase activity in urine as a tool for noninvasive detection of recurrent bladder tumors is poor and cannot be improved by timing of sampling. Clin Chem 2000;46: 2014–2015.
91. Dettlaff-Polora A, Matuszewski M and Schlichtholz B. Telomerase activity in urine sediments as a tool for noninvasive detection of bladder cancer. Cancer Lett 2005;222:83–88.
92. Yoder BJ, Skacel M, Hedgepeth R, Babineau D, Ulchaker JC, Liou LS, Brainard JA, Biscotti CV, Jones JS and Tubbs RR. Reflex Uro Vysion Testing of Bladder Cancer Surveillance Patients with Equivocal or Negative Urine Cytology: A Prospective Study With Focus on the Natural History of Anticipatory Positive Findings. Am J Clin Pathol. 2007 Feb; 127(2):295–301.
93. Shinka T, Yasunari U, Aoshi H, et al. Occurrence of uroepithelial tumors of the upper urinary tract after the initial diagnosis of bladder cancer. J Urol 1988;140:745–748.
94. Oldbring J, Glifberg I, Mikulowski P, et al. Carcinoma of the renal pelvis and ureter following bladder carcinoma: Frequency, risk factors and clinicopathological findings. J Urol 1989;141:1311–1313.
95. Holmang S, Hedelin H, Anderstrom C, et al. The relationship among multiple recurrences, progression and prognosis of patients with stages TA and T1 transitional cell cancer of the bladder followed for at least 20 years. J Urol 1995;153:1823–1827.
96. Sadek S, Soloway MS, Hook S, et al. The value of upper tract cytology after transurethral resection of bladder tumor in patients with bladder transitional cell cancer. J Urol 1999;161:77–80.
97. Herr HW, Cookson MS, Soloway SM. Upper tract tumors in patients with primary bladder cancer followed for 15 years. J Urol 1997;156:1286–1287.
98. Hurle R, Manzetti A, Losa A, et al. Intravesical instillation of mitomycin C in 242 patients with superficial bladder cancer at high risk of recurrence: Long-term results. Urol Int 1998;61:220–226.
99. Herts BR. Imaging for renal tumors. Curr Opin Urol 2003 May;13(3):181–186.
100. Miller EB, Eure GR, Schellhammer PF. Upper tract transitional cell carcinoma following treatment of superficial bladder cancer with BCG. Urology 1993;42:26–30.
101. Zincke H, Utz DC, Taylor WF, et al. Influence of thiotepa and doxorubicin instillation at time of transurethral surgical treatmentof bladder cancer on tumor recurrence: A prospective, randomized double blind, controlled trial. J Urol 1983;129:505.
102. Donat SM: Evaluation and follow-up strategies for superficial bladder cancer. Urol Clin North Am 2003; 30:765–766.
103. Jones JS and Campbell SC. Non-muscle-invasive Bladder Cancer (Stages Ta, T1 and Tis). Chapter 76, Campbell's Urology Vol 9, 2006.

2
Fluorescence Cytoscopy

Philippe E. Spiess and H. Barton Grossman

Contents

Abstract Conventional diagnostic strategies for bladder cancer have consisted of white light cystoscopy and urine markers. It is recognized that white light cystoscopy can fail to detect carcinoma in situ (CIS). Furthermore, recent experiences with fluorescence cystoscopy demonstrate that white light cystoscopy can fail to detect papillary tumors as well. Several fluorescence agents have been used for photodynamic detection of bladder cancer, including 5-aminolevulinic acid, hexylester aminolevulinate, and hypericin. These novel agents can be applied intravesically from one to several hours prior to cystoscopy with no reported systemic toxicity, resulting in improved bladder cancer detection rates, particularly for CIS.

Recent phase III trials have demonstrated that transurethral resection of bladder tumors using fluorescence reduces short-term recurrence rates. Fluorescence cystoscopy is starting to play an increasing role in our diagnostic and therapeutic armamentarium for non-muscle invasive bladder cancer.

Keywords Bladder cancer, Fluorescence cystoscopy, Diagnosis, Carcinoma in situ, Treatment

1. Introduction

Bladder cancer represents the fifth most common malignancy in the United States, with an estimated 13,180 disease-specific deaths in this past year (1, 2). The diagnosis and surveillance of nonmuscle invasive bladder cancer produces a significant cost in health-care resulting in part from frequent surveillance by cystoscopy and urinary marker evaluation. Regular surveillance is employed because up to 75% of the people with bladder cancer superficial to the muscularis propia will develop recurrent disease (3). Up to now, most practicing urologists have utilized white light cystoscopy and a urine marker as their diagnostic tools of choice for this disease. However, carcinoma in situ (CIS) and small papillary tumors can be difficult to visualize under white light cystoscopy. Failure to detect these cancers puts patients at risk of overt tumor recurrence and disease progression (4–6). A variety of alternative or adjunctive diagnostic strategies have been invcstigated in an effort to minimize this risk (5). Jocham et al. were the first to investigate the potential role of the fluorescence agent 5-aminolevulinic acid

From: *Current Clinical Urology: Bladder Cancer*, Edited by: C.T. Lee and D.P. Wood,
DOI: 10.1007/978-1-59745-417-9_2, © Humana Press, a part of Springer Science+Business Media, LLC 2010

TABLE 2.1. Overall sensitivity and specificity of fluorescence cystoscopy agents.

Study	Number of patients	Agent used	Sensitivity (%)	Specificity (%)
Zaak et al. (12)	1414	ALA	97	65
Grimbergen et al. (13)	160	ALA	97	49
Kriegmair et al. (14)	104	ALA	97	67
Schmidbauer et al. (15)	211	HAL	97	NA
Jichlinski et al. (11)	52	HAL	96	52
D'Hallewin et al. (16)	87	Hypericin	94	95
Sim et al. (17)	41	Hypericin	82	91

ALA 5-aminolevulinic acid; *HAL* hexylester aminolevulinate; *NA* not available

(ALA) as a compound that could be applied intravesically and potentially improve bladder cancer detection (7). Since this preliminary report, the technology of fluorescence cystoscopy has improved significantly with the development of newer fluorescence agents such as hexylester aminolevulinate (HAL) and hypericin.

In this chapter, we review the principles of fluorescence cystoscopy with these agents and discuss the recent literature, which suggest that it has great potential as an adjunctive tool in the diagnosis and management of nonmuscle invasive bladder cancer.

2. Fluoroscence Agents

Prior to the advent of modern fluorescence agents, compounds such as tetracycline were evaluated as potential diagnostic markers for bladder cancer. However, these agents lacked sufficient cancer detection capabilities (4, 5). Currently used fluorescence agents have been shown to enhance bladder cancer diagnosis and have minimal side-effects, which in most cases consist of lower urinary tract symptoms (i.e., urgency, frequency, and dysuria) indistinguishable from the expected side-effects associated with cystoscopy and biopsy (8–11). The reported sensitivity and specificity of these fluorescence agents in bladder cancer detection are summarized in Table 2.1 (11–17).

2.1. ALA

ALA is the first drug developed for clinical photodynamic detection of bladder cancer. Intravesical instillation of this agent results in its uptake by bladder tumors, which can be subsequently visualized using a specially designed light source (4, 6, 18). ALA fluorescence occurs because the agent is a heme precursor, and it causes protoporphyrin IX to amass within bladder cancer cells, which can be visualized as red fluorescence upon exposure to light of the appropriate wavelength. Several theories have been proposed to explain protoporphyrin accumulation in bladder cancer cells, including metabolic changes, unique chemical and structural properties, and rapid proliferation of cancer cells compared to the rest of the bladder urothelium (6, 18). The optimal dosing and duration of instillation of ALA has not been standardized. However, most urologists instill 1.5 g intravesically between 2 and 3 h before fluorescence cystoscopy. One of the major hindrances to fluorescence cystoscopy using this agent results from its net positive electrical charge, which impairs its intravesical absorption resulting in the requirement for long drug exposure.

2.2. HAL

In an attempt to improve intravesical uptake, ALA has been esterified forming the novel compound HAL. HAL is more lipophilic than ALA, facilitating its ability to cross the cell membrane and resulting in twice as rapid an absorption rate with 20 times lower concentrations required (5). Furthermore, HAL generates 2–4 times stronger fluorescence signal intensity than ALA, optimizing its bladder cancer detection. Typically, 50 ml of HAL (8 mmole/L) is instilled intravesically 1 h prior to cystoscopic evaluation (19). On 2nd March 2005, the European Union approved the use of the HAL agent Hexvix® (PhotoCure ASA) to enhance the detection of early stage bladder cancer (4, 20, 21).

2.3. Hypericin

D'Hallewin et al. were the first to report the application of hypericin as a novel agent for fluorescence cystoscopy (22). Hypericin has unique chemical and structural properties, that are quite distinct from those of ALA and HAL. Hypericin is derived from the plant extract of *Hypericum perforatum* and consists of a hydroxylated quinone compound (23). Upon excitation by fluorescence light, hypericin releases singlet oxygen molecules resulting in a bright red fluorescent signal (4, 24). Typically, hypericin is instilled at a concentration of 8 μmole/L between 1 and 2 h prior to fluorescence cystoscopy.

3. Fluorescence Cystoscopy

3.1. Rigid Cystoscopy Using Fluorescence Agents

Currently, fluorescence cystoscopy is considered an adjunctive tool to conventional white light cystoscopy for both the diagnosis and treatment of nonmuscle invasive bladder cancer. Typically, the fluorescence agent is intravesically administered via a urethral catheter 1 to several hours prior to the procedure, with the dosage and duration of instillation varying, depending on the specific agent being used. The patient is subsequently taken to the cystoscopy suite. Until recently, fluorescence cystoscopy was only conducted using rigid cystoscopes. The light source for fluorescence cystoscopy consists of a xenon lamp equipped with a light filter emitting light with frequencies between 375 and 440 nm. This fluorescence light can be activated on currently available cystoscopes via either a button on the cystoscope or by a foot pad (5). Under fluorescence cystoscopy, bladder tumors appear red, with the remaining normal urothelium having a dark blue appearance.

3.2. Flexible Cystoscopy Using Fluorescence Agents

Recently, flexible cystoscopic technology has been developed for use with fluorescence agents. Loidl et al. published a prospective study of 45 patients undergoing fluorescence cystoscopy using HAL as well as rigid cystoscopy using white light and HAL (25). Forty-one patients (91%) had exophytic papillary tumors, with 39 (95.1%) identified by HAL flexible cystoscopy and 40 (97.5%) by HAL rigid cystoscopy. In addition, CIS was identified in 17 patients, with 14 (82.3%) identified by HAL flexible cystoscopy, 15 (88.2%) by HAL rigid cystoscopy, 11 (64.7%) by white light flexible cystoscopy, and 13 (76.7%) by white light rigid cystoscopy. A phase II study by Witjes et al. similarly compared the performance of HAL flexible fluorescence cystoscopy to rigid fluorescence and white light cystoscopy (4, 26). Twenty patients participated in this study, and 27 histologically confirmed bladder tumors were detected among 19 patients. The bladder cancer detection rates for these 19 patients were 74% ($N = 14$) with HAL flexible cystoscopy, 89% ($N = 17$) with HAL rigid cystoscopy, and 79% ($N = 15$) with white light rigid cystoscopy. Overall, the fluorescence signal intensity of HAL flexible cystoscopy was 76% (30–147%) of that seen with fluorescence rigid cystoscopy. These preliminary findings suggest that the performance of flexible fluorescence cystoscopy is slightly inferior to that of rigid fluorescence cystoscopy. Future improvements in instrumentation may narrow this difference. As pointed out by Zlotta in a recent editorial, most diagnostic and surveillance cystoscopies performed today are conducted using flexible cystoscopes (27). Therefore, for fluorescence cystoscopy to be an attractive adjunctive tool in outpatient clinical practice, its merits must be demonstrated with flexible cystoscopy.

3.3. Pitfalls of Fluorescence Cystoscopy

One of the major concerns regarding fluorescence cystoscopy is its false-positive rate, which has been reported to be as high as 40% (4, 6, 13). When conducting fluorescence cystoscopy, it is essential to keep the excitation light perpendicular to the bladder urothelium. Tangential light can result in autofluorescence unrelated to bladder cancer. The experience of the surgeon and proper application of fluorescence cystoscopy can dramatically impact the performance of this test. Other causes for a false-positive test include the presence of urothelial inflammation, hyperplasia/dysplasia, and recent intravesical therapy.

4. Detection of CIS Using Fluorescence Cystoscopy

The merits of fluorescence cystoscopy are particularly evident in the detection of CIS, as illustrated in Table 2.2. As recently reported in a review by Jichlinski et al., fluorescence cystoscopy using ALA or HAL has a detection rate for CIS exceeding 90%, favoring its integration as a standard tool for the diagnosis and management of nonmuscle invasive bladder cancer (28). In a study by Zaak et al., 605 patients underwent 1,012 ALA fluorescence and white light cystoscopies as part of the diagnosis and surveillance of bladder cancer (8). Of the 142 fluorescence cystoscopies in which CIS was detected, 88 (62%) were detected on both white light and fluorescence cystoscopy, and 50 (35%) were detected solely on fluorescence cystoscopy. The remaining four cases (3%) were detected on white light cystoscopy alone. Fluorescence cystoscopy detects most CIS lesions and outperforms white light cystoscopy. In a study by Koenig et al., 55 patients with suspected cancer of the bladder underwent white light and fluorescence cystoscopy using ALA, with biopsies taken from suspected bladder lesions (29). The incorporation of fluorescence cystoscopy into their diagnostic strategy detected cancer of the bladder in six patients, two of whom had CIS. The authors concluded that fluorescence cystoscopy improved the overall diagnosis of malignant/dysplastic lesions by 18% over standard white light cystoscopy, with the improvement most notable for CIS (increased detection rate of 50% over white light cystoscopy alone). In a multicenter, prospective trial by Schmidbauer et al., 211 patients were evaluated with white light and fluorescence cystoscopy using HAL (15). Of the study population, 83 (39%) had CIS, of whom 22% were detected by HAL cystoscopy alone, 75% by white light and HAL cystoscopy, and 2% by white light cystoscopy alone. Overall, HAL fluorescence cystoscopy identified 28% more patients with CIS than white light cystoscopy. In a recent phase III, prospective trial by Jocham et al., 146 patients with known or suspected cancer of the bladder underwent white light and HAL fluorescence cystoscopy (30). Fluorescence cystoscopy improved the overall bladder cancer detection rate by 19% over white light cystoscopy alone (96 vs. 77%, respectively). This difference in bladder cancer detection capability was particularly noticeable for CIS, which was detected in 95% of cases with fluorescence cystoscopy compared to 68% with white light cystoscopy. The investigational fluorescence agent hypericin has also shown superiority over white light cystoscopy in its ability to detect CIS. In a study by D'Hallewin et al., the ability of fluorescence cystoscopy using hypericin was evaluated in 40 patients (22). Analysis of the 281 bladder biopsies revealed that hypericin fluorescence cystoscopy had a sensitivity of 93% and specificity of 98.5% in detecting CIS. In a follow-up study by D'Hallewin et al., 87 patients with papillary bladder carcinoma and/or CIS underwent white light and hypericin fluorescence cystoscopy (16). Bladder biopsies were taken from all suspected bladder lesions on fluorescence cystoscopy. Of the biopsies harvested, 165 specimens were diagnosed with CIS and 11 were consistent with normal bladder urothelium. The authors reported a sensitivity and specificity of 94 and 95%, respectively for the detection of CIS using hypericin based fluorescence cystoscopy. Seven of the false-positive biopsies were detected in patients treated with intravesical bacillus Calmette Guerin (BCG) within the first 2 months, suggesting that patients are at particular risk of false-positive tests if fluorescence cystoscopy is performed shortly after BCG treatment.

5. Detection of Papillary Tumors Using Fluorescence Cystoscopy

Although most studies have focused on the merits of fluorescence cystoscopy in the context of CIS detection, it appears that this diagnostic modality also has great potential in improving our ability to detect small papillary lesions. A multicenter study by Grossman et al. demonstrated that HAL fluorescence cystoscopy could detect an additional 19% pTa lesions and 26% pT1 bladder tumors vs. white light cystoscopy alone (31). Similarly, Durek et al. demonstrated that HAL fluorescence cystoscopy could improve the sensitivity for bladder cancer detection by 17% vs. white light cystoscopy (96 and 79%, respectively) (32). As a direct consequence of incorporating fluorescence cystoscopy into its diagnostic armamentarium, the authors reported a change in the clinical management of 25 patients (6). A study by Zaak et al. reviewed the rate of detection of bladder tumors in 1,012 consecutive ALA fluorescence cystoscopies and found that 189 additional tumors were detected by ALA fluorescence cystoscopy, with 84 of these tumors being pTa, 26 pT1, and 5 pT2 (8). Similarly, Grimbergen et al. evaluated 160 patients with suspected bladder cancer and found that ALA fluorescence cystoscopy enabled the detection of an additional 71 pTa tumors, 15 pT1 tumors, and 2 pT2 tumors (13) In the recent phase III study by Jocham et al., HAL fluorescence cystoscopy improved the bladder tumor detection rate to 96% from 77% using white light cystoscopy alone (30). Of the additional papillary tumors detected with HAL fluorescence cystoscopy, the benefits were most pronounced for pTa tumors (detection rate of 96% vs. 85%, respectively). Using the newer fluorescent agent hypericin, Sim et al. reported similar benefits for fluorescence cystoscopy over white light cystoscopy for the detection of papillary tumors (17). Of

TABLE 2.2. Detection of CIS using fluorescence cystoscopy.

Study	Number of cases with CIS	Agent used	Additional number of cases of CIS detected by FC alone (%)	Sensitivity for CIS detection using FC (%)	Specificity for CIS detection using FC (%)
Zaak et al, (8)	142	ALA	50 (35)[a]	NA	NA
Koenig et al. (29)	6	ALA	5 (83)[a]	NA	NA
Schmidbauer et al. (15)	83	HAL	18 (22)	NA	NA
Jocham et al. (30)	29	HAL	12 (41)	NA	NA
D'Hallewin et al. (22)	261	Hypericin	NA	93	98.5
D'Hallewin et al. (16)	165	Hypericin	NA	94	95

ALA 5-aminolevulinic acid; *HAL* hexylester aminolevulinate; *CIS* carcinoma in situ; *FC* fluorescence cystoscopy; *NA* not available

[a] In these studies, the number of bladder biopsies positive for CIS were reported but no mention was made of the number of patients with positive biopsies for CIS

the 41 patients evaluated, an additional 6 pTa tumors and 3 pT1 tumors were detected on fluorescence cystoscopy. The diagnostic utility of fluorescence cystoscopy extends beyond the detection of CIS, with its ability to detect papillary tumors particularly of small size and low pathologic stage. An important question is whether this enhanced sensitivity provides real benefit for the patient.

6. Transurethral Resection Using Fluorescence Agents

Fluorescence cystoscopy during transurethral resection may provide better visualization of the location and extent of bladder tumors. Better visualization improves the quality of resection and results in decreased rates of residual disease and short-term recurrence as recently reported in several series (Table 2.3) (30, 33–35). In a multicenter trial by Jocham et al., 146 patients with known or suspected bladder tumors underwent white light and HAL fluorescence cystoscopy (30). All lesions were mapped onto a bladder diagram and biopsies were taken from all suspicious areas. The tumor detection rate was 96% with HAL fluorescence cystoscopy compared to 77% with white light cystoscopy. Additional postoperative procedures were recommended in 15 patients (10%) and more extensive intraoperative treatment was performed in 10 patients (7%) as a consequence of incorporating fluorescence cystoscopy at the time of transurethral resection. In a prospective, randomized trial by Filbeck et al., 301 patients underwent white light or ALA assisted transurethral resection of bladder tumors (33). The residual tumor rate on repeat transurethral resection conducted 5–6 weeks following the initial resection was 25% in the white light arm vs. 5% in the ALA arm, with resulting 1-year recurrence-free survival rates of 74 and 90%, respectively. In a study by Babjuk et al., 122 patients with primary or recurrent Ta/T1 bladder tumors were prospectively randomized to undergo white light or ALA assisted transurethral resection (34). The 1-year recurrence-free survival rates in the white light and ALA assisted transurethral resection groups were 39 and 66%, respectively. Daniltchenko et al. recently completed a prospective randomized study comparing the long-term outcomes of 115 patients with non-muscle invasive bladder cancer randomized to undergo white light or ALA assisted transurethral resection, with a second-look resection with fluorescence 6 weeks following the initial resection in both treatment arms (35). The authors reported recurrence-free survival rates of 25 and 41% in the white light and fluorescence assisted transurethral resection groups, respectively. The median time to the first recurrence was significantly longer in the ALA assisted transurethral resection group, with a lower incidence of tumor progression (9 vs. 4 patients having tumor progression in the white light and ALA groups, respectively). Fluorescence assisted transurethral resection appears to be beneficial by increasing tumor detection and reducing recurrence rates.

7. Conclusions

Significant advances have been made in the diagnostic and therapeutic applications of fluorescence cystoscopy. Our current detection rates of CIS and small papillary lesions are clearly enhanced with the incorporation of fluorescence cystoscopy into our current diagnostic algorithm along with conventional white light cystoscopy and a cytological marker. The recently discovered fluorescence agent HAL is rapidly absorbed by the bladder urothelium and has minimal reported side-effects. Hypericin appears to have improved specificity over other fluorescence agents but is currently an investigational drug. Over the past year, major advances have been made with the application of fluorescence to flexible cystoscopy. Preliminary reports suggest that flexible fluorescence cystoscopy may perform slightly worse than rigid fluorescence cystoscopy but remains superior to conventional white light cystoscopy. Recent phase II and III trials demonstrate that the incorporation of fluorescence cystoscopy at the time of transurethral resection results in improved recurrence-free survival, more appropriate selection of treatment, and reduced morbidity.

TABLE 2.3. Transurethral resection of bladder tumors using fluorescence cystoscopy.

Study	Number of patients	Agent used	Additional tumors detected on fluorescence assisted TUR	Recurrence-free survival rate at 1 year with FC vs. WLC	Change in management due to fluorescence assisted TUR
Jocham et al. (30)	118	HAL	60 (19%)[a]	NA	22%
Filbeck et al. (33)	301	ALA	NA	90 vs. 74%	NA
Babjuk et al. (34)	122	ALA	NA	66 vs. 39%	NA
Daniltchenko et al. (35)	115	ALA	NA	57 vs. 39%	NA

ALA 5-aminolevulinic acid; *HAL* hexylester aminolevulinate; *TUR* transurethral resection; *FC* fluorescence cystoscopy; *WLC* white light cystoscopy; *NA* not available

[a]Many of the patients in the study by Jocham et al. had multifocal tumors with 60 additional tumors detected among them

The merits of fluorescence cystoscopy are convincing and it should be considered as an adjunctive tool to current diagnostic and therapeutic strategies for nonmuscle invasive bladder cancer. Further advances in the field of fluorescence cystoscopy may enhance its use in the outpatient setting.

References

1. Jemal A, Tiwari RC, Murray T, et al. Cancer statistics, 2004. CA Cancer J Clin 2004;54(1):8–29.
2. SEER cancer statistics 2005 Accessed 2005, at http://seer.cancer.goc/statistics/; 2005.
3. Kurth KH. Natural history and prognosis of untreated and treated superficial bladder cancer. Isis Medical Media; 1997.
4. Spiess PE, Grossman HB. Fluorescence cystoscopy: is it ready for use in routine clinical practice? Curr Opin Urol 2006;16:372–6.
5. Zaak D, Karl A, Knuchel R, et al. Diagnosis of urothelial carcinoma of the bladder using fluorescence endoscopy. BJU Int 2005;96(2):217–22.
6. Joudi FN, Konety BR. Fluorescence cystoscopy and bladder surveillance. Curr Opin Urol 2004;14(5):265–70.
7. Jocham D, Baumgartner R, Fuchs N, Lenz H, Stepp H, Unsold E. [Fluorescence diagnosis of porphyrin-marked urothelial tumors. Status of experimental development]. Urologe A 1989;28(2):59–64.
8. Zaak D, Kriegmair M, Stepp H, et al. Endoscopic detection of transitional cell carcinoma with 5-aminolevulinic acid: results of 1012 fluorescence endoscopies. Urology 2001;57(4):690–4.
9. Filbeck T, Wimmershoff MB, Pichlmeier U, et al. No generalized skin phototoxicity after intravesical application of 5-aminolevulinic acid for fluorescence diagnosis of superficial bladder cancer. Urol Int 2000;64(3):126–8.
10. Popken G, Schultze-Seemann W, Seiler KU, et al. Intravesical administration of 5-aminolevulinic acid (5-ALA). Safety and pharmacokinetics of 5-ALA and its metabolite protoporphyrin IX. Eur J Clin Pharmacol 2000;56(3):241–6.
11. Jichlinski P, Guillou L, Karlsen SJ, et al. Hexyl aminolevulinate fluorescence cystoscopy: new diagnostic tool for photodiagnosis of superficial bladder cancer–a multicenter study. J Urol 2003;170(1):226–9.
12. Zaak D, Hungerhuber E, Schneede P, et al. Role of 5-aminolevulinic acid in the detection of urothelial premalignant lesions. Cancer 2002;95(6):1234–8.
13. Grimbergen MC, van Swol CF, Jonges TG, Boon TA, van Moorselaar RJ. Reduced specificity of 5-ALA induced fluorescence in photodynamic diagnosis of transitional cell carcinoma after previous intravesical therapy. Eur Urol 2003;44(1):51–6.
14. Kriegmair M, Baumgartner R, Knuchel R, et al. Detection of early bladder cancer by 5-aminolevulinic acid induced porphyrin fluorescence. J Urol 1996;155(1):105–9.
15. Schmidbauer J, Witjes F, Schmeller N, et al. Improved detection of urothelial carcinoma in situ with hexaminolevulinate fluorescence cystoscopy. J Urol 2004;171(1):135–8.
16. D'Hallewin MA, Kamuhabwa AR, Roskams T, et al. Hypericin-based fluorescence diagnosis of bladder carcinoma. BJU Int 2002;89(7):760–3.
17. Sim HG, Lau WK, Olivo M, et al. Is photodynamic diagnosis using hypericin better than white-light cystoscopy for detecting superficial bladder carcinoma? BJU Int 2005;95(9):1215–8.
18. Koenig F, McGovern FJ. Fluorescence detection of bladder carcinoma. Urology 1997;50(5):778–9.
19. Lange N, Jichlinski P, Zellweger M, et al. Photodetection of early human bladder cancer based on the fluorescence of 5-aminolaevulinic acid hexylester-induced protoporphyrin IX: a pilot study. Br J Cancer 1999;80(1–2):185–93.
20. Fotinos N, Campo MA, Popowycz F, et al. 5-Aminolevulinic Acid Derivatives in Photomedicine: Basics, Application and Perspectives. Photochem Photobiol 2006;82(4):994–1015.
21. Hexyl aminolevulinate: 5-ALA, hexylester, 5-ALA hexylesther, aminolevulinic acid hexyl ester, hexaminolevulinate, hexyl 5-aminolevulinate, P 1206. Drugs R D 2005;6(4):235–8.
22. D'Hallewin MA, De Witte PA, Waelkens E, et al. Fluorescence detection of flat bladder carcinoma in situ after intravesical instillation of hypericin. J Urol 2000;164(2):349–51.
23. Lavie G, Mazur Y, Lavie D, Meruelo D. The chemical and biological properties of hypericin–a compound with a broad spectrum of biological activities. Med Res Rev 1995;15(2):111–9.
24. Yamazaki T, Ohta N, Yamazaki I, Song PS. Excited state properties of hypericin:electronic spectra and fluorescence decay kinetics. J Phys Chem 1993;97:7870–5.
25. Loidl W, Schmidbauer J, Susani M, Marberger M. Flexible cystoscopy assisted by hexaminolevulinate induced fluorescence: a new approach for bladder cancer detection and surveillance? Eur Urol 2005;47(3):323–6.
26. Witjes JA, Moonen PM, van der Heijden AG. Comparison of hexaminolevulinate based flexible and rigid fluorescence cystoscopy with rigid white light cystoscopy in bladder cancer: results of a prospective Phase II study. Eur Urol 2005;47(3):319–22.
27. Zlotta A. Fluorescence cystoscopy: is flexible scope as effective as rigid? Eur Urol 2005;47(3):318.
28. Jichlinski P, Leisinger HJ. Fluorescence cystoscopy in the management of bladder cancer: a help for the urologist! Urol Int 2005;74(2):97–101.
29. Koenig F, McGovern FJ, Larne R, et al. Diagnosis of bladder carcinoma using protoporphyrin IX fluorescence induced by 5-aminolaevulinic acid. BJU Int 1999;83(1):129–35.
30. Jocham D, Witjes F, Wagner S, et al. Improved detection and treatment of bladder cancer using hexaminolevulinate imaging: a prospective, phase III multicenter study. J Urol 2005;174(3):862–6.
31. Grossman HB, Gomella LG, Fradet Y, et al. The use of Hexvix and fluorescence cystoscopy as an adjunct in the diagnosis of stage Ta/T1 urothelial cancer in the urinary bladder (abstract 263). J Urol 2004;171:69.
32. Durek C, Wagner S, Zeylemaker B, et al. The significance of hexyl 5-aminolevulinate hydrochloride based fluorescence cystoscopy in treatment decisions- results of a prospective phase 3 multicenter study. In: European Association of Urology Annual Meeting, Vienna. Amsterdam: Elsevier BV; 2004.
33. Filbeck T, Pichlmeier U, Knuechel R, et al. Clinically relevant improvement of recurrence-free survival with 5-aminolevulinic acid induced fluorescence diagnosis in patients with superficial bladder tumors. J Urol 2002;168(1):67–71.
34. Babjuk M, Soukup V, Petrik R, et al. 5-aminolaevulinic acid-induced fluorescence cystoscopy during transurethral resection reduces the risk of recurrence in stage Ta/T1 bladder cancer. BJU Int 2005;96(6):798–802.
35. Daniltchenko DI, Riedl CR, Sachs MD, et al. Long-term benefit of 5-aminolevulinic acid fluorescence assisted transurethral resection of superficial bladder cancer: 5-year results of a prospective randomized study. J Urol 2005;174(6):2129–33.

Section 2
Understaging

3
Restaging TURBT

David Berger and Jeffrey M. Holzbeierlein

Contents

Abstract Cancer of the bladder is the fourth most common cancer in men and the eighth most common cancer in women. The majority (approximately 70–80%) of newly diagnosed bladder tumors are superficial or noninvasive. The initial diagnosis and management of bladder cancer is through the transurethral resection of the bladder tumor. This technically challenging procedure is the crux on which essentially all future therapy depends. Thus as both a diagnostic as well as a therapeutic procedure it is one of the most important urologic procedures. Unfortunately, there is a significant problem with a single TURBT providing the adequate diagnostic and therapeutic value due this procedure. Therefore, the restaging TURBT has gained favor as a method to decrease the inaccuracies of staging and to enhance treatment. In addition, the restaging TURBT plays a major role in many therapeutic options which seek to preserve the bladder. This chapter reviews the current problems with the TURBT and presents data to support the utility of a restaging TURBT.

Keywords Transurethral resection of bladder tumors, TURBT, Restaging, Chemotherapy, Bladder cancer

1. Introduction

Approximately 60 years ago the observations of Jewett and Strong demonstrated that the depth of invasion of a primary bladder tumor was predictive of the presence of extension and metastases (1). Their

From: *Current Clinical Urology: Bladder Cancer*, Edited by: C.T. Lee and D.P. Wood,
DOI: 10.1007/978-1-59745-417-9_3,

work was important particularly at the time because it often defined patients who were curable and who were not. Thus, the importance of appropriate staging with the initial transurethral resection of the bladder tumor (TURBT) was established. Jewett further correlated in a small group of patients with muscle invasive bladder cancer, that the actual depth of invasion was predictive of their 5 year survival (2). To avoid complications, Jewett divided his patients into two groups: superficial tumors and deep tumors. He found that for these two groups the 5 year survival was vastly different. Those with superficial tumors (Stage B1) survived more often (4/19) for 5 years, while the patients with deeper tumors (Stage B2) survived for a lesser period (2/61). Although, we have greater treatment options and the ability to cure some of those patients with both extravesical extension and metastases, the importance of the TURBT remains paramount in selecting the appropriate treatment option for patients today.

In 1975, Richie while at UCLA added to the foundation created by Jewett's 1952 article (2, 3) Richie showed that not only was deep muscle invasion associated with a reduced chance of survival, but that even minimal muscle invasion results in a lower survival rate. Furthermore, when Richie et al. compared the clinical and pathologic stages there was significant overstaging and understaging, which began to highlight some of the staging inaccuracies of an initial TURBT. Further adding to the problems with the initial TURBT was the data reported by Klan et al. in 1991, in which a second TURBT performed 1–2 weeks after the initial TURBT revealed residual tumor in approximately 50% of patients (4). Knowing the importance of the TURBT in predicting the stage and outcomes of patients, yet attempting to reconcile this with the inaccuracies associated with the procedure has led many to recommend that a second or "restaging" TURBT be performed in many patients with cancer of the bladder.

In this chapter we will discuss the principles of the TURBT as well as the data which support a second or "restaging" TURBT. In attempting to argue for a restaging TURBT it is necessary to highlight several points about TURBT in general. For example, how should a TURBT be performed; what are the limitations and risks of performing a TURBT; and the role of the TURBT in multimodality therapy.

2. How Should a TURBT Be Performed?

The goal of the TURBT should be to remove all visible tumor and provide the necessary information to accurately stage the patient, which typically requires the presence of muscularis propria in the pathologic specimen. As a side note, the importance of a bimanual examination both prior to the TURBT and after the TURBT can add critical additional information about the stage and resectability of the tumor. Although each individual surgeon has his or her method of performing the TURBT, there are basically two main techniques that are used. The *Staged Resection* is a operative strategy discussed by Milner in 1949 and later by Kolozsky in 1991 (5, 6). The Staged Resection promotes resection of the tumor by resecting in "layers" starting with the top or most visible portion of the tumor. The urologist then proceeds to resect the base of the lesion and the bladder beneath to access depth of invasion and deep margins, respectively. Lastly, the staged resection checks the lateral margins by removing tissue adjacent to the base. The specimens then may be sent to the pathologist as either separate specimens or as one specimen. One perceived advantage of sending them as separate specimens is that it allows the initial diagnosis to be confirmed with the superficial portion, but then alerts the pathologist to the real question of the depth of invasion by having them examine a separate second specimen.

The second technique for TURBT involves resection of the entire tumor (usually reserved for smaller tumors, 1 cm or less) or of portions of the entire tumor from superficial to deep. Proponents of this technique argue that this prevents fragmentation of the specimen, and allows preservation of the orientation of the tumor. The ability of the pathologist to observe the correct in situ orientation of the tumor is hypothesized to lead to greater ability to identify true muscularis propria invasion. However, no data to support this assertion is available.

As no direct comparison of the two techniques exists, it is primarily up to the surgeon to determine the best method of resection. However, there are some universal principles that should be applied. First avoidance of cautery artifact is critical as this may prevent the pathologist from being able to accurately identify the tumor or its depth of invasion. Cautery artifact can generally be prevented in two ways. First, a smooth rapid resection through the tumor with a cutting current helps reduce the degree of cautery damage to the specimen. Second, remove any specimen from the loop prior to the next "swipe." For carcinoma in situ (CIS) or smaller tumors that may be destroyed by the resecting loop, cold cup biopsy forceps may be used to obtain both a diagnosis and accurate staging. Many urologic surgeons will resect the top of larger tumors and then biopsy the base of the tumor with cold cup biopsy forceps. This may allow for greater control and avoidance of cautery artifact. Therefore, all this should be performed while minimizing the chance of bladder perforation, avoidance of an obturator reflex (which increases the risk of a bladder perforation), and injury to the ureteral orifice.

3. Support for a Second Or "Restaging" TURBT

3.1. Residual Tumor

As previously stated, it has long been recognized that there are significant problems with the initial TURBT both in terms of accurate staging and the ability to completely resect the original tumor. In the study by Klan et al., even experienced surgeons were often unable to predict when they had resected the entire tumor (4). Many reasons may account for this, including bleeding, edema, and fear of perforation. In this study a full 43% of patients with a T1 tumor had residual tumor detected on their repeat TURBT performed within 14 days after the initial procedure. The authors estimated that this would have accounted for 10% of their tumor recurrences, which is in accordance with a previous study, which detected a 12% recurrence rate at the initial site of resection (7). Other studies also confirm the lack of a single TURBT to successfully remove all of the tumor. Mersdorf et al. found a 31% rate of incomplete resection for Ta tumors and similarly Vogeli et al. found a 37% incidence of residual tumor on re-resection (8, 9). This obviously has great implications for several reasons. First, it puts the patient at increased risk for progression due to the presence of residual tumor. Second, the chance of recurrence is obviously greater. Third, it may adversely affect the ability of adjuvant treatment such as intravesical therapy to prevent recurrence or decrease the risk of progression. Indeed a recent publication by Herr supports this assumption when he examined the response to BCG (10). In this study, patients who received a second TURBT and then went on to receive BCG therapy had only a 29% recurrence rate and 17% rate of progression compared to a 57% recurrence rate and 34% progression rate for those who received a single resection. The theory for the decreased recurrence rate at first cystoscopy is that of the more complete resection of tumor at the second TURBT. In terms of progression, the decrease in the patients receiving a second resection is probably two-fold. First, patients with muscle invasive tumors who may have been missed on the initial resection were removed from the group (as they went to cystectomy) thus decreasing the rate of progression. Second, with less residual tumor the chance of progression was decreased.

3.2. Under-Staging

The other problem associated with a single initial TURBT is the problem of under-staging. This has been covered in the previous chapter, but a few salient studies deserve mention here to reiterate the need for a second TURBT. As mentioned previously, Richie et al. in 1975, compared the pathologic stage with the clinical stage (obtained by TURBT) and found a 40% under-staging rate (3). Klan et al. also showed significant under-staging particularly for T1 tumors (4). In 1999, Herr reported on patients who received a second TURBT after an initial resection with quite startling results (11). He found that 8% of patients who were initially staged as Ta tumors were actually found to have a T2 tumor on re-resection, and that patients with an original diagnosis of a T1 tumor were up staged to a T2 tumor 28% of the time. Most worrisome was that in those patients with an initial diagnosis of stage T1 but in whom no muscle was present, a re-resection demonstrated muscle invasion in 49%. If muscle was present the up-staging was much less at only 14%. Dutta et al., reported an even higher rate of under-staging when the clinical stage was compared to the final pathologic stage. In this study, they found that 40% of patients with clinical stage T1 tumors were actually T2 or greater at the time of cystectomy, and in patients with no muscle present who were staged as T1, there was a 69% rate of increase to invasive disease. In addition, they found that up-staging was associated with a statistically worse disease specific and recurrence free survival (12). Furthermore, the lack of muscle in the specimen on a single TURBT is not an uncommon finding, occurring in 40% of patients in a study by Dalbagni et al. (13). While after a second TURBT only 1 out of 15 patients (6%) did not have muscle in the specimen.

4. Therapeutic Value of the TURBT

An unintended recommendation that one might assume from reading the previous sections is that the only utility of the TURBT is in its staging ability. However, this is far from the truth. A well performed TURBT may be curative in many patients with superficial bladder cancer and even in highly selected patients with muscle invasive bladder cancer.

4.1. Superficial Bladder Cancer

Despite the fact that after a single TURBT there remains a chance that there is residual tumor, often manifested by a recurrence at the initial site of resection on the first follow-up cystoscopy, the vast majority of patients with stage Ta tumors may be successfully resected. Previous reports suggest that 80 to 90% of patients with low grade Ta tumors may be successfully resected (4, 7). Even for high risk superficial tumors, TUR can be used successfully to manage these tumors (14). In a study by Herr patients with Ta grade 3 tumors had only a 15 year risk of progression of 39% and a 15 year disease-specific survival of 74%; while for T1 tumors it was 56 and 62% respectively. Thus despite the high chance of recurrence, these patients can often at times be successfully managed with TURBT alone. Supporting the ability of TURBT to effectively treat many patients is the study by Lee et al. in 2004 (15). In this study, the authors stratified the patients into two groups. In the first group, the authors felt that the TURBT had been complete as evidenced by no visibly residual tumor, muscle present in the specimen, and no gross residual tumor in the cystectomy specimen. With this definition, the authors found that in patients with noninvasive disease, only 17.7% had a higher stage at cystectomy and in patients with invasive tumors 71% of patients had a lower stage at cystectomy, thus, supporting the effectiveness of TURBT.

4.2. Invasive Bladder Cancer

In certain instances, usually under the auspices of a study, patients with invasive cancer may be managed with TURBT. In one study, 217 consecutive patients with muscle invasive bladder cancer were evaluated at Memorial Sloan Kettering Cancer Center and Cornell University in 1987, and the initial TURBT gave them their first clinical stage (16). Within 2–3 weeks, all 172 were restaged using bimanual exam under anesthesia, cytologic analysis and restaging TUR. This stratified them into one of the two categories. One group required immediate cystectomy since the restaging TUR demonstrated lesions not amenable to local excision. The second group became the subjects of this study since they met the inclusion criteria for organ preservation. They were followed prospectively, and subsequent data analysis was provided which related them to the remainder of the original 172. All of the 45 patients had disease that was T2-T4, and were found to have 82% overall survival free of disease (37/45). In addition, a 67% overall survival (30/45) was found for patients with an intact bladder. This decrease is explained by the need for some patients to receive cystectomy after invasive recurrence not manageable by repeated TUR. Herr concluded from these findings that a subset of patients who had a complete response to the initial extensive TURBT, may be appropriate for organ preservation. Despite his ground breaking findings, he never refutes the need for patients with incomplete response to the initial TURBT, or those that fail bladder-sparing strategies, to ultimately receive a radical cystectomy.

What is important about the above studies in terms of restaging TURBT, is that true benefit of the TURBT is in its completeness. A restaging TURBT provides a greater chance of a complete resection.

5. Potential Complications of the Restaging TURBT?

Repetitive transurethral procedures, just like any form of medical or surgical therapy, requires careful risk vs. benefit analysis, not to mention the associated increased burden of cost on the medical care system. Another theoretical risk is an increased risk of bladder perforation, although to our knowledge no study has ever addressed whether repeat resection results in a significantly higher incidence of bladder perforation.

5.1. Risk of TURBT

More aggressive resections or restaging resections may be problematic with a bladder lesion near or at the ureteral orifice. If the surgeon chooses to resect at this site, it can be associated with an uncommon, but evident, risk of vesicoureteral reflux. If reflux ensues, a patient can experience one or more of the following: flank pain, urinary tract infection, decreased renal function, and an increased risk 15–22 times of upper tract neoplasms (17). In 2000, See reported evidence to the contrary in a small group of four patients who had lesions at the ureteral orifice or hemi-trigone (18). After having had iatrogenic distal ureteral injury from TURBT, he questioned the axiom of needing to avoid this complex bladder site. He found that at 6 weeks after the initial TURBT, each patient had cystoscopic evidence of regenerating distal ureter and no apparent reformation of cancer. Of these four patients, none of the patients had an increased need for stenting after the TURBT, but only those patients who had pre-TURBT requirement remained stent dependent. The editorial comments at the end also notated that it is important to remember to use the cutting function should be used preferentially over the coagulation at this site. This should decrease the risk of stricture formation as a result of ureteral orifice trauma.

6. Does TURBT Clinical Downstaging Confer a Survival Advantage?

6.1. Down-Staging Confers a Survival Advantage

In the early 1990s, there was significant debate about whether clinical downstaging on a restaging TURBT could confer a survival advantage for patients who may be undergoing a cystectomy. One study which examined this was by Waehre et al. who found success using clinical downstaging in a group of 227 patients in 1993 (19). Of the patients 43% were successfully down-staged to less than stage pT2 and had a survival rate of 74 vs. 46% for those without a reduction in stage. This study supported the concept that a reduction in stage by TURBT was both statistically significant ($P < 0.0001$) and clinically relevant in terms of survival.

6.2. Down-Staging Confers No Survival Advantage

Contrary to the above data, in 1994, Thrasher et al. reported on 433 cystectomy patients who underwent cystectomy (20). He compared the survival of patients who were pT0 vs. those who were pT2 but shared the same clinical stage. He found that there was no statistically significant advantage for those patients who were pT0 at the time of cystectomy and suggested that these patients had survival characteristics predicted by their clinical stage.

7. The Role of the TURBT and Restaging TURBT in Bladder Preservation

7.1. Combination TURBT and Chemotherapy

In 1998, Herr at MSKCC published his data of the 10 year outcomes for patients with T2-T3N0M0 who were treated with TUR and chemotherapy (Methotrexate, Vinblastine, Adriamycin and Cisplatin, MVAC) alone (21). Patients entered into the study were initially resected and then underwent repeat resection to confirm the presence of either T2 or T3 disease. Patients then received four cycles of MVAC and were restaged with a repeat TURBT. Of the 111 patients entered into the study 60 or 54% had a T0 response found on repeat TURBT after chemotherapy. Of these patients, 43 were then followed with TUR or a partial cystectomy alone while the remaining 17 underwent a radical cystectomy. In those patients treated with bladder sparing options 74% were alive at 10 years and 58% retained their bladder. Herr demonstrated two characteristics that favor successful bladder sparing. The first is the pretreatment tumor stage. For those patients who were T2 and underwent MVAC and TUR only, 68% survived with an intact bladder at 10 years vs. only 44% of those with T3 disease. The second factor was a post chemotherapy stage of T0 which translated into a median survival time of 79 months, vs. only 32 months if the patient had residual tumor after chemotherapy. Thus what many have inferred from this study is that the both the initial TURBT and the restaging TURBT are the critical factors in assessing the success of bladder sparing protocols.

7.2. Trimodal Therapy

Trimodal therapy involving a combination of TUR, radiation therapy and chemotherapy has emerged as the most successful bladder sparing method of treating invasive bladder cancer. In 2001, Zeitman et al. presented data on their method of trimodal therapy which is often referred to as the "Shipley Protocol"

(22). Patients with T2-T4 diseases were treated with a combination of a "complete" TUR, followed by 40Gy of external beam therapy and concurrent cisplatin chemotherapy. The majority of patients also received two cycles of neoadjuvant MVAC prior to radiation. Upon completing this induction chemoradiation (CR), a restaging TUR was used to access the level of cancer eradication. Anyone with less than a complete response was recommended for immediate cystectomy. The authors reported a 5 year disease specific survival of 63%, a survival very comparable to that of cystectomy. However, patients who had residual tumor on restaging TURBT had a decreased survival rate compared to those who were T0.

What is most interesting about these protocols, is that in these protocols as well as many others the factors that appear most important is the presence of T0 status. Those with remaining tumor regardless of stage had worse outcomes. The initial re-resection status prior to chemotherapy has also been found to be a significant predictor of the final outcome leading many researchers to hypothesize that the most effective way of managing even invasive tumors with bladder sparing options is with a complete TURBT, usually a restaging TURBT.

8. Conclusions

The TURBT is both a diagnostic and therapeutic procedure whose importance cannot be underestimated. I have often emphasized to my residents that a well performed TURBT is one of the most difficult yet important procedures that a urologist does. In addition, it is one of the more challenging procedures to teach the residents. Mounting irrefutable evidence shows that a restaging TURBT improves our diagnostic accuracy leading to more appropriate treatment. However, what remains unproven although seems intuitive is whether this translates into better survival outcomes. Several other controversies regarding restaging TURBT also remains such as the timing of the repeat TURBT. Also can the repeat TURBT really just be the re-resection of the area or base after the tumor is removed at the initial TURBT. Unfortunately, there is a lack of any objective data to answer these questions, and they are probably unlikely to be answered any time soon if ever. Despite the efforts geared towards creating a complete resection with a TURBT, there is still to this day practically no way to guarantee a complete resection. In the coming years, there is hope that new technology such as real-time intrabladder ultrasound or optical coherence tomography (OCT) will aid in the ability to resect more completely bladder tumors. These techniques may accomplish this by aiding in determining the depth of a lesion and confirming lack of residual tumor at the time of TURBT after resection. However, until the time that such technology is available and in widespread use it appears that the most accurate method of diagnosis and the most likely way to achieve pT0 status is with a restaging TURBT.

References

1. Jewett, H.J. and Strong, G.H. Infiltrating carcinoma of the bladder: relation of depth of penetration of the bladder wall to incidence of local extension and metastases. *J. Urol.*, 55: 372, 1946.
2. Jewett, H.J. Carcinoma of the bladder: influence of depth of infiltration on the 5-year results following complete extirpation of the primary growth. *J. Urol.*, 67: 672–676, 1952.
3. Richie, J.P., Skinner, D.G., and Kaufman, J.J. Radical cystectomy for carcinoma of the bladder: 16 years of experience. *J. Urol.*, 113: 188, 1975.
4. Klan, R., Loy, V., and Huland, H. Residual tumor discovered in routine second transurethral resection in patients with stage T1 transitional cell carcinoma of the bladder. *J. Urol.*, 146: 316–318, 1991.
5. Milner WA. Transurethral biopsy: an accurate method of determining the true malignancy of bladder carcinoma. *J Urol.*, 61: 917–923, 1949
6. Kolozsy Z. Histopathological "self control" in transurethral resection of bladder tumors. *Br J Urol.*, 67: 162–164, 1991.
7. National Bladder Cancer Collaborative Group A. Surveillance initial assessment and subsequent progress of patients with superficial bladder cancer in a prospective longitudinal study. *Cancer Res.*, 37: 2907, 1977.
8. Merfsdor A., Brauers A., Wolff JM., et al. Second TUR for superficial baldder cancer: a must? *J. Urol., part 3*: 159:143; abstract 542, 1998
9. Vogeli, T.A., Grimm, M., and Ackermann R. Prospective study for quality control of TUR of bladder tumors by routine second TUR (reTUR). *J. Urol., part 3*, 159:143; abstract 543, 1998
10. Herr H. Restaging transuretheral resection of high risk superficial bladder cancer improves the initial response to bacillus calmette-guerin therapy. *J. Urol.*, 174:2134–2137, 2005.
11. Herr H. The value of a second transurethral resection in evaluating patients with bladder tumors. *J. Urol.*, 162:74–76, 1999.
12. Dutta S.C., Smith J.A., Shappell S.B., et al. Clinical under staging of high risk nonmuscle invasive urothelial carcinoma treated with radical cystectomy. *J. urol.*, 166:490–493, 2001.
13. Dalbagni, G., Herr, H.W., and Reuter, V.E. Impact of a second transurethral resection on the staging of T1 bladder cancer. *Urology*, 60: 823, 2002.
14. Herr, H.W.: Tumor progression and survival of patients with high grade, noninvasive papillary (TaG3) bladder tumors: 15-year outcome. *J. Urol.*, 163: 60–61, 2000

15. Lee, S.E., Jeong, I.G., Ku, J.H., et al. Impact of transurethral resection of bladder tumor: analysis of cystectomy specimens to evaluate for residual tumor. *Urology*, 63: 873–876, 2004.
16. Herr, H.W. Conservative management of muscle-infiltrating bladder cancer: prospective experience. *J. Urol.*, 138: 1162–1163, 1987.
17. Kirkali, Z., Chan, T., and Manoharan, M., et al. Bladder cancer: epidemiology, staging and grading, and diagnosis. *Urology*, 66: 25–26, 2005.
18. See, W.A. Distal ureteral regeneration after radical transurethral bladder tumor resection. *Urology*, 55: 212–215, 2000.
19. Waehre, H., Ous, S., and Klevmark, B., et al. A bladder cancer multi-institutional experience with total cystectomy for muscle-invasive bladder cancer. *Cancer*, 72: 3044, 1993
20. Thrasher, J.B., Frazier, H.A., Robertson, J.E., et al. Does a stage pT0 cystectomy specimen confer a survival advantage in patients with minimally invasive bladder cancer? *J. Urol.*, 152: 393, 1994.
21. Herr, H.W., Bajorin, D.F., and Scher, H.I. Neoadjuvant chemotherapy and bladder sparing surgery for invasive bladder cancer: ten-year outcome. *J. Clin. Oncol.*, 16: 1298–1300, 1998.
22. Zeitman, A.L., Grocela, J., Zehr, E., et al. Selective bladder conservation using transurethral resection, chemotherapy, and radiation: management and consequences of Ta, T1, and Tis recurrence within the retained bladder. *Urology*, 58: 381–382, 2001.

4
Understaging T2: Limitations of Pelvic Imaging

Jon M. Willatt and Richard H. Cohan

Contents

Abstract Although single detector CT has been used for many years to help stage bladder cancers, the results have been disappointing. However, there is a paucity of literature evaluating the success of CT staging following the advent of multidetector CT (MDCT). The improved resolution and multiplanar reformats available with MDCT are innovations which have yet to be tested in this context.

The aims for imaging techniques to further assess patients in whom the diagnosis of bladder cancer has been made are threefold: (1) to assess for depth of tumor invasion into the bladder wall, (2) to determine the presence and extent of extravesical tumor extension, and (3) to show any local and distant sites of lymph node or other organ metastases.

Keywords CT, Bladder, Cancer, Staging, MRI

1. CT Appearance

With current scanners, CT can detect bladder cancers in over 90% of cases (1, 2). It is believed that one of the major limitations of CT is its inability to detect carcinoma-in-situ, although there are no published studies to prove this. Bladder cancers have been found to enhance more than the normal bladder wall following the administration of intravenous contrast material with peak enhancement occurring at around 60s following the injection (3, 4). This differential enhancement can facilitate tumor detection. Stage T1 tumors typically appear as focal areas of bladder-wall thickening or as pedunculated lesions or filling defects against the background of low attenuation urine or high attenuation excreted intravenous contrast which has passed into the bladder (Fig. 4.1). In contrast T2 lesions are often sessile.

It is acknowledged that CT is normally not able to determine the depth of bladder-wall invasion (i.e., to differentiate T1 from T2 disease). CT is unable to differentiate the layers of the bladder wall, which normally measures up to 3mm in thickness (Fig. 4.2). CT is therefore unable to determine the depth of tumor invasion within the wall itself: that is, it is unable to distinguish between stages T1 and T2a and stages T2a and T2b.

Both stage T1 and T2 tumors can appear as diffuse-wall thickening (Fig. 4.2). However, some of this bladder-wall thickening can be related to inflammatory change adjacent to the tumor. Detection of microscopic invasion of the perivesical tissues (T3a disease) is also challenging for CT (5). The presence of perivesical fat stranding is a poor indicator for invasion, as it is often

From: *Current Clinical Urology: Bladder Cancer*, Edited by: C.T. Lee and D.P. Wood,
DOI: 10.1007/978-1-59745-417-9_4, © Humana Press, a part of Springer Science+Business Media, LLC 2010

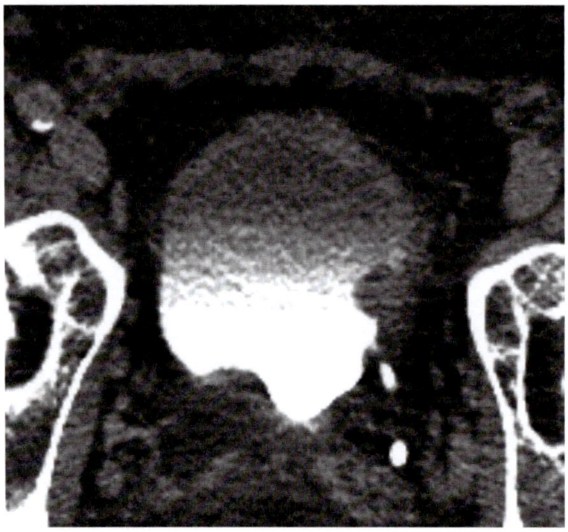

FIG. 4.1. T1 bladder tumor. Axial CT of a 68-year-old male obtained during the venous phase of enhancement. There is a 1.5 cm polypoid mass at the left bladder wall

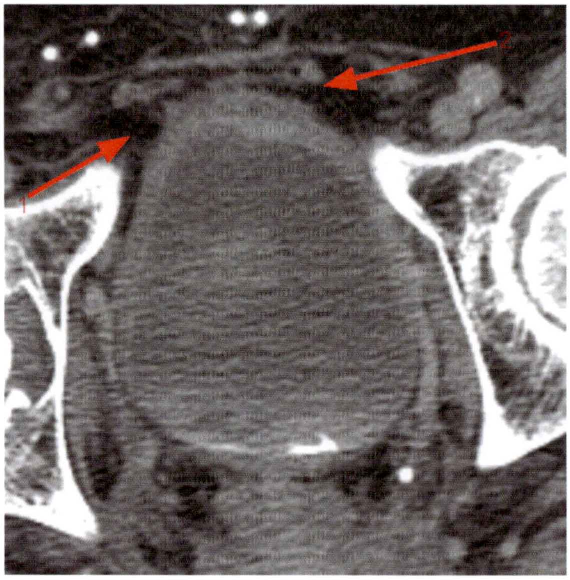

FIG. 4.3. T3 bladder tumor. There is tumor extension into the fat anterior to the bladder (*arrows*) in this 80-year-old male.

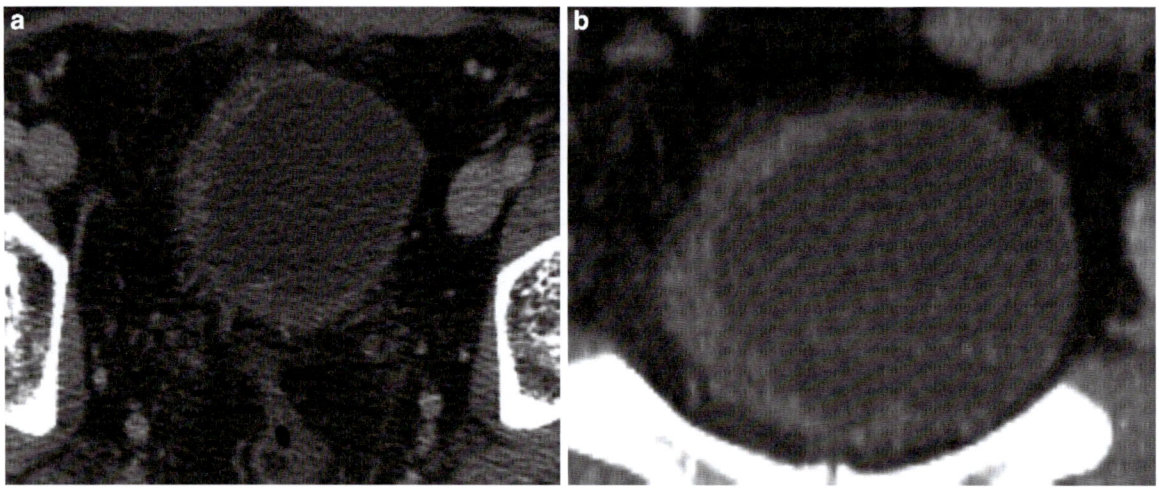

FIG. 4.2. T2 bladder tumor. Axial (**a**) and coronal CT (**b**) of a 44-year-old male. There is diffuse bladder-wall thickening, primarily on the right side laterally, without evidence of extravesical extension. It is not possible to determine the depth of invasion within the bladder wall

caused by inflammatory change or edema, particularly in the context of a recent biopsy or transurethral resection of a bladder tumor (TURBT).

Subtle stage T3b disease is also difficult to identify. Signs of mild extravesical extension include an irregular outer contour of the bladder or high attenuation soft tissue in the fat (Fig. 4.3). In comparison, gross invasion is easier to detect.

Stage T4 disease, which involves invasion of the adjacent organs including the prostate, the seminal vesicles, the uterus and the vagina, can be difficult to identify if it is microscopic or subtle because the fat planes between the bladder and these structures may be obscured even under normal circumstances. In contrast, gross invasion is seen when abnormal enhancing tumor extends directly into adjacent organs (Fig. 4.4).

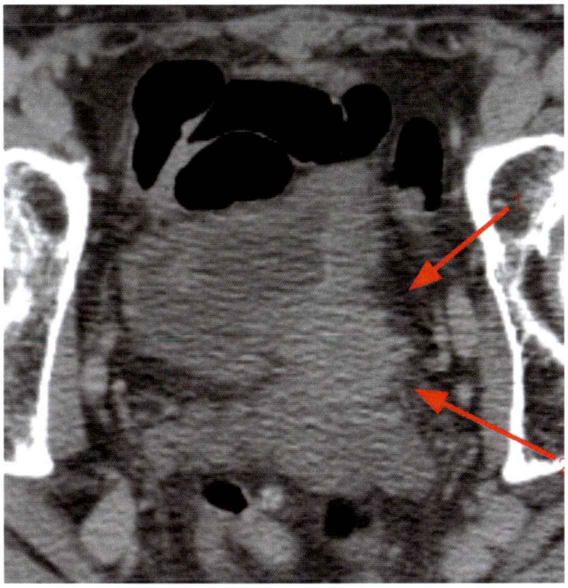

FIG. 4.4. T4 bladder tumor. 82-year-old male with bladder tumor which extends into the left seminal vesicle (*arrows*)

Still a further limitation of CT is its inability to detect microscopic tumor in lymph nodes which are not increased in size (6). The upper limits of normal for pelvic lymph nodes is generally recognized to be 1cm in short axis diameter, but this is an insensitive threshold for the detection of early lymph node involvement.

2. Accuracy of CT in Local Staging

2.1. With Single Detector CT

Despite the potential limitations of CT as described above, initially there were some encouraging studies published in the early 1980s with reported accuracies of 81% for the diagnosis of local tumor extension, and of 83–89% for the detection of lymph node metastases (7–9). In another series, Sawczuk et al. (6) showed that although CT understaged 38% of cases with pelvic lymph node metastases from carcinoma of the bladder and prostate, it overstaged patients for lymph node involvement only 6% of the time.

This early optimism was modified by later studies which appeared in the mid and late 1980s. In 1989 Voges et al. (10) reported a staging accuracy of only 32.3% with understaging noted in 28.1% and overstaging in 39.6% of tumors. There were a number of commonly encountered problems. Perivesical extension was falsely identified in 29.5% of cases, while CT failed to detect extension beyond the bladder wall in 69% of patients who had stage T3 or T4 disease. Paik et al. (11) reported an accuracy of CT in staging of only 54.9% with understaging in 39% and overstaging in 6.1%. In the subgroup of patients in which distinction of T1/T2 from T3/T4 disease was attempted, CT was particularly disappointing. The CT interpretations were incorrect in half of the cases in which the reviewers felt that it suggested the presence of extravesical involvement. In addition, there was understaging by the reviewers in 21% of tumors which involved the perivesical fat or adjacent organs. Reviewers overstaged two of six cases with lymph node metastases and understaged 21%. Finally, Yaman et al. (12) reported a CT staging accuracy of 35% with understaging in 15% and overstaging in 50%.

In summary, most studies have found that single-detector CT is not a useful tool in staging early bladder cancer, or cancer restricted to the layers of the bladder wall.

2.2. With MRI vs. Single Detector CT

When single-detector CT was compared to MRI, staging results with MRI have been either comparable or better. Bryan et al. (13) and Tanimoto et al. (14) reported staging accuracies of 40 and 58% with CT vs. 54 and 85% with MRI. Kim et al. (2) showed a staging accuracy of 55% with CT, although this accuracy improved to 83% if the tumors were grouped together as Ta through T3a and T3b through T4. The results in this study were not significantly different from those of MRI. Husband et al. (15) reported a CT sensitivity and a specificity of 94 and 62% respectively for the detection of extravesical disease. The results were similar with MRI, which demonstrated a sensitivity of 84% and specificity of 62%.

2.3. With Multidetector CT

More recently the accuracy of CT in staging bladder cancer has been reassessed using the new multi-detector CT scanners. In one of the first studies to determine the ability of four channel MDCT to differentiate stages T3a disease and below from T3b disease and above Kim et al. demonstrated an accuracy of 93% with a sensitivity of 89% and a specificity of 95% (3). The confounding factor in

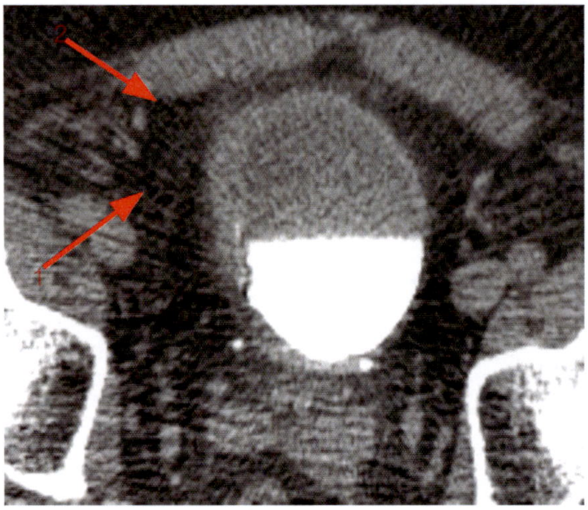

FIG. 4.5. This 58-year-old male underwent TURBT for a tumor. Extravesical extension was reported on the basis of the stranding of the fat anterior and to the right (*arrows*). The pathology report showed no evidence of invasion of the lamina propria.

those few cases which were falsely positive was believed to be inflammation from TURBT performed seven days or less prior to the staging CT. The authors therefore noted that the timing of the staging CT is important, because CT obtained subsequent to biopsy or TURBT, intravesical therapy or radiation, can lead to the appearance of confusing inflammatory stranding of the perivesical fat and false positive results (Fig. 4.5). As a result we do not recommend that staging CT is performed within seven days of biopsy or TURBT.

While previously it has been felt that the lack of fat planes between the bladder and the prostate, and the bladder and the seminal vesicles, limits the ability of CT to detect spread into adjacent organs (5, 16), it is possible that this problem may be reduced on MDCT examinations due to its ability to produce isotropic three- dimensional reformatted images in any plane, including the sagittal and coronal planes. However, this hypothesis has yet to be assessed.

3. Conclusion

CT is believed by most to be a fairly unreliable source of information with regard to many aspects of bladder tumor staging, particularly for small tumors. It cannot reliably differentiate T1 from T2 disease, and T2a from T2b disease. However, a number of recent studies suggest that CT, particularly when performed on multidetector CT scanners, can be used to differentiate T1 or T2 disease from T3 or T4 disease with good accuracy, providing the patient has not had a recent TURBT. If the only question is whether there is extravesical extension, then it appears that CT does have a role to play. Still, the difficulties of distinguishing between perivesical inflammation and local spread of cancer and between bladder wall thickening caused by carcinoma and benign conditions such as cystitis and chronic obstruction persist.

References

1. Turney BW, Willatt JM, Nixon D, Crew JP, Cowan NC. Computed tomography urography for diagnosing bladder cancer. BJU Int. 2006 Aug;98(2):345–8.
2. Kim B, Semelka RC, Ascher SM, Chalpin DB, Carroll PR, Hricak H. Bladder tumor staging: comparison of contrast-enhanced CT, T1- and T2-weighted MR imaging, dynamic gadolinium-enhanced imaging, and late gadolinium-enhanced imaging. Radiology 1994 Oct;193(1):239–45.
3. Kim JK, Park SY, Ahn HJ, Kim CS, Cho KS. Bladder cancer: analysis of multi-detector row helical CT enhancement pattern and accuracy in tumor detection and perivesical staging. Radiology 2004 Jun;231(3):725–31.
4. Xie Q, Zhang J, Wu PH, Jiang XQ, Chen SL, Wang QL, Xu J, Chen GD, Deng JH. Bladder transitional cell carcinoma: correlation of contrast enhancement on computed tomography with histological grade and tumour angiogenesis. Clin. Radiol. 2005 Feb;60(2):215–23.
5. Koss JC, Arger PH, Coleman BG. et al. CT staging of bladder carcinoma. AJR Am. J. Roentgenol. 1981;137:359.
6. Sawczuk IS, de Vere White R, Gold RP. et al. Sensitivity of computed tomography in evaluation of pelvic lymph node metastases from carcinoma of bladder and prostate. Urology 1983;21:81.
7. Colleen S, Ekelund L, Henrikson H, Karp W, Mansson W. Staging of bladder carcinoma with computed tomography. Scand. J. Urol. Nephrol. 1981;15(2):109–13.
8. Vock P, Haertel M, Fuchs WA, Karrer P, Bishop MC, Zingg EJ. Computed tomography in staging of carcinoma of the urinary bladder. Br. J. Urol. 1982 Apr;54(2):158–63.
9. Morgan CL, Calkins RF, Cavalcanti EJ. Computed tomography in the evaluation, staging, and therapy of

carcinoma of the bladder and prostate. Radiology 1981 Sep;140(3):751–61.

10. Voges GE, Tauschke E, Stockle M, Alken P, Hohenfellner R. Computerized tomography: an unreliable method for accurate staging of bladder tumors in patients who are candidates for radical cystectomy. J. Urol. 1989 Oct;142(4):972–4.
11. Paik ML, Scolieri MJ, Brown SL, Spirnak JP, Resnick MI. Limitations of computerized tomography in staging invasive bladder cancer before radical cystectomy. *J. Urol.* 2000 Jun;163(6):1693–6.
12. Yaman O, Baltaci S, Arikan N, Yilmaz E, Gogus O. Staging with computed tomography, transrectal ultrasonography and transurethral resection of bladder tumour: comparison with final pathological stage in invasive bladder carcinoma. *Br. J. Urol.* 1996 Aug;78(2):197–200.
13. Bryan PJ, Butler HE, LiPuma JP et al. CT and MR imaging in staging bladder neoplasms. *J. Comput. Assist. Tomogr.* 1987;11:96.
14. Tanimoto A, Yuasa Y, Imai Y, Izutsu M, Hiramatsu K, Tachibana M, Tazaki H. Bladder tumor staging: comparison of conventional and gadolinium-enhanced dynamic MR imaging and CT. *Radiology* 1992 Dec;185(3):741–7.
15. Husband JE, Olliff JFC, Williams MP et al. Bladder cancer staging with CT and MR imaging. *Radiology* 1989;173:435–40.
16. Lantz EJ, Hattery RR. Diagnostic imaging of urothelial cancer. *Urol. Clin. North Am.* 1984;11:567.

5
MRI Endorectal Coil

Saroja Adusumilli and Hero Hussain

Contents

Abstract Endorectal coil MRI has recently shown promise of improving the accuracy of imaging in the staging of bladder cancer. Specifically, endorectal coil MRI has demonstrated the ability to image at the submucosal and muscle layers, by overcoming limitations of insufficient spatial resolution and poor signal-to-noise that previously hindered its ability to differentiate individual layers of the bladder wall. This chapter reviews the evolution of MR-imaging techniques in bladder cancer staging over the past decade, leading to the most recently published work on endorectal coil MRI. Topics will include high resolution T2-weighted imaging, dynamic contrast-enhanced MRI, endorectal coil principles and technique, and submucosal linear enhancement, all of which have contributed to the recently improved ability of MRIs to accurately assess the relationship of bladder neoplasm to the bladder wall.

Keywords Magnetic resonance imaging, Endorectal coil, Bladder cancer staging, Gadolinium

1. Introduction

Traditionally, conventional magnetic resonance imaging (MRI) performed with external phased array coils has been useful in the detection of bladder carcinoma but has demonstrated limited accuracy in the staging of bladder tumors due to insufficient spatial resolution. The introduction of the endorectal coil in the late 1980s revolutionized MR imaging of prostate cancer by providing high signal-to-noise (SNR) and increased spatial resolution. This resulted in improved delineation of the primary tumor and better sensitivity in detecting extraprostatic spread. Similar technology has more recently been evaluated for use in the staging of bladder cancer and preliminary results are promising. This chapter reviews the evolution of MR-imaging techniques in bladder cancer staging over the past decade, leading to the more recently published work on evaluation of bladder cancer with endorectal coil MRI.

From: *Current Clinical Urology: Bladder Cancer*, Edited by: C.T. Lee and D.P. Wood,
DOI: 10.1007/978-1-59745-417-9_5,

2. Background

Staging of bladder cancer involves assessment of the degree of local tumor extension, identification of lymph node and distant metastases, and determination of the histologic tumor type as defined by the TNM (Tumor, Node, Metastasis) system (1). Conventional bladder cancer staging by MRI focuses on the detection of perivesical extension of tumor and locoregional lymph-node metastases whereas computed tomography (CT) is used primarily to identify distant metastatic disease. In general, MRI is superior to CT for local staging by virtue of its multiplanar imaging capabilities and excellent tissue contrast. However, merely answering the question of whether a bladder neoplasm is confined to the bladder wall or has spread locally in the pelvis does not fully stage tumor or allow the urologist to determine precisely the best treatment for an individual patient. Therefore, a number of radiology investigators have studied the ability of T2-weighted imaging and/or dynamic gadolinium enhanced MRI to improve staging of locally confined disease by better evaluating the depth of tumor invasion into the bladder (i.e., muscle invasion). The advantage of identifying the degree of muscle layer invasion is the ability to determine prognosis and appropriate therapeutic management. Superficial tumors that have not invaded the muscle (≤T1) can be treated by local endoscopic resection (with or without intravesical instillation of chemotherapeutic agents) whereas muscle invasive tumors (≥T2a) are usually treated by radical cystectomy (T2a–T3a) or palliative chemoradiation (T3b–T4b) (2).

For example, a Japanese study in 1995 attempted to detect muscle layer invasion with submillimeter (0.9 × 0.9 mm) pixel T2-weighted MR images to better stage bladder cancer (3). The normal bladder wall was depicted on T2-weighted images as either a single layer of low signal intensity (SI) (in 50% of patients) or a triple layer structure of varying signal intensities (in the remaining 50% of patients) (for example, low SI outer layer, intermediate SI middle layer, and low SI inner layer) (Fig. 5.1). High or intermediate signal intensity carcinomas were divided into five categories (analogous to TNM pathologic staging) based on their relationship with the different layers of the bladder wall: MR category 0 indicated that there was no detectable abnormality of the inner surface of the bladder wall. MR category I (pT1) indicated that there was a detectable high signal intensity layer over the

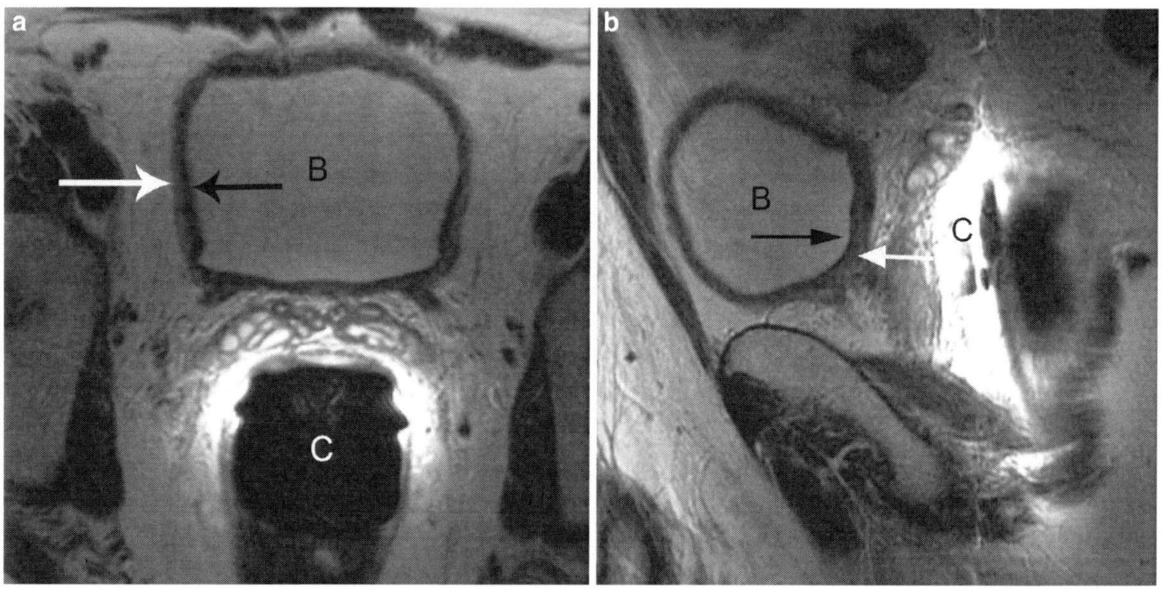

Fig. 5.1. (**a–b**) Normal bladder wall on (**a**) axial and (**b**) sagittal T2-weighted images obtained using an endorectal coil (**c**). Note the low signal intensity muscle layer (*black arrow*) relative to high signal intensity urine in the bladder-B, and the intermediate signal intensity outer serosal layer (*white arrow*). The mucosal/submucosal layer is not discernable from the muscle layer

inner surface of the bladder wall or a mass protruding into the bladder lumen without disruption of the wall. MR category II (pT2) was used when there was an identifiable mass protruding into the lumen and the inner layer of the wall was disrupted. MR category III (pT3) was applied to cases in which there was transmural disruption of the wall, and MR category IV (pT3b or pT4) was utilized when there was complete disruption of the wall (Fig. 5.2) also with an identifiable mass in the perivesicular region. The reported accuracy of this classification scheme for predicting muscle layer invasion in 26 patients was excellent at 96.2% with a sensitivity of 100% and specificity of 91.7% (3).

A number of authors found that the administration of intravenous gadolinium improves both tumor detection and staging accuracy as the bladder mucosa can be distinguished readily from the muscular layer. In addition, dynamic contrast enhanced MRI has been shown to be more accurate than unenhanced MRI in patients who are being studied after undergoing chemotherapy (4). Unfortunately, contrast-enhanced imaging protocols for assessment of bladder carcinoma are quite varied throughout the literature. Still, results have been promising. For example, Tachibana et al. were able to differentiate pT1 tumor from muscle invasive tumor on T1-weighted contrast-enhanced spin-echo sequences because when the muscle was invaded, the low signal intensity muscle layer was disrupted by high signal intensity tumor (5). European investigators have studied dynamic contrast-enhanced T1-weighted gradient-echo imaging to exploit the principle that bladder cancers develop neovascularization and therefore enhance to a greater extent than does adjacent normal muscle wall on arterial phase imaging (6, 7). These researchers found that staging for superficial tumors could be improved from 68 to 84% by using dynamic imaging that included early enhanced image acquisitions. A protocol recently published by Tekes et al. utilized axial fast multiplanar spoiled 2D gradient-echo images (TR/TE 180–300 ms/1.7–4.2 ms; 70° flip angle, 512 × 192 matrix) with fat suppression prior to and following the administration of 0.1 mmole/kg of gadopentate dimeglumine. In this report, arterial phase imaging was performed at 20 s followed by venous phase imaging with each acquisition phase lasting 52–86 s (8). This method resulted in the observation that bladder tumors demonstrate early enhancement as do the mucosa and submucosa. However, there is relatively little or no early enhancement of the muscle layer which maintains hypointensity on T1-weighted imaging (8). Nonetheless, overall accuracy in bladder cancer staging in 71 patients using this method was disappointing at 62%, although staging

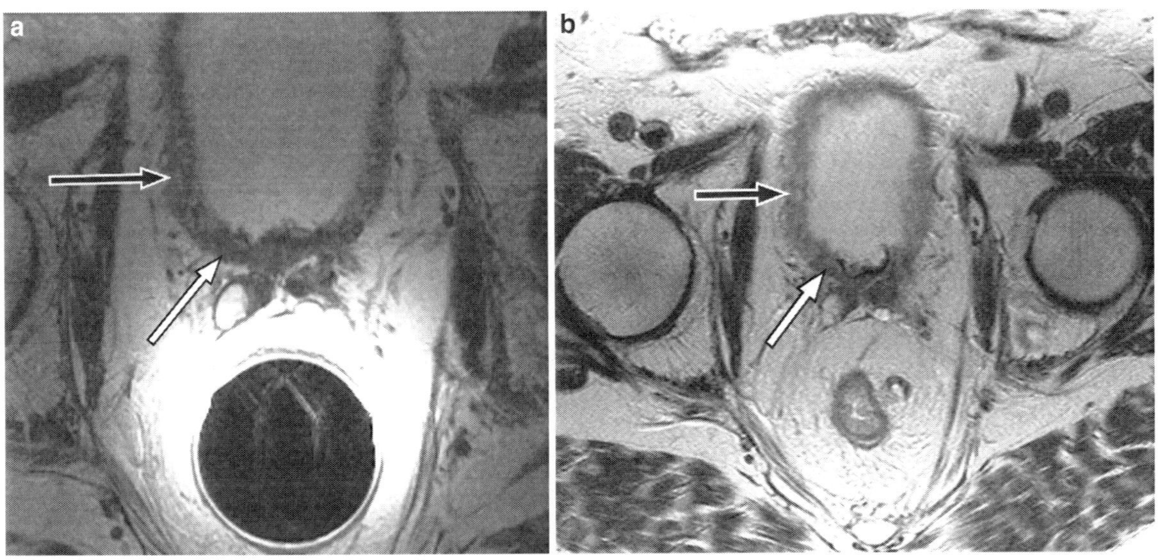

FIG. 5.2. (**a–b**) Prostate tumor invading the bladder wall on axial T2-weighted images obtained using (**a**) an endorectal coil and (**b**) a pelvic coil on a 3 T magnet. Note the complete disruption of the normal layered bladder wall (*black arrow*) by intermediate signal intensity tumor (*white arrow*)

accuracy improved to 85% when the only question to be answered was whether or not there was superficial or muscle invasive tumor.

Some investigators have shown that using these temporal differences in gadolinium enhancement is not sufficient to differentiate among enhancing tumor, scar, and postsurgical granulation tissue (9). This issue is very problematic as a substantial number of patients with bladder cancer are referred for MR staging after having undergone biopsy or transurethral resection of their bladder tumor (TURBT). As a result, investigators from the Netherlands have proposed a faster multislice dynamic contrast-enhanced study using various types of 3D gradient-echo sequences (10). The three-dimensional nature of their image acquisition allows for offline multiplanar reconstruction of high resolution images in every possible plane. Images are not just limited to a plane perpendicular to the site of tumor (11). These investigators have developed a technique that allows for much more rapid image acquisition, thereby greatly improving temporal resolution. Their protocol acquires seven slices every 2 s. The authors have shown that, as a result, they have higher specificity when evaluating bladder carcinoma (2).

3. Endorectal Coil MR Imaging Technique

3.1. Endorectal Coil

Placement of a surface coil adjacent to an organ of interest improves the resolution of an MR study by significantly increasing the signal-to-noise ratio and by reducing the field of view (FOV) (12). These principles form the basis for the development of intracavitary coils such as those used for prostate gland imaging. The proximity of the prostate gland to the rectum makes it well suited for imaging with an endorectal surface coil (13). For similar reasons, the posterolateral and posteroinferior aspects of the bladder wall as well as the bladder neck are ideally suited for imaging with an endorectal coil. The most widely available endorectal coil (Medrad, Pittsburgh, PA) consists of a receiver coil mounted on the inner surface of a balloon probe which allows for easy placement into the rectum. First, the patient is placed in the decubitus position for coil placement. Following insertion of the coil, the balloon is inflated with 60–90 cm^3 of air to seat and expand the coil (14). The patient is subsequently imaged in the supine position.

Despite the tenfold increase in SNR, there are some important disadvantages to using an endorectal coil. The coil is uncomfortable for some patients (especially, those who have severe hemorrhoidal disease) and contraindicated in patients with a history of abdominoperineal resection, radiation proctitis, and active inflammatory bowel disease. Also, with the currently available endorectal coil system, the entire bladder wall cannot be visualized clearly. While the posteroinferior half of the bladder including the bladder neck, and the posterior, posterolateral, and posteroinferior walls are clearly demonstrated (15), the anterior and superior walls of the bladder are not imaged as well. Tumors located in these regions may not be adequately visualized.

There are two patient-related factors that are also inherently important to acquiring optimal MR images of the bladder: (1) the ability of the patient to remain still and minimization of bowel peristalsis so that motion artifact is minimized and (2) the ability of the patient to be scanned while his or her bladder is optimally distended so that the entire luminal surface can be well visualized. Antiperistaltic agents such as glucagon (1 mg intramuscular; Glucagen, Bedford Laboratories, Bedford, OH), or scopolamine butylbromide (20 mg intramuscular or intravenous; Buscopan, Boehringer Ingelheim, New Zealand) are typically administered at the beginning of the examination to minimize rectal spasm and peristalsis (16, 17). An alternative regimen to reduce bowel motion has been proposed as follows: administration of 0.5 ml intravenous glucagon before the study and of 1.5 ml of intravenous glucagon by drip infusion during the MR examination (2). Optimal bladder distention can be difficult to attain depending on the patient's bladder capacity. An underdistended bladder will obscure small tumors due to resulting wall thickening. Similarly, tumors can be missed if the bladder becomes so full as to cause the patient to become restless to the point of motion or to efface subtle flat tumors stretched along the bladder wall. A useful recommendation to achieve optimal bladder filling is to have the patient void 2 h prior to the MRI and then to refrain from voiding until after completion of the study (2).

3.2. MR imaging Protocol

For optimal MR image quality, the endorectal coil is combined with an external surface phased array coil to ensure adequate signal reception from the anterior aspect of the pelvis, thereby improving visualization of tumors in the anterior and superior aspects of the bladder. Commonly employed imaging protocols will include localizer sequences to confirm adequate coil position, followed by axial T1-weighted spin-echo and high resolution T2-weighted fast spin-echo sequences in the axial, coronal, and/or sagittal planes. Optimal planes to be utilized will depend, to some extent, on the location of the tumor. Small fields of view (10–16 cm), high matrix (512 × 512, 512 × 192) and slice thicknesses of 3–5 mm can be used, maximizing image detail, without sacrificing SNR. Fat suppression is not employed for these sequences so that subtle low signal intensity tumor extension into the perivesical fat (which is normally of high signal intensity in the absence of fat suppression) can be detected (18, 19). Larger field-of-view T1- and T2-weighted sequences using the external phased array coil are also frequently used, since they may aid in evaluating the anterior aspect of the bladder and will also detect enlarged lymph nodes.

Gadolinium-enhanced MRI with an endorectal coil can be performed using a variety of different image acquisition timings. Japanese investigators with recently published data on endorectal coil imaging of bladder carcinoma perform nondynamic T1-weighted spin-echo imaging 5 min after gadolinium contrast administration using an FOV of 12 cm, slice thickness of 5 mm, and matrix of 256 × 128 (15, 20). Axial, sagittal, coronal, or oblique planes were obtained to maximize conspicuity of the various portions of the bladder wall. This method allowed for the identification of submucosal linear enhancement which divided the bladder wall into three layers (mucosal, submucosal, muscular), thus enabling the reader to differentiate superficial from muscle invasive tumors (15, 20). A faster multislice dynamic contrast-enhanced study 3D gradient-echo sequence with a temporal resolution of seven slices per 2 s (10) has been postulated as allowing for differentiation of superficial from invasive tumors, but this protocol has not yet been tested in the setting of endorectal coil use.

3.3. Staging Bladder Cancer on Endorectal Coil MRI

Two studies have been published on the topic of gadolinium-enhanced endorectal coil MRI for staging of bladder cancer, originating from Japan in 1998 and then 2000. The initial study on endorectal coil MRI by Takeda and colleagues evaluated normal bladder wall morphology on contrast-enhanced images and introduced the concept of submucosal linear enhancement (SLE) in an animal model (15). It is known that the normal bladder wall consists of four layers: mucosa, submucosal connective tissue, muscle layer, and serosa. Gadolinium has been observed to enter the submucosal layer by passive diffusion and remains in capillaries, arterioles, and small veins for a brief period of time, leading to submucosal linear enhancement. If the signal intensity of the urine is low on T1-weighted images because of early scanning (before the arrival of high SI excreted gadolinium), two layers are visualized. The innermost layer of the normal bladder wall can be seen as a linear area of low SI and the outer layer as a linear area of intermediate SI. Later, usually by the time the signal intensity of the urine is high (after arrival of excreted gadolinium contrast into the bladder lumen), three distinct layers of bladder wall are visualized on T1-weighted imaging as a low SI inner layer, an avidly enhancing middle submucosal layer, and a still intermediate SI outer layer.

On gadolinium-enhanced imaging, tumor that is limited to the mucosa (Tis) or submucosa (T1) can be differentiated from tumor extending beyond the submucosal layer (T2) based upon whether the enhancing submucosal layer is intact or not. When the SLE beneath the tumor maintains continuity, tumor is classified as superficial (≤T1), whereas, if the SLE is interrupted by tumor, disease is considered to be invasive (≥T2a) (Note: superficial muscle invasion (less than half the muscle layer) and deep muscle invasion (more than half the muscle layer) is classified as T2a and T2b, respectively). The reported accuracy for staging bladder cancer using the SLE in 71 patients has been high. Specifically, accuracy of diagnosing muscle invasion is 87% with a sensitivity of 91% and specificity of 87% (20). However, a persistent pitfall of this technique is its inability to distinguish between bladder cancer and inflammatory tissue around the tumor, a problem that can lead to overstaging.

4. Accuracy of MRI for Staging Bladder Cancer

Summarizing the accuracy of MRI in staging bladder cancer essentially reflects the evolution of imaging techniques since 1991—including improvement in both MR hardware (increasing scanner field strength, more advanced surface coils, and faster gradients) and software (faster sequences and more powerful reconstruction techniques). Early studies on low field strength (0.5 T) magnets revealed fairly poor accuracy that was not necessarily an improvement over CT. However, these advances in MR technology have resulted in greatly improved reported MR accuracy in bladder cancer staging of up 73–96% which is 10–33% higher than that obtained with CT (21). Additionally, when MRI is performed, gadolinium use is essential. A 9–14% increase in local staging accuracy has been reported with the use of intravenous gadolinium agents (2). Kim et al. documented a staging accuracy of 75% using dynamic contrast-enhanced MRI with a temporal resolution of 20–40 s in conjunction with delayed postcontrast T1-weighted images (22). Tanimoto et al. found staging accuracy improved from 58% (using unenhanced T1- and T2-weighted imaging) to 74% (using delayed enhancement) to 85% using fast dynamic contrast-enhanced imaging with one image acquired every 2 s (23). Specifically, accuracy of the intramural extent of tumor (T1–T3a) improved because the enhancing mucosa could be distinguished from the muscular layers of the bladder wall. Even faster dynamic imaging (one image per 2 s) introduced by Barentsz et al. improved staging accuracies from 67 (unenhanced T1- and T2-weighted imaging) to 84% and was able to accurately differentiate postbiopsy tissue from malignancy (9). The more recently published endorectal coil MR studies employing a nondynamic gadolinium-enhanced sequence to assess submucosal linear enhancement yielded an accuracy of 87% in diagnosing muscle invasion by tumor (20). This is in contrast to the study by Scattoni et al. which found low accuracy of staging superficial and muscle invasive tumor by using delayed T1-weighted sequences (44 and 63%, respectively). However, this last study was performed on a low field strength (0.5 T) scanner using the body coil, which did not allow for adequate resolution of the submucosal enhancement (6). No study to date has investigated the potential improvement in staging by combining an endorectal MRI with fast dynamic contrast enhanced imaging.

5. Future Developments

The emergence of higher field strength (≥3 T) clinical MR scanners has resulted in the implementation of even faster sequences with still higher resolution. Employing a 3T scanner may even obviate the need for an endorectal coil, a feature which would greatly improve patient comfort and compliance. However, the combination of a 3T scanner and an endorectal coil will probably provide the greatest amount of information. The resultant high SNR and small field of view (FOV) will facilitate the use of thin section and high matrix resolution T2-weighted imaging that could ultimately resolve the individual layers of the bladder wall with greater detail. Similarly, with 3T magnets, ultra-fast multi-slice dynamic imaging becomes feasible without sacrificing high spatial resolution. Fast dynamic contrast-enhanced MRI using a combined endorectal and external surface-phased array coil on a 3T scanner may allow for quantification of microvessel density which could be used to select patients for adjuvant therapy. Patients with tumors showing greater neovascularity may be more responsive to certain chemotherapy agents (7). Fast imaging (i.e., time resolution of at least one image every 2 s) will also help differentiate postbiopsy tissue from malignancy and identify rapidly enhancing metastatic lymph nodes and bone marrow metastases (2).

6. Conclusion

Endorectal coil MRI shows promise for improving staging of bladder cancer at the submucosal and muscle layers by overcoming previous limitations of insufficient spatial resolution and poor SNR, which has until now limited our ability to differentiate the individual layers of the bladder wall on imaging studies. However, larger prospective trials will be necessary to confirm the results of the currently published studies which are based on fairly small sample sizes. Future research will likely expand on techniques introduced by investigators reviewed in this article. For example, high resolution submillimeter pixel T2-weighted imaging is likely better achieved with an endorectal coil at 1.5 or 3T. Also, dynamic contrast-enhanced endorectal studies (1.5 and 3T) with improved temporal and spatial resolution may be combined with delayed imaging to assess the bladder for submucosal linear enhancement, thereby offering more accurate assessment of the relationship of bladder neoplasm to the bladder wall.

References

1. Greene F. *AJCC Cancer Staging Handbook*, 6th ed. New York: Springer, 2002:469.
2. Barentsz JO, Engelbrecht MR, Witjes JA, de la Rosette JJ, van der Graaf M. MR imaging of the male pelvis. Eur Radiol 1999;9:1722–1736.

3. Maeda H, Kinukawa T, Hattori R, Toyooka N, Furukawa T, Kuhara H. Detection of muscle layer invasion with submillimeter pixel MR images: staging of bladder carcinoma. Magn Reson Imaging 1995;13:9–19.
4. Barentsz JO, Berger-Hartog O, Witjes JA, et al. Evaluation of chemotherapy in advanced urinary bladder cancer with fast dynamic contrast-enhanced MR imaging. Radiology 1998;207:791–797.
5. Tachibana M, Baba S, Deguchi N, et al. Efficacy of gadolinium-diethylenetriaminepentaacetic acid-enhanced magnetic resonance imaging for differentiation between superficial and muscle-invasive tumor of the bladder: a comparative study with computerized tomography and transurethral ultrasonography. J Urol 1991;145:1169–1173.
6. Scattoni V, Da Pozzo LF, Colombo R, et al. Dynamic gadolinium-enhanced magnetic resonance imaging in staging of superficial bladder cancer. J Urol 1996;155:1594–1599.
7. Jager GJ, Ruijter ET, van de Kaa CA, et al. Dynamic TurboFLASH subtraction technique for contrast-enhanced MR imaging of the prostate: correlation with histopathologic results. Radiology 1997;203:645–652.
8. Tekes A, Kamel I, Imam K, et al. Dynamic MRI of bladder cancer: evaluation of staging accuracy. AJR Am J Roentgenol 2005;184:121–127.
9. Barentsz JO, Jager GJ, van Vierzen PB, et al. Staging urinary bladder cancer after transurethral biopsy: value of fast dynamic contrast-enhanced MR imaging. Radiology 1996;201:185–193.
10. Barentsz JO, Jager G, Mugler JP, 3rd, et al. Staging urinary bladder cancer: value of T1-weighted three-dimensional magnetization prepared-rapid gradient-echo and two-dimensional spin-echo sequences. AJR Am J Roentgenol 1995;164:109–115.
11. Narumi Y, Kadota T, Inoue E, et al. Bladder tumors: staging with gadolinium-enhanced oblique MR imaging. Radiology 1993;187:145–150.
12. Axel L. Surface coil magnetic resonance imaging. J Comput Assist Tomogr 1984;8:381–384.
13. Martin JF, Hajek P, Baker L, Gylys-Morin V, Fitzmorris-Glass R, Mattrey RR. Inflatable surface coil for MR imaging of the prostate. Radiology 1988;167:268–270.
14. Schnall MD, Lenkinski RE, Pollack HM, Imai Y, Kressel HY. Prostate: MR imaging with an endorectal surface coil. Radiology 1989;172:570–574.
15. Takeda K, Kawaguchi T, Shiraishi T, et al. Normal bladder wall morphology in Gd-DTPA-enhanced clinical MR imaging using an endorectal surface coil and histological assessment of submucosal linear enhancement using [14C]Gd-DOTA autoradiography in an animal model. Eur J Radiol 1998;26:290–296.
16. Siegelman ES. Magnetic resonance imaging of the prostate. Semin Roentgenol 1999;34:295–312.
17. Marti-Bonmati L, Graells M, Ronchera-Oms CL. Reduction of peristaltic artifacts on magnetic resonance imaging of the abdomen: a comparative evaluation of three drugs. Abdom Imaging 1996;21:309–313.
18. Mirowitz SA, Reinus WR, Hammerman AM. Evaluation of fat saturation technique for T2-weighted MR imaging of the spine. Magn Reson Imaging 1994;12:599–604.
19. Tsuda K, Yu KK, Coakley FV, Srivastav SK, Scheidler JE, Hricak H. Detection of extracapsular extension of prostate cancer: role of fat suppression endorectal MRI. J Comput Assist Tomogr 1999;23:74–78.
20. Hayashi N, Tochigi H, Shiraishi T, Takeda K, Kawamura J. A new staging criterion for bladder carcinoma using gadolinium-enhanced magnetic resonance imaging with an endorectal surface coil: a comparison with ultrasonography. BJU Int 2000;85:32–36.
21. Barentsz JO, Jager GJ, Witjes JA, Ruijs JH. Primary staging of urinary bladder carcinoma: the role of MRI and a comparison with CT. Eur Radiol 1996;6:129–133.
22. Kim B, Semelka RC, Ascher SM, Chalpin DB, Carroll PR, Hricak H. Bladder tumor staging: comparison of contrast-enhanced CT, T1- and T2-weighted MR imaging, dynamic gadolinium-enhanced imaging, and late gadolinium-enhanced imaging. Radiology 1994;193:239–245.
23. Tanimoto A, Yuasa Y, Imai Y, et al. Bladder tumor staging: comparison of conventional and gadolinium-enhanced dynamic MR imaging and CT. Radiology 1992;185:741–747.

6
PET Imaging: Advances in the Detection of Locally Advanced and Nodal Disease

Morand Piert

Contents

Abstract Promising PET tracers for the visualization of bladder wall invasion and metastastic disease in bladder cancer include [^{18}F]fluorodeoxyglucose performed with rigorous forced diuresis and [^{11}C] choline. Dedicated PET/CT imaging is preferred for better anatomical identification of suspicious lesions. Future applications may include the use of handheld intraoperative beta and high-energy gamma probes as well as endoscopic probes to detect very small-volume disease.

Keywords [^{18}F]fluorodeoxyglucose, [^{11}C]choline, [^{11}C]methionine, Intraoperative approaches, Beta probes, High-energy gamma probes

1. [^{18}F]fluorodeoxyglucose (FDG)

Although the specificity of [^{18}F]fluorodeoxyglucose (FDG) for malignant tissue is limited, positron emission tomography (PET) has undergone rapid expansion and is now well established in clinical oncology (1). FDG PET localizes malignant tissue including bladder cancer based on the upregulation of glucose transporters and subsequent phosphorylization by the hexokinase enzyme, leading to increased contrast between tumor and background tissues typically measured 1–2 h after tracer injection.

PET imaging of urological malignancies has been much slower to develop, partly because of the excretion of tracers through the renal tract with subsequent accumulation in the urinary bladder and possible uptake in ureters, hindering easy identification of suspicious pelvic structures against potentially high background levels. Since the presence of lymph node and distant metastasis are major determinants of survival in bladder cancer, initial investigations have focused on the detection of such metastatic lesions. Kosuda et al. (2) reported that PET imaging identified 17 of 17 patients with metastatic disease (lung, bone, and remote lymph nodes) as well as 2 of 3 patients with localized lymph node involvement. Similarly, Heicappell and coworkers (3) reported a 67% detection rate for local nodal disease in a small series of patients. In addition, FDG has been found useful

From: *Current Clinical Urology: Bladder Cancer*, Edited by: C.T. Lee and D.P. Wood,
DOI: 10.1007/978-1-59745-417-9_6,

for the identification of recurrent disease (2). More recently, Drieskens et al. (4) performed FDG PET and CT imaging in 55 patients with, based on conventional staging, nonmetastatic invasive bladder cancer. The imaging results were compared with the gold standard consisting of histopathology (lymphadenectomy or guided biopsy) or clinical follow-up for 12 months. The sensitivity, specificity, and accuracy of FDG PET was found to be 60, 88 and 78%, respectively, which is a modest improvement over conventional staging using CT.

High levels of FDG activity in urine can obscure low-level lesions in adjacent structures such as the kidney and urinary bladder (5). In addition, stagnant FDG in the ureter might occasionally be falsely regarded as active tumor site (6). To overcome these limitations, retrograde irrigation of the urinary bladder or forced diuresis with intravenous hydration had been advocated. Kosuda et al. (2) and Koyama et al. (7) used Foley catheterization and saline irrigation either before or during PET data acquisition. Although this technique facilitates the evaluation of bladder tumors, it may also result in substantial morbidity to the patient and increases radiation exposure to the PET personnel (8). Forced diuresis coupled with intravenous hydration, in contrast, is a safe and well-tolerated method that enhances urinary flux and allows rapid evacuation of the urinary bladder (9). By using this technique, Kamel et al. (10) recently found that any significant FDG activity from the lower urinary tract was eliminated in 31 of 32 (97%) patients after the bladder had been voided three successive times. Twelve intravesical lesions were visualized with outstanding clarity, whereas radiologic suspicion of locally recurrent bladder tumors was ruled out in three patients. Among 14 indeterminate or equivocal extravesical foci, seven were identified as clinically nonrelevant since they disappeared after furosemide challenge, whereas seven persisting foci were later proven to be true-positive PET findings. The protocol did, however, not improve the characterization of three renal lesions. On the basis of these recent findings, FDG PET imaging of bladder cancer appears to be of additional clinical value as long as rigorous forced diuresis with or without bladder irrigation is performed.

2. [^{11}C]methionine (MET)

To avoid any potential difficulties with urinary activity, PET tracers with minimal urinary excretion have been evaluated in bladder cancer patients. Most are labeled with Carbon-11, which has a short half-life of 20 min and therefore necessitates an on-site cyclotron for clinical studies.

Given an appropriate tumor size for PET imaging, primary bladder cancer could, for instance, be visualized with the carbon-11-labeled amino acid [^{11}C]methionine (MET) (11). However, no evidence was found to suggest that MET would improve local staging. Therefore, MET was not advocated for routine use.

3. [^{11}C]choline (CHOL)

Perhaps, the most promising new PET radiopharmaceutical for bladder cancer imaging was introduced in 2002. Carbon-11-labeled [^{11}C]choline (CHOL) is incorporated into tumor cells by conversion into phosphorolycholine and phosphatidylcholine, which is trapped inside the cell causing a rapid accumulation of radioactivity. Since tumor cell growth and mitotic activity demand for an increased biosynthesis of cell membranes, the key enzyme choline kinase is upregulated in a number of malignancies (12). The uptake of CHOL in tumors was found to be linked to the rate of tumor cell proliferation (13, 14), indicating its potential for monitoring of antiproliferative therapies. CHOL is cleared very rapidly from the blood and undergoes rapid uptake in bladder cancer allowing PET imaging as early as minutes after intravenous tracer injection.

De Jong and coworkers (15) were the first to study 18 patients with bladder cancer. CHOL uptake in normal bladder wall was low, and the bladder margin was only outlined by minimal urinary radioactivity. In ten patients, tumor tissues were detected correctly, while one false-positive CHOL PET scan was seen in a patient with an indwelling catheter for two weeks prior to the PET scan. Picchio et al. (16) investigated 27 patients with invasive urothelial bladder cancer referred for radical cystectomy and pelvic lymph node dissection (PLND) on the basis of a histologic evaluation after transurethral resection of bladder cancer. PET scanning was performed 5 min after intravenous tracer injection and compared with contrast-enhanced CT. The presence of residual bladder cancer (pTa-pT4) was correctly detected in 21 of 25 histologically tumor-positive patients (84%) by CT and in 24 of 25 patients (96%) by CHOL PET. Lymph node involvement was correctly detected in four of eight patients (50%) by CT and in five of eight patients (62%) by CHOL

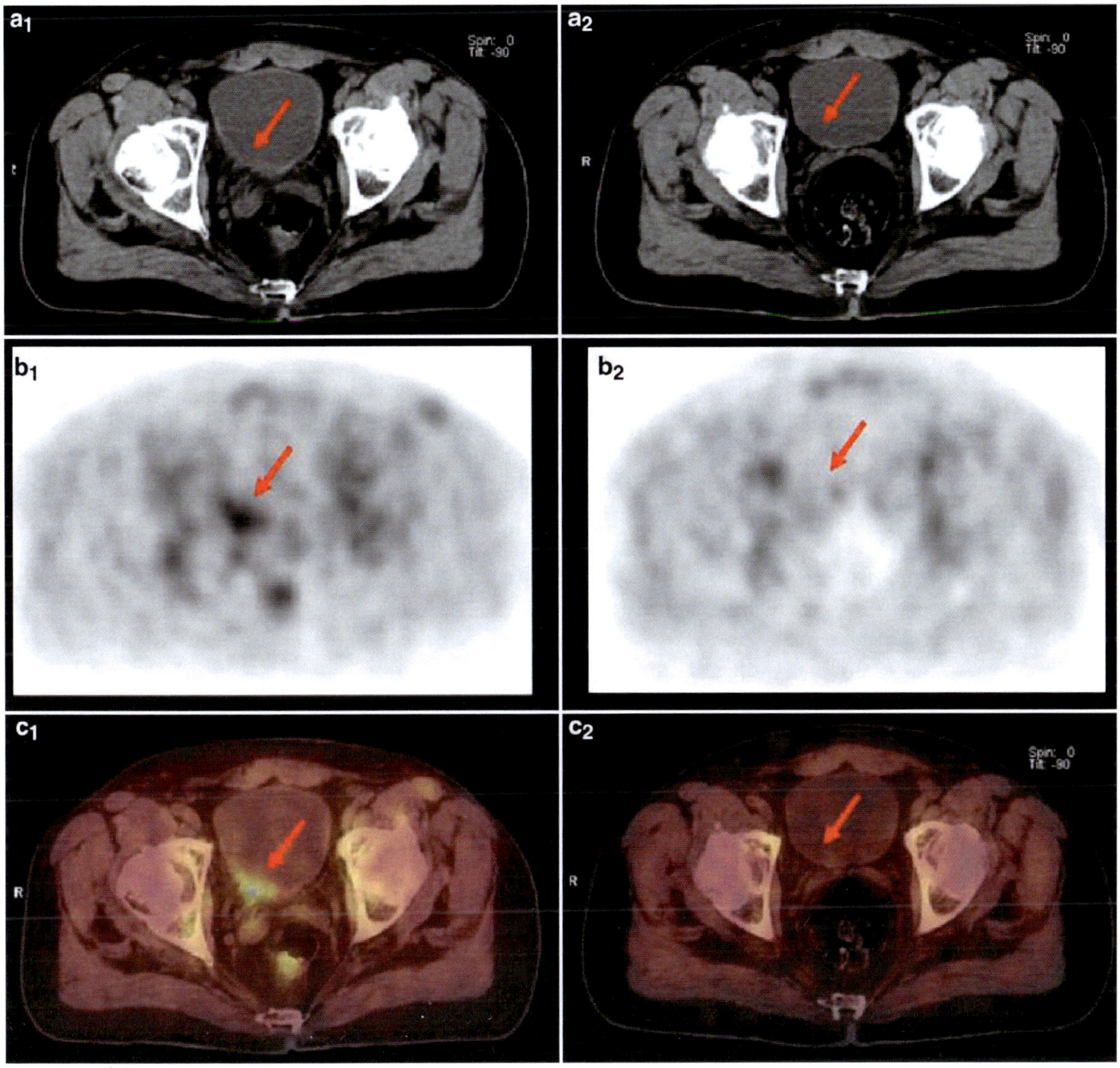

Fig. 6.1. Transaxial CT (**a**), CHOL PET (**b**) and respective PET/CT fusion (**c**) images of a patient with bladder cancer prior to and after chemotherapy with six cycles of a combination of paclitaxel, carboplatin, and gemcitabine. Before treatment (1), enhanced CHOL uptake is noted in an area of bladder wall thickening (red arrows) indicating tumor tissue on CT. After treatment (2), CHOL uptake has normalized and CT shows a normal thickness of the bladder wall, indicating that CHOL PET has potential to monitor chemotherapy of bladder cancer

PET. Interestingly, the authors provided measurements of the size of these three falsely CHOL-negative lymph nodes (median 9 mm, ranging from 6 to 21 mm), as well as the median size of the metastatic lesions within these (3 mm, range 1–15 mm). CT resulted in a high rate (22%) of false-positive lymph nodes, whereas none was demonstrated for CHOL. These data provide evidence that CHOL PET is comparable to CT for detecting residual bladder cancer after TURB but appears to be superior to CT for the evaluation of potential additional lymph node metastases.

Figure 6.1 shows a subject with bladder cancer prior to and after chemotherapy with six cycles of a combination of paclitaxel, carboplatin, and gemcitabine. While CHOL uptake in the thickened bladder wall is noted before treatment, no increased uptake is noted after successful therapy suggesting its usefulness in monitoring cytotoxic therapies of bladder cancers.

4. Intraoperative Approaches

The outcome of locally advanced bladder cancer with lymphonodal disease is poor. This, in part, can be attributed to the lack of a reliable intraoperative identification of small tumor masses such as primary tumors infiltrating neighboring structures and small lymph node metastases. Identifying vital tumor tissue visually can be especially difficult for the surgeon after neoadjuvant treatment. The ability to pinpoint vital tumor tissue, for instance with FDG or CHOL, however, opens the door to identify small tumor lesions using specifically designed handheld detectors. Such probes can either detect 511 KeV annihilation photons (high-energy gamma probes) resulting from the decay of Fluorine-18 or Carbon-11, or alternatively positron probes detect emitted beta particles (positrons). The selective detection of beta particles may be advantageous for the localization of very small amounts (mg) of tumor tissue. Beta particles resulting from the decay of Fluorine-18 have a mean range of only 0.5 mm, and a maximum range of 2.4 mm in water before annihilation into two 511-KeV photons (17, 18). If such positron probes have sufficient sensitivity, they can localize simulated tumor lesions smaller than 15 mg within the background activity. Such positron probes have been applied successfully in many cancers using FDG (19, 20). However, the short range of positrons in tissue necessitates a primary localization of suspected tumor tissue either visually by the surgeon or by using high-energy gamma detectors, which allow the detection of hot spots that are several centimeters away from the detector head. However, high-energy gamma detectors do not provide the same exquisite sensitivity as beta probes; still they are capable of detecting FDG positive tumor lesions in situ (21). Perhaps, best suited are now the commercially available detector systems that combine beta and high-energy gamma detectors in a single unit, allowing to scan the surgical bed using a gamma probe and specifically target suspicious small lesions with a positron probe (22).

Although such devices have not been tested in bladder cancer, one can speculate that it might be possible to identify tumor tissue in the bladder wall with endoscopic beta probes. Such probes may be able to guide TURB procedures using CHOL, where urinary activity is minor. Also, it can be expected that combined beta and high-energy gamma detectors are capable of detecting small tumor lesions (few mg) facilitating cystectomy procedures and lymph node explorations using either CHOL or FDG.

5. Conclusion

Imaging of bladder cancer is a particularly difficult task for any cross-sectional imaging modality including CT, MRI, and PET. On the basis of the current knowledge, either FDG imaging performed with rigorous forced diuresis with or without bladder irrigation or CHOL are promising tools for the visualization of larger vital tumor masses in the bladder wall as well as regional or distant metastases. Both methodologies allow monitoring of treatment by means of metabolic information that promise earlier detection of response to treatment compared to anatomical imaging like conventional CT and MRI. The additional utilization of dedicated PET/CT scanner will further facilitate the anatomical identification of suspicious lesions leading to increased accuracy. However, because of unavoidable resolution restriction of current state-of-the-art PET and PET/CT scanners, the successful detection of micrometastases will remain a rare event. The use of intraoperative probes that detect radioactivity derived from such tracers may, however, substantially further decrease the required size for successful detection.

References

1. Gambhir SS, Czernin J, Schwimmer J, Silverman DH, Coleman RE, Phelps ME. A tabulated summary of the FDG PET literature. J Nucl Med 2001;42(5 Suppl):1S–93S.
2. Kosuda S, Kison PV, Greenough R, Grossman HB, Wahl RL. Preliminary assessment of fluorine-18 fluorodeoxyglucose positron emission tomography in patients with bladder cancer. Eur J Nucl Med 1997;24(6):615–20.
3. Heicappell R, Muller-Mattheis V, Reinhardt M, et al.. Staging of pelvic lymph nodes in neoplasms of the bladder and prostate by positron emission tomography with 2-[(18) F]-2-deoxy-D-glucose. Eur Urol 1999;36(6):582–7.
4. Drieskens O, Oyen R, Van Poppel H, Vankan Y, Flamen P, Mortelmans L. FDG-PET for preoperative staging of bladder cancer. Eur J Nucl Med Mol Imaging 2005;32(12):1412–7.
5. Subhas N, Patel PV, Pannu HK, Jacene HA, Fishman EK, Wahl RL. Imaging of pelvic malignancies with in-line FDG PET-CT: case examples and common pitfalls of FDG PET. Radiographics 2005;25(4):1031–43.
6. Abouzied MM, Crawford ES, Nabi HA. 18F-FDG imaging: pitfalls and artifacts. J Nucl Med Technol 2005;33(3):145–55; quiz 62–3.
7. Koyama K, Okamura T, Kawabe J, et al. Evaluation of 18F-FDG PET with bladder irrigation in patients with uterine and ovarian tumors. J Nucl Med 2003;44(3):353–8.
8. Roberts FO, Gunawardana DH, Pathmaraj K, et al.. Radiation dose to PET technologists and strategies to lower occupational exposure. J Nucl Med Technol 2005;33(1):44–7.
9. Boubaker A, Prior J, Antonescu C, Meyrat B, Frey P, Delaloye AB. F + 0 renography in neonates and infants younger than 6

months: an accurate method to diagnose severe obstructive uropathy. J Nucl Med 2001;42(12):1780–8.
10. Kamel EM, Jichlinski P, Prior JO, et al. Forced diuresis improves the diagnostic accuracy of 18F-FDG PET in abdominopelvic malignancies. J Nucl Med 2006;47(11):1803–7.
11. Ahlstrom H, Malmstrom PU, Letocha H, Andersson J, Langstrom B, Nilsson S. Positron emission tomography in the diagnosis and staging of urinary bladder cancer. Acta Radiol 1996;37(2):180–5.
12. Pieterman RM, Que TH, Elsinga PH, et al. Comparison of (11)C-choline and (18)F-FDG PET in primary diagnosis and staging of patients with thoracic cancer. J Nucl Med 2002;43(2):167–72.
13. Hara T, Inagaki K, Kosaka N, Morita T. Sensitive detection of mediastinal lymph node metastasis of lung cancer with 11C-choline PET. J Nucl Med 2000;41(9):1507–13.
14. Shimizu H, Kumabe T, Shirane R, Yoshimoto T. Correlation between choline level measured by proton MR spectroscopy and Ki-67 labeling index in gliomas. AJNR Am J Neuroradiol 2000;21(4):659–65.
15. de Jong IJ, Pruim J, Elsinga PH, Jongen MM, Mensink HJ, Vaalburg W. Visualisation of bladder cancer using (11) C-choline PET: first clinical experience. Eur J Nucl Med Mol Imaging 2002;29(10):1283–8.
16. Picchio M, Treiber U, Beer AJ, et al. Value of 11C-choline PET and contrast-enhanced CT for staging of bladder cancer: correlation with histopathologic findings. J Nucl Med 2006;47(6):938–44.
17. Bai B, Ruangma A, Laforest R, Tai Y-C, Leahy RM. Positron range modeling for statistical PET image reconstruction. IEEE 2003;4:2501–5.
18. Fowler JS, Wolf AP. Positron emitter-labeled compounds: Priorities and problems. InPhelps M, Mazziotta J, Schlebert H, eds. Positron emission tomography and autoradiography Principles and applications for the brain and heart. New York: Raven Press; 1986:391–450.
19. Meisetschlaeger G, Burian M, Piert M, et al. Intraoperative Detection of Tumor Sites with increased F-18-FDG metabolism by using an intraoperative Positron Probe – Proof of principle and first experiences. J Nucl Med 2005;45(6):1413.
20. Piert M, Burian M, Meisetschläger G, et al. Positron detection for the intraoperative localisation of cancer deposits. Eur J Nucl Med Mol Imaging 2007;34:1534–44.
21. Gulec SA, Daghighian F, Essner R. PET-probe: evaluation of technical performance and clinical utility of a handheld high-energy gamma probe in oncologic surgery. Ann Surg Oncol 2006.
22. Daghighian F, Mazziotta JC, Hoffman EJ, et al. Intraoperative beta probe: a device for detecting tissue labeled with positron or electron emitting isotopes during surgery. Med Phys 1994;21(1):153–7.

7
Detection of Extravesical Disease: A Lack of Bladder Cancer Markers

Andrew A. Stec, Michael S. Cookson, and Sam S. Chang

Contents

Abstract Understaging is a significant problem in the treatment of Urothelial Carcinoma of the bladder. Up to 70% of patients with perceived organ-confined tumors have been found to be understaged by the current clinical standard at the time of cystectomy. With advances in molecular biology, tumor markers that can detect and predict prognosis of patients with bladder cancer are emerging. Both urine and serum cancer markers that aid in differentiating between superficial and invasive bladder cancer are being investigated. This chapter examines the spectrum of predictive markers including microsatellite-associated markers, proto-oncogenes/oncogenes, tumor suppressor genes, cell cycle regulators, angiogenesis-related factors, extracellular adhesion molecules, and circulating serum markers. While no marker is yet a proven gold

From: *Current Clinical Urology: Bladder Cancer*, Edited by: C.T. Lee and D.P. Wood,
DOI: 10.1007/978-1-59745-417-9_7, © Humana Press, a part of Springer Science+Business Media, LLC 2010

standard for predicting the extravesicular extension of bladder tumors, promising early data exists on bladder cancer markers that may differentiate those individuals with organ-confined disease from those with the poorer prognosis of more advanced cancer.

Keywords Bladder cancer, Tumor markers, Molecular markers, Extravesical disease, Invasive bladder cancer

1. Introduction

Bladder cancer statistics report 260,000 new cases worldwide per year with 63,210 new cases occurring in the United States alone (1). This represents the fourth most common malignancy in men and the ninth most common malignancy in women in the United States. The U.S. mortality for 2005 totalled 13,180 deaths from bladder cancer (1). The most commonly occurring bladder cancer is urothelial carcinoma (UC).

Current therapy for UC is based primarily on the initial clinical staging of the tumor, a strategy fraught with several potential pitfalls due to limitations in current diagnostic tools and prognostic parameters. Standard staging for UC consists of cystoscopy, transurethral resection (TUR), pathologic interpretation and imaging of the abdomen and pelvis including upper tracts with intravenous pyelography (IVP), computerized tomography (CT), or magnetic resonance imaging (MRI) and chest imaging with conventional chest X-ray or chest CT. CT scan, a routinely relied upon staging tool has been shown to significantly understage disease, having up to 68% false-negative rate when evaluating preoperative nodal disease in patients thought to have organ-confined UC undergoing cystectomy (2). Understaging is a significant clinical problem in the evaluation of patients with advanced UC.

To illustrate the current limitations in staging, Stein et al. reported a 43% rate of understaging in patients thought to have clinically confined tumors in a cohort of 1,054 patients who underwent cystectomy (3). Confirmed in a recent study by Ficarra et al., 70% of 140 patients thought to have clinically organ-confined (cT2) or less disease who underwent radical cystectomy were found to be understaged at the time of radical cystectomy (4). The currently accepted diagnostic approach lends itself to understaging the disease. Confounding issues include the variability of the quality and depth of the initial TUR, histopathologic interpretation difficulties, and inability of abdominal and pelvic CT scan to adequately predict extravesical disease; lack of physical exam findings to determine and appreciate disease progression, and a lack of tumor markers or blood tests to determine the lethal and metastatic potential for specific tumors. A large volume of research is being focused on evaluating and validating various molecular tumor markers in the detection of bladder cancer, while the use of markers for staging and prognosis of disease is still in its fledgling state.

Since major treatments involving bladder cancer focus on differentiating between muscle invasive and nonmuscle invasive disease, understaging disease can have lethal consequences. In this chapter, we focus on attempts to detect extravesical disease, including locally advanced pT3 disease and greater. We examine tumor markers that have implications in the staging of bladder cancer as it relates to detecting extravesical disease. No gold standard marker currently exists; the major focus is placed on tumor markers that predict the presence or likelihood of invasion. There will also be additional emphasis on tumor markers that have been found to be indicators of occult extravesical disease, rapid disease progression, or significantly decreased survival. Of note, these new prognostic markers have only been tested in a relatively limited fashion and only a few parallel studies have been performed to assess the efficacy and reproducibility of the preliminary data. However, with the advances in molecular biology and pathophysiologic development of tumors on a cellular level, much of the early data is promising.

Currently, prognostic markers for UC of the bladder, derived primarily from either urine or tissue samples, can be broken down into six major categories: microsatellite-associated markers, proto-oncogenes/oncogenes, tumor suppressor genes, cell cycle regulators, angiogenesis-related factors, and extracellular adhesion molecules (5). There are multiple genes and protein products in each of these categories. Additionally, early work is being carried out in detecting UC using traditional serum markers established for other solid tumors. This chapter emphasizes specific examples that possibly identify higher grade tumors that are more biologically aggressive. The biological role of each marker will be examined, as well as its prognostic significance in predicting advanced stages of bladder cancer.

2. Microsatellite Associated Markers

UC perpetuates along two distinct genetic pathways (6). Oxidative damage in susceptible cells causes chromosomal changes leading to DNA abnormalities that change the overall growth pattern of tumors (7). One pathway leads to carcinoma in situ (CIS), high-grade, invasive carcinoma that is more likely to progress and become invasive. The second pathway leads to recurrent, noninvasive, papillary tumors that usually do not progress. According to the work by Kiemeney et al. less than 5% of these superficial, noninvasive papillary tumors will convert to the alternate pathway of high grade, invasive UC (8). If molecular gene products and DNA analysis can predict which tumors harness these potentially lethal chromosomal alterations, it will lead to a new tool to identify those patients whose disease will progress to a more invasive and aggressive pathway.

2.1. Fluorescence In Situ Hybridization (FISH)

Different chromosomal and allelic variations that can differentiate superficial Ta tumors from those tumors with more aggressive potential have been discovered. Noninvasive papillary tumors are primarily found to have alterations of chromosome 9, specifically the loss of p16, a tumor suppressor gene found at the 9p21 locus. High-grade and more aggressive tumors exhibit a more marked genetic variation, showing a predictable yet diverse array of chromosomal additions and losses that start initially with the loss of all or a portion of chromosome 9 (7). The additional variations are primarily associated with chromosomes 7, 9, and 17 (9). Waldman et al. demonstrated that polysomy of chromosome 7 was correlated directly with increasing tumor grade and pathological stage in 27 cases of Urothelial Carcinoma (10). The allelic loss of chromosome 17p distinguishes high-grade from low-grade Urothelial Carcinoma of the bladder (11). Finally, monosomy of chromosome 9 correlates significantly with earlier tumor recurrences (12). These polymorphic genetic differences found between higher grade and stage UC open the door for clinical DNA analyses to aid in distinguishing between superficial and more aggressive forms of carcinoma.

Fluorescence in situ hybridization (FISH) utilizes fluorescently labeled DNA probes, specific for various chromosomal foci, to evaluate and detect these numerical and structural chromosomal anomalies. In 2001, the FDA approved the first test using an optimal combination of DNA probes for four specific sites on chromosomes 3, 7, 17 and locus 9p21. Cells from the urine are collected and cells with abnormal morphology, including large or irregular nuclei, are clustered and analyzed. A minimum of 25 abnormal cells are evaluated using the fluorescent probes; if at least four cells show abnormal ploidy of at least two chromosomes or at least 12 cells show loss of 9p21, the test is deemed positive (12).

A recent meta-analysis of the published FISH literature reported superior predictive capabilities of FISH compared to cytology across all stages of UC. The overall sensitivity of FISH was found to be 74%, a considerable increase from the 54% sensitivity of cytology. The most profound finding was that FISH analysis detects high-grade UC and CIS at a higher rate than conventional cytology. FISH had 96% sensitivity for Grade 3 UC compared to 71% for cytology. FISH analysis detected invasive UC 94 vs. 76% for cytology. Finally, for CIS, FISH had a sensitivity of 100 vs. 67% for cytology. Of note, most of these studies were prospective data (9). One unique study performed at the Cleveland Clinic included 82 patients with known malignancy whose cytology was negative or atypical. FISH analysis, performed on these archived tissue samples, detected 85% of the cancers including 15 invasive tumors and 23 of 24 high-grade tumors (13). While not without limitations, FISH analysis of chromosomal abnormalities in urine samples may prove to yield significant prognostic value in detecting extravesical disease, UC with increased potential to become invasive, CIS, and high-grade tumors most likely to progress.

3. Proto-Oncogenes/Oncogenes

An oncogene is a genetic sequence that can undergo a sequential or mutational change resulting in constitutive activation and gain of function. There are two major oncogenes and several minor ones being investigated in UC with varying degrees of success: epidermal growth factor (EGFR) and HER-2.

3.1. Epidermal Growth Factor Receptor (EGFR)

EGFR is a transmembrane glycoprotein which is activated by the binding of epidermal growth factor and TGFa, resulting in cellular proliferation, transformation, and cell division (14). Since a 1985 study, the overexpression of EGFR has had an association with high-grade and high-stage bladder cancer (15). Using immunohistochemistry (IHC) analysis to evaluate the expression of EGFR in UC tumors, it has been shown that invasive UC has a higher preponderance of gene overexpression when compared to superficial UC (16, 17). Overall, the prognostic results of overexpression of EGFR are mixed. One prospective study evaluating 212 patients with newly diagnosed UC found EGFR expression to be an independent predictor of survival and stage progression (18). Somewhat contrary to this study were the results when 43 patients with invasive UC were evaluated by IHC where 86% were found to have an abundance of EGFR expression, but overall this had no prognostic significance (19). Popov et al. evaluated 113 UC samples with IHC and found that EGFR overexpression was found in 6.7% of pTa, 27.7% of pT1, 80.0% of pT2, and 80.6% of pT3 and pT4 tumors (20). While the results with EGFR expression remain controversial, preliminary data suggests that its overexpression may be related to invasive tumorigenesis and worse overall prognosis.

3.2. Her-2

The Her-2 gene product is a tyrosine kinase receptor that activates intracellular phosphorylation of proteins that trigger cellular differentiation and growth (21). Lipponen et al., in 1991, used IHC to demonstrate that UC frequently overexpressed an altered product of Her-2 (22). Studies have been conducted to evaluate the prognostic significance of this oncogene with mixed results. Two separate investigations showed that Her-2 expression, when evaluated by IHC, showed no independent prognostic significance when compared with tumor stage and grade (23, 24). Sato et al. retrospectively reviewed 88 patients with muscle-invasive UC and found Her-2 to be an independent prognostic factor. It was also shown that overexpression correlated with increasing tumor grade, cancer-specific survival, and incidence of metastasis (25). This was validated by Kruger et al. who reported that increased amount of Her-2 product was found by multivariate analysis to be a prognostic factor of tumor specific survival in patients with invasive UC (26). The significance of Her-2 was further confounded by Jimenez et al. in 1991 when they performed IHC on 80 radical cystectomy specimens looking for Her-2 expression. There was no survival difference found between either the Her-2-positive or Her-2-negative groups, indicating that Her-2 overexpression may have no survival significance in invasive UC. There is uniform agreement that Her-2 overexpression is seen in urothelial carcinoma, but the data is mixed regarding its ability to predict extravesical disease, survival, or prognosis (27).

3.3. Other Oncogenes

Many other oncogenes are also under active investigation, with three showing mild potential: H-ras, bcl-2, and c-myc. It has been observed that mutations in several codons of the H-ras gene have been shown to predict progression in up to 10% of bladder cancers (28). This relatively weak correlation has met with contradiction as H-ras protein overexpression has not had any clear role in predicting prognosis (29). Another oncogene, bcl-2 was shown by Pollack et al. to be significantly associated with upstaging of tumors and overall progression of disease, but no prognostic or staging correlation was shown by Shiina et al. when they evaluated bcl-2 overexpression in patients undergoing cystectomy (30, 31). C-myc overexpression was found initially in a greater percentage of high-grade tumors (32). Unfortunately, in the limited evaluation of c-myc no significant correlation to extravesical disease, prognosis, survival, or upstaging has been found (33).

4. Tumor Suppressor Genes

Tumor suppressor genes play key roles in regulating the cell cycle as well as apoptosis. Loss of a tumor suppressor gene can ultimately result in unregulated cell growth or if it occurs in an apoptotic pathway, cellular immortality. Several tumor suppressor genes have undergone promising investigation in the disease progression of UC: p53, retinoblastoma, maspin, and survivin.

4.1. Retinoblastoma (Rb)

Rb protein interacts with chromatin, DNA-modifying enzymes and transcription factors that control the expression of genes involved in cellular proliferation, differentiation, and apoptosis (34). Rb has been under investigation, not specifically for stage or grade, but for survival and disease progression. In a small study using IHC to evaluate loss of the Rb protein, 45 patients with superficial UC were evaluated and the loss of the Rb protein correlated to a shorter period of progression-free survival (35). In two smaller studies, UC with altered Rb protein was shown to have poorer tumor-free survival in locally advanced bladder cancer treated with cystectomy and UC with normal Rb expression was shown to have greater overall patient survival in patients with muscle-invasive disease (36, 37). In a retrospective analysis of 80 patients undergoing radical cystectomy, 63% of those found to have pT2 disease or greater had altered Rb expression vs. only 22% in pathologically organ-confined disease (38). This study was the first to demonstrate that lack of Rb expression may be associated with the extravesical spread of UC.

4.2. p53

Most human cancers are caused by DNA mutations or genetic defects resulting in alterations of the cell cycle. The most common tumor suppressor gene associated with all human cancers is p53 (39). IHC analysis can be used to detect mutated p53 protein, which has a long half-life and will concentrate inside the nuclei of cells. p53 can also be detected with molecular analysis through DNA polymerase chain reactions (PCR). There is some discord between abnormal accumulation detected by IHC and defects detected through PCR. The Bladder Tumor Marker Network evaluated abnormal p53 in UC by both PCR and IHC. The two techniques had similar results when evaluating for normal levels and highly overexpressed levels of p53. In the grey zone between normal and overexpression, there was up to 20% variability when only one of the two tests was positive (40). IHC is a much more efficient cost effective means to clinically evaluate p53 while PCR is perceived as a more accurate assay.

The literature contains both positive and negative conclusions about p53 as a prognostic marker and indicator of more aggressive tumors. p53 overexpression has positively correlated with increasing tumor grade and stage in bladder cancer in some studies (41). The appropriate question is whether it has any actual prognostic significance towards disease-free survival, progression, or tumor recurrence. In a recent meta-analysis, seven trials that looked at prognosis of patients with bladder cancer and positive p53 staining by IHC were identified. Only two of the seven trials demonstrated that p53 was an independent prognostic indicator of invasion and progression of disease (42). The Bladder Tumor Marker Network evaluated 109 patients with grade 2 or higher and T2 and T3 bladder cancer, also finding no prognostic significance in detecting increases in p53 protein accumulation (43). Lipponen et al., with a larger series of 212 patients diagnosed with UC, performed a multivariate analysis that showed p53 positivity had no independent significance over traditional stage or grade (44).

There are several studies however, that support the prognostic value of p53 overexpression. Esrig et al. examined specimens from a large group of 253 patients treated with radical cystectomy for UC. An IHC analysis was performed, to look for p53 positivity in cell nuclei. Overall, they found that positive p53 expression by IHC was an independent predictor of survival and recurrence when stratified in a multivariate analysis by tumor grade, stage and lymph node status (45), although a smaller study concluded that p53 overactivity has no prognostic significance in node-positive disease treated by radical cystectomy and lymph node dissection (46). A significant finding was in a 2004 study where tumor samples from 80 patients undergoing radical cystectomy were evaluated for altered p53 expression. Sixty-five percent of patients with pT2 disease and higher were found to have p53 overexpression vs. twenty-eight percent of patients with pathologically organ-confined tumors (38). This is the first study demonstrating that p53 may definitively be overexpressed in patients with extravesical disease.

Esrig et al. assessed and validated the prognostic value of p53 overexpression in organ-confined UC in a retrospective review of 243 patients who underwent cystectomy. The likelihood of tumor recurrence in patients with pTa disease who underwent cystectomy was 7–12% in those with normal p53 expression and 56–80% in those with overexpression of p53 (45). In conclusion, it appears that p53 overactivity detected by IHC is present in higher-grade and higher-stage tumors, and several studies have found statistically significant correlations between p53 overactivity and local invasion of UC at the time of cystectomy, as well as the likelihood for UC recurrence in patients thought to have organ-confined disease after cystectomy.

4.3. Survivin

Survivin is a tumor biomarker that acts as an inhibitor of apoptosis; it has been found to be overexpressed in many human cancers leading to cellular protection from apoptosis and unregulated mitosis (47). Survivin expression in the urinary bladder is thought to cause changes in gene expression of extracellular matrix molecules and inflammatory molecules ultimately leading to potentially more invasive and aggressive tumor models. Survivin is gaining popular acceptance in the field of urology as a noninvasive urine test in the detection of bladder cancer showing potentially superior positive and negative predictive values than traditional cytology. In 2006,48 Reeves et al. reported that a positive survivin test detected tumors on an average of 3.26 months before visual detection. Their overall sensitivity for detection of UC for surviving, FISH, and cytology was 86.6, 75, and 36.6%, respectively (48). As of now, there is little data in humans indicating that survivin is capable of predicting the stage of disease or tumor invasiveness, but higher levels of survivin may be present in higher-grade UC (49).

One preliminary study has investigated the relationship between survivin expression and tumor aggressiveness in a murine model. Transgenic mouse models were created with survivin expressing and nonsurvivin expressing clones. After 12 weeks of systematic exposure to bladder carcinogens, the survivin expressing group had a considerably higher rate of tumorigenesis, 78%. All these mice had a palpable abdominal mass and a profoundly shortened survival compared to only 30% in the nonsurvivin expressing transgenic mice (50). As of now, this has not been confirmed in human tissue samples.

4.4. Maspin

Maspin is a serine protease inhibitor that shows tumor suppressing activity; it has been extensively investigated in breast cancer tumors, being shown to regulate invasiveness and metastasis (51). Reduced expression of this protein leads to uninhibited tumor cell motility, and tumor cell predilection to become invasive and metastasize. Maspin has also been implicated in the development and spread of prostate cancer (52). Sugimoto et al. evaluated 65 UC specimens from either TUR or cystectomy of which 38 were stage pT2 or greater. Of these 38 muscle-invasive samples, 64% tested positive for maspin, with 34% giving a false-negative reading. In T1 and lower stage tumors, only 7% had a positive assay for maspin and when analyzing normal urothelium, none tested positive. This was statistically significant demonstrating that a positive assay for the serine protease inhibitor maspin had a direct correlation with the presence of invasive UC (53). Maspin appears, at least initially, to be correlated with a tumor's ability to locally invade. As already shown in other human cancers, the early data in regard to UC appears quite favorable, and this may be a significant molecular marker of a UC to invade muscle.

5. Cell Cycle Regulators

Cell cycle regulator genes are quite similar to tumor suppressors, but are usually found downstream and act as gateways in the progression from one arm of the cell cycle to another. Unlike tumor suppressor products that are overexpressed, when cell cycle regulator proteins are not present, disinhibition of the normal regulatory pathways may occur with resultant tumorigenesis.

5.1. p21

p21 is a cell cycle regulator found downstream from p53. p53 has already been shown to occur in higher-stage tumors and its relationship with p21 expression may have some significance in predicting disease progression. In patients with known altered p53 tumor suppressor products, those lacking the p21 protein products have been shown to have worse survival outcomes (54). In an analysis of 242 patients, who underwent cystectomy for UC, IHC looking for p21 absence was performed. While p21 was not associated with tumor grade or stage, it was an independent predictor of prognosis and time to tumor recurrence (54). While the data on tumor behavior when p21 is absent is sparse, it represents a new arena where the cellular expression of multiple arrays of molecular markers can be combined to have more meaningful predictive value.

5.2. Cyclin E

Cyclin E, a positive regulator of the cell cycle, has also been found to be underexpressed in tissue samples from bladder tumors; 2,317 specimens were evaluated by IHC for cyclin E expression. pT2-4 disease had diminished cyclin E expression when compared to pT1 disease, indicating potential importance at the early stages of invasiveness. This correlated with poorer overall survival although no discernible prognostic significance could be found when stage and grade were controlled in the analysis (55). This data has not been duplicated and has had minimal clinical impact, but this initial data has shown some potential correlates between this marker and invasive and extravesical disease.

6. Angiogenesis-Related Factors

Many angiogenic factors are being examined in relation to various cancers. Angiogenesis, or the development of blood vessels, is instrumental in the development of the enriched vascular supply necessary for tumor propagation. Several factors have been evaluated for their relationships to bladder cancer, including vascular endothelial growth factor (VEGF), thrombospondin-1 (TSP-1), and cyclooxygenase-2 (COX-2).

6.1. COX-2

COX-2 produces prostaglandin H_2 which plays a role in the inflammatory response, development of the immune response, and tumor formation (56). COX-2 expression was evaluated by IHC and western blot, and was shown to be absent in normal urothelium, but was highly expressed in 86% of invasive UC sample and 75% of samples with CIS (57). This was confirmed with another series where COX-2 expression was found in 45% of invasive UC and 100% of tumors with CIS vs. only 20% of superficial tumors (58). Further testing in a series of 108 patients, who underwent cystectomy, demonstrated COX-2 in 64% of patients with grade 3 UC and 40% with T3 or T4 disease. An IHC analysis and univariate regression model showed a significant correlation between local invasion and expression of the COX-2 gene. Furthermore, a multivariate analysis and local invasion had a direct correlation with COX-2 expression. In this study, COX-2 demonstrated no significant prognostic factors in regard to patient survival, but the overall association with invasiveness of tumor specimens could be quite significant in regard to predicting extravesical spread of UC (59).

When a tumor invades the lamina propria and muscle wall of the bladder, it evokes a significant inflammatory response that is much more marked than that produced by the presence of noninvasive papillary tumors. Markers such as COX-2 that are present in a significantly higher level can be evaluated by simple IHC of urine samples, making it a tumor marker that has potential to predict the presence of pT3 disease and provide an additional tool to prevent understaging with traditional TUR and clinical exam.

7. Extracellular Matrix and Adhesion Molecules

Considerable molecular oncologic research is being conducted to evaluate proteins and enzymes that constitute or affect the extracellular matrix. For solid tumors to invade locally or metastasize through lymphatic or hematologic spread, they must violate this barrier in some manner. The following molecules are either degraders of the extracellular matrix, adhesion molecules that hold cells together, or regulatory molecules that modulate cell migration through the basement membrane. A breakdown in any of these steps associated with organ-confined solid tumors can ultimately lead to local invasion and extravesical spread.

7.1. Metalloproteinase-2

Matrix metalloproteinases (MMPs) are protein degraders that breakdown the basement membrane and extracellular matrix (ECM), which are associated with tumor invasiveness and metastatic spread (60). MMPs have a known role in a wide range of cancers including colon and breast cancer (61). Kanayama et al. investigated the role of a specific MMP, MMP-2 in the development of invasive UC. MMP-2 degrades type IV collagen, gelatin, and laminin, all of which are constituents of the bladder's ECM. Using reverse transcriptase-polymerase chain reaction (RT-PCR), 41 samples of UC were evaluated for expression of this proteinase and high MMP-2 expression groups demonstrated a worse cause-specific survival. A positive correlation was reported between high levels of MMP-2 expression in grade 3 tumors and in stage pT2 and higher UC when compared to MMP-2 expression in pT1 and pTa tumors (62). Another study performed on a cohort of 97 patients confirmed that high levels of MMP-2 expression measured by enzyme immunoassay was a significant and independent predictor of recurrence and advanced UC (63). Given the physiologic role of MMPs and their association with several other solid tumors, further investigation is warranted as this could be one of the prime predictors as to whether UC has the ability to invade the basement membrane and ultimately advance locally and/or metastasize.

7.2. E-Cadherin

E-cadherin is an important intraepithelial cell-to-cell adhesion molecule. Its presence provides integrity and continuity in epithelial cell layers including the epithelial lining of the bladder wall. In 1995, a study by Lipponen et al. evaluated 172 IHC-stained bladder cancer specimens. In almost all the UC specimens analyzed, E-cadherin expression was reduced and even absent in 18% of the cases. The lowest levels of E-cadherin were found in muscle-invasive and high-grade tumors. In a multivariate model, E-cadherin expression was not an independent predictor of prognosis or survival, but it was significantly underexpressed in invasive and grade III tumors. This important structural protein shows potential in that its absence may play a role in the ability of UC to be invasive with the basement membrane and ECM of the bladder (64).

7.3. Urokinase-Type Plasminogen Activator (U-PA)

Urokinase-type plasminogen activator is a serine protease that mitigates tumor invasion and metastasis by causing proteolysis, leading to less intracellular adhesion and migration of tumor cells. Fifty one patients were evaluated by Shariat et al., where preoperative levels of u-PA were obtained prior to the patient undergoing radical cystectomy. These results were analyzed to determine if they could predict cancer stage and prognosis for UC of the bladder. While they did not have enough data in their study to find a significant correlation with pathologic stage, their data suggested that increased levels of u-PA were found in pT2 and greater disease. The study did demonstrate a significant relationship between increased levels of u-PA in tumors with lymphovascular invasion and regional lymph node metastasis at the time of cystectomy (65). Overall, while not an indicator of invasive UC of the bladder, there is a correlation with metastatic UC.

7.4. Secreted Protein, Acidic and Rich in Cysteine (SPARC)

SPARC is a secreted glycoprotein that plays a regulatory role in the development of human tissues by increasing the permeability of endothelial cell layers and modulating the activity of various growth factors. Through interactions with the cell matrix it plays a role in proliferation, cell migration, remodeling, and morphogenesis (66). Many tumors have been shown to have hyperactivity of the SPARC gene with increased levels of SPARC present in cancerous tissue samples (67). Sixty-three sample of UC, surgically obtained from TUR and cystectomy, underwent RT-PCR analysis to quantify the degree os SPARC expression. A statistically significant higher level of SPARC was found in grade 2 and higher tumors when compared to grade 1. SPARC overexpression was also present in a measurable amount in pT2 UC and above when compared to T1 and Ta disease (68). SPARC is another potential molecular marker that plays a role in cellular organization and migration and is overexpressed in invasive UC.

7.5. Motility-Related Protein-1 (MRP-1/CD9)

CD9 is a cell surface glycoprotein that interacts with other transmembrane proteins forming a complex that facilitates intracellular signaling, cell growth, adhesion, and motility (69). A retrospective review was performed on 320 patients with initial pathology of pT2 or less, looking at the relation of CD9 expression to tumor grade and stage, as well as predicting the behavior of noninvasive Ta and T1 disease. In all the 320 patients, it was found that CD9 expression was altered or not present in a significantly higher number of pT2 samples than pT1 or pTa disease. The study's significant finding was when the 202 patients with pTa and pT1 disease were evaluated in the follow-up. When progression to pT2 disease or greater was evaluated in this population at a mean follow-up of 43.6 months (range 12–240 months), those original tumors that had altered or had no CD9 expression, had a relative risk of 5.59 of progressing to higher stage disease than those that had normal positive testing for CD9 expression (70). While not yet validated with additional testing or testing of extravesical, lack of CD9 expression in tissue samples could be a significant marker in delineating those patients with disease most likely to become locally advanced.

8. Serum Tumor Markers

Unlike prostate cancer with PSA, CEA, and CA 19-9 in adenocarcinoma and colon cancer, and CA-125 in gynecologic cancers, no serum marker exists for UC. Limited work has been performed, in attempting to demonstrate a serum marker that could predict extravesical extension of UC. Chang et al. looked at CA-125 as a prognostic factor in patients undergoing radical cystectomy. Elevated CA-125 was found in 11.3% of patients with pT3 disease and only 4.9% of patients with pathologically organ-confined tumors (71). A comprehensive study on markers of cellular dedifferentiation published in 2006 investigated preoperative levels of CEA in patients with pT2 UC and no evidence of extravesical disease or metastasis. Of the 91 patients in the cohort who underwent cystectomy, 49% were understaged and had pathologic evidence of extravesical extension of tumor or lymph node-positive disease. At least one of the three preoperative serum markers was elevated in 66% of the understaged patients who were found to have extravesical disease. Elevated CEA and CA-125 levels proved to be independent prognostic indicators of the presence of extravesical UC with an odds ratio of 8.6 and 29.5, respectively (72). Despite confidence intervals around these odds ratios being wide, with a 43–70% rate of understaging UC, the presence of elevated CEA or CA-125 in a patient with pT2 disease may indicate occult extravesical spread.

9. Conclusion

Clinical understaging of presumed organ-confined UC remains problematic despite refinements in staging in contemporary series. Physical examination, pathological evaluation of tissue, radiographic imaging, and cytological analysis are the main tools in the armamentarium to diagnose and monitor disease progression. Recent advances in protein and DNA technology, assays, and genetic and chromosomal analysis are making it possible to evaluate tumors at their most basic level. Considerable research is being performed, and some promising molecular markers, p53, COX-2, EGFR, MMP-2, and many others are coming to the forefront of not only bladder cancer detection, but prediction of disease progression and ultimately prognosis of individuals. While DNA hybridization techniques, FISH analysis, and IHC are becoming standard in the research arm of bladder cancer, a universally accepted and reliable test to predict which individuals at initial presentation harbor occult micrometastatic disease or will progress to extravesical disease is yet to be identified. Serum markers for UC are also being examined. With the rise of PSA, CEA, AFP, Her-2/neu, and other solid tumor markers, the search is on for one or a combination of markers that can provide additional data to identify those individuals with higher likelihood to have or progress to advanced stage bladder cancer.

References

1. American Cancer Society. Cancer Facts and Figures 2005. Atlanta: American Cancer Society; 2005.
2. Herr HW. Routine CT scan in cystectomy patients: does it change management? Urology 1996;47(3):324–5.
3. Stein JP, Lieskovsky G, Cote R, et al. Radical cystectomy in the treatment of invasive bladder cancer: long-term results in 1,054 patients. J Clin Oncol 2001;19(3):666–75.
4. Ficarra V, Dalpiaz O, Alrabi N, Novara G, Galfano A, Artibani W. Correlation between clinical and pathological staging in a series of radical cystectomies for bladder carcinoma. BJU Int 2005;95(6):786–90.
5. Habuchi T, Marberger M, Droller MJ, et al. Prognostic markers for bladder cancer: International Consensus Panel on bladder tumor markers. Urology 2005;66(6 Suppl 1):64–74.
6. Spruck CH, 3rd, Ohneseit PF, Gonzalez-Zulueta M, et al. Two molecular pathways to Urothelial Carcinoma of the bladder. Cancer Res 1994;54(3):784–8.
7. Richter J, Jiang F, Gorog JP, et al. Marked genetic differences between stage pTa and stage pT1 papillary bladder cancer detected by comparative genomic hybridization. Cancer Res 1997;57(14):2860–4.
8. Kiemeney LA, Witjes JA, Verbeek AL, Heijbroek RP, Debruyne FM. The clinical epidemiology of superficial bladder cancer. Dutch South-East Cooperative Urological Group. Br J Cancer 1993;67(4):806–12.
9. Jones JS. DNA-based molecular cytology for bladder cancer surveillance. Urology 2006;67(3 Suppl 1):35–45; discussion 7.
10. Waldman FM, Carroll PR, Kerschmann R, Cohen MB, Field FG, Mayall BH. Centromeric copy number of chromosome 7 is strongly correlated with tumor grade and labeling index in human bladder cancer. Cancer Res 1991;51(14):3807–13.
11. Olumi AF, Tsai YC, Nichols PW, et al. Allelic loss of chromosome 17p distinguishes high grade from low grade Urothelial Carcinomas of the bladder. Cancer Res 1990;50(21):7081–3.
12. Degtyar P, Neulander E, Zirkin H, et al. Fluorescence in situ hybridization performed on exfoliated urothelial cells in patients with Urothelial Carcinoma of the bladder. Urology 2004;63(2):398–401.
13. Skacel M, Fahmy M, Brainard JA, et al. Multitarget fluorescence in situ hybridization assay detects Urothelial Carcinoma in the majority of patients with bladder cancer and atypical or negative urine cytology. J Urol 2003;169(6):2101–5.
14. Partanen AM. Epidermal growth factor and transforming growth factor-alpha in the development of epithelial-mesenchymal organs of the mouse. Curr Top Dev Biol 1990;24:31–55.
15. Neal DE, Marsh C, Bennett MK, et al. Epidermal-growth-factor receptors in human bladder cancer: comparison of invasive and superficial tumours. Lancet 1985;1(8425):366–8.
16. Messing EM. Clinical implications of the expression of epidermal growth factor receptors in human Urothelial Carcinoma. Cancer Res 1990;50(8):2530–7.
17. Nguyen PL, Swanson PE, Jaszcz W, et al. Expression of epidermal growth factor receptor in invasive Urothelial Carcinoma of the urinary bladder. A multivariate survival analysis. Am J Clin Pathol 1994;101(2):166–76.
18. Mellon K, Wright C, Kelly P, Horne CH, Neal DE. Long-term outcome related to epidermal growth factor receptor status in bladder cancer. J Urol 1995;153(3 Pt 2):919–25.
19. Ravery V, Grignon D, Angulo J, et al. Evaluation of epidermal growth factor receptor, transforming growth factor alpha, epidermal growth factor and c-erbB2 in the progression of invasive bladder cancer. Urol Res 1997;25(1):9–17.

20. Popov Z, Gil-Diez-De-Medina S, Ravery V, et al. Prognostic value of EGF receptor and tumor cell proliferation in bladder cancer: therapeutic implications. Urol Oncol 2004;22 (2):93–101.
21. Schechter AL, Stern DF, Vaidyanathan L, et al. The *neu* oncogene: an erb-B-related gene encoding a 185,000-Mr tumour antigen. Nature 1984;312(5994):513–6.
22. Lipponen P, Eskelinen M, Syrjanen S, Tervahauta A, Syrjanen K. Use of immunohistochemically demonstrated c-erb B-2 oncoprotein expression as a prognostic factor in Urothelial Carcinoma of the urinary bladder. Eur Urol 1991;20(3):238–42.
23. Underwood M, Bartlett J, Reeves J, Gardiner DS, Scott R, Cooke T. C-erbB-2 gene amplification: a molecular marker in recurrent bladder tumors? Cancer Res 1995;55(11):2422–30.
24. Mellon JK, Lunec J, Wright C, Horne CH, Kelly P, Neal DE. C-erbB-2 in bladder cancer: molecular biology, correlation with epidermal growth factor receptors and prognostic value. J Urol 1996;155(1):321–6.
25. Sato K, Moriyama M, Mori S, et al. An immunohistologic evaluation of C-erbB-2 gene product in patients with urinary bladder carcinoma. Cancer 1992;70(10):2493–8.
26. Kruger S, Weitsch G, Buttner H, et al. Overexpression of c-erbB-2 oncoprotein in muscle-invasive bladder carcinoma: relationship with gene amplification, clinicopathological parameters and prognostic outcome. Int J Oncol 2002;21(5):981–7.
27. Gandour-Edwards R, Lara PN, Jr., Folkins AK, et al. Does HER2/neu expression provide prognostic information in patients with advanced urothelial carcinoma? Cancer 2002;95(5):1009–15.
28. Knowles MA, Williamson M. Mutation of H-ras is infrequent in bladder cancer: confirmation by single-strand conformation polymorphism analysis, designed restriction fragment length polymorphisms, and direct sequencing. Cancer Res 1993;53(1):133–9.
29. Ye DW, Zheng JF, Qian SX, Ma YJ. Correlation between the expression of oncogenes ras and c-erbB-2 and the biological behavior of bladder tumors. Urol Res 1993;21(1):39–43.
30. Pollack A, Wu CS, Czerniak B, Zagars GK, Benedict WF, McDonnell TJ. Abnormal bcl-2 and pRb expression are independent correlates of radiation response in muscle-invasive bladder cancer. Clin Cancer Res 1997;3(10):1823–9.
31. Shiina H, Igawa M, Urakami S, Honda S, Shirakawa H, Ishibe T. Immunohistochemical analysis of bcl-2 expression in Urothelial Carcinoma of the bladder. J Clin Pathol 1996;49(5):395–9.
32. Kotake T, Saiki S, Kinouchi T, Shiku H, Nakayama E. Detection of the c-myc gene product in urinary bladder cancer. Jpn J Cancer Res 1990;81(12):1198–201.
33. Schmitz-Drager BJ, Schulz WA, Jurgens B, et al. c-myc in bladder cancer. Clinical findings and analysis of mechanism. Urol Res 1997;25(Suppl 1):S45–9.
34. Robertson KD, Ait-Si-Ali S, Yokochi T, Wade PA, Jones PL, Wolffe AP. DNMT1 forms a complex with Rb, E2F1 and HDAC1 and represses transcription from E2F-responsive promoters. Nat Genet 2000;25(3):338–42.
35. Grossman HB, Liebert M, Antelo M, et al. p53 and RB expression predict progression in T1 bladder cancer. Clin Cancer Res 1998;4(4):829–34.
36. Logothetis CJ, Xu HJ, Ro JY, et al. Altered expression of retinoblastoma protein and known prognostic variables in locally advanced bladder cancer. J Natl Cancer Inst 1992;84(16):1256–61.
37. Cordon-Cardo C, Wartinger D, Petrylak D, et al. Altered expression of the retinoblastoma gene product: prognostic indicator in bladder cancer. J Natl Cancer Inst 1992;84 (16):1251–6.
38. Shariat SF, Tokunaga H, Zhou J, et al. p53, p21, pRB, and p16 expression predict clinical outcome in cystectomy with bladder cancer. J Clin Oncol 2004;22(6):1014–24.
39. Hollstein M, Sidransky D, Vogelstein B, Harris CC. p53 mutations in human cancers. Science 1991;253(5015): 49–53.
40. McShane LM, Aamodt R, Cordon-Cardo C, et al. Reproducibility of p53 immunohistochemistry in bladder tumors. National Cancer Institute, Bladder Tumor Marker Network. Clin Cancer Res 2000;6(5):1854–64.
41. Esrig D, Spruck CH, 3rd, Nichols PW, et al. p53 nuclear protein accumulation correlates with mutations in the p53 gene, tumor grade, and stage in bladder cancer. Am J Pathol 1993;143(5):1389–97.
42. Schmitz-Drager BJ, Goebell PJ, Ebert T, Fradet Y. p53 immunohistochemistry as a prognostic marker in bladder cancer. Playground for urology scientists? Eur Urol 2000;38(6):691–9;discussion 700.
43. Lianes P, Charytonowicz E, Cordon-Cardo C, et al. Biomarker study of primary nonmetastatic versus metastatic invasive bladder cancer. National Cancer Institute Bladder Tumor Marker Network. Clin Cancer Res 1998;4(5): 1267–71.
44. Lipponen PK. Over-expression of p53 nuclear oncoprotein in transitional-cell bladder cancer and its prognostic value. Int J Cancer 1993;53(3):365–70.
45. Esrig D, Elmajian D, Groshen S, et al. Accumulation of nuclear p53 and tumor progression in bladder cancer. N Engl J Med 1994;331(19):1259–64.
46. Fleshner N, Kapusta L, Ezer D, Herschorn S, Klotz L. p53 nuclear accumulation is not associated with decreased disease-free survival in patients with node positive Urothelial Carcinoma of the bladder. J Urol 2000;164(4): 1177–82.
47. Altieri DC. Validating survivin as a cancer therapeutic target. Nat Rev Cancer 2003;3(1):46–54.
48. Reeves M, Hamilton N, Moussa O, et al. Clinical Assessment of Survivin as a Marker for Urothelial Carcinoma (UC). SESAUA meeting; 2006: abstract.
49. Shariat SF, Casella R, Khoddami SM, et al. Urine detection of survivin is a sensitive marker for the noninvasive diagnosis of bladder cancer. J Urol 2004;171(2 Pt 1):626–30.
50. Salz W, Eisenberg D, Plescia J, et al. A survivin gene signature predicts aggressive tumor behavior. Cancer Res 2005; 65(9):3531–4.
51. Zou Z, Anisowicz A, Hendrix MJ, et al. Maspin, a serpin with tumor-suppressing activity in human mammary epithelial cells. Science 1994;263(5146):526–9.
52. Zou Z, Zhang W, Young D, et al. Maspin expression profile in human prostate cancer (CaP) and in vitro induction of Maspin expression by androgen ablation. Clin Cancer Res 2002;8(5):1172–7.
53. Sugimoto S, Maass N, Takimoto Y, et al. Expression and regulation of tumor suppressor gene maspin in human bladder cancer. Cancer Lett 2004;203(2):209–15.

54. Stein JP, Ginsberg DA, Grossfeld GD, et al. Effect of p21WAF1/CIP1 expression on tumor progression in bladder cancer. J Natl Cancer Inst 1998;90(14):1072–9.
55. Richter J, Wagner U, Kononen J, et al. High-throughput tissue microarray analysis of cyclin E gene amplification and overexpression in urinary bladder cancer. Am J Pathol 2000; 157(3):787–94.
56. Subbaramaiah K, Zakim D, Weksler BB, Dannenberg AJ. Inhibition of cyclooxygenase: a novel approach to cancer prevention. Proc Soc Exp Biol Med 1997;216(2):201–10.
57. Mohammed SI, Knapp DW, Bostwick DG, et al. Expression of cyclooxygenase-2 (COX-2) in human invasive Urothelial Carcinoma (UC) of the urinary bladder. Cancer Res 1999;59(22):5647–50.
58. Shirahama T. Cyclooxygenase-2 expression is up-regulated in Urothelial Carcinoma and its preneoplastic lesions in the human urinary bladder. Clin Cancer Res 2000;6(6): 2424–30.
59. Shirahama T, Arima J, Akiba S, Sakakura C. Relation between cyclooxygenase-2 expression and tumor invasiveness and patient survival in Urothelial Carcinoma of the urinary bladder. Cancer 2001;92(1):188–93.
60. Liotta LA, Tryggvason K, Garbisa S, Hart I, Foltz CM, Shafie S. Metastatic potential correlates with enzymatic degradation of basement membrane collagen. Nature 1980; 284(5751):67–8.
61. Grigioni WF, D'Errico A, Fiorentino M, et al. Gelatinase A (MMP-2) and its mRNA detected in both neoplastic and stromal cells of tumors with different invasive and metastatic properties. Diagn Mol Pathol 1994;3(3):163–9.
62. Kanayama H, Yokota K, Kurokawa Y, Murakami Y, Nishitani M, Kagawa S. Prognostic values of matrix metalloproteinase-2 and tissue inhibitor of metalloproteinase-2 expression in bladder cancer. Cancer 1998;82(7):1359–66.
63. Gohji K, Fujimoto N, Ohkawa J, Fujii A, Nakajima M. Imbalance between serum matrix metalloproteinase-2 and its inhibitor as a predictor of recurrence of urothelial cancer. Br J Cancer 1998;77(4):650–5.
64. Lipponen PK, Eskelinen MJ. Reduced expression of E-cadherin is related to invasive disease and frequent recurrence in bladder cancer. J Cancer Res Clin Oncol 1995; 121(5):303–8.
65. Shariat SF, Monoski MA, Andrews B, Wheeler TM, Lerner SP, Slawin KM. Association of plasma urokinase-type plasminogen activator and its receptor with clinical outcome in patients undergoing radical cystectomy for Urothelial Carcinoma of the bladder. Urology 2003;61(5):1053–8.
66. Lane TF, Sage EH. The biology of SPARC, a protein that modulates cell-matrix interactions. Faseb J 1994;8(2): 163–73.
67. Porter PL, Sage EH, Lane TF, Funk SE, Gown AM. Distribution of SPARC in normal and neoplastic human tissue. J Histochem Cytochem 1995;43(8):791–800.
68. Yamanaka M, Kanda K, Li NC, et al. Analysis of the gene expression of SPARC and its prognostic value for bladder cancer. J Urol 2001;166(6):2495–9.
69. Maecker HT, Todd SC, Levy S. The tetraspanin superfamily: molecular facilitators. Faseb J 1997;11(6):428–42.
70. Mhawech P, Herrmann F, Coassin M, Guillou L, Iselin CE. Motility-related protein 1 (MRP-1/CD9) expression in urothelial bladder carcinoma and its relation to tumor recurrence and progression. Cancer 2003;98(8):1649–57.
71. Chang A, Cai J, Miranda G, Groshen S, Skinner D, Stein JP. Usefulness of CA 125 as a preoperative prognostic marker for Urothelial Carcinoma of the bladder. J Urol 2004; 172(6 Pt 1):2182–6.
72. Margel D, Tal R, Neuman A, Konichezky M, Sella A, Baniel J. Prediction of extravesical disease by preoperative serum markers in patients with clinically organ confined invasive bladder cancer. J Urol 2006;175(4):1253–7; discussion 7.

8
Identification of Nodal Metastases: The role of Iron Oxide Enhanced MRI

Bernard H. Bochner

Contents

Abstract The natural history of invasive bladder cancer follows a pathway of progression in which tumor involving the primary tumor advances to the regional lymph nodes and then to distant sites. The overall lymph node positive rate in large radical cystectomy series is approximately 20–25%. Most of the involved lymph nodes are not suspected prior to surgery and are only found on pathologic evaluation after cystectomy. Currently size criteria alone are used to distinguish normal from potentially involved lymph nodes. Significant understaging continues to limit the overall accuracy of clinical staging. Advances in imaging techniques, particularly MRI using novel enhancing agents, have the potential for dramatically improving lymph node staging. The development of lymphotrophic iron oxide nanoparticles have provided an additional imaging option for the detection of malignant lymph nodes in bladder cancer patients.

Keywords Lymph node, Nanoparticle, MRI, Staging

1. Introduction

Invasive bladder cancer represents a potentially life threatening malignancy with a well characterized pattern of dissemination. Anatomic and clinical studies of invasive bladder cancer patients have clearly documented the propensity for regional lymphatic progression which is strongly associated with the depth of the invasion of the primary tumor (1). Involvement of the regional pelvic lymph nodes represents one of the most important adverse prognostic features for patients with bladder cancer (2). In most contemporary radical cystectomy series, approximately 20–25% of all patients demonstrate regional lymph node involvement, the majority of which were not suspected prior to surgery (2–4). Currently pretreatment staging of the pelvic and retroperitoneal lymph nodes rely on imaging evaluation using either standard magnetic resonance imaging or computerized tomography. These modalities classify nodes as abnormal when their short axis diameter is elongated and measures >1.0 cm or is rounded and

From: *Current Clinical Urology: Bladder Cancer*, Edited by: C.T. Lee and D.P. Wood,
DOI: 10.1007/978-1-59745-417-9_8,

exceeds 0.8 cm (5). Use of such anatomic criteria for establishing the presence of metastases is unreliable as many enlarged nodes are benign and many tumor bearing nodes may be smaller than the established size threshold. A significant clinical benefit would be obtained from a noninvasive pretreatment diagnostic study that was based on criteria other than size to identify smaller lymph nodes (<8 mm) that contain tumor or exclude larger (>1 cm) benign lymph nodes. Functional studies such as positron emission tomography (PET) provide a potential means to identify tumor involvement of normal sized lymph nodes. However, few studies have documented the general performance of standard PET scans for smaller lymph nodes particularly in patients with bladder cancer. The use of PET scanning in the pelvis is particularly problematic given the high levels of urinary excretion of standard PET agents which may limit the ability to identify smaller perivesical and primary drainage zone nodes.

The development of lymphotrophic iron oxide nanoparticles have provided an additional imaging option for the detection of malignant lymph nodes (6–17). Used concurrently with high resolution MRI techniques, lymphotrophic nanoparticle enhanced MRI (LNMRI) provides a potential means to accurately identify subcentimeter nodal metastases which would otherwise escape detection using standard imaging techniques. This chapter will focus on the development and clinical application of LMRI in bladder cancer.

2. Clinical Importance of Lymph Node Staging in Bladder Cancer

The presence of regional lymph node metastases in patients with bladder cancer is one of the most important prognostic indicators for recurrence and survival (2). Patients with positive lymph nodes following radical cystectomy exhibit a high rate of disease recurrence following radical cystectomy with a 5-year overall survival of 33%. Identifying patients with lymph node involvement would aid in selecting a group that would best be managed via a multimodality approach that included systemic chemotherapy. Additionally, accurate recognition of the specific sites of lymph node metastases may provide a guide as to the extent of the pelvic lymph node dissection that would be necessary at the time of radical cystectomy. Furthermore, if distant nodes, such as those located in the upper retroperitoneum, were found to be involved at presentation, definitive resection of the bladder would likely be deferred for systemic chemotherapy, thus avoiding the potential morbidity associated with surgery.

3. Anatomy of Lymphatic Drainage of the Bladder

Anatomic studies performed around the turn of the nineteenth century, provided detailed descriptions of the lymphatic drainage of the urinary bladder. The classic descriptions of the lymphatic pathways within the bladder include a rich subepithelial lymphatic plexus which provides drainage through the detrussor musculature to the exterior of the bladder. Efferent lymphatic channels drain into perivesical lymph nodes that lie on the anterior, posterior and lateral aspects of the bladder and perivesical tissues. Larger lymphatic channels then pass to nodal basins located along the external iliac vessels, hypogastric vessels and lateral sacral/sacral promontory. These basins form a ring of pelvic nodes and constitute the primary drainage sites. All primary landing sites subsequently drain into the more proximal common iliac chains which are considered secondary landing sites. Subsequent drainage progresses to the retroperitoneal nodes.

4. Current Modalities for Identification of LN Metastases in Bladder Cancer

Currently surgical staging of the pelvic lymph nodes is considered the gold standard for evaluating for regionally metastatic disease. Pelvic lymphadenectomy for bladder cancer is typically performed at the time of radical cystectomy and may include the external iliac, hypogastric, obturator, common iliac and presacral lymph node regions. An extended pelvic lymphadenectomy for bladder cancer includes all of the above listed nodal regions and is considered by some to be the standard dissection necessary to optimize outcome (18, 19). Noninvasive, pretreatment evaluation of the status of the regional pelvic lymph nodes however provides for improved planning of therapy including the rational use of preoperative chemotherapy and perhaps the extent of lymphadenectomy needed at the time of cystectomy.

Available noninvasive imaging technologies include CT, MRI and PET. Despite the relative inaccuracy of pelvic CT scanning in the staging of bladder cancer, it has emerged as the standard pelvic imaging modality of choice. Due to its technical constraints, pelvic CT understaging and overstaging of bladder cancer can be greater than 50% (20, 21). In early stage disease, clinical understaging of the primary lesion may be as high as 62% (22). Others have reported 68% of clinically organ confined bladder tumors to have pathologic evidence of extravesical tumor extension (23). More recently, the advent of multi-detector row CT has provided new advantages and potential for the delineation of small structures in the GU tract. Multidetector CT affords greater speed of acquisition and higher resolution images than the helical CT. The other advantage of multi-detector CT is the ability to reconstruct the images in any plane and view the data sets from a number of different angles and perspectives. For instance, multidetector CT data may be acquired and reconstructed to be viewed from an intraluminal perspective – a so called, virtual cystoscopy. This has been done in the colon and preliminary data exists for the bladder; which is promising (24). Virtual cystoscopy may allow for lesion localization due to its wide field of view and ability to view data from different perspectives. The size of a tumor can be measured easily and therefore, this technique may be used for the monitoring of treatment response. The source CT data may be used as well for evaluation of other structures including pelvic lymphadenopathy. Using prior CT technology, approximately 20–25% of the patients thought to have no evidence of nodal involvement are found to have regional lymph node metastases at the time of radical cystectomy (25–28). Identification of lymph node involvement characterizes a high risk patient population likely to develop disseminated distant disease and therefore in the greatest need of combination therapy.

4.1. Advances in MRI and PET

Improvements in MRI and PET have made them attractive imaging modalities for the staging of bladder cancer. Early experience with MRI demonstrated that the accuracy of primary bladder tumor staging was greater than that obtained by CT scan (75 vs. 55%) (29). Further manipulation of the imaging resolution (30) and refinements in scanning sequences (31) resulted in a better than 90% accuracy, sensitivity and specificity by MRI for the detection of muscle-invasive bladder tumors. The sensitivity, specificity, and positive predictive values for MRI were reported as 75, 98 and 94%, respectively, in identifying locoregional nodal metastasis (5). Deficiencies of these series however, include small patient size and limitations set by the equipment used. Newer technology is anticipated to provide improved imaging of the bladder wall and regional lymph nodes.

MRI, which is based on an anatomical interpretation, is useful to detect nodal involvement when the suspect nodes are enlarged. Anatomically normal sized lymph nodes that harbor low volume metastatic disease will continue to pose a diagnostic problem for standard MRI (32). In contrast, PET scanning, which detects metabolic changes in malignant cells, provides a potential complement to MRI in detecting locoregional and distant metastases. Exploiting the metabolic differences between normal and tumor cells, PET imaging with the glucose analogue fluorodeoxyglucose (FDG) was able to identify metastatic bladder tumor in the regional lymph nodes (<0.9 cm) of two of three patients (33). FDG-uptake in cancer depends in part on the activity of glucose transporters. Indeed, glucose transporters Glut1 and Glut3 are overexpressed in many tumor types including transitional cell cancer of the bladder (34, 35) and their level of overexpression correlates with FDG-PET positivity and patient prognosis (36). However, FDG undergoes renal excretion and accumulates in the urinary bladder making it unusable as an imaging agent for bladder cancer. Alternative PET agents such as 11C-acetate may prove particularly useful in patients with bladder cancer as it appears to have minimal excretion in the urine and the ability to maintain its uptake characteristics in the presence of local inflammation (such as that generated by transurethral tumor biopsy). While 18FDG has been used for cancer imaging in many studies for several years, much less is known regarding 11C acetate. There are preliminary data on the use of 11C acetate in patients with prostate and liver cancer in which good visualization of malignant lesions was reported with no artifacts related to urinary excretion (37–39).

5. Nanoparticle Enhanced MRI

Nanoparticles that preferentially localize to the lymph nodes (lymphotrophic) represent a relatively new class of imaging agents which when combined with high resolution MRI, may provide improved tumor

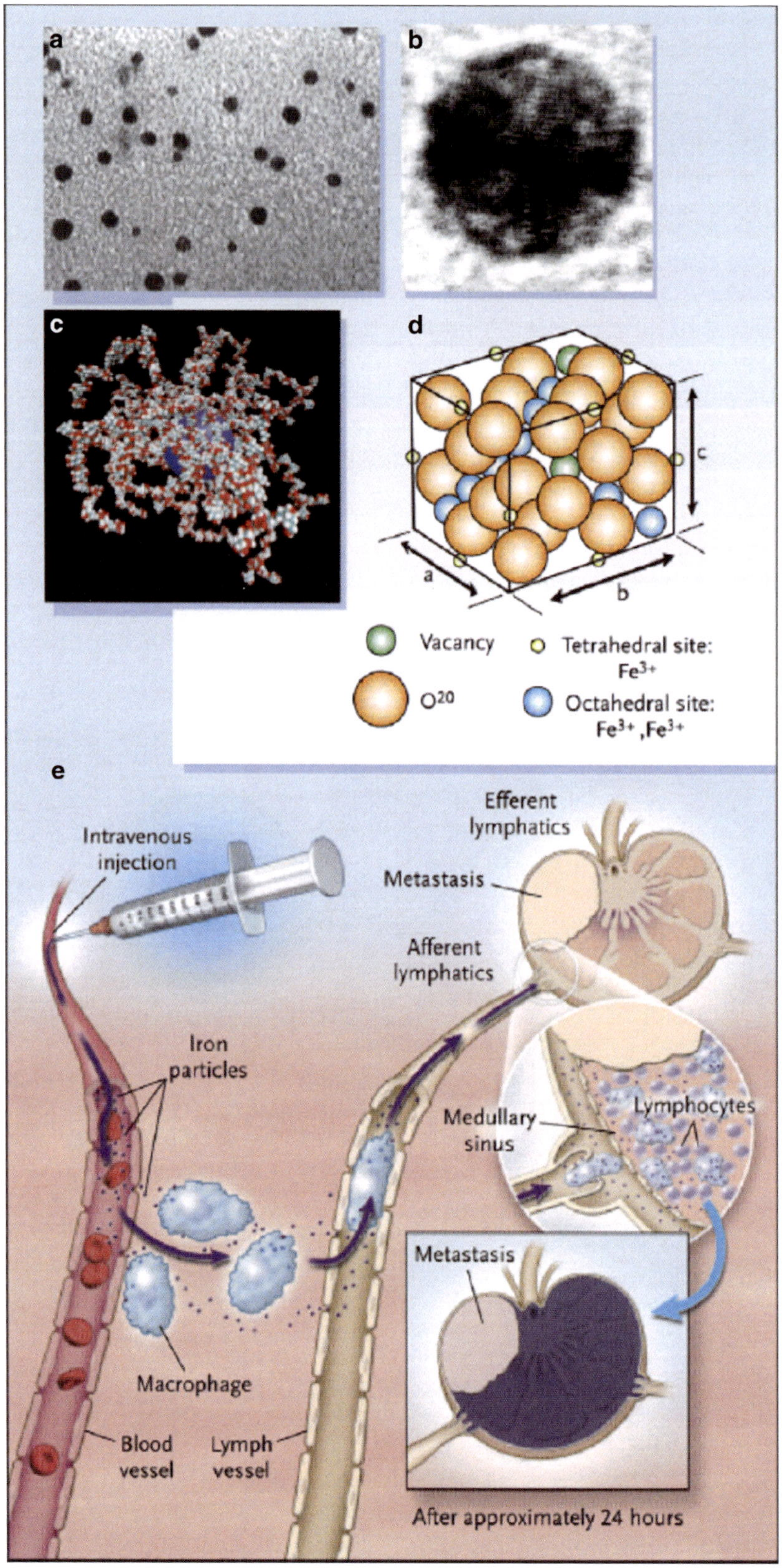
a
b
c
d
a
b
c
Vacancy
Tetrahedral site: Fe3+
O20
Octahedral site: Fe3+ ,Fe3+
e
Intravenous injection
Efferent lymphatics
Metastasis
Afferent lymphatics
Iron particles
Medullary sinus
Lymphocytes
Macrophage
Metastasis
Blood vessel
Lymph vessel
After approximately 24 hours

detection within lymph nodes. The components of lymphotrophic agents include a monocrystalline iron oxide core and a surrounding coat of low molecular weight dextran polymers to improve the molecule's bioavailability and decrease aggregation. The magnetic properties of the iron oxide core (large magnetic moment and high dipolar relaxivity) (40) makes them particularly susceptible to signal alterations ("drop out") on T2 and T2* weighted MRI and thus provides a unique visual means to potentially differentiate normal from abnormal lymph nodes (11, 41). The small particle size of these agents allows for transcapillary migration and access to the interstitial spaces within most tissues (Fig. 8.1). Transport of the nanoparticles from the interstitium into the regional draining lymph nodes occurs via the lymphatic ductal system. Addition agent access to the nodes may occur from direct transcapillary migration within the medullary sinus of the lymph nodes themselves (17, 42). After entering the lymph node, the reticuloendothelial cells (macrophages) phagocytize the nanoparticles which thus accumulate within the nodes. Any process that disrupts the normal architecture of the node, in particular alterations to the distribution of macrophages, will lead to a heterogeneity or complete loss of accumulation of the iron oxide particles and thus provide a means to differentiate abnormal from normal lymph nodes (9, 43).

Supraparamagnetic nanoparticles come as a lyophilized powder that is reconstituted in saline prior to administration. Since the particles distribute across most tissues, a systemic infusion of 2.6 mg/kg is given approximately 24 h prior to imaging the body region of interest. Lymphotrophic nanoparticle enhanced MRI consists of a precontrast and postcontrast enhanced evaluation. The precontrast study provides a standard view of the nodes of interest for comparison with the postconstrast images and identifies nodes of interest as well as characterizes the fat content and distribution within the hilar region of the nodes, which may be mistaken for a positive finding on the enhanced sequences. Previously reported studies have provided the imaging protocols and optimal acquisition techniques that should be used for LNMRI (44). Both T2 fast spin echo sequences and GRE T2* sequences (heavily T2 weighted sequences) have been used to evaluate the sensitivity and specificity of modality in the detection of tumor bearing lymph nodes in a variety of tumors. Recent studies would suggest that the T2*-weighted images with a longer TE provide improved specificity over similar sequences with shorter TE times while still maintaining a high sensitivity (45).

The administration of iron oxide nanoparticles has proven to be relatively safe with an acceptable toxicity profile. The early phase II studies of these agents on 152 patients demonstrated a 28% adverse reaction rate (7). The most frequently reported complaints were headache, back pain, vasodilation and urticaria. Most reactions were characterized as mild to moderate and of a short duration. Other reported studies have noted no serious side effects related to the administration of these agents (12). Some of the reported reactions have been related to the flow rate of contrast administration. Presently an infusion of 4 ml/cc has been established as the appropriate rate of administration for iron oxide nanoparticles suspensions.

6. Evaluation of LNMRI Evaluations of LN Metastases

The patterns of detection of lymph node involvement using LVMRI, vary from a homogenous loss of signal on T2 weighted sequences' in a completely benign node (Fig. 8.2a, b) to a complete retention of signal on T2 weighted imaging in a node completely overtaken by tumor (Fig. 8.2c, d). In between these extremes are varying gradations of signal loss corresponding to the extent of disruption of the normal macrophage cell population within the node. Tables have been constructed to guide the image reader with respect

Fig. 8.1. Electron micrograph of hexagonal lymphotropic superparamagnetic nanoparticles (*Panels* A and B), Molecular model of surface-bound 10-kD dextrans and packing of iron oxide crystals (*Panels* C and D), and mechanism of action of lymphotropic superparamagnetic nanoparticles (*Panel* E). The model lymphotropic superparamagnetic nanoparticles shown here measure 2–3 nm on average (Panels A and B). The mean overall particle size of the 10-kD dextrans is 28 nm (*Panels* C and D). In Panel E, the systemically injected long-circulating particles gain access to the interstitium and are drained through lymphatic vessels. Disturbances in lymph flow or in nodal architecture caused by metastases lead to abnormal patterns of accumulation of lymphotropic superparamagnetic nanoparticles, which are detectable by MRI (From (12), Fig. 8.1.)

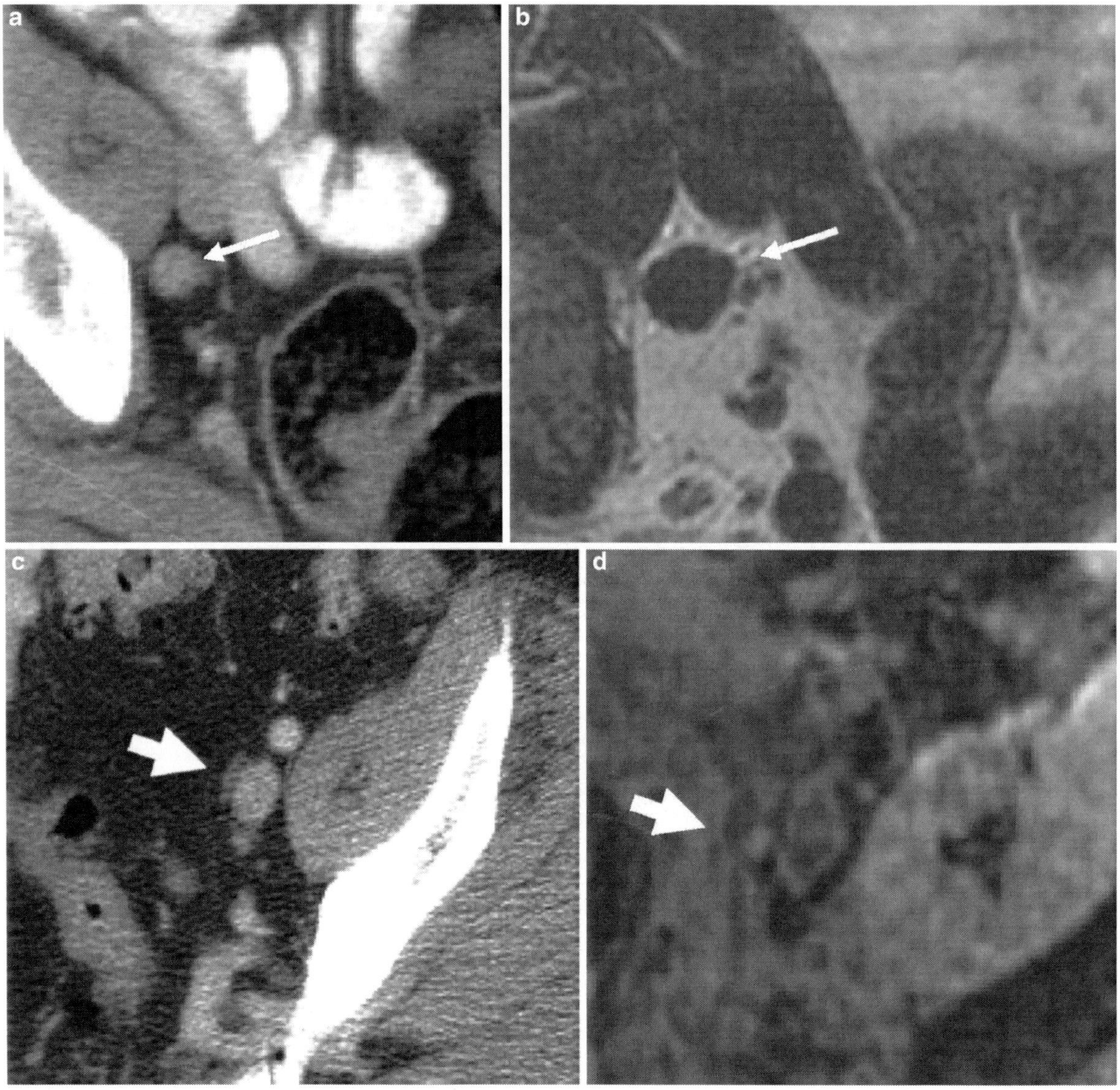

FIG. 8.2. LNMRI appearance of benign and malignant lymph nodes. (**a**) precontrast benign node, (**b**) postcontrast benign node, note loss of T2 signal. (**c**) precontrast malignant node, (**d**) postcontrast malignant node, note retention of signal on T2 weighted image (From (7))

to the gradation of changes that may be observed (Fig. 8.2). Of particular importance is the observation that several nonmalignant processes within a lymph node may look similar to a tumor bearing node and thus provide a false positive finding. Benign conditions that include focal lipomatosis, prominent fat within the hilum of the node, fibrosis due to any cause, reactive lymphoid hyperplasia and granulomatous inflammation may be characterized by a similar drop out of signal on T2* weighted enhanced imaging due to a paucity of macrophages within the effected regions. This may hold particular importance in bladder cancer patients as many patients may have been exposed to previous intravesical BCG which is associated with granulomatous changes to the regional lymph nodes. Additionally, nodal fibrosis as a reaction to tumor that has regressed following response to chemotherapy may confound the use of LNMI particularly given the documented benefits and increasing use of neoadjuvant platin-based chemotherapy.

7. LNMRI Data on Tumors Involvement of Lymph Nodes

LNMRI has been evaluated for its efficacy to detect involved lymph nodes in both the phase II and phase III settings. Since 1994 a variety of tumor types in different anatomic regions have been studied using LNMRI to determine its ability to accurately detect lymph node metastases (7, 9, 12, 14, 15, 43, 46–51). Sensitivities ranging from 33 to 100% and specificities of 37.5–100% have been reported. The wide range in the performance of LNMRI may be due to differences in the techniques used for imaging and pathologic/radiologic correlation as well as qualitative differences due to the specific anatomic location studied. Lymph node evaluations from tumors within the chest appear to have a less accurate rate of detection of lymph node disease compared to disease within the pelvis (7). This may be a result of artifact induced from respiratory movement of the thoracic structures which limits the ability to identify small (<8 mm) tumor deposits.

The techniques used to match specific lymph nodes both radiographically, surgically and histologically play an important role in these studies. Many of the reports note a "node to node" type comparative evaluation but present little detail as to how up to several hundreds of nodes identified either radiographically or histologically were specifically matched. Some investigators utilized the radiologist that read the MRI study in the operating room to guide the surgeon to the nodes of interest, while others provided 3D renderings of the lymph nodes in relation to vascular or other anatomic structures to guide the surgical resection (12). Despite these efforts many of the lymph nodes found histologically in many published studies could not be matched to a radiographic finding and therefore were not included in the subsequent analyses. In the largest study evaluating the role of LNMRI in bladder cancer, unmatched and therefore excluded nodes represented over 50% of the total lymph nodes removed (10). Based on the difficulties associated with matching multiple lymph nodes from the same anatomic region, studies have been designed on a node region basis to evaluate the accuracy of this imaging modality and many reports will thus provide a measure of the diagnostic performance on a patient by patient basis. The specific manner in which the radiographic/pathologic correlation was performed however must be considered when interpreting the results of future evaluations using LNMRI.

One of the earliest studies using LNMRI that included patients with bladder cancer was a report in 1998 that involved a total of 30 patients with various GU and other malignancies (prostate, kidney, cervix, uterine, ovary and rectum) (9). In this study little detail was given regarding the specific method of matching the nodes identified on MRI to those found at surgery. However, intraoperative guidance by the reading radiologist was used in select cases. Overall the sensitivity of LNMRI was superior to the standard MRI; however, the specificity was lower although the specific performance of LNMRI based on histologic tumor type was not detailed. Several malignant nodes in this study failed to adequately enhance after the administration of ferumoxtran-10 at a dose of 1.7 mg of iron per kilogram body weight. This information suggested that a higher dose of 2.6 mg/kg may be more advantageous. These early studies also demonstrated the potential overlap in imaging characteristics between inflammatory but benign and malignant lymph nodes. In the largest study of LNMRI designed to evaluate LN metastases, Anzai et al. reported the outcome of a multi-institutional evaluation of 147 patients including 29 with head and neck tumors, 32 with lung and mediastinal cancers, 23 with breast, 29 with abdominal malignancies and 39 with pelvic cancers (7). Of the 134 patients that underwent either surgery or biopsy, 371 nodes were identified on pre and post-contrast MRI. Only 276 nodes however were included in the matched pathology-radiographic correlation, corresponding to less than three lymph nodes/patient included in the final statistical evaluation. Overall reported accuracy varied based on the anatomic site and ranged from 73% for mediastinal tumors, to 82 and 83% for breast and pelvic tumors, respectively. Evaluation of head and neck tumors demonstrated the best correlation with an accuracy of 93% (7).

The majority of LNMRI studies of pelvic tumors have reported improved accuracy in the identification of lymph node involvement compared to conventional MRI based on anatomic criteria alone. In 2003 Harisinghana presented their findings in prostate cancer from an 80 patient evaluation (12). All patients were imaged by LNMRI using a 2.6 mg/kg dose of iron contrast agent and accuracy was compared to standard MRI using established anatomic criteria (see Fig. 8.3.) for a malignant LN which included a short axis measured diameter of greater than 1 cm for

No.	Post Dose	Description	Diagnosis
#1	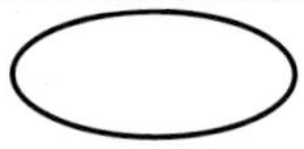	No blackening of mode or node is hyperintense to surrounding tissue; heterogeneous or homogenous architecture.	Metastatic
#2	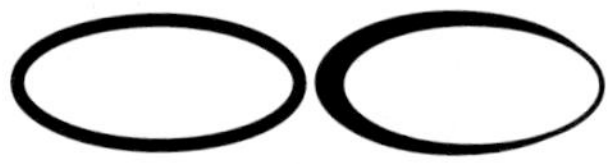	Node has central high signal with darkening along the peripheral rim; heterogeneous architecture	Metastatic
#3	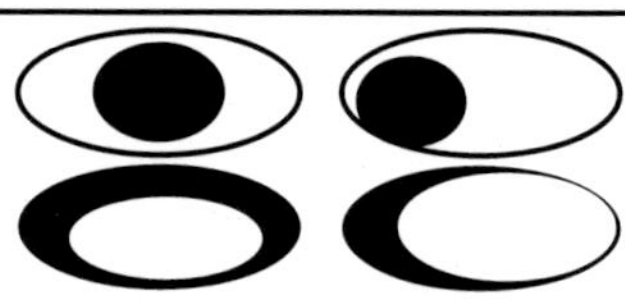	Partial darkening whereby more than 50% of the node has area of high signal intensity; heterogeneous architecture	Metastatic
#4	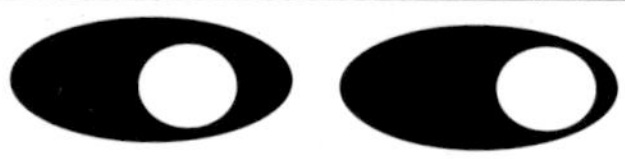	Less than 50% of node has high signal intensity; heterogeneous architecture	Possibly Metastatic
#5	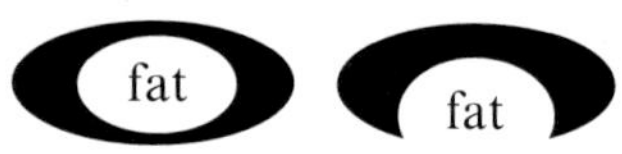	Node having an overall dark signal other than a central or hilar area of fat seen on T1 sequence; heterogeneous architecture.	Non-metastatic
#6	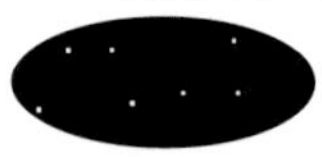	Node having an overall dark signal with speckles of subtle granularities; homogenous architecutre.	Non-metastatic
#7	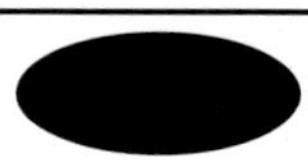	Node having an overall dark signal intensity; homogenous architecture	Non-metastatic

Fig. 8.3. Diagnostic criteria for lymphotrophic iron-oxide particle enhanced MR (From (7))

an elongated node and 8 mm for a round node. Patients then underwent either a surgical lymph node dissection or percutaneous biopsy of a suspected malignant LN identified on imaging. A total of 334 lymph nodes matched by imaging and surgical/pathologic examination were included in the analysis. A lymph node was considered malignant if it met one of three criteria including a decrease in signal intensity of less than 30% on T2-weighted fast spin–echo or gradient-echo sequences after the administration of lymphotropic superparamagnetic nanoparticles; a heterogeneous signal (giving the entire node a mottled appearance), discrete focal defects defined as isolated regions of high signal intensity within a node of interest, or both; and nodes with a central area of hyperintensity (excluding a fatty hilum) but a peripheral decrease in signal intensity (12). The reported sensitivity, specificity and accuracy for detecting tumor bearing lymph nodes, regardless of size, was 35, 90 and 76% for standard MRI alone compared to 90, 98 and 97% for feruoxtran-10 enhanced MRI. The differences in sensitivity were most notable for smaller lymph nodes between 5 and 10 mm in size, 29 vs. 96% in favor of enhanced MRI.

The largest LNMRI study to date specifically evaluating patients with bladder cancer was a multi-institutional study reported by Deserno et al. reported on 58 patients (10). All patients were studied with both pre-and postcontrast MRI using standard size criteria to identify positive nodes on nonenhanced MRI. Pre and postcontrast MRI were used to identify entire nodes or focal regions within nodes that did not demonstrate signal intensity decreases on T2* enhanced sequences. Tissue was obtained for evaluation by open lymph node dissection ($n = 44$, 76%), image guided biopsy ($n = 12$, 21%), or laporascopic LN dissection ($n = 2$, 3%). To aid in intraoperative node identification the authors reported that a preoperative schematic drawing was provided to the surgeon to locate nodes previously identified on MRI and with further aid provided by the presence of the radiologist in the operative suite at the time of dissection. Lymph nodes or lymph node packets were removed surgically from specified anatomic regions and submitted for pathologic evaluation. On an average nine lymph nodes were removed (range 2–21) per patient. Of the 404 lymph nodes identified, only 172 (43%) were matched histologically to a radiographic finding. A total of 50 nodes were found to harbor metastatic bladder cancer, 48 of which were noted to have no decrease in signal intensity after feruoxtram-10 enhanced MRI. Twelve positive lymph nodes measured below the size criteria used to detect malignancy by standard imaging (mean 7.2 mm, range 6–9 mm). No signal intensity decrease was observed focally in 10 of 12 of these smaller, tumor bearing lymph nodes on enhanced MRI. The overall reported accuracy of the precontrast studies was 92% compared to 95% for the LNMRI. The sensitivity and specificity of the precontrast MRI was 76 and 99% compared to 96 and 95% for the LNMRI, respectively. This corresponded to a significant increase in sensitivity but no statistical improvement in specificity.

There are several unique considerations for bladder cancer patients that may affect the performance of LNMRI and should be considered when evaluating past studies or designing new protocols. Patients may have received intravesical BCG therapy prior to radical cystectomy as part of their initial management of nonmuscle invasive disease. Frequent granulomatous changes within the regional lymph nodes draining the bladder could alter the nodal architecture sufficiently to lead to generalized precontrast nodal enlargement and focal postcontrast lack of signal loss on LNMRI leading to a false positive interpretation. This issue has not been addressed in previous LNMRI studies of bladder cancer patients although the phenomenon of false positive findings in the presence of inflammation or granulomatous change has been documented.

Another consideration that has been poorly documented is the potential confounding effects of neoadjuvant chemotherapy on the accuracy of LNMRI. This is a particularly relevant concern for the bladder cancer patient given that the existing data support the use of neoadjuvant systemic chemotherapy prior to radical cystectomy (52–54). A recognized reaction of tumor that responds to chemotherapy is the formation of a fibrotic or desmoplastic response. Although poorly quantitated in lymph nodes, scarring within a lymph node previously involved by metastatic tumor that has regressed in response to chemotherapy, could lead to focal regions of fibrosis that displaces the normally present macrophages. This region of scar, if large enough, could present as a focal region of lack of signal loss on a post contrast LNMRI. Both subsets of patients (previous BCG exposed or LN positive patients that receive neoadjuvant chemotherapy) should be considered in future studies on LNMRI in bladder cancer to fully understand the utility and limitations of this promising technology.

Improved imaging of the regional lymph nodes for bladder cancer would provide important clinical information that could alter treatment. Due to the powerful negative prognostic significance of regional lymph node involvement, most clinicians would recommend systemic chemotherapy prior to radical cystectomy in any cisplatin eligible patient with evidence of node positive disease. Presently node positivity is identified in approximately 20–25% of patients with invasive bladder cancer that is managed by radical cystectomy. The majority of node positive patients in contemporary surgical series have 1–2 positive lymph nodes, many of which were not suspected by standard imaging prior to surgery (19, 26, 55). Accurate identification of the location of the nodes that harbor metastatic disease would potentially be useful in surgical planning of the lymphadenectomy. Controversy exists as to the optimal extent of the lymph node dissection that should be performed at cystectomy with some recommending routine extended dissections up to the aortic bifurcation and others who limit the dissection to the nodes distal to the bifurcation of the common iliac vessels. Still others have studied the use of the sentinel node concept in bladder cancer to perhaps serve as a guide for the extent of the lymph node dissection (56–58). Regardless of present practice patterns, preoperative imaging that provides an accurate map of the involved pelvic lymph nodes could serve as a guide for the extent of the dissection necessary to remove all affected nodes and perhaps improve long term disease control.

8. Conclusions

LNMRI has demonstrated improved staging characteristics for lymph nodes compared to standard MRI techniques. Bladder cancer patients may benefit substantially from accurate nodal staging prior to definitive treatment as both medical and surgical management decisions may be affected. Unique characteristics of bladder cancer patients including the effects of prior intravesical and systemic treatments on the regional pelvic lymph nodes should be considered when evaluating the results of LNMRI studies.

References

1. Jewett H, Strong G. Infiltrating carcinoma of the bladder: relation of depth of penetration of the bladder wall to incidence of local extension and metastases. J Urol 1946; 55:366–72.
2. Bochner BH, Kattan MW, Vora KC. Postoperative nomogram predicting risk of recurrence after radical cystectomy for bladder cancer. J Clin Oncol 2006;24(24):3967–72.
3. Dalbagni G, Genega E, Hashibe M, et al. Cystectomy for bladder cancer: a contemporary series. J Urol 2001;165(4):1111–6.
4. Stein JP, Lieskovsky G, Cote R, et al. Radical cystectomy in the treatment of invasive bladder cancer: long-term results in 1,054 patients. J Clin Oncol 2001;19(3):666–75.
5. Jager GJ, Barentsz JO, Oosterhof GO, Witjes JA, Ruijs SJ. Pelvic adenopathy in prostatic and urinary bladder carcinoma: MR imaging with a three-dimensional TI-weighted magnetization-prepared-rapid gradient-echo sequence. AJR Am J Roentgenol 1996;167(6):1503–7.
6. Anzai Y, McLachlan S, Morris M, Saxton R, Lufkin RB. Dextran-coated superparamagnetic iron oxide, an MR contrast agent for assessing lymph nodes in the head and neck. AJNR Am J Neuroradiol 1994;15(1):87–94.
7. Anzai Y, Piccoli CW, Outwater EK, et al. Evaluation of neck and body metastases to nodes with ferumoxtran 10-enhanced MR imaging: phase III safety and efficacy study. Radiology 2003;228(3):777–88.
8. Bellin MF, Lebleu L, Meric JB. Evaluation of retroperitoneal and pelvic lymph node metastases with MRI and MR lymphangiography. Abdom Imaging 2003;28(2):155–63.
9. Bellin MF, Roy C, Kinkel K, et al. Lymph node metastases: safety and effectiveness of MR imaging with ultrasmall superparamagnetic iron oxide particles–initial clinical experience. Radiology 1998;207(3):799–808.
10. Deserno WM, Harisinghani MG, Taupitz M, et al. Urinary bladder cancer: preoperative nodal staging with ferumoxtran-10-enhanced MR imaging. Radiology 2004;233(2):449–56.
11. Guimaraes R, Clement O, Bittoun J, Carnot F, Frija G. MR lymphography with superparamagnetic iron nanoparticles in rats: pathologic basis for contrast enhancement. AJR Am J Roentgenol 1994;162(1):201–7.
12. Harisinghani MG, Barentsz J, Hahn PF, et al. Noninvasive detection of clinically occult lymph-node metastases in prostate cancer. N Engl J Med 2003;348(25):2491–9.
13. Harisinghani MG, Saini S, Hahn PF, Weissleder R, Mueller PR. MR imaging of lymph nodes in patients with primary abdominal and pelvic malignancies using ultrasmall superparamagnetic iron oxide (Combidex). Acad Radiol 1998;5(Suppl 1):S167–9; discussion S83–4.
14. Keller TM, Michel SC, Frohlich J, et al. USPIO-enhanced MRI for preoperative staging of gynecological pelvic tumors: preliminary results. Eur Radiol 2004;14(6):937–44.
15. Mack MG, Balzer JO, Straub R, Eichler K, Vogl TJ. Superparamagnetic iron oxide-enhanced MR imaging of head and neck lymph nodes. Radiology 2002;222(1):239–44.
16. Vassallo P, Matei C, Heston WD, McLachlan SJ, Koutcher JA, Castellino RA. AMI-227-enhanced MR lymphography: usefulness for differentiating reactive from tumor-bearing lymph nodes. Radiology 1994;193(2):501–6.
17. Weissleder R, Elizondo G, Wittenberg J, Lee AS, Josephson L, Brady TJ. Ultrasmall superparamagnetic iron oxide: an intravenous contrast agent for assessing lymph nodes with MR imaging. Radiology 1990;175(2):494–8.
18. Koppie TM, Vickers AJ, Vora K, Dalbagni G, Bochner BH. Standardization of pelvic lymphadenectomy performed at radical cystectomy: can we establish a minimum number of lymph nodes that should be removed?. Cancer 2006;107(10):2368–74.
19. Stein JP, Skinner DG. The role of lymphadenectomy in high-grade invasive bladder cancer. Urol Clin North Am 2005;32(2):187–97.
20. Paik ML, Scolieri MJ, Brown SL, Spirnak JP, Resnick MI. Limitations of computerized tomography in staging invasive bladder cancer before radical cystectomy. J Urol 2000;163(6):1693–6.
21. Yaman O, Baltaci S, Arikan N, Yilmaz E, Gogus O. Staging with computed tomography, transrectal ultrasonography and transurethral resection of bladder tumour: comparison with final pathological stage in invasive bladder carcinoma. Br J Urol 1996;78(2):197–200.
22. Ghoneim MA, el-Mekresh MM, el-Baz MA, el-Attar IA, Ashamallah A. Radical cystectomy for carcinoma of the bladder: critical evaluation of the results in 1,026 cases. J Urol 1997;158(2):393–9.
23. Lerner SP, Skinner DG, Lieskovsky G, et al. The rationale for en bloc pelvic lymph node dissection for bladder cancer patients with nodal metastases: long-term results. J Urol 1993;149(4):758–64; discussion 64–5.
24. Song JH, Francis IR, Platt JF, et al. Bladder tumor detection at virtual cystoscopy. Radiology 2001;218(1):95–100.
25. Skinner DG. Management of invasive bladder cancer: a meticulous pelvic node dissection can make a difference. J Urol 1982;128(1):34–6.
26. Vieweg J, Whitmore WF, Jr., Herr HW, et al. The role of pelvic lymphadenectomy and radical cystectomy for lymph node positive bladder cancer. The Memorial Sloan-Kettering Cancer Center experience. Cancer 1994;73(12):3020–8.
27. Wishnow KI, Johnson DE, Ro JY, Swanson DA, Babaian RJ, von Eschenbach AC. Incidence, extent and location of unsuspected pelvic lymph node metastasis in patients undergoing radical cystectomy for bladder cancer. J Urol 1987;137(3):408–10.
28. Zincke H, Patterson DE, Utz DC, Benson RC, Jr. Pelvic lymphadenectomy and radical cystectomy for transitional cell carcinoma of the bladder with pelvic nodal disease. Br J Urol 1985;57(2):156–9.

29. Kim B, Semelka RC, Ascher SM, Chalpin DB, Carroll PR, Hricak H. Bladder tumor staging: comparison of contrast-enhanced CT, T1- and T2-weighted MR imaging, dynamic gadolinium-enhanced imaging, and late gadolinium-enhanced imaging. Radiology 1994;193(1):239–45.
30. Maeda H, Kinukawa T, Hattori R, Toyooka N, Furukawa T, Kuhara H. Detection of muscle layer invasion with submillimeter pixel MR images: staging of bladder carcinoma. Magn Reson Imaging 1995;13(1):9–19.
31. Barentsz JO, Jager G, Mugler JP, 3rd, et al. Staging urinary bladder cancer: value of T1-weighted three-dimensional magnetization prepared-rapid gradient-echo and two-dimensional spin-echo sequences. AJR Am J Roentgenol 1995;164(1):109–15.
32. Strauss LG, Conti PS. The applications of PET in clinical oncology. J Nucl Med 1991;32(4):623–48; discussion 49–50.
33. Heicappell R, Muller-Mattheis V, Reinhardt M, et al. Staging of pelvic lymph nodes in neoplasms of the bladder and prostate by positron emission tomography with 2-[(18)F]-2-deoxy-D-glucose. Eur Urol 1999;36(6):582–7.
34. Kawamura T, Kusakabe T, Sugino T, et al. Expression of glucose transporter-1 in human gastric carcinoma: association with tumor aggressiveness, metastasis, and patient survival. Cancer 2001;92(3):634–41.
35. Younes M, Brown RW, Stephenson M, Gondo M, Cagle PT. Overexpression of Glut1 and Glut3 in stage I nonsmall cell lung carcinoma is associated with poor survival. Cancer 1997;80(6):1046–51.
36. Younes M, Juarez D, Lechago LV, Lerner SP. Glut 1 expression in transitional cell carcinoma of the urinary bladder is associated with poor patient survival. Anticancer Res 2001;21(1B):575–8.
37. Ho CL, Yu SC, Yeung DW. 11C-acetate PET imaging in hepatocellular carcinoma and other liver masses. J Nucl Med 2003;44(2):213–21.
38. Kotzerke J, Volkmer BG, Neumaier B, Gschwend JE, Hautmann RE, Reske SN. Carbon-11 acetate positron emission tomography can detect local recurrence of prostate cancer. Eur J Nucl Med Mol Imaging 2002;29(10):1380–4.
39. Oyama N, Miller TR, Dehdashti F, et al. 11C-acetate PET imaging of prostate cancer: detection of recurrent disease at PSA relapse. J Nucl Med 2003;44(4):549–55.
40. Koenig SH, Kellar KE. Theory of proton relaxation in solutions of magnetic nanoparticles, including the superparamagnetic size range. Acad Radiol 1996;3(Suppl 2):S273–6.
41. Clement O, Guimaraes R, de Kerviler E, Frija G. Magnetic resonance lymphography. Enhancement patterns using superparamagnetic nanoparticles. Invest Radiol 1994;29(Suppl 2):S226–8.
42. Weissleder R, Elizondo G, Wittenberg J, Rabito CA, Bengele HH, Josephson L. Ultrasmall superparamagnetic iron oxide: characterization of a new class of contrast agents for MR imaging. Radiology 1990;175(2):489–93.
43. Pannu HK, Wang KP, Borman TL, Bluemke DA. MR imaging of mediastinal lymph nodes: evaluation using a superparamagnetic contrast agent. J Magn Reson Imaging 2000;12(6):899–904.
44. Harisinghani MG, Dixon WT, Saksena MA, et al. MR lymphangiography: imaging strategies to optimize the imaging of lymph nodes with ferumoxtran-10. Radiographics 2004;24(3):867–78.
45. Saksena M, Harisinghani M, Hahn P, et al. Comparison of lymphotropic nanoparticle-enhanced MRI sequences in patients with various primary cancers. AJR Am J Roentgenol 2006;187(6):W582–8.
46. Anzai Y, Blackwell KE, Hirschowitz SL, et al. Initial clinical experience with dextran-coated superparamagnetic iron oxide for detection of lymph node metastases in patients with head and neck cancer. Radiology 1994;192(3):709–15.
47. Hoffman HT, Quets J, Toshiaki T, et al. Functional magnetic resonance imaging using iron oxide particles in characterizing head and neck adenopathy. Laryngoscope 2000;110(9):1425–30.
48. Michel SC, Keller TM, Frohlich JM, et al. Preoperative breast cancer staging: MR imaging of the axilla with ultrasmall superparamagnetic iron oxide enhancement. Radiology 2002;225(2):527–36.
49. Sigal R, Vogl T, Casselman J, et al. Lymph node metastases from head and neck squamous cell carcinoma: MR imaging with ultrasmall superparamagnetic iron oxide particles (Sinerem MR) – results of a phase-III multicenter clinical trial. Eur Radiol 2002;12(5):1104–13.
50. Memarsadeghi M, Riedl CC, Kaneider A, et al. Axillary lymph node metastases in patients with breast carcinomas: assessment with nonenhanced versus uspio-enhanced MR imaging. Radiology 2006;241(2):367–77.
51. Curvo-Semedo L, Diniz M, Migueis J, et al. USPIO-enhanced magnetic resonance imaging for nodal staging in patients with head and neck cancer. J Magn Reson Imaging 2006;24(1):123–31.
52. Neoadjuvant chemotherapy in invasive bladder cancer: update of a systematic review and meta-analysis of individual patient data advanced bladder cancer (ABC) meta-analysis collaboration. Eur Urol 2005;48(2):202–5; discussion 5–6.
53. Grossman HB, Natale RB, Tangen CM, et al. Neoadjuvant chemotherapy plus cystectomy compared with cystectomy alone for locally advanced bladder cancer. N Engl J Med 2003;349(9):859–66.
54. Neoadjuvant chemotherapy in invasive bladder cancer: a systematic review and meta-analysis. Lancet 2003; 361(9373):1927–34.
55. Bochner BH, Cho D, Herr HW, Donat M, Kattan MW, Dalbagni G. Prospectively packaged lymph node dissections with radical cystectomy: evaluation of node count variability and node mapping. J Urol 2004;172(4 Pt 1):1286–90.
56. Liedberg F, Chebil G, Davidsson T, Gudjonsson S, Mansson W. Intraoperative sentinel node detection improves nodal staging in invasive bladder cancer. J Urol 2006;175(1):84–8; discussion 8–9.
57. Leissner J, Ghoneim MA, Abol-Enein H, et al. Extended radical lymphadenectomy in patients with urothelial bladder cancer: results of a prospective multicenter study. J Urol 2004;171(1):139–44.
58. Sherif A, De La Torre M, Malmstrom PU, Thorn M. Lymphatic mapping and detection of sentinel nodes in patients with bladder cancer. J Urol 2001;166(3):812–5.

9
Presence and Significance of Micrometastases

Stephen Boorjian and Douglas S. Scherr

Contents

Abstract Micrometastases may be defined as the presence of cancer cells detected by molecular techniques in patients with no demonstratable evidence of disease by conventional radiographic and pathologic staging. To date, the detection of micrometastases in bladder cancer has primarily involved evaluating the expression of several urothelial-marker genes from the lymph nodes, serum, and bone marrow of patients with urothelial carcinoma. Uroplakin II (UP II) has been the most widely investigated of these genes, as UP II mRNA expression has been consistently detected in lymph nodes considered to be negative for carcinoma by conventional histology. UP II expression has thus shown promise as a molecular marker of micrometastatic disease, although correlation with patient outcome has been limited, and thus the ability to determine the clinical significance of detecting such molecular, or micro-metastases remains to be established.

In addition to detecting micrometastases, efforts have also been made to predict the presence of micrometastases in patients with urothelial cancer, based on the molecular characteristics of the primary bladder tumor. Here, investigators have focused mainly on evaluating the expression of cell-cycle regulatory genes, specifically the p53 and retinoblastoma (pRb) genes. The expression of these targets in primary bladder tumors has been found to correlate with disease recurrence and patient survival, independent of tumor stage, grade, and nodal status, suggesting their potential role as molecular predictors of micrometastatic disease. Future efforts are likely to utilize high-throughput techniques such as proteomics and microarrays to determine patients' risk of disease progression from the molecular expression pattern of the primary tumor. Here, we review the current status of the detection, prediction, and clinical significance of micrometastases in bladder cancer.

From: *Current Clinical Urology: Bladder Cancer*, Edited by: C.T. Lee and D.P. Wood,
DOI: 10.1007/978-1-59745-417-9_9, © Humana Press, a part of Springer Science+Business Media, LLC 2010

Keywords Micrometastases, Lymph node dissection, Uroplakin, Cytokeratin, p53, pRB, Oligonucleotide microarray

1. The Detection of Micrometastatic Disease

1.1. Background

Micrometastases may be defined as the presence of cancer cells in the lymph nodes, circulation, or distant sites in patients with no demonstratable evidence of disease spread by conventional radiographic and pathologic staging. The detection of micrometastases has previously been explored in a variety of malignancies, including melanoma (1–2), gastrointestinal (3–4), breast (5), and prostate (6–9) cancer. In prostate cancer, for example, PSA mRNA has been detected in up to 40% of histologically negative lymph nodes using reverse transcription polymerase chain reaction (RT-PCR) (6). However, while lymph-node PSA RT-PCR detection has been correlated with Gleason score (6), no clinical follow-up data has been provided to correlate PSA detection with clinical or biochemical recurrence. Indeed, although several other studies have suggested a clinical relevance for detecting PSA mRNA (7–8), the value of "molecular staging" in prostate cancer has been questioned elsewhere (9).

In patients with urothelial carcinoma of the bladder, the potential significance of micrometastatic disease is suggested in part by the fact that up to 25% of patients with lymph-node negative, organ-confined tumors experience systemic relapse after radical cystectomy (10). Disease recurrence in these patients may result from metastases not detected by conventional radiologic and pathologic staging. In addition, studies have shown an improved survival for patients who have a greater number of lymph nodes removed at the time of radical cystectomy, even when the nodes are pathologically negative, as well as for patients with a lower calculated lymph node density who have pN+ disease (11–14). The removal of occult, micrometastatic disease in lymph nodes classified as negative by conventional histology may explain the improved outcomes in these cases.

The prospective value of being able to identify micrometastases, moreover, is several-fold. For one, the ability to detect micrometastases may guide early adjuvant therapies, particularly if clinical correlation demonstrates a high rate of disease recurrence in patients with histologically negative but molecularly positive nodes. In addition, as molecular techniques evolve, the presence of micrometastases may be able to be determined intraoperatively, thereby guiding surgical management, as for example in the extent of lymph node dissection to employ (15). Here, then, we review the detection, prediction, and clinical significance of micrometastases in bladder cancer.

1.2. Micrometastases in Lymph Nodes

Initial attempts to detect micrometastases from bladder cancer evaluated cytokeratin (a marker of epithelial cells) protein expression in the lymph nodes of patients using immunohistochemistry demonstrated no advantage in the ability to detect metastases over conventional H&E-stained sections (16). However, subsequent studies have investigated mRNA expression of bladder-cancer-specific genes using RT-PCR. The most widely investigated of these urothelial markers have been the uroplakins, a group of proteins present on the apical membrane of terminally-differentiated urothelial cells that serve as a part of the bladder epithelium's barrier mechanism (15, 17–18). Four uroplakin (UP) genes exist: UPIa, UPIb, UPII, and UPIII, of which the UPIa and UPII genes are highly specific to urothelium, while UPII has been most frequently detected in advanced urothelial carcinomas and metastases (18).

Seraj et al. (19) utilized RT-PCR to evaluate UP II mRNA expression in the perivesical tissue and lymph nodes of patients who underwent radical cystectomy for urothelial carcinoma. Interestingly, UP II mRNA was detected in the perivesical tissue from 42% of patients with pathologically organ-confined tumors, and was found in the lymph nodes in 25% of patients with pathologically node negative disease (19). Moreover, UPII mRNA was present in 100% of the patients with pathologically positive nodes. Although no clinical follow-up was provided in the study, the findings suggest that UP II may serve as a marker for micrometastatic disease.

A subsequent study comparing the mRNA expression of UP II to cytokeratin 20 (CK 20) in lymph node specimens from patients with bladder cancer detected UP II in 10% of histologically negative lymph node samples, while CK 20 was found in none (20). In addition, UP II was detected in 93.8% of pathologically-proven metastases, while CK 20 was detected in only 56.6% of nodal metastases (20). Again, however, correlation with patient outcome wasnot provided, thus limiting the potential extrapolation of the detection of micrometastases to clinical significance.

Kurahashi and associates (21) used real-time PCR to evaluate CK19 and UP II expression in lymph nodes from patients who underwent radical cystectomy; here, however, expression was then correlated with disease recurrence and cancer-specific survival. UP II expression was detected in all histologically-positive lymph nodes, and either UP II or CK 19 mRNA was found in 35% of histologically negative nodes (21). The presence of such micrometastases was significantly associated with the pathological tumor stage and the presence of microvascular invasion in the primary lesion. Moreover, 33% of pN0 patients with mRNA evidence of micrometastases experienced recurrence of disease, versus 4.5% of pN0 patients without micrometastases (21). In addition, the cause-specific survival for patients with histologically negative lymph nodes that were positive for CK 19 or UP II mRNA was significantly lower than for patients with histologically negative lymph nodes without detectable CK 19 or UP II (Fig. 9.1) (21). These findings suggest a potential clinical relevance for the detection of micrometastases. However, in this small (40 patients) study, with limited follow-up (median 22 months), the presence of micrometastases was not an independent predictor of cause-specific survival on multivariate Cox proportional hazards regression analysis (21).

Copp et al. (22) prospectively evaluated UP II mRNA expression in the perivesical tissue and lymph nodes from patients undergoing radical cystectomy. All patients with pathologically positive nodes had positive UP II RT-PCR signals, and no patient with a negative RT-PCR for UP II had pathologically-positive lymph nodes. In addition, 33% of pathologically node-negative patients had detectable UPII mRNA in the nodes. Again here, UP II expression correlated with an increased disease recurrence rate, as 91% of patients with pathologically-negative but UP II-positive lymph nodes experienced disease recurrence, versus 5% of patients with lymph nodes negative by both histology and RT-PCR (Fig. 9.2) (22). In addition, 32% of

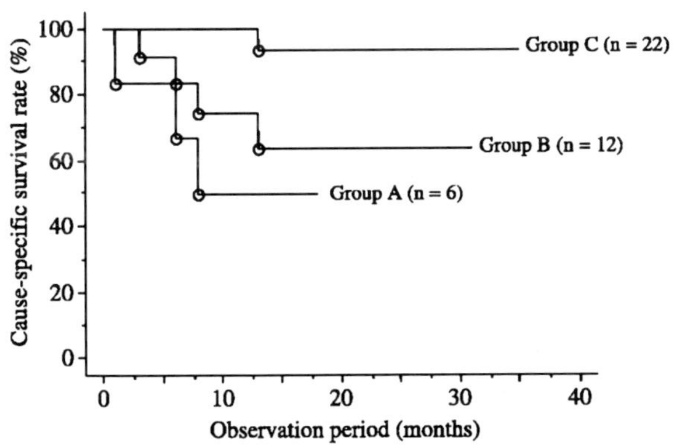

FIG. 9.1. Comparison of cause-specific survival rates in groups A, B, and C by the Kaplan-Meier method. The cause-specific survival rates in groups A and B were significantly lower than that in group C ($P < 0.005$, group A vs. group C; $P < 0.05$, group B vs. group C by the log-rank test). (Legend from Kurahashi T, Hara I, Oka N, Kamidono S, Eto H, Miyake H. Detection of micrometastases in pelvic lymph nodes in patients undergoing radical cystectomy for focally invasive bladder cancer by real-time reverse transcriptase-PCR for cytokeratin 19 and uroplakin II (21)

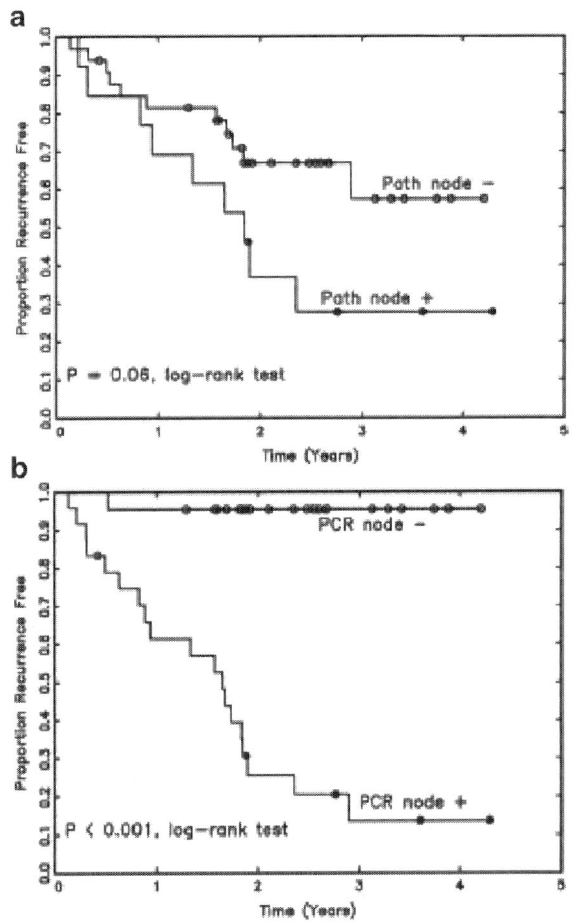

FIG. 9.2. Kaplan-Meier estimates for overall recurrence-free survival based on node positivity defined by (**a**) conventional pathologic analysis and (**b**) Uroplakin II (UPII) reverse-transcriptase polymerase chain reaction (RT-PCR). *P* values for comparing curves based on the log-rank test (from (22))

patients with pathologically organ-confined tumors experienced disease recurrence, and all had UP II RT-PCR positive lymph nodes, a rate which is roughly in accordance with published outcome for patients with organ-confined disease (10), further suggesting micrometastases as a possible mechanism for the recurrences noted in such cases. Moreover, unlike in the study by Kurahashi et al. (21), UP II RT-PCR positivity was found, on multivariate analysis, to be a significant predictor of tumor recurrence here, with a hazard ratio of 37.0 (22).

Another gene which has been investigated as a potential marker of lymph node micrometastases in bladder cancer patients is mucin 7 (MUC7). MUC7, a high molecular weight glycoprotein, is expressed in invasive urothelial cell carcinomas, but not in superficial tumors or in normal bladder urothelium (23). Retz and colleagues (24), using nested RT-PCR (a technique which may improve the sensitivity of conventional RT-PCR), found MUC7 mRNA in 29% of histologically negative lymph nodes and in 5/6 histologically positive nodes from patients undergoing radical cystectomy, suggesting MUC7 may be a sensitive and specific marker for occult metastatic disease, although clinical follow-up was not provided.

1.3. Circulating Micrometastases

In addition to analyzing lymph nodes removed at cystectomy for molecular markers of micrometastatic disease, investigators have also looked at the serum and bone marrow of patients with bladder cancer for occult metastases. Potentially, detection of a circulating marker of micrometastases would offer an even earlier and less invasive method of identifying patients at high risk for disease progression who would benefit from multimodal treatment. For example, Li and colleagues (25) performed RT-PCR for UP II on peripheral blood samples from patients with urothelial cell carcinoma of the bladder. They detected UP II in 2/2 patients with metastatic bladder cancer who were chemotherapy naïve and 1/8 patients with metastatic bladder cancer who had received chemotherapy, but in 0/50 patients with nonmetastatic urothelial carcinoma, and thereby suggested that the detection of UP II may be associated with metastatic bladder cancer (25).

Lu et al. (26) then utilized nested PCR to detect circulating UP II-positive cells in the peripheral blood of patients with urothelial carcinoma. Their study found that the presence of circulating UP II-expressing cells correlated with the tumor stage (with nearly 30% of muscle-invasive cancers positive for circulating UP II-positive cells), lymph node status (circulating UPII was detected in 40% of patients with pathologically-positive lymph nodes), and distant metastases (75% of patients with metastases had UPII detected in the blood). Although no correlation with recurrence or survival was provided in the study, the investigators did report evidence that UP II expression may correlate with patients' response to chemotherapy, as 2/3 patients with metastatic disease had a disappearance of circulating UP II expression after a favorable response to treatment (26).

Matsumoto and associates (27) evaluated plasma levels of soluble E-cadherin, and found that higher preoperative E-cadherin levels correlated with regional lymph node metastases and postoperative disease progression independent of stage and grade in patients who underwent radical cystectomy. Similarly, Hofmann et al. (28), using a monoclonal antibody assay, demonstrated a significant correlation between the detection of cytokeratin 18 (CK18) positive cells in bone marrow aspirates from patients with bladder cancer and lymph node involvement as well as tumor progression.

Fujii and colleagues (29), meanwhile, detected mRNA transcripts of CK20 in the peripheral blood from 22.5% of bladder cancer patients, and found that detection correlated with tumor stage and clinical metastases. On the other hand, Ribal et al. (30) found no correlation between peripheral blood or bone marrow expression of CK20 mRNA transcripts and pathologic tumor stage, although they reported that CK20 expression in the lymph nodes of patients with invasive bladder cancer did correlate with stage.

However, despite the promise of being able to detect micrometastases from these studies, several important limitations currently exist. First, correlation of the *detection* of micrometastases with the *clinical outcome* of patients remains to be validated in large, prospective series. That is, the detection of cells expressing bladder-specific antigens may not inevitably lead to clinical disease recurrence, as current molecular techniques may be sensitive enough to detect circulating cells that have not yet achieved a critical number to establish metastases, or have not yet undergone the cellular adaptations necessary to develop into clinical metastases (6). In addition, other molecular targets need to be identified for study as potential predictors of micrometastatic disease. Furthermore, no established protocols have been developed yet for the collection of tissue or for the analysis of patient specimens, specifically regarding the technique of RT-PCR to be used (real-time vs. semi-quantitative), the number of cycles to establish a threshold for detection, and the type of primers (nested vs. non-nested) which are most appropriate (15).

2. Molecular Predictors of Micrometastatic Disease

In addition to the *detection* of micrometastases, research has also focused on the ability to *predict* micrometastases in bladder cancer. Specifically, efforts have been made to correlate the expression of selected genes from primary bladder tumors in patients with urothelial carcinoma with the patients' clinical outcome, after controlling for tumor stage, grade, and lymph node status. The conceptual approach here has been that for pathologically-matched patients, the heterogeneity in clinical outcome reported (10) may be the result of molecular discrepancies in the primary tumors which confer differing risks of disease recurrence. Disease recurrence in these cases, furthermore, particularly in those patients without clinical, pathologic, or radiographic evidence of disease spread, may be through micrometastases. This potential correlation of micrometastases with disease recurrence, as discussed in the previous section, awaits validation in large clinical series. Until these studies have been reported, however, the association of marker expression in primary bladder tumors with the clinical outcome of patients in the studies to date may be seen as an indirect link between marker expression and micrometastases. Thus, we will discuss here several molecular markers analyzed in primary bladder tumors that have been shown to independently predict clinical outcome (and which therefore, as explained above, may potentially be seen as markers for micrometastases as well).

2.1. Cell-Cycle Regulatory Targets

The molecular changes involved in bladder cancer recurrence and progression have been previously reviewed (31–33). Research on molecular predictors of bladder cancer outcome has focused primarily on cell-cycle regulatory and apoptosis-related genes. The most widely investigated of these genes has been p53, a tumor-suppressor gene which mediates growth arrest and apoptosis in response to DNA damage and cellular stress (Fig. 9.3) (33–34). Esrig and colleagues (35) analyzed p53 expression using immunohistochemistry in 243 patients treated with radical cystectomy for urothelial carcinoma, and found on multivariate analysis that p53 status (specifically, nuclear accumulation of the p53 protein) predicted tumor recurrence and overall survival independent of tumor stage, grade, and lymph-node status. The strongest association of p53 immunoreactivity with survival was in fact noted for patients with organ-confined disease without pathological evidence of lymph node metastases (35), suggesting a role for p53 as a marker of micrometastatic disease. While a separate study demonstrated that overexpression of p53 did not have independent prognostic value on multivariate analysis (36), Sarkis and associates (37) found that p53 nuclear overexpression correlated with a significantly lower progression-free interval in patients with clinical T1 bladder cancer.

Another potential molecular marker of micrometastases in urothelial cancer is the retinoblastoma (pRb) gene, a tumor-suppressor gene that inactivates transcription factors responsible for DNA replication (32). pRB regulates cell growth by controlling exit from the G1 phase of the cell cycle (34). Both Cordon-Cardo and colleagues (38) and Logothetis et al. (39) have reported the independent prognostic value of pRB expression in bladder cancer. Specifically, both groups have reported significantly decreased survival in patients with muscle invasive urothelial carcinoma, who have altered Rb protein expression on immunohistochemical analysis (38–39). The predictive value of pRB expression for disease progression and overall survival in patients with superficial bladder tumors has also been demonstrated (40).

In addition to evaluating the prognostic value of these markers individually, researchers have also studied the expression pattern of combinations of these markers to predict the likelihood of micrometastases and disease progression. For example, Cordon-Cardo et al. (40) demonstrated increased progression and decreased overall survival rates in patients whose tumors had alterations in both p53 and Rb protein expression, after controlling for stage, grade, and vascular invasion. The potential cooperative effect of p53 and pRb mutations was also supported by a separate study, where it was found that patients with tumors altered in both p53 and pRb had significantly increased rates of recurrence and decreased survival after radical cystectomy (41).

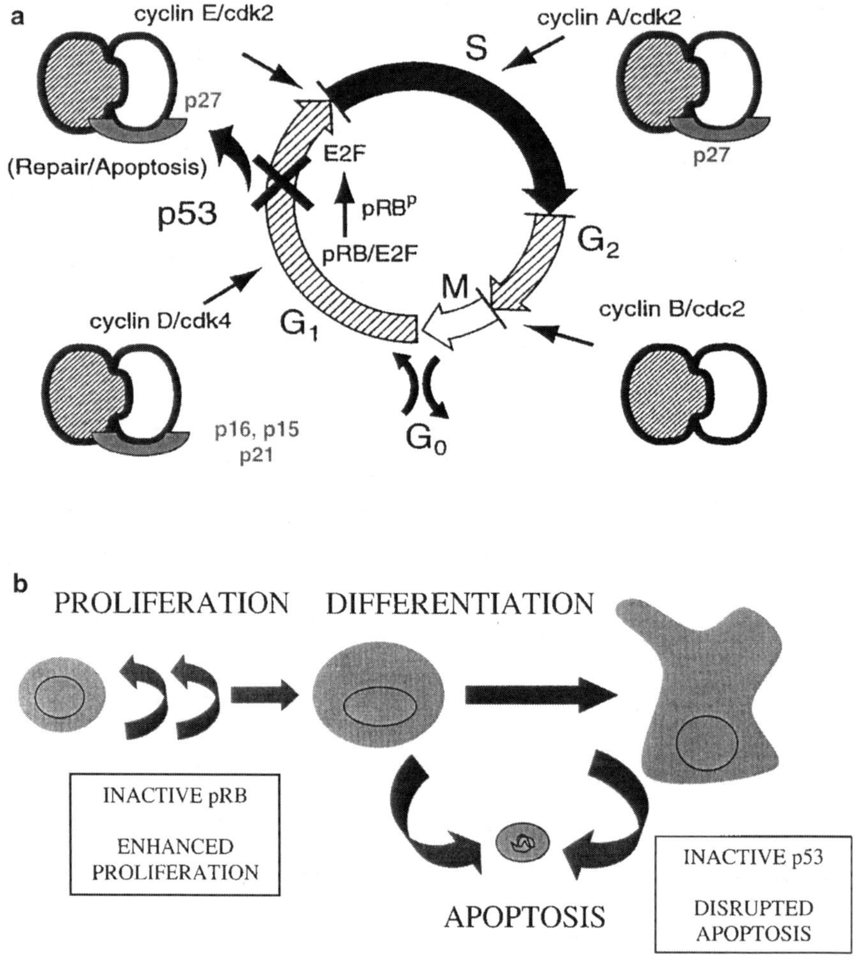

Fig. 9.3. (**a**) Cell cycle transitions and checkpoints. The product of the retinoblastoma gene (pRB) is the main regulator of cell cycle progression, while p53 exerts its functions as the DNA damage checkpoint, triggering growth arrest or apoptotic processes in response to DNA aberrations and cellular stress. (**b**) Tissue homeostasis and tumorigenesis. pRB and p53 serve collaborative roles in tumorigenesis. Deactivation of a p53-dependent cell suicide program is needed to abolish an apoptotic response to unchecked cellular proliferation resulting from RB deficiency. Tumor cells that spurn apoptotic responses are likely to be deficient in mechanisms of cell killing, such as those imposed by certain chemotherapeutic regimens (from (34))

p53 has in addition been analyzed as a potential marker for micrometastatic disease in combination with HER-2/neu, a transmembrane glycoprotein with tyrosine kinase activity. In an immunohistochemical analysis of radical cystectomy specimens, Tsai et al. (42) found that coexpression of p53 and HER-2/neu significantly correlated with nodal metastases, time to relapse, and overall survival, although HER-2/neu expression did not have independent prognostic significance.

Another gene which has been evaluated as a potential marker of micrometastatic disease alone and in combination with other markers is the cyclin-dependent kinase inhibitor p21WAF/CIP1 (p21), which mediates the action of p53 on cell cycle regulation. Stein and colleagues (43) analyzed tumor specimens from 242 patients who underwent cystectomy for bladder cancer and found that p21 protein expression was an independent predictor of tumor recurrence and survival on multivariate analysis. Specifically, patients with p21-positive tumors had a decreased probability of tumor recurrence and increased overall survival. Moreover, patients with p53 altered/p21 negative tumors demonstrated a higher rate of recurrence and worse survival rates compared to those with p53-altered/p21-positive tumors (43). Lipponen et al. (44), on the other hand, found that p21 protein expression did not independently predict survival on a univariate analysis of 186 patients, although 93/186 patients in their study had superficial (pTa/pT1) disease. The inability of p21 immunostaining to predict survival in superficial bladder cancer was confirmed on a subsequent study (45). However, the combined expression of p53 and p21 was found to be independently associated with disease recurrence, progression, and cancer-specific survival in patients with carcinoma in situ of the bladder (46).

p21 expression was also recently analyzed in combination with p53, pRB, and p16 expression using immunohistochemistry on archival specimens from 80 patients who underwent radical cystectomy, with a median follow-up of 101 months (47). On multivariate analysis, the alteration of each marker was independently associated with disease progression and disease-specific survival, while the incremental number of altered markers was associated with an increased risk of bladder cancer progression and decreased disease-specific survival (47). These findings suggest a potentially synergistic effect for alterations in multiple cell cycle regulators on the risk of developing clinical disease progression. As these associations were independent of stage, grade, lymphovascular invasion, and lymph node status, the effect of these markers on clinical outcome may be through micrometastases.

Chatterjee and associates (48), in an immunohistochemical study of p53, p21, and pRb expression from archived radical cystectomy specimens similarly found that alterations in expression of each of the three proteins was independently associated with time to recurrence and overall survival. Moreover, after stratifying by stage, the number of altered markers was also significantly associated with time to recurrence and overall survival. In fact, when patients were categorized as having no alterations, one marker alteration, two marker alterations, or all three markers altered, the 5-year recurrence rates were 23, 32, 57, and 93%, respectively ($p < 0.001$), while the 5-year survival rates were 70, 58, 33, and 8%, respectively ($p < 0.001$) (Table 9.1) (48). These findings further support the value of evaluating the expression of a combination of markers.

Survivin, an inhibitor of apoptosis has also been investigated for its prognostic value in bladder cancer. Ku et al. (49) investigated survivin expression using immunohistochemistry on superficial urothelial carcinomas, and found that survivin expression independently predicted disease-free survival on multivariate analysis.

2.2. Cytoskeletal/Angiogenic Markers of Micrometastases

Another group of molecular targets which have been investigated as potential predictors of micrometastases are the Rho family of GTPases, together with Rho-associated serine-threonin protein kinase (ROCK). These proteins regulate actin cytoskeleton reorganization, and thereby contribute to cell migration and cancer progression. Kamai et al. (50) investigated Rho and ROCK protein expression using Western blotting

TABLE 9.1. Increased hazard of recurring or dying according p53, p21, pRB status (Table from (48)).

	No of patients	Recurrence			Survival		
		Hazard ratio[a]	95% CI	*P*[b]	Hazard ratio[a]	95% CI	*P*[b]
p53 wt	102	1		0.001	1		0.004
p53 alt	62	2.50	1.49–4.18		1.86	1.23–2.82	
p21 wt	110	1		.005	1		0.104
p21 alt	54	2.04	1.24–3.35		1.41	0.94–2.14	
pRb wt	73	1		0.009	1		0.014
pRb alt	91	2.00	1.17–3.43		1.68	1.10–2.56	
p53/p21/pRB							
I: all wt	47	1		<0.001	1		0.008
II: onc alt	51	1.36	0.60–3.08		1.42	0.79–2.54	
III: two alt	42	2.69	1.24–5.82		2.25	1.26–4.01	
IV: all alt	24	4.57	2.05–10.16		2.67	1.39–5.13	

p53 wt ≤10% nuclear reactivity; *p53 alt* >10% nuclear reactivity; *p21 wt* >10% nuclear reactivity; *p21 alt* ≤10% nuclear reactivity; *pRb wt* 1–50% nuclear reactivity; *pRb alt* 0 or >50% nuclear reactivity
wt wild-type; *alt* altered phenotype
[a]Hazard ratios based on univariate analysis using Cox proportional hazards model and stratifying by stage
[b]*P* value based on the likelihood ratio test

in tumors from patients with urothelial carcinoma of the bladder, and found that high Rho C expression independently predicted disease-free survival on multivariate analysis, while Rho C and Rho A were significantly associated with overall survival. When the analysis was then restricted to patients with muscle-invasive disease, Rho C expression remained a significant predictor of overall survival (50).

The prognostic significance of molecular effectors of the angiogenesis pathway have similarly been investigated. For example, Grossfeld and colleagues (51–52) investigated the expression of thrombospondin-1 (TSP), a p53 dependent inhibitor of angiogenesis, in bladder tumors from 163 patients with invasive urothelial carcinoma using a monoclonal antibody. They found that TSP expression was an independent predictor of disease recurrence and overall survival after stratifying for tumor stage, grade, and lymph node status. Specifically, patients with low TSP expression had increased recurrence rates and shorter overall survival (52).

In the future, efforts to identify patients at risk for micrometastases and disease progression are likely to shift from the study of single targets or even combinations of markers using techniques such as RT-PCR and immunohistochemistry to high-throughput analyses such as proteomics and cDNA/tissue microarrays. Such techniques have already been applied in bladder cancer to identify gene expression changes along the progression from superficial to invasive urothelial cancers (53–55), and, of particular relevance for the prediction of micrometastases, to stratify patients with similarly-staged tumors based on risk of disease progression (54–55). A recent study by Sanchez-Carbayo et al. (56) from Memorial Sloan-Kettering used hierarchical clustering of oligonucleotide arrays to stratify patients with bladder cancer on the basis of clinical outcome. These investigators were able to predict overall survival in patients with invasive disease with an accuracy of 90%. Moreover, they created a genetic profile of 174 probes from patients with positive lymph nodes and poor overall survival, and were able to confirm the association of this profile with lymph node metastases and overall survival (56). Thus, the study provided a mechanism for stratifying the lymph node status and clinical outcome of invasive tumors. Interestingly, altered expression of these probes was also noted in the grossly normal urothelium adjacent to the invasive tumors, suggesting the possibility for early identification of a "molecular signature" of aggressive disease in patients who may benefit from early multimodality treatment (56).

References

1. Mellado B, Colomer D, Castel T, et al. Prognostic significance of the detection of circulating malignant cells by reverse transcriptase-polymerase chain reaction in long-term clinically disease-free melanoma patients. Clin Cancer Res 1999;5:1843–1848.
2. Mellado B, Colomer D, Castel T, et al. Detection of circulating neoplastic cells by reverse-transcriptase polymerase chain reaction in malignant melanoma: association with clinical stage and prognosis. J Clin Oncol 1996;14:2091–2097.
3. Weitz J, Kienle P, Magener A, et al. Detection of disseminated colorectal cancer cells in lymph nodes, blood, and bone marrow. Clin Cancer Res 1999;5:1830–1836.
4. Liefers GJ, Cleton-Jansen AM, van de Velde CJ, et al. Micrometastases and survival in stage II colorectal cancer. N Engl J Med 1998;339:223–228.
5. Peley G, Toth J, Csuka, Sinkovics I, Farkas E, Koves I. Immunohistochemistry and reverse transcriptase polymerase chain reaction on sentinel lymph nodes can improve the accuracy of nodal staging in breast cancer patients. Int J Biol Markers 2001;16:227–232.
6. Martínez-Piñeiro L, Rios E, Martínez-Gomariz M, et al. Molecular staging of prostatic cancer with RT-PCR assay for prostate-specific antigen in peripheral blood and lymph nodes: comparison with standard histological staging and immunohistochemical assessment of occult regional lymph node metastases. Eur Urol 2003;43:342–350.
7. Edelstein RA, Zeitman AL, de las Morenas A, et al. Implications of prostate micrometastases in pelvic lymph nodes: an archival tissue study. Urology 1996;47:370–375.
8. Okegawa T, Nutahara K, Higashihara E. Detection of micrometastatic prostate cancer cells in the lymph nodes by reverse transcriptase polymerase chain reaction is predictive of biochemical recurrence in pathological stage T2 prostate cancer. J Urol 2000;163:1183–1188.
9. de la Taille A, Olsson CA, Katz AE. Molecular staging of prostate cancer: dream or reality? Oncology 1999;13:187–194.
10. Stein JP, Lieskovsky G, Cote R, et al. Radical cystectomy in the treatment of invasive bladder cancer: long-term results in 1,054 patients. J Clin Oncol 2001;19:666–673.
11. Stein JP, Cai J, Groshen S, Skinner DG. Risk factors for patients with pelvic lymph node metastases following radical cystectomy with en bloc pelvic lymphadenectomy: concept of lymph node density. J Urol 2003;170:35–41.
12. Herr HW, Bochner BH, Dalbagni G, Donat SM, Reuter VE, Bajorin DF. Impact of the number of lymph nodes retrieved on outcome in patients with muscle invasive bladder cancer. J Urol 2002;167:1295–1298.
13. Herr H. Superiority of ratio based lymph node staging for bladder cancer. J Urol 2003;169:943–945.
14. Herr HW. Surgical factors in cancer: more (nodes) + more (pathology) = less (mortality). BJU Int 2003;92:187–188.
15. Theodorescu D, Frierson HF. When is a negative lymph node really negative? Molecular tools for the detection of lymph node metastasis from urologic cancer. Urol Oncol 2004;22:256–259.
16. Yang XJ, Lecksell K, Epstein JI. Can immunohistochemistry enhance the detection of micrometastases in pelvic lymph

nodes from patients with high-grade urothelial carcinoma of the bladder. Am J Clin Pathol 2000;112:649–653.
17. Lobban ED, Smith BA, Hall GD, et al. Uroplakin gene expression by normal and neoplastic human urothelium. Am J Pathol 1998;153:1957–1967.
18. Olsburgh J, Harnden P, Weeks R, et al. Uroplakin gene expression in normal human tissues and locally advanced bladder cancer. J Pathol 2003;199:41–49.
19. Seraj MJ, Thomas AR, Chin JL, Theodorescu D. Molecular determination of perivesical and lymph node metastasis after radical cystectomy for urothelial carcinoma of the bladder. Clin Cancer Res 2001;7:1516–1522.
20. Wu X, Kakehi Y, Zeng Y, Taoka R, Tsunemori H, Inui M. Uroplakin II as a promising marker for molecular diagnosis of nodal metastases from bladder cancer: comparison with cytokeratin 20. J Urol 2005;174:2142–2143.
21. Kurahashi T, Hara I, Oka N, Kamidono S, Eto H, Miyake H. Detection of micrometastases in pelvic lymph nodes in patients undergoing radical cystectomy for focally invasive bladder cancer by real-time reverse transcriptase-PCR for cytokeratin 19 and uroplakin II. Clin Cancer Res 2005;11:3773–3777.
22. Copp HL, Chin JL, Conaway M, Theodorescu D. Prospective evaluation of the prognostic relevance of molecular staging for urothelial carcinoma. Cancer 2006;107:60–66.
23. Retz M, Lehmann J, Roder C, et al. Differential mucin MUC7 gene expression in invasive bladder carcinoma in contrast to uniform MUC1 and MUC2 gene expression in both normal urothelium and bladder carcinoma. Cancer Res 1998;58:5662–5666.
24. Retz M, Lehmann J, Szysnik C, et al. Detection of occult tumor cells in lymph nodes from bladder cancer patients by MUC7 nested RT-PCR. Eur Urol 2004;45:314–319.
25. Li SM, Zhang ZT, Chan S, et al. Detection of circulating uroplakin-positive cells in patients with transitional cell carcinoma of the bladder. J Urol 1999;162:931–935.
26. Lu JJ, Kakehi Y, Takahashi T, et al. Detection of circulating cancer cells by reverse transcription-polymerase chain reaction for uroplakin II in peripheral blood of patients with urothelial cancer. Clin Cancer Res 2000;6:3166–3171.
27. Matsumoto K, Shariat SF, Casella R, Wheeler TM, Slawin KM, Lerner SP. Preoperative plasma soluble E-cadherin predicts metastases to lymph nodes and prognosis in patients undergoing radical cystectomy. J Urol 2003;170:2248–2252.
28. Hofmann T, Riesenberg R, Buchner A, Zimmermann W, Hofstetter A, Oberneder R. Disseminated tumor cells in bone marrow of patients with transitional cell carcinoma: immunocytochemical detection and correlation with established prognostic indicators. J Urol 2003;169:1303–1307.
29. Fujii Y, Kageyama Y, Kawakami S, Kihara K, Oshima H. Detection of disseminated urothelial cancer cells in peripheral venous blood by a cytokeratin 20-specific nested reverse transcriptase-polymerase chain reaction. Jpn J Cancer Res 1999;90:753–757.
30. Ribal MJ, Mengual L, Marin M, et al. Molecular staging of bladder cancer with RT-PCR assay for CK-20 in peripheral blood, bone marrow and lymph nodes: comparison with standard histological staging. Anticancer Res 2006;26:411–419.
31. Quek ML, Quinn DI, Daneshmand S, Stein JP. Molecular prognostication in bladder cancer–a current perspective. Eur J Cancer 2003;39:1501–1510.
32. Duggan B, Williamson K. Molecular markers for predicting recurrence, progression and outcomes of bladder cancer (do the poster boys need new posters?). Curr Opin Urol 2004;14:277–286.
33. Mitra AP, Datar RH, Cote RJ. Molecular staging of bladder cancer. BJU Int 2005;96:7–12.
34. Cordon-Cardo C. p53 and RB: simple interesting correlates or tumor markers of critical predictive nature? J Clin Oncol 2004;22:975–977.
35. Esrig D, Elmajian D, Groshen S, et al. Accumulation of nuclear p53 and tumor progression in bladder cancer. N Engl J Med 1994;331:1259–1264.
36. Lipponen PK. Over-expression of p53 nuclear oncoprotein in transitional-cell bladder cancer and its prognostic value. Int J Cancer 1993;53:365–370.
37. Sarkis AS, Dalbagni G, Cordon-Cardon C, et al. Nuclear overexpression of p53 protein in transitional cell bladder carcinoma: a marker for disease progression. J Natl Cancer Inst 1993;85:53–59.
38. Cordon-Cardo C, Wartinger D, Petrylak D, et al. Altered expression of the retinoblastoma gene product: prognostic indicator in bladder cancer. J Natl Cancer Inst 1992;84:1251–1256.
39. Logothetis CJ, Xu HJ, Ro JY, et al. Altered expression of retinoblastoma protein and known prognostic variables in locally advanced bladder cancer. J Natl Cancer Inst 1992;84:1256–1261.
40. Cordon-Cardo C, Zhang ZF, Dalbagni G, et al. Cooperative effects of p53 and pRB alterations in primary superficial bladder tumors. Cancer Res 1997;57:1217–1221.
41. Cote RJ, Dunn MD, Chatterjee SJ, et al. Elevated and absent pRb expression is associated with bladder cancer progression and has cooperative effects with p53. Cancer Res 1998;58:1090–1094.
42. Tsai YS, Tzai TS, Chow NH, et al. Prognostic values of p53 and HER-2/neu coexpression in invasive bladder cancer in Taiwan. Urol Int 2003;71:262–270.
43. Stein JP, Ginsberg DA, Grossfeld GD, et al. Effect of p21WAF1/CIP1 expression on tumor progression in bladder cancer. J Natl Cancer Inst 1998;90:1028–1029.
44. Lipponen P, Aaltomaa S, Eskelinen M, Ala-Opas M, Kosma VM. Expression of p21(waf1/cip1) protein in transitional cell bladder tumours and its prognostic value. Eur Urol 1998;34:237–243.
45. Liukkonen T, Lipponen P, Raitanen M, et al. Evaluation of p21WAF1/CIP1 and cyclin D1 expression in the progression of superficial bladder cancer. Urol Res 2000;28:285–292.
46. Shariat SF, Kim J, Raptidis G, Ayala GE, Lerner SP. Association of p53 and p21 expression with clinical outcome in patients with carcinoma in situ of the urinary bladder. Urology 2003;61:1140–1145.
47. Shariat SF, Tokunaga H, Zhou J, et al. p53, p21, pRB and p16 expression predict clinical outcome in cystectomy with bladder cancer. J Clin Oncol 2004;22:1014–1024.
48. Chatterjee SJ, Datar R, Youssefzadeh D, et al. Combined effects of p53, p21, and pRb expression in the progression of bladder transitional cell carcinoma. J Clin Oncol 2004;22:975–977.
49. Ku JH, Kwak C, Lee HS, Park HK, Lee E, Lee SE. Expression of survivin, a novel inhibitor of apoptosis, in

superficial transitional cell carcinoma of the bladder. J Urol 2004;171:631–635.

50. Kamai T, Tsujii T, Arai K, et al. Significant association of Rho/ROCK pathway with invasion and metastasis of bladder cancer. Clin Cancer Res 2003;9:2632–2641.
51. Grossfeld GD, Shi SR, Ginsberg DA, et al. Immunohistochemical detection of thrombospondin-1 in formalin-fixed, paraffin-embedded tissue. J Histochem Cytochem 1996;44:761–766.
52. Grossfeld GD, Ginsberg DA, Stein JP, et al. Thrombospondin-1 expression in bladder cancer: association with p53 alterations, tumor angiogenesis, and tumor progression. J Natl Cancer Inst 1997;89:219–227.
53. Sanchez-Carbayo M, Cordon-Cardo C. Applications of array technology: identification of molecular targets in bladder cancer. Br J Cancer 2003;89:2172–2177.
54. Sanchez-Carbayo M, Socci ND, Lozano JJ, et al. Gene discovery in bladder cancer progression using cDNA microarrays. Am J Pathol 2003;163:505–516.
55. Dyrskjot L, Thykjaer T, Kruhoffer M, et al. Identifying distinct classes of bladder carcinoma using microarrays. Nat Gen 2003;33:90–96.
56. Sanchez-Carbayo M, Socci N, Lozano J, Saint F, Cordon-Cardo C. Defining molecular profiles of poor outcome in patients with invasive bladder cancer using oligonucleotide microarrays. J Clin Oncol 2006;24:778–789.

Part II
Optimizing Treatment of Localized Disease

Section 1
Intravesical Theraphy

10
Perioperative Intravesical Therapy

Ralph Madeb and Edward Messing

Contents

Abstract For well over a decade, the results of prospective, randomized, controlled clinical trials performed primarily outside the United States have shown that intravesical instillation of chemotherapeutic agents immediately after transurethral resection of bladder tumor (TURB) decreases the likelihood of tumor recurrence, particularly for patients with newly diagnosed bladder cancers. Despite this, guidelines by the American Urological Association do not advocate its use as standard of care for the treatment of superficial bladder cancer while the European Association of urology does. We have reviewed the world literature and feel that there is ample evidence to recommend the routine use of intravesical mitomycin C after transurethral resection of bladder tumors in the United States.

Using a health-care based medical research database there is significant under-utilization of perioperative intravesical chemotherapy by American urologists. Reasons for this policy not being incorporated into standard practice, including barriers to its acceptance and performance, are unclear. Furthermore, an analysis for potential cost savings with its incorporation in routine care of patients with low-grade superficial bladder cancer revealed a $24.8 million cost savings to the American health care system per year. We therefore conclude that there is ample evidence to show that immediate intravesical chemotherapy can decrease the likelihood of tumor recurrence and adopting this policy would significantly lower the cost of care for bladder cancer in the U.S.

Keywords Immediate intravesical chemotherapy, Mitomycin C, Tumor recurrence, Cost effectiveness, Clinical trials

1. Introduction

Bladder cancer is the fourth most commonly diagnosed cancer in men and the eighth most common in women in the United States. An estimated 61,420 new cases of bladder cancer will be diagnosed in 2006 and 13,060 patients will die of this disease (1).

From: *Current Clinical Urology: Bladder Cancer*, Edited by: C.T. Lee and D.P. Wood,
DOI: 10.1007/978-1-59745-417-9_10,

Low grade, superficial urothelial cancer has a high likelihood of recurrence after initial transurethral resection (TURB). While a variety of approaches for treating such patients exist, including immediate post-TURB intravesical instillation chemotherapy, a series of intravesical immuno – or chemotherapy instillations, and/or use of fluorescence cystoscopy, the major form of management in the United States has remained repeat surveillance cystoscopic examinations and TURBs for recurrences. Although these patients are at low risk for tumor progression, they carry a significant risk for tumor recurrence and the morbidity of repeat resections. In this chapter we review current data and urologic literature in order to evaluate the efficacy, utilization, and cost effectiveness of using immediate intravesical chemotherapy after TURB.

1.1. Natural History of Superficial Bladder Cancer

Urothelial cancer can be roughly broken down into superficial (Stages Ta, Tis, T1) and muscle invasive disease (Stage T2 or greater), with low grade (grade 1 and 2) vs. high-grade (grade 3) lesions (2, 3). Seventy-five percent of newly diagnosed TCCs are superficial, of which 10–25% progress to muscle invasive disease (Stage T2+) upon subsequent recurrences (2–4). The majority of those superficial cancers that progress are high grade, yet these only represent 25–30% of all superficial cancers at diagnosis. Because virtually all patients who die from bladder cancer do so from metastatic disease, it is important to note that almost all patients with metastases have concomitant or prior muscle invasive cancers (i.e., it is extremely rare for a patient who has never had a stage T2 cancer to develop metastases (5). Moreover, if one eliminates patients with superficial grade 3 (high-grade) cancer or carcinoma-in-situ (CIS), the risk of recurrence after endoscopic resection alone, is quite high, but that of progression to muscle invasion relatively low (3, 6–8). The data indicate that recurrences of seemingly completely resected stage Ta and T1 tumors occur because of new tumor development at other regions of the urothelium, implantation of tumor cells derived from the original tumor in other sites of the urothelium (presumably occurring spontaneously as well as because of perturbations induced by instrumentations such as cystoscopy and TURB), and because of failure to resect the original malignancy (9, 10). While recurring, well and moderately differentiated superficial bladder cancers only rarely progress to a life-threatening condition, repeated transurethral resections and intravesical instillations are associated with considerable inconvenience, expense and morbidity.

1.2. History and Efficacy of Transurethral Resection of Bladder Tumors

A milestone in the treatment of bladder cancer occurred in 1910, when Edwin Beer of the Mount Sinai Hospital in New York, became the first surgeon to successfully remove bladder cancer through a transurethral approach under direct vision. He used a high frequency current derived from an Oudin resonator made by Reinhold Wappler (11–16). The resonator was attached to an X-ray machine and the current flowed between insulated electrodes channeled through the Nitze cystoscope (11, 12). His success was published in the Journal of American Medical Association (JAMA) in 1910 (11), and was quickly embraced by many urologists interested in treating bladder cancer. Its importance can best be summarized in the urology textbooks of the early twentieth century edited by Hugh Hampton Young and Frank Hinman of the John Hopkins institute (15, 16);

> Only 20 years ago, tumor of the bladder presented an almost hopeless situation. Surgery was the only recourse and most cases were too far advanced even for surgery when first seen. Snare excisions then in common use were followed by recurrences which quickly became malignant. In 1910, Edwin Beer introduced fulguration...Since then, the use of radium has undergone a rise and fall, but preserves a certain usefulness, so that today with fulguration, surgery, and irradiation, the picture has changed materially and we are now getting results that we can be proud of even though we are far from the goal at which we are aiming.

This method was quickly adapted by all urologists, and today remains the first line of therapy for the diagnosis and treatment of bladder cancer. Interestingly, its clinical efficacy has not changed. In a review of 400 cases, Beer reported that he had cured 40% of bladder cancer cases with fulguration alone (12, 15, 16). This also was shown in Young's and Hinman's series (11, 12, 15, 16). Although much has been learned about the genetics and pathophysiology of bladder cancer, the clinical efficacy of transurethral resection of superficial bladder tumors, if one includes both low and high grade, stage Ta and T1 cancers that are newly diagnosed or recurrent, is probably still 40%. This has been shown in a variety of current day follow-up studies of superficial bladder cancer as well as in placebo arms of randomized trials using BCG and other agents (17–27).

1.3. Rationale for Immediate Intravesical Instillation of a Chemotherapeutic Agent

As stated earlier, recurrence of completely resected bladder cancers represent new tumor occurrence elsewhere in the urothelium, implantation of clones from the index tumor, and/or incomplete resection of the original tumor. Evidence to support implantation includes differences in locations of newly diagnosed tumors compared to recurrences with the former primarily located on the lateral bladder walls (70%) and trigone (20%), while recurrences frequently arise on the dome and anterior bladder wall (28–32). Animal models also indicate that both spontaneous and mechanically facilitated implantation occurs (28, 32). Sites of urothelial injury are preferential sites of recurrence. To reduce the frequency of early recurrences in individuals at high risk for disease recurrence, courses of intravesical therapy with a variety of chemo- and immunotherapeutic agents have been used. Agents have included BCG, mitomycin C, doxyrubicin, thiotepa, epirubicin and epodil. Courses of instillation therapy starting days to weeks after TURB have been reported to reduce recurrences in up for 50% compared with controls (7, 10, 33, 33, 34, 34–40). In addition, randomized trials have demonstrated that adjuvant intravesical therapy for superficial bladder cancer with BCG has further reduced short-term recurrence by 15–20% and long term recurrence by 6% (41). Because intravesical BCG therapy has also been found to reduce rates of disease worsening (to requiring cystectomy and/or developing muscle invasive disease (22)), it is recognized as the treatment of choice for patients with intermediate-and high-risk superficial bladder cancer. These treatments, however, are not without considerable inconvenience, expense, and morbidities for patients with side effects including severe thrombocytopenia and leukopenia with thiotepa in 9% of patients, genital rash due to mitomycin in 6% of patients, and bladder contracture in as many as 16% of patients treated with doxyrubicin and a smaller percentage of those treated with mitomycin. Side effects of BCG therapy occur in 20–45% of patients and can include high fever, granulomatous prostatitis, pneumonitis, and hepatitis. Furthermore, virtually all patients who receive intravesical instillation therapy courses experience transient dysuria and urinary frequency. To reduce these sources of morbidity, inconvenience, and expense, immediate post-TURB intravesical instillations of a variety of chemotherapeutic agents have been tested in prospective randomized studies (7, 10, 33–40). The theory behind a single, immediately post-TURB intravesical instillation of chemotherapy is that such treatment should primarily reduce the rate of tumor implantation, decreasing the likelihood of disease recurrence and the need for long courses of intravesical therapy and repeat TURB.

1.4. Clinical Trials Using Immediate Intravesical Therapy

Table 10.1 reviews the randomized studies of same day intravesical instillation of a chemotherapeutic agent after TURB. While patients, drug dosages, times of instillation after resection, and durations of follow-up have varied, most studies have shown between 25 and 50% reduction in tumor recurrences with active agents. In some studies, patients with newly diagnosed cancers were particularly advantaged, while in others those with recurrent tumors were advantaged. The largest of the studies is that reported by Oosterlinck et al. in 1993, carried out by the European Organization for Research and Treatment of Cancer (EORTC) (7). In this study 80 mg of epirubicin in 50cc of saline was compared with 50cc of sterile water immediately after TURB of stage Ta and T1 completely resected tumors in 399 patients. Roughly 80% had new tumors and experienced a reduction of recurrence by over 50%, from 31% recurrences per year in control patients to less than 15% in treated patients. Patients whose index tumors were recurrent cancers experienced a non-statistically significant reduction of recurrence rates compared to controls (p value = 0.38). The reductions in recurrences were primarily achieved during the first 12 months, but these differences persisted in each arm up to four years of follow up. Tolley et al. (38) and Rajala et al. (36), obtained similar results using single or multiple instillations of mitomycin and epirubicin, respectively. Others have found similar results in smaller series (10, 33–36, 39, 40, 42). Recently, a meta-analysis by Sylvester et al. confirmed the benefits of using immediate post-TURB intravesical chemotherapy (37). They showed that this treatment has decreased the risk of recurrence by 39% in patients with stage Ta and T1 bladder cancer. Virtually

TABLE 10.1. World literature of randomized studies for immediate post-TURB intravesical instillation of a chemotherapeutic agent.

<table>
<tr><th>Reference</th><th>Agent [dose]/control</th><th>No. of patients</th><th>Type of patient</th><th>Stage</th><th>Interval of follow-up</th><th colspan="4">Recurrence rate outcome (study arm vs. control)</th></tr>
<tr><td>MRC (33)</td><td>Thiotepa [30 mg/50 ml]/observation</td><td>256</td><td>100% New</td><td>Ta and T1</td><td>Recurrence rate at 2 years</td><td colspan="4">35.4 vs. 41.3% ($p = 0.7$)</td></tr>
<tr><td>MRC (34)</td><td colspan="9">Follow up of above study at 8.75 year showed no difference of time to primary recurrence, recurrence rate, or failure free interval</td></tr>
<tr><td rowspan="2">Solsona (10)</td><td rowspan="2">Mitomycin C [30 mg/50 ml of NS]/ observation</td><td rowspan="2">121</td><td>90% New</td><td rowspan="2">Ta and T1</td><td rowspan="2">Recurrence rate at 1 year</td><td colspan="4" rowspan="2">22 vs. 59%($p < 0.005$)</td></tr>
<tr><td>10% Recurrent</td></tr>
<tr><td rowspan="3">Oosterlinck (7)</td><td rowspan="3">Epirubicin[80 mg in50ccNS]/50cc of H_2O</td><td rowspan="3">399</td><td>80% New</td><td rowspan="3">Ta and T1</td><td rowspan="3">Recurrence rate per year</td><td colspan="4">New: 15 vs. 31% ($p < 0.0001$)</td></tr>
<tr><td>20% Recurrent</td><td colspan="4">Recur: 26 vs. 35% ($p = 0.38$)</td></tr>
<tr><td>Overall</td><td colspan="4">Overall: 17 vs. 32% ($p < 0.0001$)</td></tr>
<tr><td>Burnand (42)</td><td>Thiotepa [90 mg/100cc]/observation</td><td>51</td><td>Unknown</td><td>Ta and T1</td><td>Recurrences at 2–5 year follow – up</td><td colspan="4">57.9 vs. 96.8% ($p < 0.005$)</td></tr>
<tr><td rowspan="2">Ali-el-dein (35)</td><td rowspan="2">Epirubicin [50 mg/50 ml NS]/observation</td><td rowspan="2">109</td><td>55% New</td><td rowspan="2">Ta and T1</td><td rowspan="2">Recurrence rate at mean of 2.5 years</td><td colspan="4" rowspan="2">24 vs. 52% ($p < 0.002$)</td></tr>
<tr><td>45% Recurrent</td></tr>
<tr><td rowspan="4">Rajala (36)</td><td rowspan="4">Epirubicin [100 mg] vs. interferon a2b[50 M units] vs. observation (3-arm study)</td><td rowspan="4">200</td><td rowspan="4">100% New</td><td rowspan="4">Ta and T1</td><td rowspan="4">Recurrence rate at 2 years</td><td></td><td>Epi (%)</td><td>INF-a (%)</td><td>Obs (%)</td></tr>
<tr><td>Overall</td><td>32</td><td>62</td><td>60 $p < 0.05$</td></tr>
<tr><td>1-tumor</td><td>27</td><td>63</td><td>55</td></tr>
<tr><td>Multiple</td><td>56</td><td>67</td><td>74</td></tr>
<tr><td>Tolley (38)</td><td>Mitomycin C [40 mg/40ccH_2O]/ Observation</td><td>306</td><td>100% New</td><td>Ta and T1</td><td>Recurrence rate at 2 years</td><td colspan="4">42 vs. 55% ($p = 0.01$)</td></tr>
<tr><td rowspan="4">Zincke (39)</td><td rowspan="4">Thiotepa [60 mg/60 ml H_2O] vs. doxir [50 mg/60 ml H_2O] vs. H_2O (3-arm Study)</td><td rowspan="4">45</td><td>21% New</td><td rowspan="4">Ta, T1, Tis</td><td rowspan="4">Recurrence rate at 3–4 months</td><td></td><td>Ttp (%)</td><td>Doxir (%)</td><td>H_2O (%)</td></tr>
<tr><td rowspan="3">79% Recurrent</td><td>Overall</td><td>30</td><td>32</td><td>71</td></tr>
<tr><td>New</td><td>43</td><td>0</td><td>43</td></tr>
<tr><td>Recurrent</td><td>26</td><td>38</td><td>81</td></tr>
</table>

all series report minimal complications, although in most, investigators could elect to withhold the instillation if they had concerns about bleeding (and the need for continuous bladder irrigation) or perforation of the bladder during TURB. Most studies do not report the number of patients eligible for such therapy who did not receive it because of these concerns, although in our experience it is below 10%.

1.5. Who Should Receive Immediate Post-TURB Intravesical Therapy, and What Agent Should be Used?

As can be seen, immediate post-TURB reduces the rate of recurrence but does not eliminate it (Table 10.1). While studies vary, the greatest benefit appears to be for patients with newly diagnosed cancers (Table 10.1). Because patients with high grade cancers are at considerable risk for stage progression, and BCG has been shown to significantly reduce that likelihood (25), it is probable that such patients, while they are unlikely to be hurt by immediate post-resection instillation chemotherapy, should also receive additional treatment. These cancers can usually be recognized by their endoscopic appearance from low grade superficial papillary cancers by experienced cystoscopists (43), and can obviously be distinguished based on pathologic inspection. Additionally, because a course of mitomycin C instillation was found to be more effective than a single instillation in a randomized prospective trial, it is our belief, that patients with frequently recurring and/or large numbers of low grade superficial cancers should not have their therapy limited to a single post-TURB instillation of chemotherapy (36, 38–40). Therefore, based on clinical history and inspection, at the time of diagnostic cystoscopy, most urologists can identify suitable candidates for immediate post-TURBT intravesical instillation therapy and arrange for the agent to be given in the operating or recovery room. While randomized controlled evidence supports use of mitomycin, doxyrubicin, or thiotepa vs. placebo, large controlled studies with adequate follow-up testing one of these agents vs. another have not been done. However, because of the serious hematologic side effects reported in as many as 9% of patients receiving courses of thiotepa intravesical instillations (10, 36, 40), and the risk of systemic absorption of an agent placed into a bladder with a fresh resection bed, this agent should probably not be the one chosen.

1.6. Utilization of Immediate Intravesical Therapy in the Unites States

Despite the evidence supporting the effectiveness and safety of immediate post-TURB intravesical therapy, there have been no reports on its actual utilization in the United States. Currently, the AUA has not yet established immediate intravesical therapy as standard of care although it recommends its use as an option for therapy (44). The European Association of Urology does consider this treatment to be standard of care for superficial bladder cancer (45–47). We therefore set out to determine whether American urologists have adopted this evidence-based practice into standard care by using large commercial insurance claims and Medicare database, and to ascertain whether there is potential cost-effectiveness with implementing post-TURB intravesical instillation.

Despite compelling evidence for its efficacy we found that post-TURB instillation of a chemotherapeutic agent is rarely employed in the United States. Only 0.33% of a large cohort of patients diagnosed with, and treated for bladder cancer were identified as receiving postsurgical intravesical instillation of a chemotherapeutic agent (48). The study was based on the analysis of individual medical claims provided by Medstat, a healthcare information company that provides market intelligence and benchmark databases and research services for managing costs and quality of healthcare in the United States. We used Medstat's Commercial Claims and Encounters (CCAE) and Medicare Supplemental Coverage claims databases. These include claims from patients enrolled into health plans provided by large employers, nationwide plans such as Blue Cross/Blue Shield, third party administrators, and patients with primary or Medicare Supplemental coverage through privately insured fee-for-service, point of service, or capitated health plans. Medstat currently follows over seven million covered lives. The databases have been validated and used for oncological and non-oncological research studies throughout the nation (49–54). The databases contain claims for inpatient admissions and services, outpatient services, and all inpatient and outpatient prescriptions filled, which is directly linked to medical and surgical data from 1989 onward. Each prescription drug filled by each patient could be identified by its unique NDC(National Drug Code) or CPT(Current Procedure Terminology) code and could be linked to the individual patient's medical and surgical histories and claims.

Using both the CCAE and medicare databases from 1997 (the first full calendar year following publication of results of a large randomized prospective clinical trial supporting use of immediate post-TURB instillation therapy with an agent available in the U.S.) through 2004, we identified 16,748 patients who had a new diagnosis of bladder cancer as their primary or secondary diagnosis upon visiting their physicians and who had never had a prior bladder cancer or bladder tumor diagnosis. (This represents 4% of all patients in the U.S. who were newly diagnosed with bladder cancer during the same time interval.) From those patients 14,677 (87.6%) subsequently underwent cystoscopy with biopsy or TURB of their newly diagnosed bladder cancer (Table 10.2). Of these 14,677 patients, only 49 (0.33%) patients received same or following day instillation therapy after their surgical procedure (Table 10.3). The majority of these patients received mitomycin C (48 of the 49; 98%), while one patient (2%) received interferon alpha-2B (Table 10.4). No patient received intravesical doxorubicin or thiotepa. When analyzed from 1997 through 2004, there have been no significant fluctuations in the yearly rate of new diagnosis, treatment of bladder cancer, or the use of same day intravesical therapy after TURB in the analyzed cohort (Table 10.5).

We therefore concluded that although there is ample evidence based data for the incorporation of immediate intravesical therapy after TURB it is not routinely used in the United States.

1.7. Reasons Why Immediate Post-TURB Intravesical Therapy is Not Performed

One obvious reason for failure to perform immediate post-TURB intravesical therapy is a technical matter involving dispensing and administering chemotherapeutic medications. Many American centers require special chemotherapy nurses and ancillary staff to handle and instill these agents, which prevents most operating room or recovery room nurses from administering them. In the current situation of a national/international shortage of nurses, requiring additional training and/or personnel for routine management of a very frequently performed operation would increase the cost of care and restructuring of current day recovery units. A solution which urologists currently resort to in order to offer their patients this treatment is to instil the medication and oversee its dispensing and handling by themselves. The inconvenience of ordering, instilling, and waiting for the chemotherapy to dwell for 1–2 h for a busy practitioner is clearly a deterrent to its use.

Another barrier to its acceptance is the economic burden placed on the hospital or surgicenter without any financial gain. Currently the additional expenses of using intravesical chemotherapy in an operating room setting, are borne by the facility without reimbursement for matters such as longer time in the recovery room (as a Foley catheter remains clamped for 1–2 h after surgery while the agent dwells in the

TABLE 10.2. Counts of patients undergoing cystoscopy with biopsy (CPT code 52204) or transurethral resection of bladder tumor (CPT code 52224, 52234, 52235, 52240) among patients with newly diagnosed bladder cancer.

Index year	1997	1998	1999	2000	2001	2002	2003	2004	Total
CC&E									
Bx (CPT 52204)	133	87	145	98	207	171	169	121	1,131
TURB (CPT 52224, 52234, 52235, 52240)	324	275	350	303	637	557	697	564	3,707
Total CC&E									4,838
Medicare									
Bx (CPT 52204)	156	273	207	161	448	245	267	193	1,950
TURB (CPT 52224, 52234, 52235, 52240)	453	1,033	714	632	1,832	1,201	1,121	903	7,889
Total Medicare									9,839
Total CC&E and Medicare									14,677

TABLE 10.3. Counts of patients with a service date for an intravesical instillation of a chemotherapeutic agent (CPT code 51720) on the same day or the day after their procedure.

	Same day or next day chemotherapy	Total	Percentage of all bladder cancer (188.9)	Percentage With Cysto, Bx, TURB
CC&E	16	16	0.10	0.10
MDCR	33	33	0.20	0.22
Total	49	49	0.29	0.33

TABLE 10.4. Frequency of same day intravesical chemotherapeutic agent used after their procedure.

Drug	CC&E (n)	Medicare (n)	Total (n)
Doxorubicin	0	0	0
Interferon alfa-2B, recombinant	0	1	1
Mitomycin (5 mg)	2	7	9
Mitomycin (20 mg)	5	4	9
Mitomycin (40 mg)	9	21	30
Total	16	33	49

TABLE 10.5. Frequency and percentages of intravesical instillation between the years of 1997–2004.

Index year	1997	1998	1999	2000	2001	2002	2003	2004	Total
Total no. of intravesical instillations post TURB	1	7	5	3	9	9	9	6	49
Procedures per year	1,066	1,668	1,416	1,194	3,124	2,174	2,254	1,781	14,677
% of instillations/per year	0.093	0.420	0.353	0.251	0.288	0.413	0.39	0.336	0.333

bladder), increased monitoring by specially trained nursing staff because of the small risk of bladder perforation, and the expenses of disposing of the chemotherapeutic agent. Alternatively, cost savings resulting from decreased recurrence and decreased subsequent intervention primarily benefit the insurance company and patient.

Another possible reason for not performing this treatment deals with the ways new scientific data are transmitted to, and incorporated into practice by practicing physicians. Although, numerous clinical trials have shown its effectiveness, these data have not been widely accepted by urologists to the extent that clinical practice has changed. Whether this is because urologists in America are not aware of the published data, or because these trials have largely been performed outside the U.S. without the inclusion of American centers, The reason's why American urologists appear to be resistant to embracing these results and incorporating them into their daily practices are unknown.10.

1.8. Cost-Effectiveness of Immediate Intravesical Instillation of Mitomycin C

Despite its low adoption rate, processes that can decrease the possibility of, and prolong the time of recurrence can theoretically have savings on medical health care costs. We therefore, implemented a theoretical model in order to determine whether a post-TURB intravesical instillation would be cost-effective (Fig. 10.1). On the basis of multiple prospective randomized studies, we identified the standard of care and likely outcomes for bladder cancer patients with newly diagnosed grade 1 and 2 superficial (stage Ta and T1) bladder cancer after initial TURBT with zero, one, two, or three episodes of recurrence over a 3-year period (Table 10.6) (5, 17, 22–27, 55–59). To assign cost values to the typical utilization associated with each of the recurrence patterns, with and without intravesical instillations of chemotherapy, we used Medicare reimbursement fees for the related procedures and medications (including reimbursement for one intravesical instillation procedure in the operating room) (Table 10.6). These analyses are conducted from a health insurance perspective, in order to determine whether a post-TURB intravesical instillation would be cost-effective.

The results are presented as an average cost per patient for the population without recurrences during a 3-year period (60% all low grade superficial bladder cancer patients), patients with one recurrence (30% of all low grade superficial bladder cancer patients), with two (4%) and with three recurrences (6%) (17, 22–27, 55–59). For the base case analysis, we assumed that same day intravesical therapy will reduce the proportion of patients with recurrences by 25% so that 22.5% would have one, 3% would have two, and 4.5% would have three recurrences over a 3-year period. The remaining 70% of patients will experience no recurrences.

Since there is a wide variation in the reported efficacy of intravesical instillation therapy, we conducted a threshold analysis to estimate the minimal (threshold)

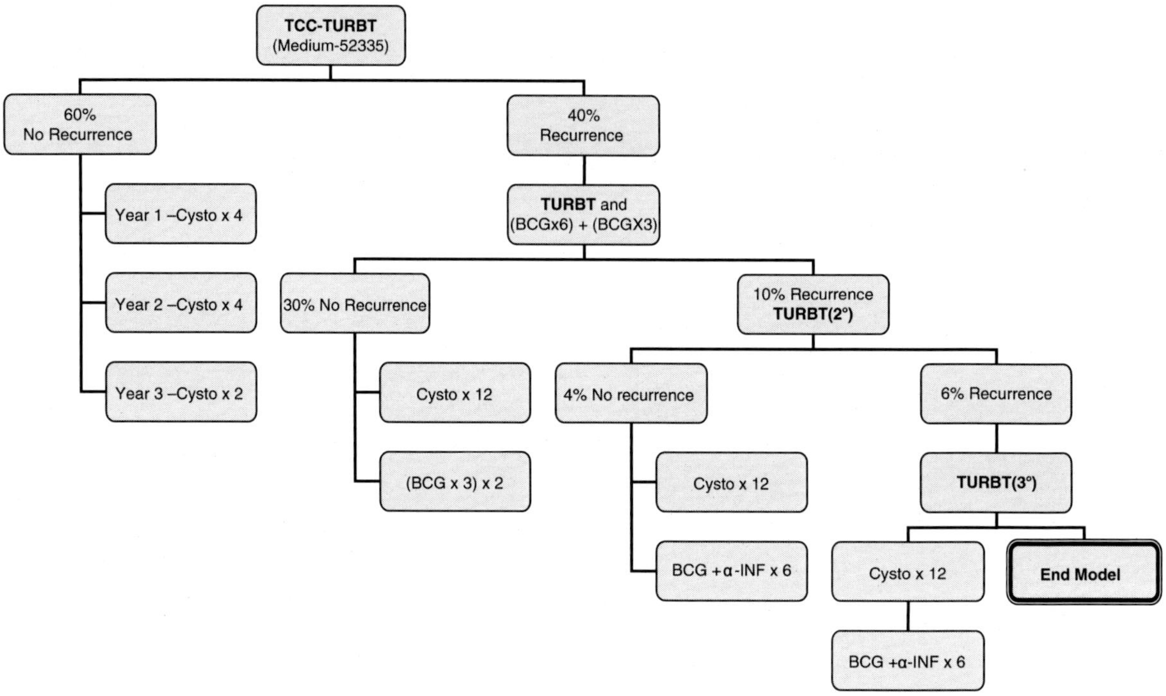

60%	30%	4%	6%
Cysto x 10	TURBT	TURBT x 2	TURBT x 3
	Cysto x 12	Cysto x 12	Cysto x 12
	BCG x 15	BCG x 9	BCG x 9
		BCG-αINF x 6	BCG-αINF x 6

FIG. 10.1. Algorithm for the treatment of superficial bladder cancer over a 3-year period

TABLE 10.6. Standard care for bladder cancer, over 3 year period.

	Costs, ($. USD)	No recurrence, (*n*)	One recurrence, (*n*)	Two recurrence, (*n*)	Three recurrences, (*n*)
Cystoscopy	196	12	12	12	12
TURB	1,595		1	2	3
BCG instillation	392		15	9	9
BCG and INF instillation	1,055			6	6
TURB with intravesical instillation	1,856				
Medication cost (Mitomycin C)	260				

effectiveness of an intravesical chemotherapeutic agent required to balance off the added costs of the medication and procedures to perform same-day intravesical instillation of chemotherapeutic agents compared to the standard TURBT. Using the utilization rates and population case-mix as above, we estimated that if no intravesical agent is used, it costs on average $5,760 to treat one patient with superficial bladder cancer, or $5,760,090 per 1,000 patients (Table 10.7). If all patients were to receive an intravesical chemotherapeutic agent, the average per patient cost of 3 years of care goes down to $5,070. We estimated cost savings

TABLE 10.7. Average 3-year cost of treating recurrent bladder cancer (for a cohort of 1,000 bladder cancer patients).

	No recurrence	One recurrence	Two recurrence	Three recurrences
Percentage of patients, without intravesical instillation	60	30	4	6
Costs ($)	11,764	29,480	6,160	10,197
Average ($)	5,760			
Percentage of patients, after intravesical instillation (with 25% efficacy)	70	22.5	3	4.5
Cost ($)	13,985	22,370	4,880	7,908
Average ($)	5,070			

After intravesical instillation there is a decrease in recurrence by 25%

of $689 (12%) per patient treated with chemotherapy agent after TURBT compared with those who did not receive same day intravesical therapy. Nationally, this would reflect a $24.8 million in saved resources. Moreover our threshold analysis demonstrated that the addition of a chemotherapy instillation after TURB has to improve outcomes (e.g., reduce the rate of cancer recurrence) by at least 7% to cover the additional cost of medical services and medication. It should be noted that these estimates are extremely conservative in that we assumed no progression to muscle invasive disease, cystectomy, or death from bladder cancer, and a low reduction in the rate of tumor recurrence (by only 25%).

2. Conclusion

In review of this topic we feel that there is ample evidence to show that immediate intravesical instillation with mitomycin C and several other agents can prevent (and/or delay the time of recurrence) of bladder cancer. Despite wide acceptance of same day intravesical instillation of chemotherapy after TURB by many practitioners outside the United States, this policy has not been widely embraced by American urologists and unlike the European Association for Urology, the AUA has not considered this therapy as standard of care in its present guidelines. Reasons for this policy not being incorporated into standard practice including barriers to its acceptance and performance, are unclear. It is possible that an American study showing its efficacy will popularize this approach and increase acceptance. Moreover, we have shown that assuming very conservative parameters for efficacy, adopting this policy would significantly lower the cost of care for bladder cancer in the United States.

References

1. Jemal A, Siegel R, Ward E et al. Cancer statistics, 2006. CA Cancer J Clin 2006; 56(2):106–130.
2. Madeb R, Messing EM. Gender, racial and age differences in bladder cancer incidence and mortality. Urol Oncol 2004; 22(2):86–92.
3. Messing EM. Urothelial tumors of the urinary tract. In: Walsh PC et al. editor. Campbell's Urology. Philadelphia: WB Saunders; 2002, pp. 2732–2784.
4. Malkowicz S. Management of Superficial Bladder Cancer. In: Walsh PC et al. editor. Campbell's Urology. Phildaelphia: WB Saunders; 2002, pp. 2785–2802.
5. Marshall VF. Symposium on bladder tumors: Current clinical problems regarding bladder tumors. Cancer 1956; 9:543–550.
6 Borhan A, Reeder JE, O'Connell MJ et al. Grade progression and regression in recurrent urothelial cancer. J Urol 2003; 169(6):2106–2109.
7. Oosterlinck W, Kurth KH, Schroder F, Bultinck J, Hammond B, Sylvester R. A prospective European Organization for Research and Treatment of Cancer Genitourinary Group randomized trial comparing transurethral resection followed by a single intravesical instillation of epirubicin or water in single stage Ta, T1 papillary carcinoma of the bladder. J Urol 1993; 149(4):749–752.
8. Shuin T, Kubota Y, Noguchi S et al. A phase II study of prophylactic intravesical chemotherapy with 4ć-epirubicin in recurrent superficial bladder cancer: comparison of 4ć-epirubicin and adriamycin. Cancer Chemother Pharmacol 1994; 35 Suppl:S52–S56.
9. Klan R, Loy V, Huland H. Residual tumor discovered in routine second transurethral resection in patients with stage T1 transitional cell carcinoma of the bladder. J Urol 1991; 146(2):316–318.
10. Solsona E, Iborra I, Ricos JV, Monros JL, Casanova J, Dumont R. Effectiveness of a single immediate mitomycin C instillation in patients with low risk superficial bladder cancer: short and long-term followup. J Urol 1999; 161(4):1120–1123.
11. Beer E. Removal of neoplasms of the urinary bladder: a new method employing high frequency (Oudin) currents through a catheterizing cystoscope. JAMA 1910; 54:1768–1769.
12. Beer E. Tumors of the Urinary Bladder. Baltimore: William Wood; 1935.

13. Bransford Lewis. AUA Histroy of Urology. McAllen, Texas: Wilkins and Wilkins; 1933.
14. Chinegwundoh F. The Early Surgical Histroy of Bladder Cancer. In: Mattelaer J, editor. de Historia Urologiae Europaeae, 4 ed. Belgium: European Association of Urology; 1997, pp. 163–174.
15. Hinman F. The Principles and Practice of Urology, 1st ed. Philadelphia: W.B. Saunders; 1937.
16. Young HH, Davis D. Young's Practice of Urology, 1st ed. Philadelphia: W.B. Saunders; 1926.
17. Heney NM. Natural history of superficial bladder cancer. Prognostic features and long-term disease course. Urol Clin North Am 1992; 19(3):429–433.
18. Herr HW. Intravesical therapy. A critical review. Urol Clin North Am 1987; 14(2):399–404.
19. Herr HW, Badalament RA, Amato DA, Laudone VP, Fair WR, Whitmore WF, Jr. Superficial bladder cancer treated with bacillus Calmette-Guerin: a multivariate analysis of factors affecting tumor progression. J Urol 1989; 141(1):22–29.
20. Herr HW, Wartinger DD, Fair WR, Oettgen HF. Bacillus Calmette-Guerin therapy for superficial bladder cancer: a 10-year followup. J Urol 1992; 147(4):1020–1023.
21. Herr HW. Natural history of superficial bladder tumors: 10- to 20-year follow-up of treated patients. World J Urol 1997; 15(2):84–88.
22. Lamm DL, Blumenstein BA, Crawford ED et al. Randomized intergroup comparison of bacillus calmette-guerin immunotherapy and mitomycin C chemotherapy prophylaxis in superficial transitional cell carcinoma of the bladder. Urol Oncol 1995; 1:119–126.
23. Lamm DL. Long-term results of intravesical therapy for superficial bladder cancer. Urol Clin North Am 1992; 19(3):573–580.
24. Lamm DL. Bladder cancer: twenty years of progress and the challenges that remain. CA Cancer J Clin 1998; 48(5):263–268.
25. Lamm DL, Blumenstein BA, Crissman JD et al. Maintenance bacillus Calmette-Guerin immunotherapy for recurrent TA, T1 and carcinoma in situ transitional cell carcinoma of the bladder: a randomized Southwest Oncology Group Study. J Urol 2000; 163(4):1124–1129.
26. Lamm DL. Management of bladder cancer. J Urol 2004; 171(6 Pt 1):2482–2483.
27. Messing E, Kim KM, Sharkey F et al. Randomized prospective phase III trial of difluoromethylornithine vs placebo in preventing recurrence of completely resected low risk superficial bladder cancer. J Urol 2006; 176(2):500–504.
28. See WA, Miller JS, Williams RD. Pathophysiology of transitional tumor cell adherence to sites of urothelial injury in rats: mechanisms mediating intravesical recurrence due to implantation. Cancer Res 1989; 49(19):5414–5418.
29. See WA, Chapman PH, Williams RD. Kinetics of transitional tumor cell line 4909 adherence to injured urothelial surfaces in F-344 rats. Cancer Res 1990; 50(8):2499–2504.
30. See WA, Crist SA, Williams RD. Single-dose cyclophosphamide for the prevention of bladder tumor implantation in F344 rats: site of drug activity. Cancer Res 1991; 51(5):1378–1383.
31. See WA, Crist SA, Boileau MA, Williams RD. Single-dose preoperative systemic cyclophosphamide for the prevention of bladder tumor implantation in F344 rats. Cancer Res 1991; 51(5):1373–1377.
32. See WA. Intravesical recombinant tissue plasminogen activator for the prevention of implantation-mediated bladder tumor recurrence. Clin Exp Metastasis 1992; 10(2):99–109.
33. The effect of intravesical thiotepa on the recurrence rate of newly diagnosed superficial bladder cancer. An MRC Study. MRC Working Party on Urological Cancer. Br J Urol 1985; 57(6):680–685.
34. The effect of intravesical thiotepa on tumour recurrence after endoscopic treatment of newly diagnosed superficial bladder cancer. A further report with long-term follow-up of a Medical Research Council randomized trial. Medical Research Council Working Party on Urological Cancer, Subgroup on Superficial Bladder Cancer. Br J Urol 1994; 73(6):632–638.
35. Ali-El-Dein B, Nabeeh A, el-Baz M, Shamaa S, Ashamallah A. Single-dose versus multiple instillations of epirubicin as prophylaxis for recurrence after transurethral resection of pTa and pT1 transitional-cell bladder tumours: a prospective, randomized controlled study. Br J Urol 1997; 79(5):731–735.
36. Rajala P, Liukkonen T, Raitanen M et al. Transurethral resection with perioperative instilation on interferon-alpha or epirubicin for the prophylaxis of recurrent primary superficial bladder cancer: a prospective randomized multicenter study–Finnbladder III. J Urol 1999; 161(4):1133–1135.
37. Sylvester RJ, Oosterlinck W, van der Meijden AP. A single immediate postoperative instillation of chemotherapy decreases the risk of recurrence in patients with stage Ta T1 bladder cancer: a meta-analysis of published results of randomized clinical trials. J Urol 2004; 171(6 Pt 1):2186–90, quiz.
38. Tolley DA, Parmar MK, Grigor KM et al. The effect of intravesical mitomycin C on recurrence of newly diagnosed superficial bladder cancer: a further report with 7 years of follow up. J Urol 1996; 155(4):1233–1238.
39. Zincke H, Utz DC, Taylor WF, Myers RP, Leary FJ. Influence of thiotepa and doxorubicin instillation at time of transurethral surgical treatment of bladder cancer on tumor recurrence: a prospective, randomized, double-blind, controlled trial. J Urol 1983; 129(3):505–509.
40. Zincke H, Benson RC, Jr., Hilton JF, Taylor WF. Intravesical thiotepa and mitomycin C treatment immediately after transurethral resection and later for superficial (stages Ta and Tis) bladder cancer: a prospective, randomized, stratified study with crossover design. J Urol 1985; 134(6):1110–1114.
41. Lamm DL. Intravesical therapy for superficial bladder cancer: slow but steady progress. J Clin Oncol 2003; 21(23):4259–4260.
42. Burnand KG, Boyd PJ, Mayo ME, Shuttleworth KE, Lloyd-Davies RW. Single dose intravesical thiotepa as an adjuvant to cystodiathermy in the treatment of transitional cell bladder carcinoma. Br J Urol 1976; 48(1):55–59.
43. Herr HW, Donat SM, Dalbagni G. Correlation of cystoscopy with histology of recurrent papillary tumors of the bladder. J Urol 2002; 168(3):978–980.
44. Smith JA, Jr., Labasky RF, Cockett AT, Fracchia JA, Montie JE, Rowland RG. Bladder cancer clinical guidelines panel summary report on the management of nonmuscle invasive bladder cancer (stages Ta, T1 and TIS). The American Urological Association. J Urol 1999; 162(5):1697–1701.
45. Oosterlinck W, Lobel B, Jakse G, Malmstrom PU, Stockle M, Sternberg C. Guidelines on bladder cancer. Eur Urol 2002; 41(2):105–112.
46. Oosterlinck W, Lobel B, Jackse G, Malmstrom PU, Stockle M, Strenberg C. [EAU Recommendations 2001. "Guidelines on bladder cancer"]. Prog Urol 2002; 12(5):1161–1163.
47. Oosterlinck W. Guidelines on diagnosis and treatment of superficial bladder cancer. Minerva Urol Nefrol 2004; 56(1):65–72.

48. Madeb R, Golijanin D, Noyes K, et al. Utilization and cost-effectiveness of same day intravesical chemotherapeutic instillation following transurethral resection of newly diagnosed bladder cancer. J Urol 175[4], 13. 2006.
49. Briesacher B, Kamal-Bahl S, Hochberg M, Orwig D, Kahler KH. Three-tiered-copayment drug coverage and use of non-steroidal anti-inflammatory drugs. Arch Intern Med 2004; 164(15):1679–1684.
50. Chang S, Long SR, Kutikova L et al. Estimating the cost of cancer: results on the basis of claims data analyses for cancer patients diagnosed with seven types of cancer during 1999 to 2000. J Clin Oncol 2004; 22(17):3524–3530.
51. Cohen FJ, Neslusan CA, Conklin JE, Song X. Recent anti-hyperglycemic prescribing trends for US privately insured patients with type 2 diabetes. Diabetes Care 2003; 26(6):1847–1851.
52. Hillman AL, Schwartz JS, Willian MK et al. The cost-effectiveness of terazosin and placebo in the treatment of moderate to severe benign prostatic hyperplasia. Urology 1996; 47(2):169–178.
53. Lyman GH, Berndt ER, Kallich JD et al. The economic burden of anemia in cancer patients receiving chemotherapy. Value Health 2005; 8(2):149–156.
54. Ozminkowski RJ, Marder WD, Hawkins K et al. The use of disease-modifying new drugs for multiple sclerosis treatment in private-sector health plans. Clin Ther 2004; 26(8):1341–1354.
55. Lamm DL. Efficacy and safety of bacille Calmette-Guerin immunotherapy in superficial bladder cancer. Clin Infect Dis 2000; 31 Suppl 3:S86–S90.
56. Kamat AM, Lamm DL. Intravesical therapy for bladder cancer. Urology 2000; 55(2):161–168.
57. Young MJ, Soloway MS. Office evaluation and management of bladder neoplasms. Urol Clin North Am 1998; 25(4):603–611.
58. Kamat AM, Lamm DL. Intravesical therapy for bladder cancer. Urology 2000; 55(2):161–168.
59. Sylvester RJ, van der MEIJDEN AP, Lamm DL. Intravesical bacillus Calmette-Guerin reduces the risk of progression in patients with superficial bladder cancer: a meta-analysis of the published results of randomized clinical trials. J Urol 2002; 168(5):1964–1970.

11
BCG Refractory Disease

Tara Allen and Graham F. Greene

Contents

Abstract For the last 30 years, we have depended upon Bacillus Calmette-Guerin (BCG) therapy to reduce the recurrence of non invasive urothelial carcinoma of the bladder and prevent the progression to muscle invasive disease. Since Morales first reported the efficacy of BCG in 1976, no other form of systemic or intravesical therapy has produced comparable response rates especially with carcinoma in-situ or high grade disease (1, 2). Our confidence in this proven treatment is humbled by the fact that we lack the ability to identify those tumors which will be unresponsive to BCG and express a malignant phenotype for invasion and metastasis. While most patients with noninvasive urothelial tumors can preserve their bladders, a delay in cystectomy for some may put them at risk of developing incurable metastatic disease. In this chapter we will attempt to define BCG refractory disease, identify the risks with salvage therapy, report on biological markers of progression, introduce new therapies and suggest a treatment algorithm for approaching urothelial carcinomas that fail BCG therapy.

Keywords Bladder neoplasm, BCG failure, Risk, Intravesical, Cystectomy

1. Introduction

Urothelial carcinoma of the bladder is the second most common urologic malignancy. It affects an estimated 600,000 Americans and will claim the lives of nearly 15,000 men and women in 2006. Bladder cancer is the fourth most common cancer diagnosed and the eighth most common cause of cancer related deaths in men. Women are less affected then men (male to female incidence ratio of 3:1) and have better survival (male to female mortality ratio of 2:1). The lifetime risk of bladder cancer in Caucasians is twice that found in African Americans. Two thirds of patients present after the age of 65 with rare occurrences seen in patients younger than age 35. Younger patients tend to have low grade disease (3). The etiology of bladder cancer is multi-factorial with the strongest associated risk being cigarette smoking. Cigarette smokers increase their lifetime risk for bladder cancer two to three times that of nonsmokers (4, 5). While the exact mechanism of carcinogenesis due to cigarette smoking is unknown 4-amino biphenyl, acrolien and oxygen free radicals have been implicated in the literature (6). The impact of smoking cessation on tumor recurrence and progression

From: *Current Clinical Urology: Bladder Cancer,* Edited by: C.T. Lee and D.P. Wood,
DOI: 10.1007/978-1-59745-417-9_11,

TABLE 11.1. Risk factors for tumor recurrence and progression.

Tumor size > 3 cm
Multifocality
Sessile or solid shape
Stage T1
High grade histology
Carcinoma in situ
Urothelial cancer in the upper tracts or prostate

and whether it interferes with BCG therapy remains unknown (7–9).

Seventy to 80% of those patients presenting with urothelial carcinoma of the bladder will have non-muscle invasive disease. Within 5 years, 50–70% will experience recurrences and 15–20% progress to muscle invasive disease (10). It is important to obtain complete tumor resection with muscularis propria in the specimen for accurate staging. If there is no muscle in the specimen or there is ambiguity over whether the few smooth muscle cells seen are of the muscularis mucosa or muscularis propria, repeat resection is mandatory. Repeat resection has demonstrated residual tumor as high as 75% (11). At presentation 1/3 of patients will exhibit features known to be associated with increased risk of recurrence and progression (Table 11.1). These features have formed the basis for individualized treatment strategies.

The goals of intravesical therapies have been threefold: first, to decrease tumor recurrences due to implantation or affecting field change within the urothelial cells, second to augment transurethral resection, and third to prevent muscle invasion. When compared to intravesical chemotherapies, only intravesical BCG has been shown to reduce tumor progression from superficial to muscle invasive disease. BCG therapy remains the standard initial treatment for preventing both recurrence and progression in newly diagnosed noninvasive bladder cancer, especially carcinoma in situ, with response rates of 60–70%. An induction cycle of BCG involves 6 weekly intravesical instillations (12). Interruption of these treatments in absence of significant toxicity may compromise an optimal immune response. The addition of subcutaneous BCG administration has not been shown to improve response rates (13, 14). Of the various strains of BCG available, none have been proven better than the other.

Fifty percent of patients receiving BCG therapy will experience recurrence or progression at 5 years with only 30% achieving long term disease free status (15). Half of those patients that have recurrence after the first induction cycle of BCG will respond to a second course (16). Maintenance BCG therapy consisting of 3 weekly instillations at 3 months post induction cycle and every 6 months thereafter up to 3 years has improved response rates at the expense of increased toxicity and decreased compliance (17). Salvage intravesical therapies yield variable and inconsistent response rates of around 20% (18). While attempting to achieve disease free status with intravesical BCG therapy it is important to recognize its limitations and signs of nonresponsiveness as not to expose the patient to muscle invasive and potentially incurable metastatic disease (19–21).

2. BCG Failure

The term BCG failure implies that the patients' exposure to BCG therapy has failed in preventing tumor recurrence or progression to invasive disease. Within the literature, the terms BCG failure and BCG refractory disease lack clear definition. One interpretation is that BCG failure refers to any tumor recurrence after the initial induction cycle of BCG and that BCG refractory disease refers to tumor recurrence after two cycles of BCG or while on maintenance treatments. This ambiguity may be due to a number of factors including inconsistent reporting methods, combinations of patients receiving one or two induction cycles, mixing of various risk groups and lack of reporting time to disease recurrence. Regardless of the terminology the clinician has the responsibility to individualize each patient's treatment regimen and decide when the therapy has lost it benefit.

Some of the proposed mechanisms for tumor recurrence after BCG therapy are listed in Table 11.2. While BCG has achieved its best results with carcinoma in situ, it does not perform as well when used for cytoreduction for residual papillary or T1 disease. Complete resection of tumor is an important therapeutic goal prior to intravesical BCG. Residual tumor has been implicated for high recurrence rates. Herr reported a residual tumor rate of 75% in 96 patients undergoing a repeat resection for Ta, Tis

TABLE 11.2. Potential causes of tumor recurrence after BCG treatment.

Incomplete resection
Understaging
Tumor implantation
Extravesical disease in prostate or upper tracts
Inadequate exposure to BCG
Inability to maintain an immune response

or T1 with 29% being upstaged to invasive disease (11). Divrik et al. suggested that high tumor grade was the strongest predictor of residual tumor on second transurethral resection (22). Prostatic urethral involvement with bladder carcinoma in situ has been reported to be as high as 60% (23). Abnormal urine cytology after apparent tumor control within the bladder may indicate unrecognized carcinoma within the bladder or somewhere else within the urinary tract warranting evaluation of the upper tracts, prostate urethra and re-resection of tumor base (24).

The dosing schedule of 6 weekly instillations of BCG as an induction cycle has proven its efficacy in the literature. Attempts to prolong the regimen to 8 weeks by Talic et al. did not improve complete response rates beyond 70%, and more than one fourth of patients did not complete all treatments due to severe bladder irritability (25). Sarosdy and Lamm evaluated 120 patients over 5 years and noted that initial response rates of 79% could be increased to 89% after retreatment of early failures, suggesting that a single induction cycle may be inadequate for some patients (26). A randomized prospective trial by the South West Oncology Group comparing of a single induction cycle to an induction cycle followed by 3 weekly instillations at 3 months in 150 patients reported an improvement in response rates from 56 to 82% (27). Another trial by the South West Oncology Group evaluating the benefits of an aggressive maintenance program involving a total of 27 treatments of BCG did in fact produce an excellent response rate of 83%, yet only 16% of patients were able to tolerate an entire course (17). Urinary cytokine data would suggest the immune response elicited by an induction cycle peeks at 6 weeks and lasts for approximately 6 months (28, 29). These studies lend support for additional treatments beyond an induction cycle of a single 3 week treatment at 3 months in responders and a full 6 week reinduction cycle for patients with tumor recurrences. The benefits of maintenance therapy and the optimal regimen remain undefined.

The time from the induction cycle of BCG till tumor recurrence has helped define the biology of the urothelial carcinoma. Early failures, defined as tumors that recur within 6 months are at high risk of failing salvage intravesical therapy and usually go on to radical cystectomy as compared to those late failures in which retreatment with BCG can incite an adequate immune and clinical response (30). A clinical concern in delaying cystectomy for early failures is the potential for unrecognized invasion and metastasis which ultimately impacts on survival. Catalona et al. reported that the risk of invasion and metastasis, after one failed induction cycle of BCG, was 11 and 14% respectively. After two or more cycles of BCG therapy the rates of invasion and metastatsis increased to 30 and 50% respectively (31). In a series of 90 patients followed up to 20 years, Herr and Sogani reported an improvement in survival with early cystectomy for either superficial (92 vs. 56%) or invasive disease (54 vs. 36%) after failed BCG therapy (32). The majority of cancer related deaths are associated with high risk disease of which the worst combination is high grade T1 with multi-focal carcinoma in situ. It is not unreasonable to offer these patients radical cystectomy without a trial of BCG. For those patients that have persistent T1 or progress to T1 disease after one cycle of BCG, radical cystectomy is recommended (33).

TABLE 11.3. Definition of BCG refractory disease.

Recurrence within 6 months
Recurrence after two cycles of BCG
Recurrence while on maintenance therapy
Recurrence after one cycle BCG with T1 tumor

In summary, the most compelling definition of BCG failure would include those tumor recurrences within 6 months of an initial complete response, recurrence after two courses of BCG therapy, recurrent disease while on maintenance therapy, and recurrent T1 tumor after one course of BCG (Table 11.3).

3. Risk Stratification

There is a broad spectrum of malignant potential in noninvasive urothelial carcinomas ranging from a single small papillary TA, low grade tumor with less than 10% lifetime recurrence to carcinoma in situ presenting with occult metastatic disease. In 1983, Heney et al. reported on the natural history of bladder cancer in 249 patients after tumor resection without adjuvant therapy. They demonstrated that tumor stage, grade, multiplicity, and size influenced the risk of recurrence. Progression varied significantly between TA and T1, and Grades I, II and III: 4, 30, 2, 11, and 45% respectively (34). Although tumor grade is known to be an important prognostic factor pathologists have been inconsistent in distinguishing a papilloma from a Ta low grade tumor (papillary neoplasm of low malignant potential), and defining an intermediate grade between low and high grades. In 2004, the World Health Organization (WHO) and the International

TABLE 11.4. Risk stratification of noninvasive urothelial carcinomas.

Low risk	Solitary Ta tumor, low grade
	Papilloma
	Papillary neoplasm of low malignant potential
	Size ≤ 3 cm
Intermediate risk	Ta, high grade
	T1, low grade
	Multifocal tumors
	Size > 3 cm
High risk	T1, high grade
	Carcinoma in situ (CIS)
	T1 with CIS
	Recurrence within 6 months
	Recurrence on maintenance BCG therapy

Society of Urologic Pathologists (ISUP) agreed on a classification system that graded superficial urothelial carcinomas as either a papilloma, papillary neoplasm of low malignant potential, low grade tumor or high grade tumor (35).

Since being first described by Melicow in 1952, carcinoma in situ has been recognized for its aggressive and unpredictable nature (36). The average incidence of invasive disease associated with carcinoma in situ was reported by Lamm to be 54% in 349 patients. Overall the natural history of untreated superficial bladder cancer is associated with a 3 year recurrence rate of 35–40% in low risk disease and 70–80% in high risk disease, with an average 10% progression rate to muscle invasive disease (37, 38). These results have helped to identify the risk factors useful in establishing the risk groups for patients listed in Table 11.4.

Risk adapted therapy is important to consider when individualizing treatment regimens. Millan-Rodríguez et al., identified risk groups for recurrence, progression and mortality in 1,529 patients. Recurrence was influenced by tumor size, multiplicity, BCG exposure, and presence of CIS. Tumor grade was the main predictor of progression and survival. The rates of recurrence, progression, and mortality were 37, 0, and 0% in the low-risk group; 45, 1.8, 0.73% in the intermediate group; and 54, 15 and 9.5% in the high-risk group respectively (39). The incorporation of intravesical therapies has influenced the natural history of bladder cancer requiring the addition of treatment failure and time to recurrence or progression as prognostic factors. Scientists are actively seeking biological markers either secreted in the urine or expressed in urothelial cells that will help predict response to therapy and indicate a change in the malignant potential within urothelium before it is detected by conventional means (40).

4. Markers of Progression

Mapping of the human genome along with advances in genomics and proteomics has allowed scientists to explore the process of urothelial oncogenesis. As in most cancers, bladder cancer is a multi step process involving alterations in growth regulation, programmed cell death, angiogenesis, cell adhesion and DNA repair. Certain defects can be seen in early bladder cancer and others later, while some are expressed throughout the disease. By understanding the genetic profile of a patient's tumor and its altered metabolic pathways, we hope to better predict the tumor phenotype and individually tailor their therapy.

The most common chromosomal abnormalities seen in bladder cancer involve chromosomes 9, 17 and 13. Sixty to sixty-five percent of urothelial tumors have loss of heterozygosity (LOH) on chromosome 9 with the majority of deletions occurring at 9p21 locus where three suppressor genes (INK4a/ARF and INK4b) encode for negative cell cycle regulatory proteins $p16^{INK4A}$, $p14^{ARF}$ and $p15^{INK4B}$. These alterations are found exclusively in early disease and carry a favorable prognosis. In contrast, the allelic loss or mutation on 17p13 which is the locus of the well known *p53* suppressor gene is associated with high grade tumors, CIS and more aggressive tumor behavior (41). One third of bladder tumors will have Rb gene mutations on chromosome 13q which encodes for cell cycle regulatory Rb protein. Loss of pRb function has been implicated in bladder cancer progression (42).

Normal genes can react to various genetic insults to become oncogenes which over express normal protein or produce aberrant protein. The two most implicated in bladder cancer are cH-*ras* and HER2/*neu*. Fontana et al. suggested that in the absence of p53, the over expression of cH-*ras* was correlated with early recurrence in superficial bladder cancer (42). HER2/*neu* encodes a transmembrane glycoprotein that stimulates cell growth through the tyrosine kinase pathway. Over expression of HER2/*neu* has been reported with higher grade tumor, metastasis and reduced overall survival. While these conclusions remain controversial in bladder cancer we await the results of targeted therapies towards HER2/*neu* over expression in other cancers (43).

In order for malignant cells to metastasize they need to loosen their cell–cell attachments, dissolve extracellular matrix and access new tumor vessels. The cadherin family of molecules helps anchor cells to their basement membrane and each other. Reduced expression of E-cadherin has been associated with an aggressive phenotype of bladder cancer (44). CD44, another cell surface adhesion molecule has been shown to have increased expression in superficial disease with decreased expression at the time of invasion (45). Metalloproteinases (MMP-2, MMP-9) are enzymes that degrade extracellular matrix and have been found to have elevated levels in serum and urine of patients with invasive bladder cancer (46). Vascular endothelial growth factor (VEGF) and basic fibroblast growth factor (bFGF) are the most relevant angiogenic factors in bladder cancer that in turn are inhibited by thrombospondin-1 (TSP-1). This potent inhibitor of angiogenesis requires transcriptional activation by p53. Low TSP-1 expression has been associated with higher recurrence rates and reduced overall survival in patients with invasive bladder cancer (47).

As we search for the molecular phenotypes of early superficial urothelial tumors that progress to invasive disease, we must also look for expression profiles that help select effective therapies for patients and evaluate treatment response. In the area of muscle invasive bladder cancer, Cote et al. have initiated a large multi-institutional trial comparing the progression free survival of patients with p53 alterations following cystectomy randomized to MVAC chemotherapy or observation (48). Currently, there have been no studies which have identified reliable predictive markers for treatment response with intravesical BCG therapy for noninvasive bladder cancer. Soon it should be possible for us to better define BCG failure and guide patients either to cystectomy or to a salvage bladder preserving regimen.

5. Treatment of BCG Failure

The standard treatment of BCG-refractory bladder cancer is cystectomy. The uncertainty of recognizing treatment failures and delaying radical cystectomy threatens to compromise on patient survival. Better patient selection through risk stratification and identifying markers of treatment failure will help select those most suitable for bladder preservation. The search continues for therapeutic agents or combinations of therapies that will improve upon the treatment response rates achieved with BCG therapy. Many common daily medications such as mega-dose vitamins, oral antibiotics and anti-inflammatory COX-2 inhibitors have been suggested to augment BCG response; yet await confirmation in clinical trials (49–51). Currently, the most promising agents include gemcitabine, docetaxel, valrubicin, interferon and photodynamic therapy. These will be briefly discussed here, with gemcitabine and docexatel being reviewed in more detail in subsequent chapters.

The role of immediate postresection intravesical chemotherapy instillation and sequential maintenance therapy alternating with BCG has been evaluated using the antibiotic mitomycin (52). Encouraged by a European trial that demonstrated the efficacy of another antibiotic epirubicin given as a single dose post tumor resection, mitomycin has likewise been evaluated by many groups and has been found to decrease recurrence rates in Ta and T1 cancers (53–57). When mitomycin was evaluated in sequential therapy with BCG, recurrence-free and progression-free survival was found to be inferior to BCG treatment alone (58). Interest has turned toward agents with improved efficacy in the salvage setting after failed BCG therapy.

Valrubicin, an analogue of adriamycin, is the only agent that has received FDA approval for use in patients with recurrent CIS after BCG therapy or refusal of cystectomy. A phase II trial by Steinberg et al. evaluated the efficacy of 800 mg of valrubicin given weekly for 6 weeks in 90 patients with CIS after multiple intravesical therapies including at least one cycle of BCG. They reported a 21% complete response rate at 6 months with most patients experiencing mild to moderate symptoms of urgency and frequency and no undue risk in survival in those patients that went on to cystectomy (59). A cost analysis for administering valrubicn in these 90 patients was performed and reported a 6 week course of valrubicin was six times as expensive as an induction cycle of BCG. Valrubicin has been shown to be safe and well tolerated when given post resection with negligible systemic absorption (60). Its expense and availability have limited its use.

Gemcitabine is a deoxycytidine analogue that interferes with DNA synthesis and possesses a broad spectrum of antitumor activity. A randomized phase III trial of metastatic bladder cancer patients treated with gemcitabine and cisplatin demonstrated similar survival rates with less toxicity when compared to standard MVAC chemotherapy (61). Its success in treating advanced urothelial cancer as well as its safety profile has lead to gemcitabine being evaluated as an intravesical agent. Phase I studies have confirmed the safety of intravesical gemcitabine at a dose of 2 gm twice weekly for 6 weeks (62–64). Dalbagni et al. reported their results of salvage gemcitabine therapy in 30 patients with BCG-refractory disease. Fifteen patients did not respond. Twelve patients recurred with a median freedom from recurrence of 3.6 months (65). Further trials will define the durability of responses and the roles of perioperative and maintenance therapy with gemcitabine (66). Docetaxal is another chemotherapeutic agent that has demonstrated efficacy in metastatic urothelial cancer and which is now being applied to superficial disease. Intrasvesical administration of docetaxel of up to 75 mg weekly for 6 weeks has been shown to be tolerable (67). Early results suggest favorable response rates in BCG refractory disease, yet they require future verification in phase II studies.

Interferons are glycoproteins that mediate immune responses and have antiproliferative and antiangiogenic properties. Intravesical IFN-α has demonstrated efficacy and safety both alone and in combination with low dose BCG for the treatment of noninvasive bladder cancer (68). In a series of 490 patients with intermediate risk disease, O'Donnell et al. reported a 42% response rate in BCG refractory patients treated with low-dose BCG and INF-α. and an associated reduction in BCG toxicity of 50% (69). Other series have suggested that two thirds of these patients will have a durable response of at least 1 year (70, 71). All this comes at a price, for INF-α therapy can cost over ten times that of an induction cycle of BCG (59). The role of maintenance therapy with low dose BCG and IFN-α in treating high risk disease is unclear.

Photodynamic therapy (PDT) of urothelial carcinomas includes the administration of a photosensitizing agent and its subsequent activation with light of the appropriate wave length. It has potential not only in treatment of noninvasive disease but also in identifying occult disease at surveillance (72, 73). Porfimer

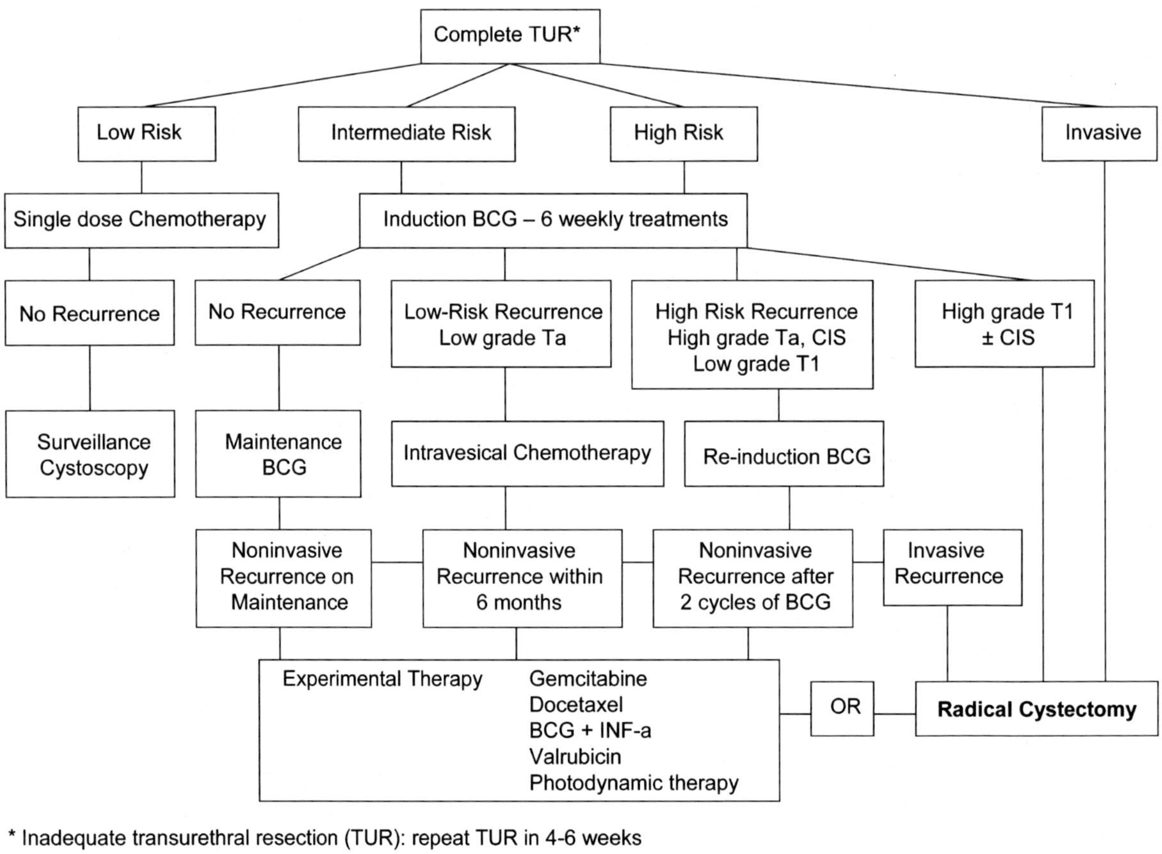

FIG. 11.1. Algorithm for treating noninvasive urothelial carcinoma of the bladder

sodium and 5-aminolevulinic acid (5-ALA) are the most common photo-sensitizers being evaluated. The wavelength of the activating light has variable depth of penetration and resultant injury to the muscle fibers. Severe irritative bladder symptoms and bladder contracture are potential outcomes with this therapy. Manyak and Ogan reported on 34 patients with BCG refractory disease treated with PDT. The complete response rate at 3 months was 44% with a mean time to recurrence in responders of 9.8 months. With a mean follow up of 52 months, 68% of the 22 surviving patients of were alive with their bladders intact, with no evidence of disease in nine and superficial disease only in six (74). The ideal photo-sensitizer is yet to be found. The utility of PDT in upper tract and prostatic involvement is also being evaluated.

Conclusion

While BCG has served our patients well, we must continue to test new agents and search for those markers in urothelial carcinogenesis that will identify an invasive phenotype and predict for subsequent failure of intravesical therapy. A clear definition of BCG failure will help distinguish those patients most suitable for a radical cystectomy from patients in whom bladder preservation remains a possibility. Figure 11.1 illustrates our systematic approach to noninvasive bladder cancer. Advances in technology and the development of new intravesical chemotherapeutic agents will only increase our ability to offer patients effective salvage therapies and alternatives to BCG therapy.

References

1. Morales A, Eidinger D, Bruce AW. Intracavitary Bacillus Calmette-Guerin in the treatment of superficial bladder tumors. J Urol 1976;116:180–3.
2. Lamm DL. In F. Pagano and W. Fair (eds.), Carcinoma-in-situ. Superficial Bladder Cancer. Oxford: Isis Medical Media, 1997.
3. American Cancer Society. Cancer Facts and Figures 2006. Atlanta:American Cancer Society; 2006.
4. Ross RK, Jones PA, Yu MC. Bladder cancer epidemiology and pathogenesis. Semin Oncol 1996;23:536–545.
5. Wynder EL, Goldsmith R. The epidemiology of bladder cancer. A second look. Cancer 1977;40:1246–1268.
6. Lower GM, Jr. Concepts in causality: chemically induced human urinary bladder cancer. Cancer 1982;49:1056–1066.
7. Carpenter AA. Clinical experience with bladder cancer with special reference to smoking. J Urol 1989;141:527–528.
8. Thompson IM, Peek M, Rodriguez FR. The impact of cigarette smoking on stage, grade and number of recurrences of transitional cell carcinoma of the bladder. J Urol 1987;187:401–403.
9. Hartge P, Silverman D, Hoover R, et al. Changing cigarette habits and bladder cancer risk: A case controlled study. J Natl Cancer Inst 1987;78:1119–1125.
10. Heney NM. Natural History of superficial bladder cancer. Prognostic features and long-term disease course. Urol Clin North Am 1992;19:429–433.
11. Herr HW. The value of a second transurethral resection in evaluating patients with bladder tumors. J Urol 1999; 162:74–76.
12. Morales A, Nichol JC, Wilson JWL. Dose response of Bacillus Calmette-Guerin in the treatment of superficial bladder cancer. J Urol 1992;147:1256–1258.
13. Lamm DL, Dehaven JI, Shriver J, et al. Randomized prospective comparison of oral versus intravesical and percutaneous BCG for superficial bladder cancer. J Urol 1990;144:65–67.
14. Lüftenegger W, Ackermann DK, Futterlieb A, et al. Intravesical versus intravesical plus intradermal Bacillus Calmette-Guerin: a prospective randomized study in patients with recurrent superficial bladder tumors. J Urol 1996;155:483–487.
15. Herr HW, Schwalb DM, Zhang ZF, Sogani PC, Fair WR, Whitmore WF Jr., et al. Intravesical Bacillus Calmette-Guerin therapy prevents tumor progression and death from superficial bladder cancer: Ten-year follow-up of a prospective randomized trial. J Clin Oncol 1995;13:1404–1408.
16. Bretton PR, Herr HW, Kimmel M, et al. The response of patients with superficial bladder cancer to a second course of intravesical Bacillus Calmette-Guerin. J Urol 1990;143:710–713.
17. Lamm DL, Blumenstein B, Crissman JD, et al. Maintanance BCG immunotherapy for recurrent Ta, T1 and carcinoma in situ transitional cell carcinoma of the bladder: a randomized Southwest Oncology Group study. J Urol 2000;163:1124–1129.
18. Joudi FN, O'Donnell MA. Second-line intravesical therapy versus cystectomy for Bacilli Calmette-Guerin (BCG) failures. Curr Opin Urol 2004;14:271–275.
19. Hudson MA. When intravesical measures fail. Indications for cystectomy in superficial disease. Urol Clin North Am 1992;19:601–609.
20. Luciani LG, Neulander E, Murphy WM, et al. Risk of continued intravesical therapy and delayed cystectomy in BCG refractory superficial bladder: an investigational approach. Urology 2001;58:376–379.
21. Kim JC, Steinberg GD. The limits of bacillus Calmette-Guerin for carcinoma in situ of the bladder. J Urol 2001;165:745–756.
22. Divrik T, Yildirim U, Eroglu AS, et al. Is second transurethral resection necessary for newly diagnosed pT1 bladder cancer? J Urol 2006;175:1258–1261.
23. Schellhammer PF, Bean MA, Whitmore WF, Jr. Prostatic involvement by transitional cell carcinoma: pathogenesis, patterns and prognosis. J Urol 1977;118:399–403.
24. Solsona E, Iborra I, Ricos JV, et al. Extravesical involvement in patients with bladder carcinoma in situ: biological and therapeutic implications. J Urol 1996;895–899.
25. Talic RF, Hargreave TB, Bishop MC, et al. Intravesical Evans bacille Calmette-Guerin for carcinoma in situ of the urinary bladder. Br J Urol 1994;73:645–648.

26. Sarosdy MF, Lamm DL. Long-term results of intravesical bacillus Calmete-Guerin therapy for superificial bladder cancer. J Urol 1989;142:719–722.
27. Lamm DL, Crawford ED, Blumenstein B, et al. Maintanance BCG immunotherapy of superficial bladder cancer: a randomized prospective Southwest Oncology Group study. J Urol Suppl 1992; 147:274A, abstract 242.
28. DeBoer EC, De Jong WH, Steerenberg PA, et al. Induction of urinary IL1, IL2, IL6, and TNF during intravesical immunotherapy with BCG in superficial bladder cancer. Cancer Immunol Immunother 1991;33:306–312.
29. Prescott S, James K, Hargreave TB, et al. Immunopathological effects of intravesical BCG therapy. Prog Clin Biol Res 1989;310:93–105.
30. Herr HW and Dalbagni G. Defining bacillus Calmette-Guerin refractory superficial bladder tumors. J Urol 2003;169:1706–1708.
31. Catalona WJ, Hudson MA, Gillen DP, Andriole GL, Ratliff TL. Risks and benefits of repeated courses of intravesical bacillus Calmette-Guerin therapy for superficial bladder cancer. J Urol 1987;187:220–204.
32. Herr HW, Sogani PC. Does early cystectomy improve the survival of patients with high risk superficial bladder tumors. J Urol 2001;166:1296–1299.
33. Herr HW, Jakse G, Sheinfeld J. The T1 bladder tumor. Semin Urol 1990;8:254–261.
34. Heney NM, Ahmed S, Flanagan MJ, et al. Superficial bladder cancer: progression and recurrence. J Urol 1983;130: 1083–1086.
35. Reuter VE. The pathology of bladder cancer.Urology 2006;67(suppl 3a):11–17; discussion 17–18.
36. Melicow MM, Hollowell JW. Intraurothelial cancer:carcinoma in situ, Bowen's disease of urinary system: discussion of 30 cases.J Urol 1952;68:763–773.
37. Lamm DL. Carcinoma in situ. Urol Clin North Am 1992;19:499–508.
38. Schrier BPH, Hollander MP, van Rhijn BWG, et al. Prognosis of muscle invasive bladder cancer: difference between primary and progressive tumors: possible implications for therapy. Eur Urol2004;45:292–296.
39. Millan-Rodriguez F, Chechile-Toniolo G, Salvador-Bayarri J, et al. Primary superficial bladder cancer risk groups according to progression, mortality and recurrence.J Urol 2000;164:680–684.
40. Grossman BH, Blute ML,Dinney CPN, et al. The use of urine-based biomarkers in bladder cancer. Urol 2006;67 (suppl 3a):62–64.
41. Buscarini M, Quek ML,Gill P, et al. Molecular prognostic factors in bladder cancer. BJU Int 2005;95:739–742.
42. Grossman HB, Liebert M, Antelo M, et al. p53 and RB expression predict progression in T1 bladder cancer. Clin Cancer Res 1998;4:829–834.
43. Sato K, Moriyama M, Mori S, et al. An immunohistologic evaluation of C-erbB-2 gene product in patients with urinary bladder cancer. Cancer 1992;70:2493–2498.
44. Shariat SF, Pahlavan S, Baseman AG, et al. E-cadherin expression predicts clinical outcome in carcinoma in situ of the urinary bladder. Urol 2001;57:60–65.
45. Miyake H, Eto H, Arakawa S, et al. Over expression of CD44V8-10 in urinary exfoliated cells as an independent prognostic predictor in patients with urothelial cancer. J Urol 2002;167:1282–1287.
46. Gohji K, Fujimoto N, Ohkawa J, et al. Imbalannce between serum matrix metalloproteinase-2 and its inhibitor as a predictor of recurrence of urothelial cancer. Br J Cabcer 1998;77:650–655.
47. Grossfeld GD, Ginsberg DA, Stein JP, et al. Thrombospondin-1 expression in bladder cancer: association with p53 alterations, tumor angiogenesis, and tumor progression. J Natl Cancer Inst 1997;89:219–227.
48. Cote RJ, Lerner SP, Datar RH. Molecular biology and prognostic markers in bladder cancer. In Vogelzang N, Scardino PT, Shipley WU (eds.), Comprehensive Textbook of Genitourinary Oncology 3rd ed. Philadephia: Lippincott Williams & Wilkins, 2006:385–401.
49. Kamat AM. BCG combination therapy: other agents. Supple. Urol Renal News 2004;3:14–15.
50. Lamm DL, Riggs DR, Shriver JS, et al. Megadose vitamins in bladder cancer: a double-blind clinical trial. J Urol 1994;151:21–26.
51. Kamat AM, Lamm DL. Antitumor activity of common antibiotics against superficial bladder cancer. Urol 2004;63: 457–460.
52. Sylvester RJ, Oosterlink W, van der Meijden AP. A single immediate post-operative instillation of chemotherapy decreases the risk of recurrence in patients with stage Ta/T1 bladder cancer: ameta-analysis of published results of randomized clinical trials. J Urol 2004;171:2186–2190.
53. Kaasinen E, Wijkstrom H, Malmstrom PU, et al. Alternating mitomycin C and BCG instillations versus BCG alone in treatment of carcinoma in situ of the urinary bladder: a Nordic Study. Eur Urol 2003;43:637–645.
54. Tolley DA, Parmer MKB, Grigor KM, et al. The medical research council superficial bladder cancer working party. The effect of intravesical mitomycin C on recurrence of newly diagnosed superficial bladder cancer: a further report with 7 years of followup. J Urol 1996;155:1233–1228.
55. Au JL, Badalament RA, Wientjes MG, et al. Methods to improve efficacy of intravesical mitomycin-C: results of randomized phase III trial. J Natl Cancer Inst 2001;93:597–604.
56. Bohle A, Bock PR. Intravesical bacillus Calmette-Guerin versus mitomycin C in superficial bladder cancer: formal meta-analysis of comparative studies on tumor progression. Urol 2004;62:682–686.
57. Freidrich MG, Conrad S, Pichlmeier U, et al. Long term prophylaxis with mitomycin-C significantly reduces tumor recurrence compared to short term prophylaxis with mitomycin-C or BCG in non-muscle invasive bladder cancer. J Urol 2006;175(suppl:abstr 836):270.
58. Di Stasi SM, Giannantoni A, Giurioli A, et al. Sequential BCG and electromotive mitomycin-C versus BCG alone for high risk superficial bladder cancer: long-term follow-up results of a prospective controlled study. J Urol 2006;175 (suppl:abstr 830):268.
59. Steinberg G, Bahnson R, Brosman S, et al. Efficacy and safety of valrubicin for the treatment of bacillus Calmette-Guerin refractory carcinoma in situ of the bladder. J Urol 2000;163:761–767.
60. Marchetti A, Wang L, Magar R, et al. Management of patients with bacilli Calmette-Guerin refractory carcinoma

in situ of the urinary bladder: cost implications of a clinical trial for valrubicin. Clin Ther 2000;22:422–438.
61. von der Maase H, Hansen SW, Roberts JT, et al. Gemcitabine and cisplatin versus methotrexate, vinblastine, doxorubicin, and cisplatin in advanced or metastatic bladder cancer: results of a large, randomized, multicenter, phase III study. J Clin Oncol 2000;18:3068–3077.
62. Dalbagni G, Russo P, Sheinfeld J, et al. Phase 1 trial of intravesical Gemcitabine in bacillus Calmette-Guerin refractory transitional cell carcinoma of the bladder. J Clin Oncol 2002;20:3193–3198.
63. Bassi P, De Marco V, Tavolini IM, et al. Pharmacokinetic study of intravesical Gemcitabine in carcinoma in situ of the bladder refractory to bacillus Calmette-Guerin therapy. Urol Int 2005;75:309–313.
64. Brocks CP, Buttner H, Bohle A. Inhibition of tumor implantation by intravesical gemcitabine in a murine model of superficial bladder cancer. J Urol 2005;174:1115–1118.
65. Dalbagni G, Russo P, Ben-Porat L, et al. Phase II trail of intravesical Gemcitabine in BCG refractory transitional cell carcinoma of the bladder. J Urol 2006;175(suppl:abstr 839):270.
66. Bartoletti R, Cai T, Gacci M, et al. Intravesical gemcitabine therapy for superficial transitional cell carcinoma: results of a phase II prospective multicenter study. Urol 2005;66:726–731.
67. Masson P, Murphy AM, Goetzl MA, et al. Long-term follow up of intravesical docetaxel for the treatment of superficial bladder cancer resistant to standard intravesical therapy. J Urol 2006;175(suppl:abstr 846):273.
68. O'Donnell MA. Combined bacillus Calmette-Guerin and interferon use in superficial bladder cancer. Expert Rev Anticancer Ther 2003;3:809–821.
69. O'Donnell MA, Lilli K, Leopold C. Interim results from a national multicenter phase II trial of combination BCG plus interferon-α-2B for superficial bladder cancer. J Urol 2004;172:888–893.
70. Stricker P, Pryor K, Nicholson T, et al. Bacillus Calmette-Guerin plus intravesical interferon alpha-2B in patients with superficial bladder cancer. Urology 1996;48:957–961; discussion 961–962.
71. O'Donnell MA, Krohn J, DeWolf WC. Salvage intravesical therapy with interferon alpa-2B plus low dose bacillus Calmette-Guerin is effective in patients with superficial bladder in whom bacillus Calmette-Guerin alone previously failed. J Urol 2001;166:1300–1304; discussion 1304–1305.
72. Nseyo UO, B Shumaker, EA Klein and K Sutherland. Photodynamic therapy using porfimer sodium as an alternative to cystectomy in patients with refractory transition cell carcinoma in situ of the bladder. J Urol 1998;60: 39–44.
73. Jain S, Kockelbergh RC. The role of photodynamic diagnosis in the contemporary management of superficial bladder cancer. BJU Int 2005;96:17–21.
74. Manyak MJ, Ogan K. Photodynamic therapy for refractory superficial bladder cancer: long-term clinical outcomes of single treatment using intravesical diffusion medium. J Endourol 2003;17:633–639.

12
Beyond BCG: Gemcitabine

Ganesh V. Raj and Guido Dalbagni

Contents

Abstract Currently, recurrence of carcinoma in situ (CIS) after intravesical BCG mandates a radical cystectomy, as BCG-refractory CIS is aggressive with a high propensity for progression. Novel intravesical agents are needed to salvage refractory disease. Gemcitabine is an antimetabolite with proven single agent efficacy against metastatic bladder cancer. In this review, the ability of gemcitabine to treat BCG-refractory CIS is examined in preclinical, phase I and phase II trials. Future studies with intravesical gemcitabine are also examined.

Keywords Bladder cancer, Carcinoma in situ, BCG-refractory, Intravesical therapy, Gemcitabine, Efficacy, Clinical trials

1. Rationale for Intravesical Approaches

Cancer of the urinary bladder is the fourth most common cancer in men and the ninth in women. Approximately 61,420 people develop bladder cancer each year in the United States with 13,060 associated deaths from disease (1). While the spectrum of bladder cancer encompasses superficial, invasive, and metastatic disease, a majority of patients with bladder cancer have superficial disease that has not yet invaded the muscularis propria. Superficial bladder cancer includes CIS (carcinoma in situ), Ta tumors that are confined to the urothelium above the basement membrane and T1 tumors that extend into the underlying lamina propria, but superficial to the muscularis propria (2).

The standard initial treatment is a complete cystoscopic resection of visible tumor (TURBT), and selected biopsies of the bladder mucosa and prostatic urethra (3). An examination under anesthesia should also be performed, since the presence of a palpable mass suggests muscle invasive disease. Even with complete resection of visible lesions by TURBT, the propensity for recurrence is high; 80–90% will recur within 12 months (2). Because of these high recurrence rates, adjuvant intravesical instillation of cytotoxic or immunomodulatory agents has gained widespread use in this patient population. Intravesical administration permits high local concentrations of a cytotoxic agent to be achieved within the bladder, potentially destroying viable tumor cells that remain following TURBT, preventing tumor implantation

From: *Current Clinical Urology: Bladder Cancer*, Edited by: C.T. Lee and D.P. Wood,
DOI: 10.1007/978-1-59745-417-9_12,

and theoretically recurrences. The decision to proceed with intravesical therapy depends on the number and size of the bladder lesions, their histologic type and grade, and whether the tumor is primary or recurrent.

2. Intravesical Therapy with BCG

Currently, the most commonly used agent for intravesical therapy is Bacillus Calmette-Guerin (BCG), a live attenuated form of Mycobacterium bovis (4). Although the exact mechanism of its antitumor action is unknown, a 6-week course of intravesical BCG reduces the recurrence rate by 30–40%. In a Cochrane review of six randomized trials involving 585 eligible patients, there were significantly fewer recurrences at 12 months (odds ratio 0.30; 95% confidence interval [CI], 0.21–0.43) among patients treated with BCG and TURBT in comparison to those undergoing TURBT only (5).

Further, BCG decreases the need for later cystectomy, and improves overall and disease-specific survival. In a landmark study, Herr *et al.* randomly assigned 86 high-risk patients with superficial bladder cancer to receive TURBT with or without intravesical BCG for 6 weeks, followed by reevaluation every 3–6 months. Patients receiving intravesical BCG had a significantly higher 10-year progression-free survival (61 vs. 37%), and disease-specific survival rate (75 vs. 55%) than those undergoing TURBT alone (6).

3. Rationale for Alternative Intravesical Approaches

Although BCG represents the most effective current intravesical therapeutic option for superficial bladder cancer, several factors point to the need for alternative prophylactic intravesical chemotherapeutic agents, including:

- Up to a third of patients with superficial bladder cancer will not respond to BCG (7, 8). While this may be, in part, attributed to clinical understaging and completeness of resection by TURBT alone, not all superficial bladder cancer responds equally to BCG. Indeed, patients who have tumor present at the first posttreatment cystoscopy have higher recurrence and stage progression rates than those with negative first cystoscopy findings (8, 9).
- Intravesical BCG is effective in all stages of superficial bladder cancer, including Tis: but its effect on recurrence and progression is dependent on grade, stage, multifocality of the primary tumor. For example, BCG reduces the recurrence rate for Tcis by 70% at 1-year, but its effect on T1 tumors is less profound with a 30–40% reduction in the 1-year recurrence rate (10).
- BCG may be associated with significant toxicity that may limit its use. Systemic invasion of BCG after intravesical administration may occur, if there is a breach of integrity of the urogenital mucosa. "BCG"-osis and disseminated infections can ensue, and, while rare, deaths have resulted. In the Cochrane review, most common toxicities associated with intravesical BCG administration included urinary frequency (71%), cystitis (67%), fever (25%), and hematuria (23%) (5).
- Even patients who initially respond to BCG may become BCG-refractory (11). Additional effective intravesical approaches may provide alternatives to radical cystectomy for these patients with BCG-refractory bladder cancer.

In this chapter, we explore the utility of a potential alternative intravesical chemotherapeutic agent, Gemcitabine.

4. Gemcitabine (Gemzar)

Gemcitabine (2′,2′-difluoro-2′-deoxycytidine; Gemzar, Eli Lilly and Co, Indianapolis, IN) is a pyrimidine nucleoside antimetabolite that is structurally analogous to cytarabine (12, 13). Gemcitabine is sequentially phosphorylated intracellularly by nucleoside kinases to two active metabolites, gemcitabine diphosphate (dFdCDP) and gemcitabine triphosphate (dFdCTP) and by cytidine deaminase to inactive metabolite difluorodeoxyuridine (dFdU) (Fig. 12.1). Gemcitabine inhibits ribonucleotide reductase, stimulates deoxycytidine kinase, and inhibits cytidine deaminase (14). The cytotoxic effects of gemcitabine are exerted through incorporation of the triphosphate form dFdCTP into DNA with the assistance of its diphosphate form dFdCDP, resulting in inhibition of DNA synthesis and induction of apoptosis (15). Gemcitabine thus specifically works on S and G_1/S phases of the cell-cycle. Gemcitabine has a broad spectrum of activity against tumor cells (16), and is FDA-approved as a primary chemotherapeutic agent for induction and radiosensitizing chemotherapy against:

- Adenocarcinoma of the pancreas: First-line therapy in locally-advanced (nonresectable stage II or stage III) or metastatic (stage IV) pancreatic adenocarcinoma (17)

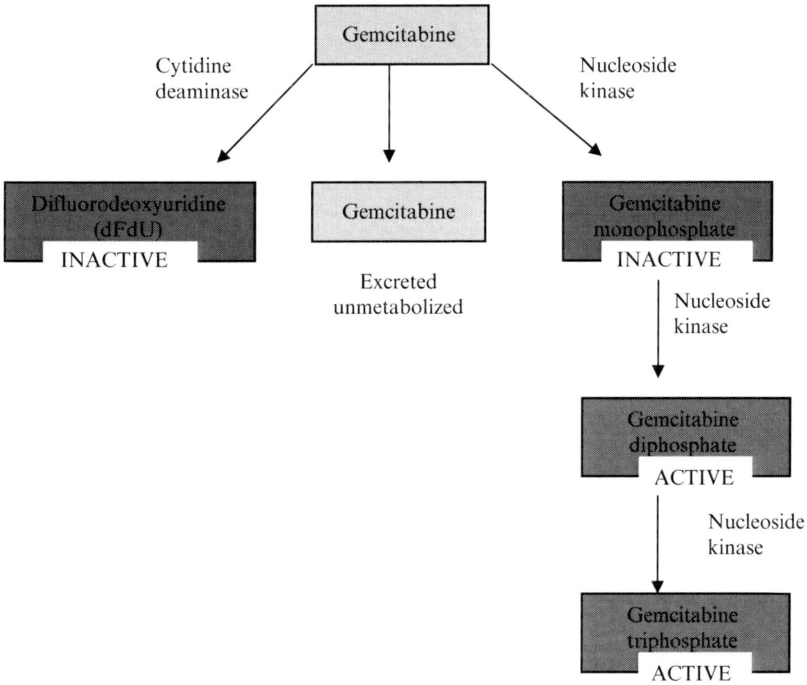

FIG. 12.1. Metabolism of gemcitabine. Pathway of metabolism of gemcitabine into inactive and active metabolites

- Breast cancer: First-line therapy in metastatic breast cancer (18)
- Non small-cell lung cancer: First-line therapy in locally-advanced (stage IIIA or IIIB) or metastatic (stage IV) non small-cell lung cancer
- Ovarian cancer: Second line therapy for tumors that have relapsed at least 6 months after completion of platinum-based therapy (19)

Intravenous infusion of gemcitabine is generally well tolerated. Gemcitabine is metabolized in the liver and virtually always excreted in the urine either as intact drug or inactive uridine metabolite (20). Toxicity associated with Gemcitabine includes myelosuppression, paresthesias, and severe rash. Patients should be typically monitored prior to each dose with a complete blood count (CBC), including differential and platelet count.

5. Gemcitabine and Bladder Cancer

Gemcitabine (1,000 mg/m^2 i.v. infusion once weekly for 3 weeks; repeat cycle every 4 weeks) is highly effective (overall response rates ranging from 22.5 to 28%) and well tolerated as both first- and second-line single-agent therapy for the treatment of metastatic transitional cell carcinoma (TCC) (21, 22). In a randomized, multicenter, phase III study, patients with unresectable or metastatic disease treated with gemcitabine plus cisplatin had a similar survival to patients treated with the MVAC (methotrexate, vinblastine, doxorubicin, and cisplatin) regimen. In contrast to MVAC, the combination of gemcitabine and cisplatin had a better safety profile and tolerability (23, 24).

Several factors served as the impetus for examining gemcitabine in an intravesical setting including

- Efficacy in an intravenous setting against metastatic urothelial carcinoma as outlined above (23–25).
- Efficacy in *in vitro* cell culture studies: Gemcitabine was an effective cytotoxic agent against variety of bladder cancer cell lines (26).
- Small molecular weight (299.66 D), (13) which is larger than thiotepa (189 D) and may potentially avoid the exposure toxicity associated with thiotepa.
- Excellent liposolubility which facilitates transport across cell membranes and intracytoplasmic penetration without the use of active calcium channel pumps and activation of the multidrug resistance channels (13).

- Even when systemically administered, gemcitabine is rapidly deaminated by cytidine deaminase, resulting in the inactive metabolite 2′,2′-difluorodeoxyuridine (dFdU) which is excreted in the urine (15).
- Gemcitabine has a high total body clearance with 98% of drug excreted in the urine (15).
- Favorable toxicity profile even when administered as a systemic agent.

The utility of intravesical gemcitabine was first examined in preclinical animal models and then investigated in phase I and phase II studies as outlined below.

6. Animal Studies Using Intravesical Gemcitabine

The first animal study evaluating the safety profile with toxicology and pharmacokinetics of administration of intravesical gemcitabine was performed in beagles by Cozzi et al. (27). Intravesical instillation of gemcitabine at a dose equivalent to the recommended human systemic dose of 1,000 mg/m^2, was well tolerated with no adverse clinical effects and no demonstrable effect on the bone marrow or bladder. However, significant systemic absorption of gemcitabine was detected after intravesical treatment, even at lower doses (see Fig. 12.2). Further, the half life of the drug was markedly prolonged following intravesical administration (T1/2 = 5.5 h) when compared with intravenous administration (T1/2 = 1.5 h). These findings were confirmed by studies performed in the rabbit (28) and pigs (29). These animal studies established the basis for phase I studies in humans.

7. Phase I Studies for Intravesical Gemcitabine

The first study in patients with bladder cancer to evaluate the safety profile and toxicity of intravesical gemcitabine was a dose escalation protocol reported by Dalbagni et al. (30). Eighteen high-risk BCG-refractory patients were treated with increasing doses of intravesical gemcitabine and reported excellent tolerability, with no instances of therapy-limiting or dose-limiting toxicity. None of the 18 patients had Grade 4 toxicity (Table 12.1). Grade 3 systemic

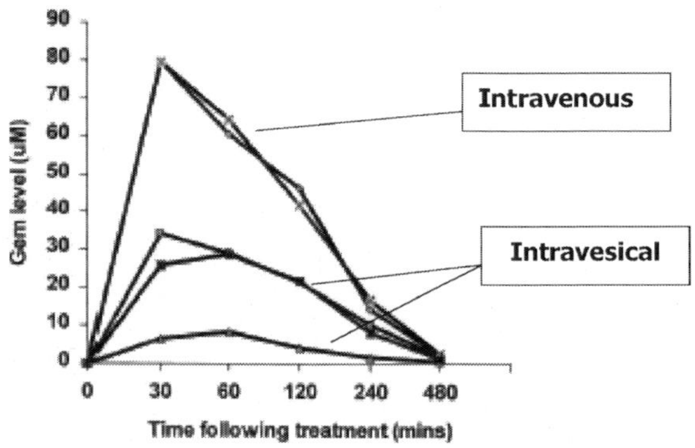

FIG. 12.2. Metabolism of gemcitabine. Serum gemcitabine levels after administration of the equivalent of 1,000 mg of drug via intravenous and intravesical administration, respectively. From (27)

TABLE 12.1. Grade 2 or greater toxicity in 18 patients receiving intravesical gemcitabine. From (30).

	Dose						
	500 mg (5 mg/ml)	1,000 mg (10 mg/ml)		1,500 mg (15 mg/ml)		2,000 mg (20 mg/ml)	
		$n = 6$		$n = 3$		$n = 6$	
	$n = 3$	Grade 2	Grade 3	Grade 2	Grade 3	Grade 2	Grade 3
Urinary frequency	0	4	1	1	1	0	0
Hematuria	0	3	0	1	0	1	0
UTI	0	0	0	1	0	0	0
Hand-foot syndrome	0	0	1	0	0	0	0
Neutropenia	0	0	0	0	0	0	1
Thrombocytopenia	0	0	0	0	0	0	1
Asthenia	0	1	0	0	0	1	0
Nausea	0	0	0	0	0	1	0
Vomiting	0	0	0	0	0	1	0

No patients experienced Grade 4 toxicity
UTI urinary tract infection

manifestations included a hand-foot syndrome in one patient at the 1,000 mg dosage and neutropenia and thrombocytopenia in one patient at the 2,000 mg dose level. The excellent tolerability of intravesical gemcitabine has been confirmed in several additional phase I and phase II studies.

Concerns about the systemic absorption of intravesical gemcitabine prompted several evaluations of serum levels of gemcitabine and its metabolites. Consistently, serum levels of gemcitabine have been undetectable up to 1,500 mg dosage (30–33). At the 2,000 mg dosage level, low levels of gemcitabine (≤–1 μg/ml) have been transiently detected in the serum. In the first phase I study, Dalbagni et al. detected gemcitabine in the serum of 2 of 6 patients treated with 2,000 mg of intravesical gemcitabine (30). Laufer *et al.* identified plasma levels of the inactive metabolite dFdU in patients given intravesical gemcitabine at doses ≥1,500 mg (31). Serum dFdU concentrations increased until 90–120 min, implying an absorption rate of 0.5–5.5% of instilled dose. Between 61 and 100% of the gemcitabine dose was accounted for in voided urine (30–33).

In patients for whom a single intravesical instillation of gemcitabine was administered immediately after complete transurethral resection, Palou observed systemic levels of gemcitabine at ≥1,500 mg (34). Intravesical administration of gemcitabine was associated with higher serum levels but well tolerated even in patients with a suspected bladder perforation. Absorbed gemcitabine was rapidly metabolized and degraded within 2 h.

Overall, the data from seven phase I trials (30–32, 34–37), which involved distinct dosing schedules, variant dwell times, drug concentrations, indicated that intravesical gemcitabine at concentrations up to 40 mg/ml was relatively well tolerated (Table 12.2). Intravesical gemcitabine administration was consistently associated with some systemic absorption that is minimal and transiently detectable. Even with systemic absorption of gemcitabine, the systemic side effect profile was tolerable, with no reported clinically significant adverse events (Table 12.2). Of the 90 patients cumulatively evaluated in phase I trials, only two had Grade 3 toxicity attributable to systemic absorption.

In addition, the phase I studies hinted at the potential utility of intravesical gemcitabine for patients with recurrent bladder cancer (30–32, 34–37). Even though most of the phase I studies evaluated cohorts of patients who had been heavily pretreated with BCG and other intravesical therapies, intravesical gemcitabine demonstrated efficacy (Table 12.2). Taken together, phase I studies have so far demonstrated that intravesical Gemcitabine has a substantial ablative activity on high-risk bladder cancer, including BCG-refractory cancer. These data set the stage for the phase II studies with intravesical gemcitabine (38).

8. Phase II Studies for Intravesical Gemcitabine

Studies evaluating the utility of intravesical gemcitabine in Phase II studies typically involve an examination of the ablative effect of gemcitabine on a "marker lesion" and its ability to prevent tumor recurrence and progression (Table 12.3).

Gontero evaluated the efficacy of intravesical Gemcitabine at a concentration of 40 mg/ml (2,000 mg in 50 ml saline solution) on a single marker tumor left in the bladder after a complete TUR of all other lesions in 39 patients, a majority (77%) of whom had recurred after prior intravesical therapy (39). A complete response was noted at 3 months in 22 out of 39 patients (56%). No progression was observed among the 17 nonresponders at the time of the TUR. These data indicated that intravesical gemcitabine has a tumor ablative or cytoreductive activity even in patients with recurrences after prior intravesical therapy.

These findings have been confirmed in separate evaluations (Table 12.3). Serreta observed a lower CR rate (23%) in his dose escalation study on the effect of intravesical gemcitabine on 1–3 papillary markers (40). However, among the patients receiving the higher dose (2,000 mg) of gemcitabine, CR rates were higher at 33% (3/9).

In an evaluation of patients with BCG-refractory bladder cancer, a subgroup with a high risk of recurrence and progression, Dalbagni noted that 15 of 30 patients, (50; 95% CI, 32–68%) receiving 2,000 mg of intravesical gemcitabine achieved a complete response (CR) (Table. 12.3) (41). Twelve of these patients with CR at 3 months had recurrence of tumor with a median recurrence-free survival time of 3.6 months from the date of CR. Only two patients maintained a CR at 23 and 29 months, respectively. The 1-year recurrence-free survival rate for patients with a CR was 21%. Two patients progressed to a higher stage while on gemcitabine therapy while another 11 (37%)

TABLE 12.2. Summary of phase I clinical trials with gemcitabine.

References	Dosage	Schedule	Patients	Toxicity	Response
(30)	4 doses – 500, 1,000, 1,500 and 2,000 (20 mg/ml)	Two courses: twice weekly × 3 weeks: 1 week off 1 h dwell time	18 pts with BCG-refractory TCC	500 mg – no G3/G4 toxicity 1,000 mg – 50% hematuria, 17% G3 1,500 mg – no G3/G4 toxicity 2,000 mg – 17% G3 (neutropenia)	100% completed course 7/18 CR 4/18 PR 7/18 NR
(31)	Four doses – 500, 1,000, 1,500 and 2,000	2–4 weeks after complete TUR: Once weekly for 6 weeks 2 h dwell time	15 pts with recurrent TCC who had failed prior intravesical therapies	2/15 had G3 toxicity 500 mg – no G3/G4 toxicity 1,000 mg – 1/3 had G3 (retention) 1,500 mg – no G3/G4 toxicity 2,000 mg – 1/6 had G3 (frequency)	9/13 recurrence-free at 12 weeks
(32)	Three doses – 1,000, 1,500 and 2,000	Once weekly for 6 weeks 1 h dwell time	Ten patients with Ta and T1	7 with side effects 4 with dysuria 3 with headache/fatigue	5/10 recurred within 12 months, including 5/6 high-risk
(33)	Four doses – 500, 1,000, 1,500 and 2,000	Once weekly for 6 weeks 2 h dwell time	12 pts with recurrent TCC who had failed prior intravesical therapies	No systemic toxicity Minimal local toxicity	NA
(35)	One dose 2,000 mg (40 mg/ml)	Once weekly for 4 weeks 1 h dwell time	26 pts with recurrent Ta-T1 G1-G2 TCC	G3 in 1 pt G2 in 5 pts All six had tx discontinued	10/20 CR
(37)	One dose 2,000 mg (40 mg/ml)	Once weekly for 4 weeks 1 h dwell time	Nine pts with recurrent Ta-T1 G1-G2 TCC	No systemic toxicity 3/9 local toxicity	5/9 CR
(36)	Three doses– 1,000, 1,250 and 1,500	Once weekly for 6 weeks 1 h dwell time	Nine pts with BCG-refractory TCC	No G2–4 toxicity G1 neutopenia 1 pt G1 frequency 1 pt G1 hematuria 3 pts	5/10 with recurrence within 12 months, including 5/6 with high-risk of recurrence

TUR transurethral resection; *G* grade; *pts* patients; *BCG* Bacille-Camille Guerin; *TCC* transitional cell carcinoma; *NA* not available; *CR* complete response; *PR* partial response; *NR* no response

underwent a radical cystectomy following therapy (Fig. 12.4). Overall, incidence of progression at 1 year was 3.5% (95% CI, 0.5–24.8%), and the incidence of cystectomy at 1 year was 20.5%. These data confirm that intravesical gemcitabine has activity in this high-risk patient population but its effect is not durable.

While the above reported studies generally involved a marker lesion to examine the ability of gemcitabine to ablate the tumor, insight into recurrence outcomes following complete resection by TUR of bladder lesions comes from a study by Bartoletti (42). In a study of 116 patients with intermediate-risk and high-risk bladder cancer, who had undergone a complete TUR with no residual marker lesion and then received intravesical gemcitabine including maintenance therapy, recurrences were noted in 29 patients (25.4%) at an average of 7 months after TUR. Among the subgroup of patients with BCG-refractory bladder cancer, recurrences were noted in 38% (15/40). Recurrences were less commonly noted following intravesical gemcitabine among patients without prior tumors or prior exposure to any intravesical therapy.

In all the reported phase II studies (39–43), gemcitabine was generally very well tolerated: neither the systemic nor local side effects typically exceeded Grade 2 toxicity. Overall the data suggest that administration of intravesical gemcitabine has significant efficacy in ablating bladder cancer, including those tumors at high-risk of recurrence such as BCG-refractory bladder cancer. The durability

TABLE 12.3. Summary of phase II clinical trials evaluating the efficacy of intravesical gemcitabine.

References	Dosage	Schedule	Patients	Response@ 3 months	Recurrence and progression
(39)	2,000 mg (40 mg/ml)	Once weekly for 6 weeks 1 h dwell time	26 pts with recurrent Ta-T1 G1-G2 TCC with single, 0.5–1 cm marker lesion	56% (22/39) CR 44% (17/39) NR	No progression among 17 NR noted at TUR
(41)	2,000 mg (20 mg/ml)	Two courses: twice weekly × 3 weeks: 1 week off 1 h dwell time	30 pts with BCG-refractory TCC	50% (15/30) CR 23% (7/30) PR 27% (8/30) NR	12/14 pts with CR recurred with a median recurrence-free interval of 3.6 months after CR. 1 y recurrence-free survival 21% 1 y progression incidence 3.5% 1 y incidence of RC 20.5%
(40)	Three doses-500, 1,000 and 2,000 mg	Once weekly for 6 weeks 2 h dwell time	27 patients with Ta tumors and 1–3 marker lesions	23% (6/26) CR 8% (2/26) PR 69% (18/26) NR	2/6 patients with CR recurred.
(43)	2,000 mg (20 mg/ml)	Single dose, or Two doses/ wk for 3 weeks or Once weekly for 6 weeks 1 h dwell time	32 pts with multiple recurrent Ta G1-2 TCC with single 1 cm marker lesion	Overall CR 31% (9/30) 10% (1/11) single dose 44% (4/9) once weekly 40% (4/10) twice weekly	
(42)	2,000 mg (40 mg/ml)	Once weekly for 6 weeks 1 h dwell time Maintenance schedule at 3, 6, 12, 18, 24, 30 and 36 months	116 pts with Ta, T1 or Tis TCC after complete resection by TUR Including 40 pts with BCG-refractory TCC		25% had recurrent tumors within 12 months Among pts with BCG-refractory tumors, 33% (13/40) had recurrence

TUR transurethral resection; *G* grade; *pts* patients; *BCG* Bacille-Camille Guerin; *TCC* transitional cell carcinoma; *NA* not available; *CR* complete response; *PR* partial response; *NR* no response; *RC* radical cystectomy

of a complete response to a 6-week course of intravesical gemcitabine is typically short: durable complete responses are generally rare.

9. Gemcitabine: Optimization of Therapy

Optimization of gemcitabine therapy includes an ongoing evaluation of the toxicity, dosage and schedules, timing of intravesical installation, patient selection criteria, efficacy responses in terms of recurrences and progression, durability of response and the need for maintenance therapy. Each of these criteria is detailed below.

Toxicity: The Phase I and II studies have indicated an excellent safety profile up to intravesical concentrations of 40 mg/ml and doses of 2,000 mg. Systemic absorption has been noted in doses above 1,500 mg. Detectable levels of serum gemcitabine are temporally limited due to its rapid metabolism by cytidine deaminase into dFdU. Toxicity is limited primarily to low grade dysuria symptoms and mild systemic symptoms. Overall, intravesical gemcitabine is well tolerated with a favorable side-effect profile.

Dosage, schedules, and dwell times: Dosages above 2,000 mg have not been evaluated in phase I studies and may be worth evaluating especially for patients at a high-risk for recurrence and progression.

Since the initial application of BCG by Morales, the 6 weekly instillations scheme has become the standard for intravesical instillations, and the basis for a number of phase I and II trials outlined above (4). *In vitro* and *in vivo* animal studies indicating that the cytotoxic effect of gemcitabine was maximal when given every third day represented the rationale

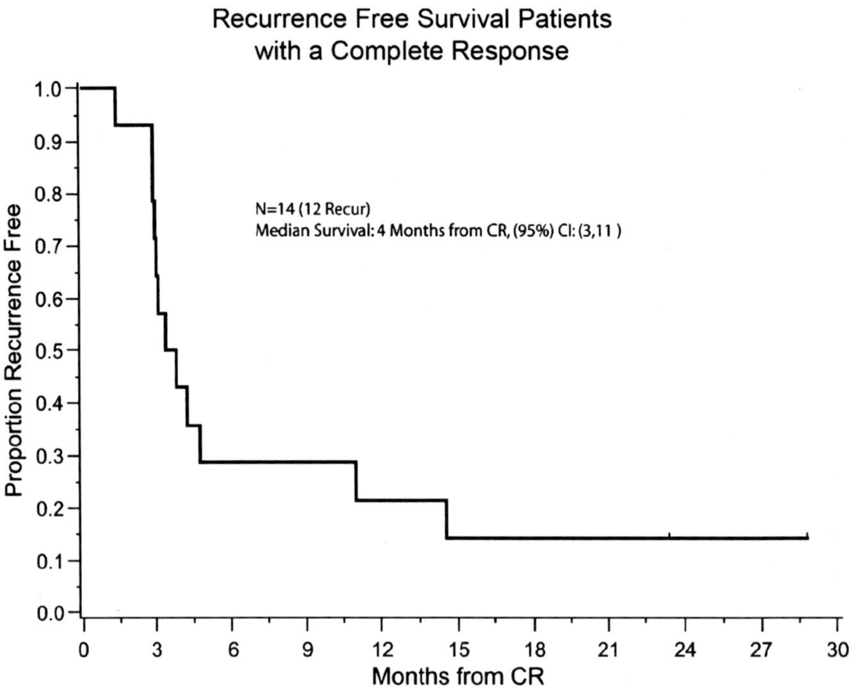

Fig. 12.3. Efficacy of gemcitabine. Recurrence-free survival among patients with a complete response. From (41)

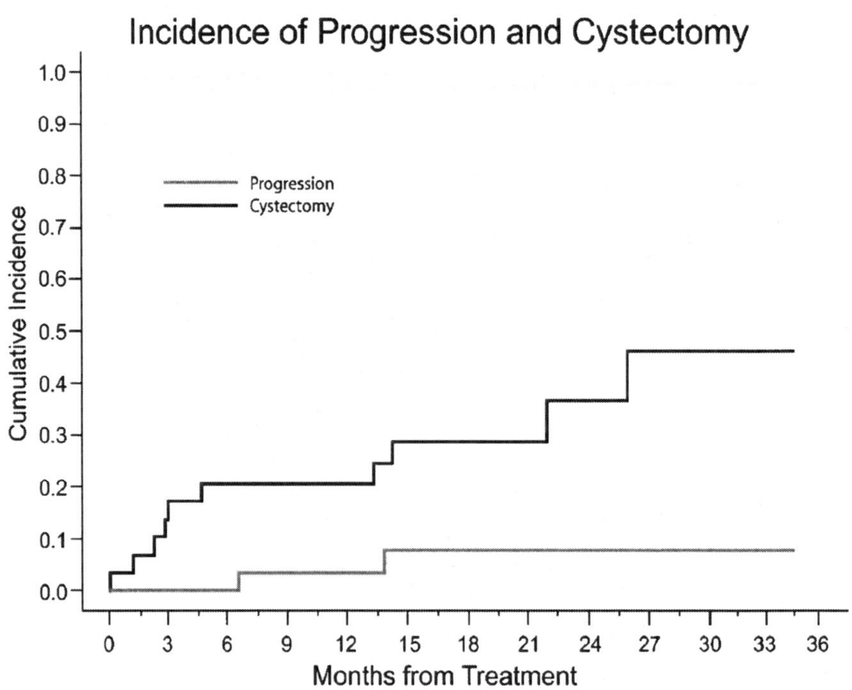

Fig. 12.4. Efficacy of gemcitabine. Incidence of progression and cystectomy. From (41)

for studies employing a twice-weekly schedule of gemcitabine administration. Gardmark evaluated the effect of dosing schedules on the efficacy of 2,000 mg of intravesical gemcitabine: in his study, respective subgroup response rate was 10% in the single-dose group, 44% in the once-weekly group, and 40% in the twice-weekly group (43).

Theoretically longer chemotherapeutic dwell times increase the likelihood of cell kill: however, issues standard with any intravesical therapy are applicable including patient tolerance of urgency symptoms, bladder compliance, hydration status and bladder reactivity to instilled chemotherapy. Both 1 and 2-h dwell times have been examined with intravesical gemcitabine: no direct comparison has been performed. Improvement in therapeutic efficacy can be achieved by restricting fluid intake prior to the procedure and emptying the bladder prior to administration of intravesical agent in order to minimize dilution of the active agent.

Timing of intravesical administration: Most of the studies reported herein examined the utility of administration of intravesical gemcitabine 2 weeks after a transurethral resection (30, 32, 33, 36, 40, 41, 43, 44). In an elegant animal study, Brocks noted that a single intravesical instillation of gemcitabine could prevent iatrogenically induced tumor implantation and resulting tumor outgrowth (45). Palou demonstrated the safety and tolerability of the administration of gemcitabine immediately after TUR, even in cases of suspected bladder perforation (34). In these patients, the systemic absorption of gemcitabine was more profound. The optimal timing of gemcitabine administration deserves further attention.

Patient selection criteria: The utility of intravesical gemcitabine has primarily been evaluated for a heavily pretreated population of patients with recurrent bladder tumors who have failed primary intravesical approaches, including BCG.

Further, the study by Bartoletti has shown that recurrences were less frequent in patients who received primary intravesical gemcitabine indicates that gemcitabine may be useful as primary intravesical therapy and not just in a BCG-refractory setting (42).

Efficacy: The various phase II studies conducted thus far indicate a moderate efficacy of intravesical gemcitabine in a typically heavily pretreated population, with a 50–56% CR (41, 44). Importantly, not all patients respond to gemcitabine. Most of these studies are small and from single institution and do not permit analyses of factors that predict response to gemcitabine. Factors that may influence the efficacy of intravesical gemcitabine include the number of recurrent tumors, tumor multifocality, concurrent presence of CIS, expression of markers such as cytidine deaminase or nucleoside kinase and prior intravesical therapy. A study by a large cohort, such as that proposed by SWOG may help identify risk factors to predict gemcitabine response in patients with BCG-refractory bladder cancer and thus identify patients who may benefit from intravesical gemcitabine.

Durable response: Although a significant rate of CR was achieved at 3 months following intravesical administration of gemcitabine, the majority of patients experienced a relapse within 12 months. Durable complete response to intravesical gemcitabine is rare. Unlike BCG which induces a host response against the tumor, the cytotoxic effect of gemcitabine is direct and transient. As is the paradigm with many other cytotoxic drugs, recurrent treatment may be necessary. Repeated administration of intravesical gemcitabine may replicate log-cell-kill obtained with chemotherapy agents, provided that chemoresistance does not develop. Although the role of maintenance therapy for intravesical chemotherapeutic agents is controversial, in a meta-analysis of 11 randomized trials, chemotherapy for 2 years had the greatest effect on decreasing the recurrence rates (46). Thus, the role of maintenance therapy for intravesical gemcitabine should be explored.

Combinations: Future directions: In order to improve the efficacy of intravesical gemcitabine in treating patients with superficial bladder cancer, combinations of gemcitabine with other intravesical agents may be explored. Syngergistic interactions between intravesical gemcitabine and other agents like mitomycin-C epidoxorubicin paclitaxel or novel antisense olignocleotides may help increase the cell kill and effectiveness of intravesical gemcitabine (47–50). Combinations with other intravesical agents may improve the efficacy of intravesical gemcitabine and minimize recurrence and progression.

10. Conclusions

Data from the phase I and phase II studies thus far indicate that intravesical gemcitabine has an excellent safety profile, significant but transient systemic absorption, minimal local or systemic toxicity, excellent tolerability and efficacy against bladder cancer in a primary, recurrent and BCG-refractory setting.

These findings are promising and indicate a possible role for intravesical gemcitabine as a safe effective therapeutic option in the management of superficial bladder cancer. Additional Phase II and Phase III studies are warranted prior to optimize and to establish gemcitabine as a standard therapeutic strategy.

References

1. Jemal A, Siegel R, Ward E, Murray T, Xu J, Smigal C, and Thun MJ. Cancer statistics, 2006. *CA Cancer J Clin* 56: 106–30, 2006.
2. Herr HW. Tumor progression and survival of patients with high grade, noninvasive papillary (TaG3) bladder tumors: 15-year outcome. *J Urol* 163: 60–1; discussion 61–2, 2000.
3. Herr HW. Transurethral resection of muscle-invasive bladder cancer: 10-year outcome. *J Clin Oncol* 19: 89–93, 2001.
4. Morales A, Eidinger D, and Bruce AW. Intracavitary Bacillus Calmette-Guerin in the treatment of superficial bladder tumors. *J Urol* 167: 891–3; discussion 893–5, 2002.
5. Shelley MD, Court JB, Kynaston H, Wilt TJ, Coles B, and Mason M. Intravesical bacillus Calmette-Guerin versus mitomycin C for Ta and T1 bladder cancer. Cochrane Database Syst Rev CD003231, 2003.
6. Herr HW, Wartinger DD, Fair WR, and Oettgen HF. Bacillus Calmette-Guerin therapy for superficial bladder cancer: a 10-year followup. *J Urol* 147: 1020–3, 1992.
7. Herr HW, Badalament RA, Amato DA, Laudone VP, Fair WR, and Whitmore WF, Jr. Superficial bladder cancer treated with bacillus Calmette-Guerin: a multivariate analysis of factors affecting tumor progression. *J Urol* 141: 22–9, 1989.
8. Herr HW 2005 Restaging transurethral resection of high risk superficial bladder cancer improves the initial response to bacillus Calmette-Guerin therapy. *J Urol* 174: 2134–7.
9. Dalbagni G, Rechtschaffen T, and Herr HW. Is transurethral biopsy of the bladder necessary after 3 months to evaluate response to bacillus Calmette-Guerin therapy? *J Urol* 162: 708–9, 1999.
10. Cookson MS, Herr HW, Zhang ZF, Soloway S, Sogani PC, and Fair WR. The treated natural history of high risk superficial bladder cancer: 15-year outcome. *J Urol* 158: 62–7, 1997.
11. Herr HW and Dalbagni G. Defining bacillus Calmette-Guerin refractory superficial bladder tumors. *J Urol* 169: 1706–8, 2003.
12. Mini E, Nobili S, Caciagli B, Landini I, and Mazzei T. Cellular pharmacology of gemcitabine. *Ann Oncol* 17 Suppl 5: v7–v12, 2006.
13. Hui YF and Reitz J. Gemcitabine: a cytidine analogue active against solid tumors. *Am J Health Syst Pharm* 54: 162–70; quiz 197–8, 1997.
14. Plunkett W, Huang P, and Gandhi V. Preclinical characteristics of gemcitabine. *Anticancer Drugs* 6 Suppl 6: 7–13, 1995.
15. Plunkett W, Huang P, Searcy CE, and Gandhi V. Gemcitabine: preclinical pharmacology and mechanisms of action. *Semin Oncol* 23: 3–15, 1996.
16. Storniolo AM, Allerheiligen SR, and Pearce HL. Preclinical, pharmacologic, and phase I studies of gemcitabine. *Semin Oncol* 24: S7-2–S7-7, 1997.
17. Michael M and Moore M. Clinical experience with gemcitabine in pancreatic carcinoma. *Oncology (Williston Park)* 11: 1615–22; discussion 1622, 1625–7, 1997.
18. Heinemann V. Gemcitabine in metastatic breast cancer. *Expert Rev Anticancer Ther* 5: 429–43, 2005.
19. Bookman MA. Gemcitabine monotherapy in recurrent ovarian cancer: from the bench to the clinic. *Int J Gynecol Cancer* 15 Suppl 1: 12–7, 2005.
20. Plunkett W, Huang P, Xu YZ, Heinemann V, Grunewald R, and Gandhi V. Gemcitabine: metabolism, mechanisms of action, and self-potentiation. *Semin Oncol* 22: 3–10, 1995.
21. Advanced Bladder Cancer (ABC) Meta-analysis Collaboration. Adjuvant chemotherapy in invasive bladder cancer: a systematic review and meta-analysis of individual patient data Advanced Bladder Cancer (ABC) Meta-analysis Collaboration. *Eur Urol* 48: 189–199; discussion 199–201, 2005.
22. Advanced Bladder Cancer (ABC) Meta-analysis Collaboration. Neoadjuvant chemotherapy for invasive bladder cancer. Cochrane Database Syst Rev CD005246, 2005.
23. von der Maase H, Hansen SW, Roberts JT, Dogliotti L, Oliver T, Moore MJ, Bodrogi I, Albers P, Knuth A, Lippert CM et al, 2000Gemcitabine and cisplatin versus methotrexate, vinblastine, doxorubicin, and cisplatin in advanced or metastatic bladder cancer: results of a large, randomized, multinational, multicenter, phase III study. *J Clin Oncol* 18: 3068–77.
24. von der Maase H, Sengelov L, Roberts JT, Ricci S, Dogliotti L, Oliver T, Moore MJ, Zimmermann A, and Arning M. Long-term survival results of a randomized trial comparing gemcitabine plus cisplatin, with methotrexate, vinblastine, doxorubicin, plus cisplatin in patients with bladder cancer. *J Clin Oncol* 23: 4602–8, 2005.
25. von der Maase H. Current and future perspectives in advanced bladder cancer: is there a new standard? *Semin Oncol* 29: 3–14, 2002.
26. Kilani RT, Tamimi Y, Karmali S, Mackey J, Hanel EG, Wong KK, and Moore RB. Selective cytotoxicity of gemcitabine in bladder cancer cell lines. *Anticancer Drugs* 13: 557–66, 2002.
27. Cozzi PJ, Bajorin DF, Tong W, Nguyen H, Scott J, Heston WD, and Dalbagni G. Toxicology and pharmacokinetics of intravesical gemcitabine: a preclinical study in dogs. *Clin Cancer Res* 5: 2629–37, 1999.
28. Matera M, Costantino G, Clementi G, Lempereur L, Vasta D, and Vasquez E. Experimental study on the

toxicity and the local and systemic tolerability of gemcitabine after topical treatment of the rabbit bladder. *Oncol Rep* 11: 1145–51, 2004.
29. Witjes JA, Vriesema JL, van der Heijden AG, Peters GJ, and Schalken JA. Pharmacokinetics of intravesical gemcitabine: a preclinical study in pigs. *Eur Urol* 44: 615–9, 2003.
30. Dalbagni G, Russo P, Sheinfeld J, Mazumdar M, Tong W, Rabbani F, Donat MS, Herr HW, Sogani P, dePalma D et al, 2002. Phase I trial of intravesical gemcitabine in bacillus Calmette-Guerin-refractory transitional-cell carcinoma of the bladder. *J Clin Oncol* 20: 3193–8.
31. Laufer M, Ramalingam S, Schoenberg MP, Haisfield-Wolf ME, Zuhowski EG, Trueheart IN, Eisenberger MA, Nativ O, and Egorin MJ. Intravesical gemcitabine therapy for superficial transitional cell carcinoma of the bladder: a phase I and pharmacokinetic study. *J Clin Oncol* 21: 697–703, 2003.
32. Witjes JA, van der Heijden AG, Vriesema JL, Peters GJ, Laan A, and Schalken JA. Intravesical gemcitabine: a phase 1 and pharmacokinetic study. *Eur Urol* 45: 182–6, 2004.
33. De Berardinis E, Antonini G, Peters GJ, Loves WJ, Van der Born K, Codacci-Pisanelli G, and Di Silverio F. Intravesical administration of gemcitabine in superficial bladder cancer: a phase I study with pharmacodynamic evaluation. *BJU Int* 93: 491–4, 2004.
34. Palou J, Carcas A, Segarra J, Duque B, Salvador J, Garcia-Ribas I, and Villavicencio H. Phase I pharmacokinetic study of a single intravesical instillation of gemcitabine administered immediately after transurethral resection plus multiple random biopsies in patients with superficial bladder cancer. *J Urol* 172: 485–8, 2004.
35. Campodonico F and Maffezzini M. Gemcitabine in intravesical treatment of Ta-T1 transitional cell carcinoma of the bladder. *Urology* 66: 1141–2; author reply 1142, 2005.
36. Bassi P, De Marco V, Tavolini IM, Longo F, Pinto F, Zucchetti M, Crucitta E, Marini L, and Dal Moro F. Pharmacokinetic study of intravesical gemcitabine in carcinoma in situ of the bladder refractory to bacillus Calmette-Guerin therapy. *Urol Int* 75: 309–13, 2005.
37. Mattioli F, Curotto A, Manfredi V, Gosmar M, Garbero C, Ambruosi C, Carmignani G, and Martelli A. Intravesical gemcitabine in superficial bladder cancer: a phase II safety, efficacy and pharmacokinetic study. *Anticancer Res* 25: 2493–6, 2005.
38. Gontero P and Frea B. Actual experience and future development of gemcitabine in superficial bladder cancer. *Ann Oncol* 17 Suppl 5: v123–8, 2006.
39. Gontero P, Casetta G, Maso G, Sogni F, Pretti G, Zitella A, Frea B, and Tizzani A. Phase II study to investigate the ablative efficacy of intravesical administration of gemcitabine in intermediate-risk superficial bladder cancer (SBC). *Eur Urol* 46: 339–43, 2004.
40. Serretta V, Galuffo A, Pavone C, Allegro R, and Pavone-MacAluso M. Gemcitabine in intravesical treatment of Ta-T1 transitional cell carcinoma of bladder: Phase I-II study on marker lesions. *Urology* 65: 65–9, 2005.
41. Dalbagni G, Russo P, Bochner B, Ben-Porat L, Sheinfeld J, Sogani P, Donat MS, Herr HW, and Bajorin D. Phase II trial of intravesical gemcitabine in bacille Calmette-Guerin-refractory transitional cell carcinoma of the bladder. *J Clin Oncol* 24: 2729–34, 2006.
42. Bartoletti R, Cai T, Gacci M, Giubilei G, Viggiani F, Santelli G, Repetti F, Nerozzi S, Ghezzi P, and Sisani M. Intravesical gemcitabine therapy for superficial transitional cell carcinoma: results of a Phase II prospective multicenter study. *Urology* 66: 726–31, 2005.
43. Gardmark T, Carringer M, Beckman E, and Malmstrom PU. Randomized phase II marker lesion study evaluating effect of scheduling on response to intravesical gemcitabine in recurrent Stage Ta urothelial cell carcinoma of the bladder. *Urology* 66: 527–30, 2005.
44. Gontero P, Marini L, and Frea B. Intravesical gemcitabine for superficial bladder cancer: rationale for a new treatment option. *BJU Int* 96: 970–6, 2005.
45. Brocks CP, Buttner H, and Bohle A. Inhibition of tumor implantation by intravesical gemcitabine in a murine model of superficial bladder cancer. *J Urol* 174: 1115–8, 2005.
46. Huncharek M and Kupelnick B. Impact of intravesical chemotherapy versus BCG immunotherapy on recurrence of superficial transitional cell carcinoma of the bladder: metaanalytic reevaluation. *Am J Clin Oncol* 26: 402–7, 2003.
47. Miyake H, Eto H, Hara I, So A, Li D, and Gleave ME. Synergistic antitumor activity by combined treatment with gemcitabine and antisense oligodeoxynucleotide targeting clusterin gene in an intravesical administration model against human bladder cancer kotcc-1 cells. *J Urol* 171: 2477–81, 2004.
48. Perabo FG, Lindner H, Schmidt D, Huebner D, Blatter J, Fimmers R, Muller SC, and Albers P. Preclinical evaluation of gemcitabine/paclitaxel-interactions in human bladder cancer lines. *Anticancer Res* 23: 4805–14, 2003.
49. Perabo FG and Muller SC. New agents in intravesical chemotherapy of superficial bladder cancer. *Scand J Urol Nephrol* 39: 108–16, 2005.
50. Zoli W, Ricotti L, Tesei A, Ulivi P, Gasperi Campani A, Fabbri F, Gunelli R, Frassineti GL, and Amadori D. Schedule-dependent cytotoxic interaction between epidoxorubicin and gemcitabine in human bladder cancer cells in vitro. *Clin Cancer Res* 10: 1500–7, 2004.

13
Beyond BCG: Taxanes

James M. McKiernan and Phillip M. Pierorazio

Contents

Abstract Many patients undergoing intravesical therapy for superficial bladder cancer will fail initial treatment; therefore additional bladder-sparing options are needed for these patients. The taxanes are potentially ideal agents for intravesical therapy as they have demonstrated efficacy as systemic agents and have little systemic absorption due to a large molecular weight. Early clinical research indicates minimal toxicities associated with the use of taxanes as an intravesical treatment. These agents may yet play an important role in the intravesical treatment of bladder cancer.

Keywords Bladder neoplasm, Carcinoma, Transitional cell, Administration, Intravesical, Taxoids, Neoplasm recurrence, Local

1. Introduction

As discussed earlier in this publication, the standard of care for superficial transitional cell cancer (TCC) of the bladder is intravesical therapy. Upwards of 50% of patients treated with intravesical therapies will recur (1). For those patients that recur, second-line treatments and salvage intravesical therapies have demonstrated response rates between 20 and 40% (2, 3) indicating a substantial population of patients diagnosed with superficial bladder cancer that do not respond to the standard of care. The only remaining option for definitive treatment is radical cystectomy with urinary diversion. Many patients are not candidates for this complex surgery and many more refuse the procedure with a reluctance to live with the consequences of urinary diversion (catheterization most commonly) and a desire to maintain their current quality of life. In addition, multiple trials have demonstrated significant short- and long-term morbidity associated with radical cystectomy (4–7) that highlight the importance of novel intravesical therapies for the treatment of superficial bladder cancer.

2. The Taxanes: Paclitaxel (TAXOL) and Docetaxel (TAXOTERE)

Docetaxel (Taxotere) is a semisynthetic antineoplastic agent similar to paclitaxel (Taxol), which together form the taxane family of chemotherapeutic drugs. Paclitaxel was isolated from the bark of the Pacific yew tree (*Taxus brevifolia*) in 1971 as part of the National Cancer Institute (NCI) screening program for

From: *Current Clinical Urology: Bladder Cancer*, Edited by: C.T. Lee and D.P. Wood,
DOI: 10.1007/978-1-59745-417-9_13,

natural cytotoxic products. A result of the same NCI program, docetaxel was isolated from the needles of the European Yew Tree (*Taxus baccata*) in 1986.

Taxanes share a similar chemical structure and are antimicrotubule agents that bind to tubulin. By binding to tubulin, they promote the assembly of microtubules and stabilize the formed structures by inhibiting depolymerization. Microtubules rely on continuous polymerization and depolymerization to assemble and mobilize the components of the spindle apparatus during cell division as well as to continue proper function of cellular motility, intracellular transport and the maintenance of cellular shape. The extremely stable microtubules, reinforced by the influence of the taxanes, are unable to cycle between polymerization and depolymerization and become nonfunctional. This effectively prevents cell division, specifically centrosome organization, as well as mechanisms of motility, attachment, and intracellular transport essential components of S-phase and of mitosis (8, 9). These effects are believed to explain the radiosensitizing effects of the taxanes, especially paclitaxel, when used in other cancers and organ systems due to the ability of these drugs to stop the cell cycle at points where the cell is most vulnerable to radiation – the premitotic G2 and mitotic phases.

The taxanes therefore, when administered systemically, have demonstrated antitumor activity in a number of cancer lines. Paclitaxel currently carries FDA approval for treatment of breast cancer, ovarian and non-small cell lung cancer; docetaxel for breast, gastric, nonsmall cell lung cancer and metastatic prostate cancer.

As clinical use and scientific knowledge regarding the taxanes has advanced, these agents have been regarded as potentially "ideal" intravesical treatments for TCC of the bladder. As an ideal therapy for intravesical treatment, an agent should be: (a) highly efficacious anticancer therapy, specifically targeting bladder tumor cells, (b) demonstrate minimal to no systemic absorption (and therefore systemic side effects) and (c) exhibit little if any local side effects from treatment.

The taxanes have demonstrated efficacy as anti-TCC agents both in vitro and in vivo. Rangel et al. demonstrated docetaxel to be a potent inhibitor of human bladder cancer cell lines at concentrations as low as 0.1 μm in vitro (10). In the treatment of metastatic TCC of the bladder, systemic formulations of both paclitaxel and docetaxel have demonstrated efficacy as single agents and components of multiple-agent regimens. The Eastern Cooperative Oncology Group (ECOG) trial administering systemic paclitaxel to 26 previously untreated patients, demonstrated a 42% response rate and was generally well tolerated, establishing paclitaxel as an active agent in the treatment of metastatic TCC (11). In phase II study using systemic docetaxel as a single-agent for the treatment of metastatic TCC, deWit et al. observed a 31% overall response rate with 14% of patients achieving complete response (12). To date, several studies have evaluated the efficacy of both paclitaxel and docetaxel in double- and triple-regimens, most often coupled with platinum-based agents and gemcitabine. These studies of combination systemic chemotherapy regimens have demonstrated response rates from 33.3 to 66.7% (13–16).

The advantages of intravesical therapy allow direct contact between cancer cells and chemotherapeutic medications, and theoretically sequester the antineoplastic agents away from normal and healthy tissues. The chemical nature of the taxanes makes them excellent candidates for intravesical treatment. It is believed that molecules greater than 300 Da are unlikely to enter the systemic circulation through the bladder urothelium, as molecules this large require active transport to enter the bloodstream (7). The large molecular weight of the taxanes (861.9 Da for docetaxel, 853 Da for paclitaxel) is believed to provide protection against systemic absorption. Current intravesical agents mitomycin C and doxorubicin, 334 and 580 Da respectively, demonstrated little systemic absorption (17). Conversely, thiotepa (198 Da), when used as an intravesical treatment, is readily absorbed systemically with a high associated incidence of side effects (18).

In addition, the highly lipophilic nature of the taxanes is believed to provide these drugs with the ability to penetrate effectively into the urothelial layers of bladder tissue. In a study of the effects of intravesical paclitaxel (Taxol) in dogs, Song et al. demonstrated penetration of the drug into the urothelium at a greater rate than mitomycin C or doxorubicin, concluding that a much smaller dose of paclitaxel was needed to deliver therapeutic concentrations to bladder tissues than other drugs. In addition, the same study demonstrated minimal systemic absorption of paclitaxel, a level <0.05% of the maximal tolerated dose, indicating a large tissue-targeting advantage with paclitaxel – on the order of 6,000 times the targeting advantage of previously established intravesical therapies (19). Although the study was not repeated with docetaxel, similar biochemical natures of the taxanes allow extrapolation that similar results would be observed and that taxanes, when used intravesically, would demonstrate little systemic absorption and side effects.

Clinical trials using taxanes as intravesical agents are necessary to determine local toxicities resulting from treatment. Results from a Phase I clinical trial using intravesical docetaxel are discussed in the next section.

3. Results of Phase I Trial of Intravesical Docetaxel

Columbia University Medical Center recently completed the first phase I trial investigating docetaxel as an intravesical agent for the treatment of TCC refractory to prior intravesical agents (20). Enrolled patients had a histologically confirmed diagnosis of superficial TCC – Ta, T1, or Tis disease – and were either medically ineligible for or refused cystectomy. Patients had all visible disease resected prior to enrollment and then underwent intravesical docetaxel infusions weekly for 6 weeks. The docetaxel was infused over 5 min and patients were required to retain medication without voiding for 2 h.

The primary objective of this study was the definition of the maximum tolerated dose (MTD) of intravesical docetaxel as well as the dose-limiting toxicity. The initial cohort started with 5 mg of docetaxel in 40 mL of normal saline (NS). The concentration of docetaxel was increased in each of five cohorts to a maximum of 75 mg docetaxel in 100 mL NS (0.75 mg/mL). The nature of docetaxel prevents concentrations of greater than 0.75 mg/mL, and as the 2 h dwell time prevented the infusion of larger volumes of medication, the target MTD was set at 75 mg docetaxel.

Toxicity was monitored through several modalities and was defined as measurable plasma levels of docetaxel or the presence of any systemic or local toxicity symptoms. Plasma docetaxel levels were measured by high-pressure liquid chromatography (HPLC) at weekly visits 2 h following the intravesical infusion. The National Cancer Institute (NCI) common toxicity criteria (version 2.0) were used to assess both systemic and local toxicities. Local toxicities were defined as hematuria, dysuria, urinary retention, urinary frequency, urgency or bladder spasms. Following the third treatment, each patient underwent cystoscopy to assess any local erythema or ulceration secondary to docetaxel. A final cystoscopic exam under anesthesia was performed 4 weeks after completion of the study protocol, at which time patients underwent visual examination and bladder biopsy as a final assessment of local toxicity and evaluate efficacy of the treatment.

Eighteen patients were enrolled and completed the study. The cohort was comprised of sixteen men and two women of median age 75 years; all patients were BCG-refractory with a mean of three prior intravesical treatments, nine patients undergoing only BCG therapy and nine undergoing BCG-interferon therapy (Table 13.1). Over the course of 108 intravesical treatments, 108 HPLC serum measurements demonstrated undetectable levels of docetaxel. Eight patients (44%) experienced grade 1 or 2 local toxicities. Ten patients (56%) experienced no toxicity, and no toxicities were encountered at the highest dose of docetaxel. No systemic toxicities were observed.

Although the study was not formally designed to evaluate efficacy and was therefore not powered to make any clear conclusions regarding efficacy, cancer control response rates were promising. Ten patients (56%) demonstrated a complete response to the combination of bladder resection and intravesical docetaxel; two patients (11%) achieved a partial response defined as a negative final biopsy but persistent positive cytology; six patients (33%) had no clinical response to the treatment protocol (Table 13.2). Four of the six patients with no response proceeded to cystectomy without progression to muscle-invasive disease. Figure 13.1 illustrates the long-term results in this population; 39% of patients remained free of disease recurrence without further intravesical therapy or cystectomy.

TABLE 13.1. Cohort characteristics.

Characteristic	Patients (*n*)
Mean age (range)	75 (39–89)
Sex	
Male	16
Female	2
Clinical stage	
Tis	5
Ta	7
T1	1
Ta + Tis	1
T1 + Tis	4
Prior therapy with BCG	18
BCG alone	9
BCG + IFN	9
Prior BCG + chemotherapy	4
Mitomycin	2
Valrubicin	1
Thiotepa	1

TABLE 13.2. Clinical response to intravesical taxotere.

Patient #	Dose (mg)	Pretrial Stage	Response
1	5	HG Ta	Complete
2	5	Tis	Complete
3	5	T1 + Tis	Complete
6	10	HG Ta	Complete
7	20	HG Ta	Complete
8	20	Tis	Complete
9	20	HG Ta	Complete
13	60	HG Ta	Complete
15	60	T1	Complete
18	75	Tis	Complete
12	40	Tis	Partial
17	75	T1 + Tis	Partial
4	10	HG Ta + Tis	No
5	10	Tis	No
10	40	HG Ta	No
11	40	HG Ta	No
14	60	T1 + Tis	No
16	75	T1	No

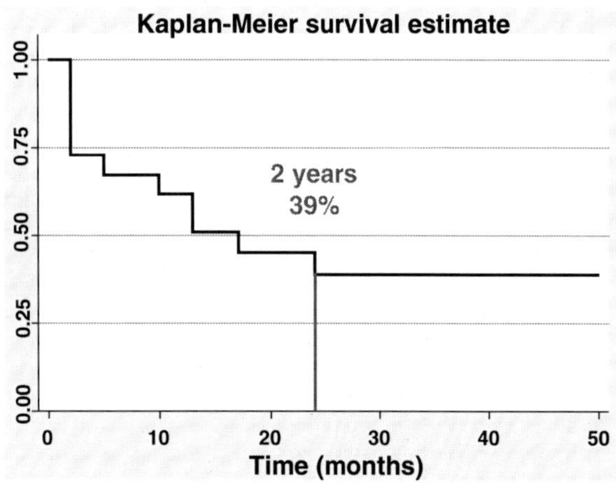

FIG. 13.1. Disease-free survival maintained without further intravesical treatment or cystectomy

The phase I trial, despite investigating a heavily pretreated population, demonstrated promising results for patients failing BCG treatments. First, a low percentage of patients experienced side effects and those side effects were of relatively low consequence. In contrast, patients receiving BCG as first-line treatment have experienced local and systemic toxicity rates of 19 and 44% respectively, with a significant number of patients experiencing the severe complications of BCG sepsis and pneumonitis (21). Second, as stated earlier in this chapter, response rates following failure of initial intravesical therapy often portends response rates to secondary treatment between 20 and 40%. Therefore the response rate of 67% although inconclusive, is promising for future studies.

4. The Future of Taxanes

The taxanes are steadily improving our treatment of bladder cancer. Systemic chemotherapy regimens have demonstrated efficacy in the treatment of advanced bladder cancer and the promising results of early studies of intravesical therapy are capable of changing the course of BCG-refractory superficial bladder cancers. Future areas of investigation may include an additional phase I study of protein-bound paclitaxel (Abraxane) at concentrations five times those achieved in the previous phase I trial, as well as subsequent phase II trials to determine the role that taxanes will assume in the treatment of superficial bladder cancer.

References

1. Kim SC, Steinberg GD. Medical management of patients with refractory carcinoma in situ of the bladder. Drugs Aging 18:335–344, 2001.
2. Malmström P-U, Wijkström, Lundholm C, et al. 5-year followup of a randomized prospective study comparing mitymycin C and bacillus Calmette-Guérin in patients with superficial bladder carcinoma. J Urol 161:1124–1127, 1999.
3. Steinberg G, Bahnson R, Brosman S, et al. Efficacy and safety of valrubicin for the treatment of bacillus Calmette-Guérin refractory carcinoma in situ of the bladder. Valrubicin Study Group. J Urol 163:761–767, 2000.
4. Palapattu GS, Haisfield-Wolfe ME, Walker JM, et al. Assessment of perioperative psychological distress in patients undergoing radical cystectomy for bladder cancer. J Urol 172:1814–1817, 2004.
5. Parkinson JP, Konety BR: Health related quality of life assessments for patients with bladder cancer. J Urol 172:2130–2136, 2004.
6. Babaian RJ, Smith DB. Effect of ileal conduit on patients' activities following radical cystectomy. Urology 37:33–35, 1991.
7. Crawford ED. Intravesical therapy for superficial cancer: need for more options. J Clin Oncol 20:3185–3186, 2002.
8. Bissey MC, Nohynek G, Sanderink GJ, et al. Docetaxel (Taxotere(R)): a review of preclinical and clinical experience. Part I: preclinical experience. AntiCancer Drugs 6:339–355; 363–8, 1995.
9. Hennequin C, Fiocanti N, Favaudon V. S-phase specificity of cell killing of docetaxel (Taxotere) in synchronised HeLa cells. Br J Cancer 71:1194–1198, 1995.
10. Rangel C, Niell H, Miller A, et al. Taxol and taxotere in bladder cancer: in vitro activity and urine stability. Cancer Chemother Pharmacol 33:460–464, 1994.

11. Roth BJ, Dreicer R, Einhorn LH et al. Significant activity of paclitaxel in advanced transitional cell carcinoma of the urothelium: a phase II trial of the Eastern Cooperative Oncology Group. J Clin Oncol 12: 2264–70, 1994.
12. deWit R, Kruit WH, Stoter G, et al. Docetaxel (Taxotere): an active agent in metastatic urothelial cancer; results of a phase II study in non-chemotherapy-pretreated patients. Br J Cancer 78:1342–1345, 1998.
13. Gitlitz BJ, Baker C, Chapman Y, et al. A phase II study of gemcitabine and docetaxel therapy in patients with advanced urothelial carcinoma. Cancer 98:1863–1869, 2003.
14. Pectasides D, Glotsos J, Bountouroglou N, et al. Weekly chemotherapy with docetaxel, gemcitabine and cisplatin in advanced transitional cell urothelial cancer: a phase II trial. Ann Oncol 13:243–250, 2002.
15. Garcia del Muro X, Marcuello E, Guma J, et al. Phase II multicentre study of docetaxel plus cisplatin in patients with advanced urothelial cancer. Br J Cancer 86:326–330, 2002.
16. Pectasides D, Visvikis A, Aspropotamitis A, et al. Chemotherapy with cisplatin, epirubicin and docetaxel in transitional cell urothelial cancer. Phase II trial. Eur J Cancer 36:74–79, 2000.
17. Uchio EM, Linehan WM, Figg WD, et al. A phase I study of intravesical suramin for the treatment of superficial transitional cell carcinoma of the bladder. J Urol 169:357–360, 2003.
18. Messing E, Catalona. Urothelial tumors of the urinary tract. In: Walsh PC, Retik AB, Vaughan ED, Wein AJ (eds.) Campbell's Urology, 7rd Ed., vol. 3. PhiladelphiaP: WB Saunders Company, 2327–2410, 1998.
19. Song D, Wientjes MG, Au JL. Bladder tissue pharmacokinetics of intravesical taxol. Cancer Chemother Pharmacol 40:285–292, 1997.
20. McKiernan JM, Masson P, Murphy AM, Goetzl M, Olsson CA, Petrylak DP, Desai M, Benson MC. Phase I trial of intravesical docetaxel in the management of superficial bladder cancer refractory to standard intravesical therapy. J Clin Oncol 24(19):3075–80, 2006.
21. Shelley MD, Wilt TJ, Court J, Coles B, Kynaston H and Mason MD. Intravesical bacillus Calmette-Guerin is superior to mitomycin C in reducing tumour recurrence in high-risk superficial bladder cancer: a meta-analysis of randomized trials. BJU International 93:485–90, 2004.

Section 2

Cystectomy: Cancer Control and Organ Preservation

14
Extended Lymph Node Dissection

Michael E. Woods and Marcus L. Quek

Contents

Abstract Radical cystectomy with pelvic lymphadenectomy remains the standard therapy for high-grade invasive bladder cancer with well-documented oncological outcomes. Several studies have demonstrated the prognostic and therapeutic benefits of an appropriately performed lymph node dissection. While the need for pelvic lymphadenectomy in the management of bladder cancer is clear, the optimal template or number of lymph nodes that should be removed remains controversial. The historical evolution and current role of an extended pelvic lymphadenectomy in the management of bladder cancer is the focus of this chapter.

Keywords Bladder neoplasms, Lymphadenectomy, Lymph nodes, Prognosis, Cystectomy, Lymph node dissection

1. Introduction

Urothelial carcinoma of the bladder is the fifth most common malignancy in the United States. It is estimated that during 2006, approximately 61,420 new cases of bladder cancer will be diagnosed and nearly 13,060 deaths will result from the disease (1).

From: *Current Clinical Urology: Bladder Cancer*, Edited by: C.T. Lee and D.P. Wood,
DOI: 10.1007/978-1-59745-417-9_14,

Most cases are superficial at diagnosis, although 20–40% will present with or progress to muscle invasion (2). Invasive bladder cancer is a lethal disease with survival rates less then 15% at 2 years if left untreated (3). Radical cystectomy remains the standard therapy for clinically-localized bladder cancer with well-documented oncological outcomes (2, 4).

Despite improvements in radiographic imaging, about 25% of patients will have pathologic evidence of lymph node metastases at the time of radical cystectomy (4–7). The inclusion of a pelvic lymphadenectomy at the time of cystectomy provides both prognostic information and potential therapeutic benefit. Since patients with lymph node involvement are known to have worse survival rates (4, 7–9), accurate pathologic staging of these patients will identify those who may benefit most from adjuvant therapy. In addition, some node positive patients achieve long-term disease-free survival from cystectomy and pelvic lymphadenectomy alone, suggesting that the procedure may be curative in select patients (4, 8, 10–12). Improvements in surgical technique and perioperative care have decreased the morbidity and mortality rates of contemporary radical cystectomy (13, 14). The development of orthotopic lower urinary tract reconstruction has improved the quality of life for many patients and appears to be a viable option even for those with node positive disease (15). For these reasons, an appropriate pelvic lymph node dissection continues to be an integral part of the comprehensive management of muscle-invasive bladder cancer.

Lymphadenectomy is performed in the surgical management of many genitourinary malignancies. The benefit of a regional lymph node dissection has been clearly established in the management of testis and penile cancer. Several reports have also addressed its role in both renal cell and prostate carcinoma (16–21). The need for pelvic lymphadenectomy in the management of bladder cancer is clear, given the incidence of and adverse prognosis associated with lymph node involvement, but the optimal template or number of lymph nodes that should be removed has not been established. The rationale for an "extended" lymph node dissection in bladder cancer is to improve pathologic staging and potentially improve survival without increasing morbidity (4, 22). The historical evolution and current role of an extended pelvic lymphadenectomy in the management of bladder cancer is the focus of the remainder of this chapter.

2. Evolution of Lymphadenectomy in Bladder Cancer

The benefits of including a regional lymphadenectomy in addition to primary tumor excision were initially described for the management of locally-advanced breast cancer (23, 24). The uniformly poor outcomes of patients with subsequent local pelvic recurrences following simple cystectomy led to the initial reports on the role of a pelvic lymph node dissection in conjunction with wide excision of the bladder (25, 26). Colston and Leadbetter reported a cadaveric study involving 98 bladder cancer patients and found that 25% had metastatic disease localized to the lymphatic tissue of the pelvis and retroperitonium (27). This prompted a careful evaluation of the lymphatic drainage of the bladder to define the technique of pelvic lymphadenectomy for bladder cancer (25). Using this original template with the cephalad extent at the aortic bifurcation, a 26.6% incidence of node positive disease was found (25).

Whitmore and Marshall later reported on the long-term survival of two lymph node positive bladder cancer patients, demonstrating that a survival benefit was possible when lymphadenectomy was combined with cystectomy (28). They demonstrated a 16% survival at 5 years in a subset of patients with metastatic disease confined to the pelvis without local extension of the primary tumor into adjacent organs. In addition, there was no increased mortality for those 230 patients treated with pelvic lymph node dissection at the time of cystectomy, compared to their previous 113 simple cystectomies (28).

Dretler further confirmed the survival benefit of cystectomy with lymphadenectomy in a report on 35 patients who had pelvic lymph node metastases without evidence of distant spread or invasion of adjacent organs by the primary tumor (29). The patients were divided into two groups; those with 1–2 positive nodes and those with >2 positive nodes. A difference in 5-year survival of 33 vs. 8.7% was seen between the two groups, representing one of the first reports demonstrating the prognostic significance of lymph node tumor burden. A final point from the Dretler study worth mentioning is the 2.8% mortality rate. This confirmed the safety of routinely including pelvic lymphadenectomy during cystectomy (29).

In 1982, Skinner reported his experience with 153 patients undergoing radical cystectomy with a meticulous pelvic lymph node dissection (30). Thirty-six patients (24%) were found to have positive lymph nodes. This report further supported the therapeutic benefits of lymphadenectomy in the face of node positive disease as these patients experienced a 5-year survival of 36%. The dissection used by Skinner extended proximally 2 cm above the aortic bifurcation. Only in 2 of 22 patients with tumor relapse was the recurrence in the pelvis, thus demonstrating the excellent local control rates possible with radical cystectomy and extended lymphadenectomy. He also noted within this analysis that patients with <3 positive lymph nodes compared to patients with >3 had improved survival. These findings suggest that patients with clinically undetectable micrometastases might benefit most from a meticulous pelvic lymph node dissection (30).

Despite improvements in radiographic staging techniques, there has been little stage migration observed over time for invasive bladder cancer. The chance of finding positive nodes at cystectomy has remained relatively stable at about 25% since Colston and Leadbetter's report in 1936 (27). Novel molecular markers and imaging modalities may some day allow for improved detection of nodal disease and select appropriate patients for neoadjuvant or adjuvant targeted therapies. Until then, an extended pelvic lymph node dissection will continue to play an important prognostic role in the overall management of invasive urothelial cancer.

3. Anatomic Basis for an Extended Pelvic Lymphadenectomy

An appreciation of the lymphatic drainage of the bladder is critical if one is to understand the anatomic rationale for an extended lymph node dissection. Lymphatic involvement with tumor will typically (though not always) follow a stepwise pattern through the following lymphatic channels and nodal groups (25)

- Visceral lymphatic plexus: Complex of lymphatic channels within the submucosal layer of the bladder that penetrates the detrusor to involve the serosal surface.
- Intercalated lymph nodes – nodes that lie within perivesical fat and receive drainage from the visceral plexus.
- Pelvic collecting trunks – lymphatic channels that coalesce after receiving drainage from the intercalated nodes and course toward the external iliac and hypogastric region.
- Regional pelvic lymph nodes – external iliac, internal iliac / hypogastric, and presacral lymph nodes.
- Lymphatic trunks- channels that drain from the regional pelvic lymph nodes to the common iliac lymph nodes.
- Common iliac lymph nodes – nodal group surrounding the common iliac vessels. These groups of nodes also serve to connect the pelvic to aortocaval (and upper retroperitoneal) lymph nodes (the second and third tier in the lymphatic echelon for the bladder).

Surgical series since the 1980s have described the local spread of bladder cancer further illustrating the lymphatic drainage of the bladder. Smith and Whitmore reported their outcomes in 134 patients with node positive disease from a series of 662 patients undergoing cystectomy and lymphadenectomy (31). The most common location for metastases was the obturator and external iliac lymph nodes, 74 and 65%, respectively. There was a 16–17% incidence of involvement of the hypogastric and perivesical nodes and nearly 20% involvement of the common iliac chain. This relatively high incidence of common iliac involvement highlights the need to include this region during lymphadenectomy. The template of dissection from this series included tissue extending 2 cm above the bifurcation of the iliac vessels, and there was a 25% incidence of isolated local recurrence in the node positive group. Stein et al. reported 13% local recurrence in a similar group of patients in whom the cephalad extent of the lymphadenectomy was at the level of the inferior mesenteric artery (IMA), suggesting that a benefit exists by further cephalad extension of the template (4).

A multi-center, prospective study from Leissner and colleagues evaluated the lymphatic spread and distribution of metastases in lymph node positive patients (32). An extended lymphadenectomy template to the level of the IMA, including presacral nodal tissue, was divided into 12 regions to evaluate the incidence and pathway of tumor spread within the template. By correlating these results with the location of the primary tumor within the bladder, the laterality of spread was further defined. The study involved 290 patients over a 3-year period with reported incidence of positive nodal disease ranging from 14% in the right obturator to 2.9% in the paracaval nodes. Even for unilaterally-confined primary tumors, contralateral spread was found at all levels (32). Although a unilateral dissection or sentinel node excision has been advocated in the past (33), this study further supported the importance of routinely performing a bilateral dissection, regardless of the location of the primary tumor (5, 11).

This study also classified lymph node metastases into three levels – distal to the bifurcation of the iliac vessels, between aortic bifurcation and bifurcation of the iliac vessels, and between the IMA and the bifurcation of the aorta. Based on this classification, if the dissection was performed in "standard" fashion (proximal extent being the bifurcation of the common iliac vessels), 6.9% of patients would not have been diagnosed with node positive disease and 43.7% of all positive lymph nodes would have been left behind. Of all patients with a single positive node, 10% of the cases were located above the bifurcation of the common iliac vessels.

Bochner et al. published a report prospectively, evaluating the factors affecting lymph node counts in 144 patients. They noted that 4 of 12 patients with grossly negative lymph nodes had metastatic disease present in the common iliac lymph nodes, supporting these authors' belief of routinely extending the lymphadenectomy to include the common iliac chain (34). This pattern of spread suggests that skip lesions are possible and that a sentinel node may not be readily identifiable for bladder cancer, as has been defined in other malignancies (35).

This is in contrast to a report by Abol-Enein et al., in which there was no nodal involvement above the bifurcation of the iliac vessels without the involvement of the obturator or internal iliac nodal groups (5). In this single-center, prospective evaluation of lymphadenectomy specimens, the authors concluded that the obturator/internal iliac lymph nodes do represent a sentinel nodal region and that if these nodes are negative on frozen section then more cephalic dissection can be avoided.

Vazina et al. reported a retrospective study evaluating the incidence and location of lymph node metastases by pathologic T-stage (36). The incidence of positive lymph nodes did increase with T stage, but involvement of common iliac, presacral, and distal paraaortic nodes was seen in all T-stages (T2–T4). This study lends additional support to the view that an extended lymphadenectomy may benefit patients undergoing radical cystectomy regardless of the extent of the primary tumor.

4. Incidence of Node Positive Bladder Cancer

4.1. Autopsy Series

The malignant potential of bladder cancer was reported by Cunningham in a large autopsy series in the early 1900s (37). The series included 411 patients with an overall rate of local and distant metastases of 32.4%. Colston and Leadbetter evaluated 98 patients post mortem who died from bladder cancer to determine the extent of metastases. They determined that 25% of patients had direct lymphatic spread to pelvic and retroperitoneal lymph nodes (27). In 1946, Jewett and Strong published an autopsy study correlating the depth of invasion of the primary tumor with the incidence of metastatic spread (38). There were no lymph node metastases for tumors isolated to the submucosa. With muscular infiltration there was a 7% incidence of metastases and this increased to 58% with the presence of perivesical fat infiltration. This study was significant for being one of the first to correlate the depth of invasion of the primary tumor with metastases. Another interesting aspect of this report was the number of patients with limited local nodal involvement alone, suggesting that for select node positive patients, pelvic lymphadenectomy could be curative.

4.2 Surgical Series

The incidence of lymph node metastases in patients undergoing radical cystectomy ranges from 14 to 32.4% (4, 7, 9, 14, 31–33, 36). Jewett and Strong's autopsy observation of increasing lymph node involvement with depth of invasion has been confirmed by many radical cystectomy series. The incidence of lymph node metastases for superficial (Tis,Ta,T1), T2, T3, and T4 disease has been reported to be 1.8–9.6%, 15.6–19.4%, 38.8–49%, and 42–75%, respectively (4, 7, 9, 14, 32, 36). These series are summarized in Table 14.1.

5. Factors Affecting Lymph Node Counts During Lymphadenectomy

The identification of both positive and negative lymph nodes appears to provide important prognostic information and potential therapeutic benefit. Several factors play a role in the absolute number of lymph nodes evaluated in lymphadenectomy specimens following radical cystectomy.

TABLE 14.1. Incidence of lymph node metastasis by pathologic T stage after radical cystectomy.

Study	Total number of patients	Percentage with lymph node metastasis	pTis, pTa, pT1	pT2	pT3	pT4
Stein et al. (4)	1,054	24	5	18	38.8	42
Vazina et al. (36)	176	24.4	3.6	15.6	40	50
Abdel-Latif et al. (9)	418	26.3	3.9	18	47.8	65
Leissner et al. (32)	290	27.9	1.8	18.3	44.2	50
Leissner et al. (7)	447	32.4	9.6	19.4	49	75
Poulsen et al. (14)	194	26	2.6	18	43	44

These factors are related to inherent patient variability, pathologic evaluation, surgeon's characteristics, as well as the template used for lymph node dissection. Patient factors such as age, obesity, prior treatment, and comorbidities affect lymph node counts (39).

5.1. Pathologic Evaluation

The role of the pathologist is central in lymph node identification. The diligence to locate small, grossly negative nodes will vary among and within institutions. The use of fat clearing techniques may alter pathologists' ability to locate lymph nodes. The effect of submitting specimens en bloc or in separate packets has been evaluated prospectively. It was demonstrated that lymph node counts increased from 2.4 to 8.5 in a standard template and from 22.6 to 36.5 lymph nodes with an extended template when the specimens were submitted as separate packets as opposed to an "en bloc" fashion (40). The authors concluded that with bulky en bloc specimens it was more likely that only palpable or grossly positive nodes would be identified. However, with individual, less bulky packets, it was easier for the pathologist to dissect and identify smaller lymph nodes. This approach has been adopted by others to improve pathologic accuracy (41).

Nodal counts have been shown to vary among surgeons with similar training and experience, despite using the same boundaries of dissection (7, 39). It can be assumed that the cause is multi-factorial. The contrary was seen in a report by Bochner et al., as they did not demonstrate any significant difference among four surgeons in a prospective study of 144 patients (40). Interestingly, the method of pathologic evaluation was standardized during the study, which included 20 different pathologists, a fact that may have contributed to the consistency of nodal counts within this study.

5.2. Surgical Boundaries

Skinner described the template for an "extended" lymph node dissection (42). The distal extent is the circumflex iliac vein and lymph node of Cloquet (or Rosenmuller), including all lymphatic tissue posterior to the obturator nerve lying between the pelvic sidewall and the bladder and rectum. The lateral extent is the genitofemoral nerve bilaterally. Bilateral presciatic and presacral tissue is included. The cephalad extent of the extended dissection is the IMA, including distal paracaval and paraaortic tissue. A "standard" dissection template shares similar distal and lateral borders but the cephalad extent is typically up to the bifurcation of the iliac vessels and presacral tissue is not routinely included.

The boundaries of dissection have a significant impact on lymph node counts. In a multicenter study by Herr et al. the number of lymph nodes removed increased from 13 to 26 when an extended dissection was performed (39). Poulsen et al. found that by extending their dissection to the bifurcation of the aorta, the average lymph node counts increased from 14 to 25 (14). This was also reported by Bochner who experienced a greater than fourfold increase in lymph nodes removed (8.5–36.5) using an extended dissection (40). Similar results were reported by Gill and co-workers with laparoscopic pelvic lymphadenectomy, in which extension of the dissection to the proximal common iliacs, increased the number of lymph nodes removed from 3 to 21 (43). Since adopting the "extended" template and routinely submitting individual lymph node packets to the pathologist from 13 sites (Table 14.2), we have also noted a greater than fivefold increase in average node counts from 10 (range: 1–44) to 55 (range: 26–105) (unpublished data).

It is clear that many factors affect the absolute number of lymph nodes evaluated at the time of radical

TABLE 14.2. Lymph node packets submitted during extended pelvic lymphadenectomy.

Distal paracaval
Right common iliac
Distal paraaortic
Left common iliac
Right external iliac
Right lymph node of Cloquet
Right obturator/hypogastric
Left external iliac
Left lymph node of Cloquet
Left obturator/hypogastric
Right presciatic
Presacral
Left presciatic

cystectomy. Unfortunately, many of these factors are out of the surgeons' control. This being the case, the urologist needs to perform a careful dissection of all potentially involved lymph nodes and follow a set template regardless of the number of nodes reported by the pathologist to ensure that a complete and meticulous lymphadenectomy is consistently performed.

6. How many Lymph Nodes Should be Removed?

There is no consensus on the minimum number of lymph nodes that should be removed during lymphadenectomy for bladder cancer. Several authors have evaluated the lymph node counts following extended lymphadenectomy, with reported ranges from 14.7 to 50.6 (5, 7, 14, 32, 44). The wide variation within these studies is partially due to the fact that several are retrospective in nature (7, 14, 44). Abol-Enein et al. performed a prospective study evaluating a meticulous dissection with the proximal extent at the IMA, including presacral tissue (5). The average number of lymph nodes evaluated was 50.6 (range 21–99). The high yield experienced by these authors is largely due to the extended template and thorough dissection, but having been evaluated prospectively likely played a role as well. This is a fact that needs to be kept in mind when comparing outcomes and node counts in the literature.

Although there is no consensus on the optimum number of lymph nodes to be removed, several groups have made recommendations on the minimum number that should be evaluated. Leissner et al. stated that removal of 20 lymph nodes would be a reasonable goal (7). This was based on the fact that when <16 lymph nodes were removed, 60% of node positive patients were identified, whereas if 20 lymph nodes were removed, 80% of node positive patients were included. A large retrospective, multi-center study was conducted to evaluate radical cystectomy and pelvic lymph node dissection in an attempt to develop pathologic goals for the procedure (39). The study group included four high volume institutions and concluded that 10–14 lymph nodes should be removed during pelvic lymphadenectomy. A similar recommendation was made by Konety et al. in a retrospective review of the SEER database (Surveillance, Epidemiology, and End Results program) to determine the effect of lymph node dissection on the outcome of patients undergoing radical cystectomy (2). This study involved many institutions and surgeons and was subsequently more heterogeneous then the previous study (39). The authors concluded that the removal of 10–14 lymph nodes was a minimum to demonstrate adequacy of dissection and pathologic evaluation to obtain appropriate staging. This range was chosen based on the improved survival in this group of patients. As previously stated, caution should be taken when interpreting these reports as they are based on retrospective studies.

Herr analyzed the surgical factors within a multi-institutional prospective study designed to evaluate the role of neoadjuvant chemotherapy. The study enrolled 317 patients who were randomized to cystectomy alone or chemotherapy followed by cystectomy (45). Two hundred and seventy patients underwent cystectomy. There was variability in the extent of lymphadenectomy, with 24 patients receiving no dissection at all. The survival was significantly different between patients with >10 vs. <10 lymph nodes removed. Further analysis of surgical factors demonstrated that the extent of lymph node dissection, number of lymph nodes removed, and surgeon experience were significant factors affecting survival. Interestingly, these factors were more important than if preoperative chemotherapy was given or not (46). He hypothesized that increased node counts resulted in improved survival for the following reasons: a diminished risk of local and regional recurrence by removal of micrometastatic disease, more complete dissection with wider margins, and a more thorough evaluation by the pathologist that can improve staging. This report highlights the role of surgery in the comprehensive management of muscle-invasive bladder cancer.

7. Morbidity of Pelvic Lymphadenectomy

Modern anesthetic and perioperative care, along with improved surgical techniques, have greatly reduced the mortality rate of patients undergoing radical cystectomy. Despite these improvements, overall complication rates are still significant. This patient population is at particularly high risk for postoperative complications given their age and commonly associated comorbidities. There exists little debate that a pelvic lymph node dissection should be performed at the time of cystectomy, although the extent of dissection has not been defined. An extended lymph node dissection may provide improved staging accuracy and survival, but does it cause any additional morbidity and mortality? Mortality rates of 1–2.5% and complication rates of 17–28% have been reported in radical cystectomy series using extended lymph node dissections (4, 5). In a recent analysis of mortality following radical cystectomy and extended pelvic lymphadenectomy from a single high volume center, Quek et al. noted an overall mortality rate of 2% (47). Of note, this rate dropped to 1% in the last 10 years of this series. This is comparable with other large cystectomy series employing a standard lymph node dissection (48–51). Obviously, certain factors may affect the ability to perform a pelvic lymph node dissection, such as prior pelvic radiotherapy, surgery, and individual anatomy. The urologic surgeon should consider such factors on an individual basis when determining the feasibility and extent of lymphadenectomy.

Brössner et al. specifically evaluated this question in a contemporary retrospective review of 92 patients (22). They found no difference in short-term complications for patients undergoing an extended lymphadenectomy, although the operative time was on average 63 min longer. In a single center study, Poulsen et al. did not experience any increase in morbidity when they changed to an extended template after their first 68 patients (14). The rate of lymphoceles and lymphedema was evaluated in a series of 447 patients by the number of lymph nodes removed. An extended template was used in all patients. In patients with <16 lymph nodes removed there was a 2% incidence of lymphocele and lymphedema formation versus 1.1% in patients with ≥16 lymph nodes removed (7). Despite the fact that there does not exist any prospective trial comparing the outcomes of a standard versus an extended pelvic lymph node dissection with radical cystectomy, from the available data there does not appear to be any increased morbidity associated with an extended lymphadenectomy in appropriately selected patients.

8. Pathologic Factors Associated with Prognosis and Therapeutic Benefit in Bladder Cancer

The routine use of an extended pelvic lymph node dissection in bladder cancer is a debated topic despite reports to suggest improved clinical outcomes (52). Although, there exist an abundance of retrospective reviews that have correlated the extent of lymphadenectomy with patient survival, there are currently no prospective, randomized trials to assess this issue with regard to cancer specific and overall survival.

8.1. Total Number of Lymph Nodes Removed

The number of lymph nodes removed during pelvic lymphadenectomy can be used as a surrogate marker for the thoroughness of the dissection performed. In 1998 Poulsen reported a small 5-year recurrence-free survival benefit of 6% between patients who underwent an extended versus a standard lymph node dissection (25 vs. 14 lymph nodes removed). This difference did not reach statistical significance for the entire cohort, although for the subset of patients with ≤T3a primary tumors the survival benefit did reach significance (14). A large, single-center study from Germany involving 447 patients demonstrated a significant improvement in 5-year disease-free survival in patients who had greater then 15 lymph nodes evaluated (65 vs. 51%) (7). Herr et al. noted that evaluation of <10 vs. ≥10 nodes resulted in decreased overall survival, 44 vs. 61% (53). In the review of the SEER database, Konety et al. demonstrated improved cancer-specific survival if patients had greater then three lymph nodes removed, but the greatest risk reduction was seen in patients with 10–14 lymph nodes removed (2). In 2002, Herr et al. reported their single-center experience on the effect of the number of lymph nodes removed in both node negative and node positive patients (6). The study included 322 patients who had not received either neoadjuvant or adjuvant therapy and who had been followed for 10 years. Five-year overall survival was improved in node negative patients when ≥8 compared to <8 lymph nodes were removed, 82 vs. 41%. A significant overall survival was seen in node positive patients as well. The cutoff for removed lymph nodes in this group was ≥11 or <11, with survival rates of 44 vs. 20%, respectively.

One possible explanation for the improved survival seen in these studies is improved staging. A more extensive lymphadenectomy may be detecting nodal metastases more accurately and creating bias within these retrospectives studies, although this cannot completely explain the survival benefit. Herr et al. noted a significant benefit in survival within the node positive cohort when a greater number of lymph nodes was removed (6). Since all of these patients were considered stage IV there should be no effect seen by more accurate staging and the survival benefit may in part be attributed to decreasing the tumor burden. This finding was confirmed by Stein et al. in a subset analysis of 244 patients with lymph node metastases from a series of 1,054 patients undergoing radical cystectomy (44). They noted a significant improvement in 10-year recurrence-free survival for patients with >15 vs. ≤15 lymph nodes removed, 36 vs. 25%, respectively. The survival benefit seen in this large cohort of node positive patients lends further support to the therapeutic role of an extended lymphadenectomy in bladder cancer.

8.2. Number of Positive Lymph Nodes Removed

As early as 1973, Dretler and colleagues noted a relationship between the number of positive lymph nodes removed and survival (29). They reported outcomes from a series of 35 lymph node positive patients following radical cystectomy. Patients with 1–2 positive nodes demonstrated a 33% 5-year survival compared to 8.7% for patients with >2 positive lymph nodes. Nearly a decade later Skinner reported his experience with a series of 153 patients, of which 36 were found to have lymph node metastasis (30). He found that patients with 1–5 vs. >5 positive lymph nodes experienced a 5-year overall survival of 46 and12.5%, respectively. Stein et al. recently updated this group's experience using a cut-off of ≤8 or >8 positive lymph nodes (44). The 10-year disease-specific survival was 40 and 10%, respectively. A study from Memorial Sloan Kettering of 686 patients demonstrated a 10-year disease-specific survival of 42 and 22% for patients who were pathologically N1 and N2, respectively (10). A single-center report from Mills et al. demonstrated improved overall survival for patients with <5 vs. ≥5 positive lymph nodes. There was a total of 83 node positive patients and the survival difference was 27 vs. 15 months (11). In a large contemporary series from Egypt, Abdel-Latif et al. reported 3-year overall survival at 59, 32, and 7% for patients with 1, 2–5, and >5 positive lymph nodes following radical cystectomy (9). From these studies with a collective experience of over 650 patients with lymph node metastases, there is compelling data that surgery alone may be curative for some patients with low volume metastatic disease. Clearly, the surgeon cannot control the number of lymph nodes that are positive, but a diligent excision of all lymphatic tissue draining the bladder will increase the probability that metastatic disease will be identified and removed.

8.3. Lymph Node Density

Several authors have evaluated the concept of lymph node density, which simply refers to the number of positive nodes divided by the total number removed. In early 2003, Herr published a report evaluating lymph node density in a cohort of 162 lymph node positive patients who were followed for 7.5 years (54). There was a significant improvement in 5-year survival for patients with <20 vs. >20% positive lymph nodes, 64 vs. 8% respectively. This was corroborated by Stein et al., also using a cutoff of 20% for lymph node density (44). This series evaluated the outcomes of 244 patients with lymph node metastases. They found that patients with <20% had a 10-year recurrence-free survival of 43 vs. 17% for patients with >20%. Abdel-Latif evaluated lymph node density using the following cutoffs; <10, 10–20, and >20% (9). The 3-year overall survival was 56, 39, and 16%, respectively. This survival advantage reached significance on univariate analysis, but not in multivariate analysis. The survival benefit seen with lower lymph node density is not surprising given that it is a ratio of positive lymph nodes and total lymph nodes removed, both of which have demonstrated prognostic significance as independent variables.

8.4. Extracapsular Extension of Lymph Node Metastases

Extracapsular extension of nodal metastases has also been evaluated as a possible prognostic marker in bladder cancer. This was first reported by Mills et al. in 2001. They demonstrated an overall survival of

93 vs. 16 months for patients without versus patients with lymph node capsule penetration with tumor (11). This group updated this series in 2005, which included 124 patients with lymph node positive disease (55). They again demonstrated that lymph node capsular penetration resulted in significantly worse 5-year recurrence-free survival on multivariate analysis. A similar trend was reported by Abdel-Latif et al., which showed a significantly worse 3-year overall survival with capsular penetration, 44 vs. 66% (9). Although on multivariate analysis the survival difference no longer reached significance, the significance of this pathologic finding clearly needs to be evaluated further. The reason for disease relapse and progression in these patients needs to be defined. The approach of lymphadenectomy may affect the outcomes in these patients as a more meticulous dissection may help negate the detrimental effects seen by lymph node capsular penetration.

9. Conclusion

Radical cystectomy remains the standard of care for muscle-invasive bladder cancer. There is no argument over the need for concurrent lymphadenectomy given the approximate 25% incidence of lymph node metastases and the long-term survival seen in select node-positive patients with surgery alone. Controversy does exist over the benefits of an extended pelvic lymph node dissection versus a standard approach. No prospective, randomized trial exists to evaluate this question. Multiple studies were presented throughout this chapter to support the benefit of an extended lymph node dissection. These studies used different parameters (lymph node counts, lymph node density) but fundamentally they represent thoroughness of dissection. Though retrospective in nature, these studies collectively represent a large number of patients and draw very similar conclusions regarding the benefits of a meticulous lymphadenectomy. The onus is on the surgeon to provide each patient with the best chance of cure from bladder cancer. With multiple factors contributing to node counts (many of which are beyond the control of the surgeon), one should focus on the dissection template to assure an adequate resection. As there appears to be little difference in morbidity compared to a more limited dissection, it is the authors' belief that a lymphadenectomy with the cephalad extent to the IMA should be considered in all patients undergoing radical cystectomy.

References

1. Jemal A, Siegel R, Ward E, Murray T, Xu J, Smigal C, Thun MJ. Cancer Statistics, 2006. CA Cancer J Clin 2006;56:106–130.
2. Konety BR, Joslyn SA, O'Donnell MA. Extent of pelvic lympadenectomy and its impact on outcome in patients diagnosed with bladder cancer: analysis of data from the surveillance, epidemiology, and end results program data base. J Urol 2003;169:946–950.
3. Prout GR, Marshall VF. The prognosis with untreated bladder tumors. Cancer 1956;9:551–558.
4. Stein JP, Lieskovsky G, Cote R, Groshen S, Feng A, Boyd S, Skinner E, Bochner B, Thangathurai D, Mikhail M, Raghavan D, Skinner DG. Radical Cystectomy in the treatment of invasive bladder cancer: long-term results in 1,054 patients. J Clin Oncology 2001;19:666–675.
5. Abol-Enein H, El-Baz M, Abd El-Hameed MA, Abdel-Latif M, Ghoneim MA. Lymph node involvement in patients with bladder cancer treated with radical cystectomy: a patho-anatomical study-a single center experience. J Urol 2004;172:1818–1821.
6. Herr HW, Bocher BH, Dalbagni G, Donat SM, Reuter VE, Bajorin DF. Impact of the number of lymph nodes retrieved on outcome in patients with muscle invasive bladder cancer. J Urol 2002;167:1295–1298.
7. Leissner J, Hohenfellner R, Thuroff JW, Wolf HK. Lymphadenectomy in patients with transitional cell carcinoma of the urinary bladder; significance for staging and prognosis. BJU Int 2000;85:817–823.
8. Roehrborn CG, Sagalowsky AI, Peters PC. Long-term patient survival after cystectomy for regional metastatic transitional cell carcinoma of the bladder. J Urol 1991;146:36–39.
9. Abdel-Latif M, Abol-Enein H, El-Baz M, Ghoneim MA. Nodal involvement in bladder cancer cases treated with radical cystectomy: incidence and prognosis. J Urol 2004;172:85–89.
10. Vieweg J, Gschwend JE, Herr HW, Fair WR. Pelvic lymph node dissection can be curative in patients with node positive bladder cancer. J Urol 1999;161:449–454.
11. Mills RD, Turner WH, Fleischmann A, Markwalder R, Thalmann GN, Studer UE. Pelvic lymph node metastases form bladder cancer: outcome in 83 patients after radical cystectomy and pelvic lymphadenectomy. J Urol 2001;166:19–23.
12. Dretler SP, Ragsdale BD, Leadbetter WF. The value of pelvic lymphadenectomy in the surgical treatment of bladder cancer. J Urol 1973;109:414–416.
13. Cookson MS, Chang SS, Wells N, Parekh DJ, Smith JA. Complications of radical cystectomy for nonmuscle invasive disease: comparison with muscle invasive disease. J Urol 2003;169:101–104.
14. Poulsen AL, Horn T, Steven K. Radical cystectomy: extending the limits of pelvic lymph node dissection improves survival for patients with bladder cancer confined to the bladder wall. J Urol 1998;160:2015–2020.
15. Lebret T, Herve J, Yonneau L, Molinie V, Barre P, Lugagne P, Butreau M, Laurent M, Botto H. After cystectomy, is it justified to perform a bladder replacement for patients with lymph node positive bladder cancer. Eur Urol 2002;42:344–349.
16. Allaf ME, Palapattu GS, Trock BJ, Carter HB, Walsh PC. Anatomic extent of lymph node dissection: impact on men with clinically localized prostate cancer. J Urol 2004;172:1840–1844.

17. Heidenreich A, Varga Z, Von Konbloch R. Extended pelvic lymphadenectomy in patients undergoing radical prostatectomy: high incidence of lymph node metastasis. J Urol 2002;167:1681–1686.
18. Schafhauser W, Ebert A, Brod J, Petsch S, Schrott KM. Lymph node involvement in renal cell carcinoma and survival chance by systematic lymphadencetomy. Anticancer Res 1999;19:1573–1578.
19. Terrone C, Guercio S, De Luca S, Poggio E, Castelli E, Scoffone C, Tarabuzzi R, Scarpa RM, Fontana D, Rocca Rossetti S. The number of lymph nodes examined and staging accuracy in renal cell carcinoma. BJU Int 2003;91:37–40.
20. Pantuck AJ, Zisman A, Dorey F, Chao DH, Han K, Said J, Gitlitz BJ, Figlin RA, Belldegrun AS. Renal cell carcinoma with retroperitoneal lymph nodes: role of lymph node dissection. J Urol 2003;169:2076–2083.
21. Barth PJ, Gerharz EW, Ramaswamy A, Reidmiller H. The influence of lymph node counts on the detection of pelvic lymph node metastasis in prostate cancer. Path Res Prac 1999;195:633–636.
22. Brössner C, Pycha A, Toth A, Mian C, Kuber W. Does extended lymphadenectomy increase the morbidity of radical cystectomy?. BJU Int 2004;93:64–66.
23. Halsted WS. The treatment of wounds. Johns Hopkins Hosp Rep 1891;2:279.
24. Taylor GW, Wallace RH. Carcinoma of the breast. End results: Massachusetts general hospital 1933–1935. N Engl J Med 1947;237:475–477.
25. Leadbetter WF, Cooper JF. Regional gland dissection for carcinoma of the bladder: a technique for one-stage cystectomy, gland dissection, and bilateral uretero-enterostomy. J Urol 1950;63:242–226.
26. Kerr WS, Colby FH. Pelvic lymphadenectomy and total cystectomy in the treatment of carcinoma of the bladder. J Urol 1950;63:842–851.
27. Colston JA, Leadbetter WF. Infiltrating carcinoma of the bladder. J Urol 1936;36:669–689.
28. Whitmore WF, Marshall VF. Radical total cystectomy for cancer of the bladder: 230 consecutive cases five years later. J Urol 1962;87:853–868.
29. Dretler SP, Ragsdale BD, Leadbetter WF. The value of pelvic lymphadenectomy in the surgical treatment of bladder cancer. J Urol 1973;109:414–416.
30. Skinner DG. Management of invasive bladder cancer: a meticulous pelvic lymph node dissection can make a difference. J Urol 1982;128:34–36.
31. Smith JA, Whitmore WF. Regional lymph node metastasis from bladder cancer. J Urol 1981;126:591–593.
32. Leissner J, Ghoneim MA, Abol-Enein H, Thuroff JW, Franzaring L, Fisch M, Schulze H, Managadze G, Allhaoff EP, El-Baz MA, Kastendieck H, Buhtz P, Kropf A, Hohenfellner R, Wolf HK. Extended radical lymphadenectomy in patients with urothelial bladder cancer: results of a prospective multicenter study. J Urol 2004;171:139–144.
33. Wishnow KI, Johnson DE, Ro JY, Swanson DA, Babian RJ, von Eschenbach AC. Incidence, extent and location of unsuspected pelvic lymph node metastasis in patient undergoing radical cystectomy for bladder cancer. J Urol 1987;137:408–410.
34. Bochner BH, Cho D, Herr HW, Donat M, Kattan MW, Dalbagni G. Prospectively packaged lymph node dissections with radical cystectomy: evaluation of node count variability and node mapping. J Urol 2004;172:1286–1290.
35. Cochran AJ, Roberts AA, Saida T. The place of lymphatic mapping and sentinel node biopsy in oncology. Int J Clin Oncol 2003;8:139–150.
36. Vazina A, Dugi D, Shariat SF, Evans J, Link R, Lerner SP. Stage specific lymph node metastasis mapping in radical cystectomy specimens. J Urol 2004;171:1830–1834.
37. Cunningham JH. Tumors of the Bladder. J Urol 1931;25:559–587.
38. Jewett HJ, Strong GH. Infiltrating carcinoma of the bladder: relation of depth of penetration of the bladder wall to incidence of local extension and metastases. J Urol 1946;55:366–372.
39. Herr H, Lee C, Chang S, Lerner S. for the bladder cancer collaborative group. Standardization of radical cystectomy and pelvic lymph node dissection for bladder cancer: a collaborative group report. J Urol 2004;171:1823–1828.
40. Bochner BH, Herr HW, Reuter VE. Impact of separate versus en bloc pelvic lymph node dissection on the number of lymph nodes retrieved in cystecomy specimens. J Urol 2001;166:2295–2296.
41. Quek ML, Sanderson KM, Daneshmand S, Stein JP. The importance of an extended lymphadenectomy in the management of high-grade invasive bladder cancer. Expert Rev Anticancer Ther 2004;4:1007–1016.
42. Skinner DG. Technique of radical cystectomy. Urol Clin N Am 1981;3:353–366.
43. Finelli A, Gill IS, Desai MM, Moinzadeh A, Magi-Galluzzi C, Kaouk JH. Laparoscopic extended pelvic lymphadenectomy for bladder cancer: technique and initial outcomes. J Urol 2004;172:1809–1812.
44. Stein JP, Cai J, Groshen S, Skinner DG. Risk factors for patients with pelvic lymph node metastases following radical cystectomy with en bloc pelvic lymphadenectomy: the concept of lymph node density. J Urol 2003;170:35–41.
45. Grossman HB, Natale RB, Tangen CM, Speights VO, Vogelzang NJ, Trump DL, deVere White RW, Sarosdy MF, Wood DP, Raghaven D, Crawford ED. Neoadjuvant chemotherapy plus cystectomy compared with cystectomy alone for locally advanced bladder cancer. N Engl J Med 2003;349:859–866.
46. Herr HW. Surgical factors in bladder cancer: more (nodes) + more (pathology) = less (mortality). BJU Int 2003;92: 187–188.
47. Quek ML, Stein JP, Daneshmand S, Miranda G, Thangathurai D, Roffey P, Skinner EC, Lieskovsky G, Skinner DG. A critical analysis of perioperative mortality from radical cystectomy. J Urol 2006;175:886–890.
48. Chang SS, Cookson MS, Baumgartner RG, Wells N, Smith JA. Analysis of early complications after radical cystectomy: results of a collaborative care pathway. J Urol 2002;167:2012–2016.
49. Ghoneim MA, El-Mekresh MM, El-Baz MA, El-Attar IA, Ashamallah A. Radical cystectomy for carcinoma of the bladder: critical evaluation of the results of 1,026 cases. J Urol 1997;158:393–399.
50. Rosario DJ, Becker M, Anderson JB. The changing pattern of mortality and morbidity from radical cystectomy. BJU Int 2000;85:427–430.
51. Frazier HA, Robertson JE, Paulson DF. Complications of radical cystectomy and urinary diversion: a retrospective review of 675 cases in 2 decades. J Urol 1992;148:1401–1405.

52. Herr HW, Donat M. Outcome of patients with grossly node positive bladder cancer after pelvis lymph node dissection and radical cystectomy. J Urol 2001;165:62–64.
53. Herr HW, Faulkner JR, Grossman B, Natale RB, deVere White R, Sarosdy MF, Crawford ED. Surgical factors influence bladder cancer outcomes: a cooperative group report. J Clin Oncology 2004;22:2781–2789.
54. Herr HW. Superiority of ratio based lymph node staging for bladder cancer. J Urol 2003;169:943–945.
55. Fleischmann A, Thalmann GN, Markwalder R, Studer UE. Extracapsular extension of pelvic lymph node metastases from urothelial carcinoma of the bladder is an independent prognostic factor. J Clin Oncology 2005;23: 2358–2365.

15
Prostate Capsule Sparing Cystectomy

Alon Z. Weizer and Timothy Schuster

Contents

Abstract While an effective local therapy for organ confined bladder cancer, radical cystoprostatectomy is also associated with significant morbidity in terms of urinary and sexual function in addition to body image. Orthotopic urinary diversion addresses some but not all of these issues. Prostate capsule sparing is an alternative approach which leaves the peripheral zone capsule for anastomosis to a neobladder. While the literature has reported excellent functional outcomes for this approach, concerns over residual prostate cancer, local recurrence and metastatic disease necessitate appropriate selection of the patient for this procedure. However, careful selection has the potential to improve functional outcomes without compromising cancer control.

Keywords Bladder neoplasms, Prostatic neoplasms, Cystectomy, Prostate, Urinary incontinence

1. Introduction

Radical cystoprostatectomy (Radical Cystetomy) remains the predominant treatment for muscle invasive and high grade nonmuscle invasive cancer of the bladder refractory to intravesical chemotherapy. While an effective local treatment for these selected patients, RADICAL CYSTETOMY significantly impacts the patient's urinary and sexual function. Several modifications have been proposed to improve these functions in patients following RADICAL CYSTETOMY. A major advance has been the development of the orthotopic urinary diversion. While this allows the patient to void normally through his or her native urethra, problems may exist with diurnal or nocturnal continence as well as hypercontinence necessitating intermittent catheterization (1).

In an attempt to improve urinary control and preserve sexual function, several additional modifications have

From: *Current Clinical Urology: Bladder Cancer,* Edited by: C.T. Lee and D.P. Wood,
DOI; 10.1007/978-1-59745-417-9_15,

been proposed. Experience with nerve-sparing radical retropubic prostatectomy has lead to the development of a similar procedure for men undergoing RADICAL CYSTETOMY with orthotopic neobladder (2) with improved urinary continence and potency as reported (2–4). Prostate capsule sparing cystectomy represents another alternative to standard RADICAL CYSTETOMY for preservation of urinary and sexual function. Several retrospective studies have evaluated preservation of part or all of the prostate gland to improve urinary control and preserve the neurovascular bundles that control erectile function (5–7). With this technique, the prostate adenoma is separated from the prostate peripheral zone/capsule (PZC) that is then left *in situ* for anastomosis to the neobladder.

Despite these promising functional results, concerns have been raised about leaving prostate cancer or urothelial cancer in the prostate PZC (8). In addition, some studies have raised concern regarding an increased risk of local recurrence in the pelvis and of metastatic disease with less radical surgery. This chapter will review the surgical approach to prostate capsule sparing cystectomy. The oncologic concerns as well as the sexual and urinary outcomes will be reviewed in order to suggest possible indications and contraindications to this surgical approach in the management of the cancer of the bladder.

2. Surgical Approach

The primary goal of prostate capsule sparing cystectomy is to remove the bladder while preserving the external urethral sphincter and avoid damaging the neurovascular bundles that contribute to sexual function. After standard surgical preparation and scrub, an infraumbilical midline incision is made, the peritoneum is entered at the superior portion of the incision and the urachus is identified and ligated. The peritoneum on either side of the bladder is incised to the level of the vas deferens which are mobilized and preserved in select patients.

The peritoneum is mobilized along the line of Toldt cephalad bilaterally and the ureters are identified and mobilized towards the bladder inferiorly. The obliterated umbilical arteries are then ligated when identified. In addition the superior vesical arteries on either side are identified and ligated. A distal ureteral margin is sent for frozen section analysis.

The posterior peritoneum is divided in the pouch of Douglas. The plane of dissection is closer to the bladder (several centimeters above the most dependent portion Fig. 15.1) here than the standard RADICAL CYSTETOMY in order to identify the seminal vesicles which are preserved and mobilized away from the base

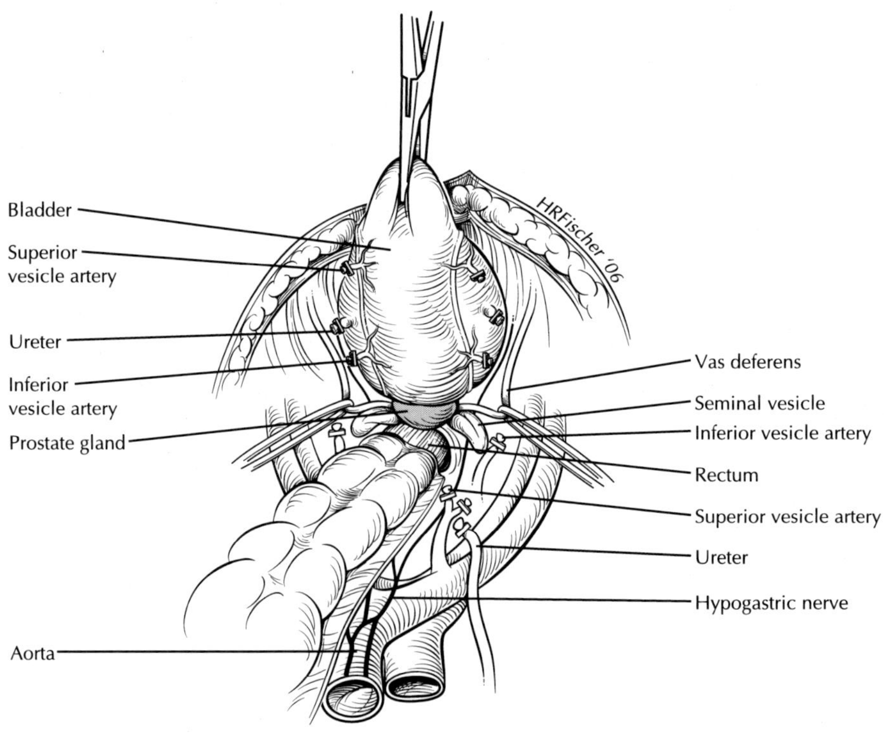

FIG. 15.1. Antegrade dissection for prostate capsule sparing cystectomy

of the bladder. This maneuver is performed in order to preserve the neurovascular bundles which can be injured at this point. The antegrade plane of dissection is performed until the endopelvic fascia is reached laterally and the seminal vesicals are identified medially.

Following antegrade dissection, the endopelvic fascia is opened on either side of the prostate. A single absorbable suture line is placed parallel to the bladder neck similar to a Millin retropubic prostatectomy (9). The prostate capsule is then entered proximal to the suture line using electrocautery or thermal energy (Fig. 15.2). The prostate adenoma is then separated from the capsule using a combination of blunt and sharp dissection. The urethra is identified and divided and the adenoma is then separated from the posterior prostate capsule. The posterior bladder neck is identified and divided removing the bladder and prostate adenoma intact and leaving the prostate capsule/peripheral zone in situ (Fig. 15.3). A distal urethral margin from the adenoma is obtained for a frozen section followed by hemostasis. The adenoma is also sent for frozen section analysis.

An extended lymph node dissection is performed bilaterally to the level of the common iliac vessels (10). A neobladder is then fashioned as described by

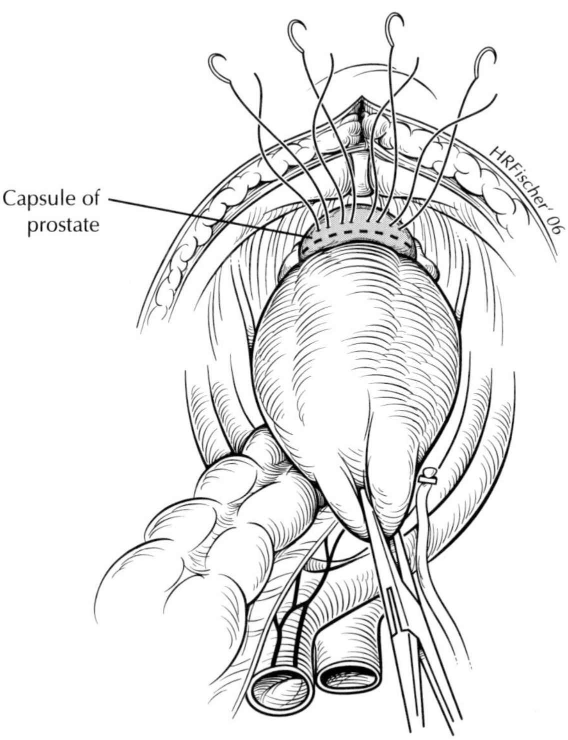

Fig. 15.2. Hemostasis prior to capsular incision for prostate capsule sparing cystectomy

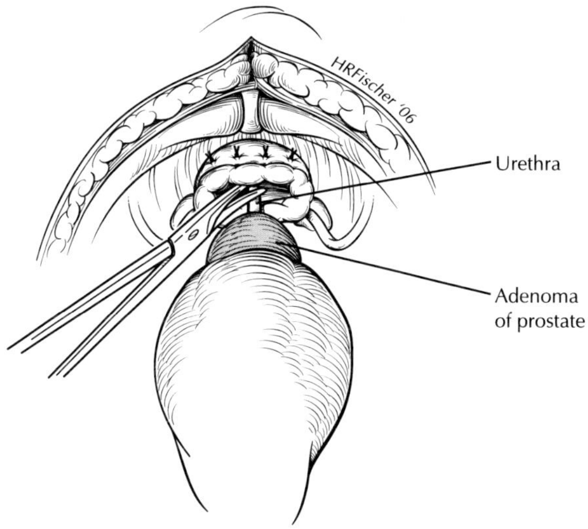

Fig. 15.3. Prostate adenoma is separated with bladder from prostate peripheral zone/capsule

Hautmann (11). The neobladder is anastomosed to the prostate peripheral zone/capsule using absorbable suture in a running fashion closing the posterior anastomosis first (Fig. 15.4). The ureteral stents are brought through the neobladder wall and the bladder is drained with a 20 French foley catheter. Patient management postoperatively is similar to that described for a RADICAL CYSTETOMY/neobladder (12).

2.1. Alternative Approaches to Prostate Capsule Sparing Cystectomy

1. In addition to the standard open approach that we use at our institution, several alternatives have been reported in the literature. Several authors have described performing a standard transurethral resection (TURP) prior to a prostate capsule sparing cystectomy. Vallancien and colleagues performed a TURP under the same anesthetic or a few days prior to surgery from the bladder neck to the verumontanum avoiding capsular penetration. The mucosal and transitional zone chips are examined by frozen section to identify transitional cell carcinoma. The cystectomy is then performed. A foley balloon is used to identify the prostatovesical junction and the prostate is divided 3–5 mm distal to that area. A frozen section of the prostate capsule is sent to ensure negative margins (5).
2. A similar procedure has been described by the same group utilizing a laparoscopic technique. Five transperitoneal trocars are placed along the level of

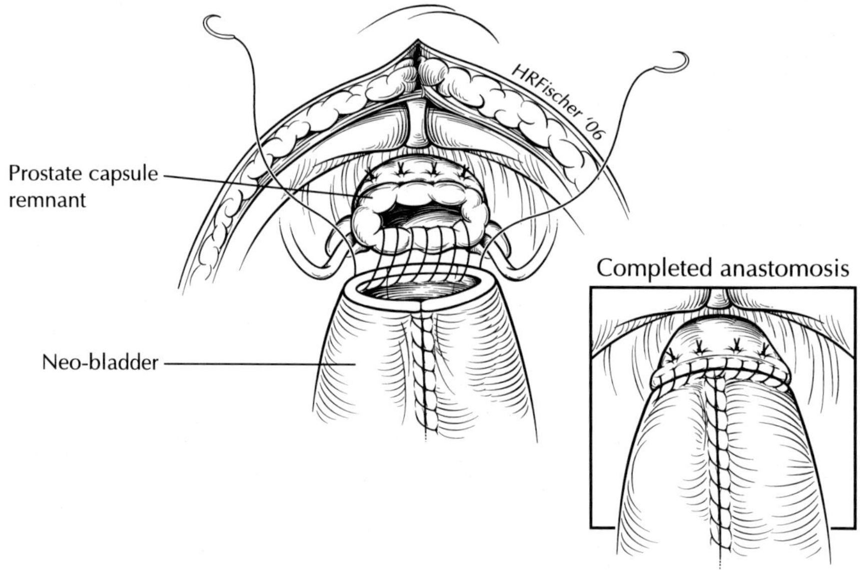

FIG. 15.4. Neobladder is anastomosed to prostate peripheral zone capsule

the umbilicus. A bilateral pelvic lymph node dissection is performed first. The ureters are ligated distally with Hem-o-lock clips and margins are sent for frozen section analysis. The peritoneum in the pouch of Douglas is incised and the vasa and seminal vesicals are identified and mobilized. The space of Retzius is then developed releasing the bladder from the anterior abdominal wall. The prostate capsule is incised distal to the bladder neck and the adenoma is removed using monopolar and bipolar energy. The bladder neck is closed to avoid tumor spillage. The anterior and posterior bladder pedicles are divided. A small infraumbilical incision is made and the bladder is removed. The neobladder and anastomosis to the prostate capsule are performed extracorporeally through the inicision (13).

3. Finally, although not technically "prostate capsule sparing," several authors have described leaving part (apex) or the entire prostate in situ removing only the bladder. Descriptions of these procedures can be found in the literature and will not be described in this chapter.

3. Oncologic Concerns and Outcomes

Several concerns have been proposed regarding prostate capsule sparing cystectomy. As this is a "less" radical surgery, opponents have suggested that there is a risk of leaving both urothelial carcinoma as well as prostate cancer behind which would both be difficult to treat.

3.1. Urothelial Carcinoma Involving Prostate

An estimated 17–48% of patients with urothelial carcinoma of the bladder have concominant transitional cell carcinoma (TCC) of their prostate/prostatic urethra (8). We reviewed a series of 35 patients at our institution who underwent radical cystectomy for bladder cancer. Once the cystoprostatectomy specimen was removed from the patient, the prostate peripheral zone/capsule was separated from the rest of the specimen to evaluate the risk of urothelial and prostate cancer in both the adenoma and peripheral zone. Through prospective review, 26% of patients had TCC involving the prostate including three men with involvement of the PZC. As anticipated (14), pre-cystectomy prostatic urethral biopsy identified all of the patients with urothelial carcinoma involving the prostate. Due to the retrospective nature of this study, not all patients had a pre-cystectomy biopsy of the prostatic urethra performed. As a consequence, the identification of all patients by preoperative biopsy may have been due to a selection bias.

However, in a previous study, Wood and colleagues performed step sections on 84 cystoprostatectomy specimens. Forty-three percent of patients had TCC involving the prostate including 17% with stromal involvement. However, their study demonstrated that preoperative biopsy would identify patients with TCC involving the prostate (14). In a similar study Revelo and colleagues performed step section analysis on 121 patients in order to determine whether the prostate apex could be spared to improve continence in patients undergoing neobaldder. They identified 58 men (48%) with TCC of the prostate (predominantly dysplasia) including 16 patients with involvement at the apex (15). Other studies reported similar rates of prostatic urethral involvement.

While it is likely that stromal involvement could be identified preoperatively and the patient offered alternative treatments, there is a risk of superficial recurrence within the retained prostatic fossa. However, the same surveillance as patients with a neobladder or ileal conduit with a retained urethra could be applied to patients undergoing prostate capsule sparing cystectomy. In their series of 100 patients, Vallancien and colleagues had two superficial recurrences in the prostatic urethra at a mean follow-up of 38 months (5). Pinthus and colleagues have suggested that the same management options for urethral recurrence following neobladder could be applied to patients with superficial recurrence following prostate capsule sparing cystectomy including resection, intravesical therapy, and undiversion/no diversion (16).

3.2. Prostate Cancer

The relatively high incidence of prostate cancer in patients undergoing RADICAL CYSTETOMY is well established. In our study described above, we found that 46% of the patients had prostate cancer. Fifteen prostate cancers were in the peripheral zone/capsule; the same location that would be left in situ for a prostate capsule sparing cystectomy. However, unlike transitional cell carcinoma which was identified by preoperative prostatic urethral biopsy, identification of prostate cancer was more problematic. Prostate specific antigen, prostate volume, family history, and body mass index were equivalent between those patients with and without prostate cancer. Although not significant, 4/7 patients with cancer in peripheral zone/capsule only and 2/4 patients with clinically "significant" prostate cancer had abnormal digital rectal exams suggesting that this group may warrant a more aggressive search for prostate cancer by extended biopsy techniques. Patients with peripheral zone/capsule prostate cancer were more likely to be older than those without cancer. While focusing this procedure on younger patients might reduce the likelihood of leaving prostate cancer behind in the peripheral zone/capsule, it is difficult to draw conclusions from our small cohort. In addition, there is no consensus as to the impact of leaving clinically "insignificant" prostate cancer behind in younger patients. As a consequence, caution could dictate that every effort to identify all prostate cancer preoperatively should be made and if prostate cancer was found, the entire prostate should be removed. We would recommend an extended core transrectal ultrasound guided prostate biopsy regardless of prostate specific antigen or digital rectal exam for anyone considered for prostate capsule sparing cystectomy.

Our results are similar to other published series (15, 17). Ruffion et al. reviewed 100 patients undergoing radical cystectomy over a 10 year period and found that 51% of patients had prostate cancer. Twenty-two patients had clinically significant prostate cancers. Similar to our series, digital rectal exam and prostate specific antigen could not distinguish between clinically significant or insignificant cancers (18).

Hautmann reported on 133 patients who had a sextant biopsy of the prostate and prostate needle aspiration immediately following removal of the bladder and prostate. Of the 58 patients with prostate cancer, sextant biopsy detected seven cancers and needle aspiration detected seven cancers with overlap in only one case for a total detection rate of 22%.As a majority of these patients had clinically insignificant cancers and the biopsies were as likely to detect the significant as the insignificant cancers, the authors concluded that screening was not justified (19). However, it is likely that their detection rate might have been improved by using an extended biopsy pattern rather than the traditional sextant biopsy pattern (20).

However, many clinical series of prostate capsule sparing cystectomy have reported that rigorous preoperative screening can help appropriately select candidates for the procedure. Table 15.1 summarizes the number of patient identified or developing prostate cancer who underwent prostate capsule sparing cystectomy. Nieuwenhuijzen et al. evaluated all patients preoperatively with transurethral resection of the prostatic urethra, prostate specific antigen, digital rectal exam, and sextant prostate biopsy. In their series of 44 patients, only one patient developed prostate cancer 5 years after the cystectomy utilizing their rigorous screening method (23). In another series of 68 patients utilizing a similar screening method, three patients with high grade prostatic intraepithelial neoplasia and one patient with prostate cancer were identified at the time of prostate capsule preservation. These four

TABLE 15.1. Oncologic outcomes of prostate capsule sparing cystectomy.

References	No. patients	Mean Age (range)	Follow-up (months, range)	Clinical Stage T1	Clinical Stage T2	Clinical Stage >T2	Path stage T1	Path stage T2	Path stage T3	Path stage T4	Path stage N+	Recurrence Local	Recurrence Distant	Prostate cancer
Martis (6)	32	59 (52–72)	32 (6–60)	9	14	9	4	11	15	2	2	0	0	0
Colombo (21)	27	52 (36–61)	32	21	5		22	5			1	0	1	0
Muto (22)	61	49 (36–68)	68	55	5		48	5	1		1	0	5	1, 3 HGPIN
Terrone (2004)	27	51 (23–65)	90.5 (10–228)	24	2	1	24		3		1	2	4	0
Ghanem (2002)	4	47	36		3	1		3	1			1	0	0
Girgin (2006)	4	39 (36–43)	25 (6–35)	3	1		3	1				0	1	0
Vallancien (5)	100	64 (48–82)	38 (2–111)				24	48	28		13	5	31	3
Arroyo (13)	25	60	9.7 (3–27)	8	8	9					0	1	2	1
Nieuwenhuijzen (23)	44	57	42	13	18	13 (neoadj)	12	12	6		14	3	13	1
Botto (7)	34	61	26		all		6	16	7		2	1	6	1
Saidi (24)	25	57 (47–75)	53.4									6	6	1

patients had normal prostate specific antigen values prior to surgery and at a mean follow-up of 19 months, all patients had a prostate specific antigen <0.2 ng/ml (22). Saidi et al. had one patient develop prostate cancer 36 months following prostate capsule sparing cystectomy who was treated with external beam radiation successfully (24). Martis et al. identified 85 patients who were deemed candidates for prostate capsule sparing cystectomy over a 5-year period. Again, using rigorous preoperative screening, 18 patients were excluded due to positive prostate biopsy; 11 due to PSA > 10, and seven due to a prostate specific antigen ratio <15% with a prostate specific antigen between 4 and 10 ng/ml. With rigorous screening, none of the patients treated with prostate capsule sparing cystectomy had prostate cancer in the prostate peripheral zone/capsule (6).

3.3. Local Recurrence and Metastatic Disease

Another major concern of prostate capsule sparing cystectomy is the potential risk of increased local recurrence and metastatic disease. Several series with at least a 3 year follow-up have reported low rates of local recurrence that are similar to those found for radical cystoprostatectomy. Nieuwenhuijzen reported a 6.9% local recurrence rate at a mean follow-up of 42 months (23). Vallancien in his series of 100 patients reported a 5% rate of local recurrence (5). Other series in which patients selected for prostate capsule sparing cystectomy had superficial disease in their bladder have reported no pelvic recurrence. In an attempt to avoid local recurrence, Martis et al. excluded patients with a positive prostatic urethral biopsy (6), tumor involving the bladder trigone (7), and nonorgan confined patients (25) from prostate capsule sparing cystectomy (6). Although retrospective, these studies suggest that prostate capsule sparing cystectomy does not increase the risk of local recurrence in properly selected patients.

One small series suggested an increased risk of metastatic disease. Of 34 patients undergoing prostate capsule sparing cystectomy, six patients developed metastatic disease without local recurrence suggesting the presence of micrometastatic disease prior to intervention (7). Of 100 patients who had prostate capsule sparing cystectomy in another series, 31 patients developed distant metastases. However, of these patients, 17 had T3 disease and/or nodal disease suggesting that it was stage and not the procedure driving the outcome. Based on these small series, it does not appear that prostate capsule sparing cystectomy increases the risk of either local recurrence or metastases (5). The rates of local recurrence and metastatic disease described in the literature are summarized in Table 15.1.

4. Outcomes of Prostate Capsule Sparing Cystectomy

The goal of prostate capsule sparing cystectomy is to improve upon the functional outcomes of radical cystectomy with neobladder without compromising disease control. Below, we outline the results of the literature on prostate capsule sparing cystectomy. A major limitation of these results is the retrospective nature of these series and the physician reported outcomes of urinary and sexual function. However, these results suggest that preservation of the prostate PZC may improve functional outcomes in highly selected patients compared to conventional radical cystectomy. Table 15.2 summarizes the urinary and sexual function outcomes of prostate capsule sparing cystectomy.

4.1. Sexual Function

Unlike standard radical cystoprostatectomy, prostate capsule sparing cystectomy avoids dissection of the posterolateral prostate. As a consequence, the cavernosal nerves are not identified, mobilized, or manipulated. While the anticipation would be that this procedure would result in preservation of potency in all men with adequate baseline sexual function, the manipulation of the seminal vesicles risks injury to the neurovascular tissue as it travels near the seminal vesicle tip. While the goal of nerve-sparing radical cystectomy is preservation of erectile function, an added role of prostate capsule sparing cystectomy is the preservation of ejaculatory function, especially in young men who continue to desire fertility.

4.1.1. Potency

Table 15.2 outlines the results of the published series on prostate capsule sparing cystectomy. Variable methods have been used to assess potency in these series ranging from validated instruments (International Index of Erectile Function (IIEF), IIEF-15, other instruments) to more quantitative measures such as Rigiscan device (Dacomed Corporation, Minneapolis, Minnesota)

TABLE 15.2. Functional outcomes following prostate capsule sparing cystectomy.

		Sexual function			Urinary function		
References	No. patients	Evaluation method	Potency	Ejaculation	Evaluation method	Daytime continence	Nightime continence
Martis (6)	32	IIEF-15, penetration	80%	–	Voiding diary, 1-h pad test, IPSS	98%	83%
Spitz (25)	4	Not specified	100%	100%	Not specified	100%	100%
Colombo (21)	27	IIEF, penile Doppler, Rigiscan, survey	100%	100%	Voiding diary, Urodynamics	100	100
Muto (22)	61	Not specified	95%	100%	Not specified	95% (1 ISC)	31%
Terrone (2004)	27	Questionnaire	92.8%	54	UDS, no pads	100% (20 ISC)	100%
Ghanem (2002)	4	Questionnaire	75%		UDS, questionnaire	100%	100%
Girgin (2006)	4	Not specified	100	50	≤1 pad	100% (1 ISC)	100%
Vallancien (5)	100	Penetration	82	100	No pads	97%	95%
Arroyo (13)	25	Intercourse	84	100	Pads	100%	100%
Guazzoni (2003)	3	IIEF, Rigiscan, Doppler	100		UDS	100%	100%
Nieuwenhuijzen (23)	44	IIEF, questionnaire	77.5	45%	No pads	95.3 (ISC 10)	74.4
Botto (7)	27	IIEF	90	100	No pads	80	80
Saidi (24)	25	IIEF	37.5		Ditrovie	93.7	75

results and dynamic penile Doppler ultrasound studies to assess blood flow. In these studies, reported rates of potency were 37.5–100% with most studies reporting return of adequate sexual function (erection adequate for penetration) in 80–90% of patients (8).

In one of the more rigorous assessments, Colombo and colleagues evaluated their patients pre and postoperatively with Rigiscan device (Dacomed Corporation, Minneapolis, Minnesota), dynamic penile Doppler ultrasound, and IIEF. In all elements, at 12 month follow-up there was no significant difference in IIEF scores, peak systolic velocity, or erectile episodes/rigidity compared to baseline levels (21).

While the results of these studies do indeed appear promising, there are several aspects to sexual function that these measures do not consider. A more standardized evaluation of baseline sexual function and its recovery is needed to evaluate the benefit of this procedure similar to the validated surveys used for the assessment of sexual recovery following radical prostatectomy. In addition, while the recovery of sexual function may be important for younger patients requiring surgical intervention for their bladder cancer, majority of our patients in the United States are older and have poor baseline sexual function and will likely derive very little benefit from this aspect of prostate capsule sparing cystectomy.

4.1.2. Ejaculation

Some younger men requiring cystectomy may desire continued fertility following surgical treatment of their bladder cancer. In addition to preservation of sexual function, prostate capsule sparing cystectomy also attempts to preserve ejaculatory function by preserving both the seminal vesicles as well as the vas deferens. Rates of ejaculation range from 45 to 100%. For the most part, retrograde ejaculation is the most common occurrence following surgery, especially if a transurethral resection of the prostate was performed as part of the procedure as opposed to adenoma enucleation (8).

Spitz and colleagues reported on four patients who underwent prostate capsule sparing cystectomy for nonurothelial bladder cancers. They reported antegrade ejaculation in 3 of 4 of their patients with a steady improvement in ejaculate volume 1 year following surgery. One patient was able to father a child following the surgery (25).

For the select few patients who are candidates for the procedure and desire to preserve fertility, preservation of the vas deferens and seminal vesicles is still likely to result in retrograde ejaculation. Colombo et al. demonstrated variable rates of antegrade and retrograde ejaculation in his series. While masturbation resulted in low counts from the ejaculate, an average of 8 × 10 (6) sperm were collected from the urine with motility ranging from 20 to 50% opening the possibility of in vitro fertilization for the motivated patient. This, however, has not been reported to this date (21). For the rare individual who desires future fertility following radical cystectomy and neobladder, we continue to advocate preoperative sperm cryopreservation until postoperative sperm retrieval has been documented.

4.2. Urinary Function

A likely more meaningful outcome for patients undergoing radical cystectomy with orthotopic neobladder is improvement in urinary function and control. While proponents of orthotopic neobladder report reasonable rates of daytime continence, nighttime continence continues to be a major problem for patients undergoing this procedure with roughly 30% of patients experiencing nocturnal incontinence (range 0–70%) (1). In addition, a recent quality of life instrument for cancer of the bladder (Bladder Cancer Index) developed at our institution demonstrated a reduced satisfaction with urinary function in patients undergoing orthotopic neobladder compared to ileal conduit (26). While this outcome may be related in differential expectations of patients undergoing orthotopic urinary diversion vs. ileal conduit, the fact is there is room for improvement.

Unlike the prostatectomy literature which has adopted the use of validated quality of life instruments, the literature on prostate capsule sparing cystectomy uses various measures to evaluate urinary function including questionnaires, voiding diaries, urodynamic studies, and pad tests as a measure. As a result it is difficult to compare studies and know what constitutes continence as some studies use a rigorous definition of 0 pads while others rely on other instruments.

That being said, most studies report daytime continence rates of 60–100% with most series reporting continence in the 90% + range. Colombo and colleagues reported a 100% daytime continence rate 15 days after catheter removal (21). Vallancien reported a 97% daytime continence rate in his series of 100 patients undergoing prostate capsule sparing cystectomy (5).

The rates of nighttime continence are more variable. While most studies report continence rates between 80 and 100%, Muto and colleagues reported a nighttime continence rate of only 31% (22). Hypercontinence may be a more significant issue with this procedure compared to standard radical cystectomy and orthotopic neobladder. In a study by Colombo and colleagues, urodynamic evaluation revealed adequate neobladder volumes of low pressure with high outlet resistance (21). In patients who cannot generate an adequate Valsalva or adequately relax their pelvic floor, this may translate into a need for intermittent self catheterization. Horenblas demonstrated that IPSS scores were higher in these patients postoperatively likely due to the need to strain to complete micturation (23). However, without standardized reporting it is unclear if more patients undergoing prostate capsule sparing cystectomy require intermittent self catheterization (ISC) compared to patients undergoing radical cystectomy with neobladder. In addition Table 15.1 demonstrates the ISC rate for prostate capsule sparing cystectomy demonstrating/stating that only a handful of studies reported more than one patient requiring ISC suggesting that this may be no more of a problem than standard orthotopic neobladder patients.

5. Indications, Contraindications and Algorithm for Patient Selection

Based on the information and limitations of the retrospective literature, we have recently initiated a prospective randomized study comparing Prostate Capsule Sparing Cystectomy and Nerve-Sparing Cystectomy at

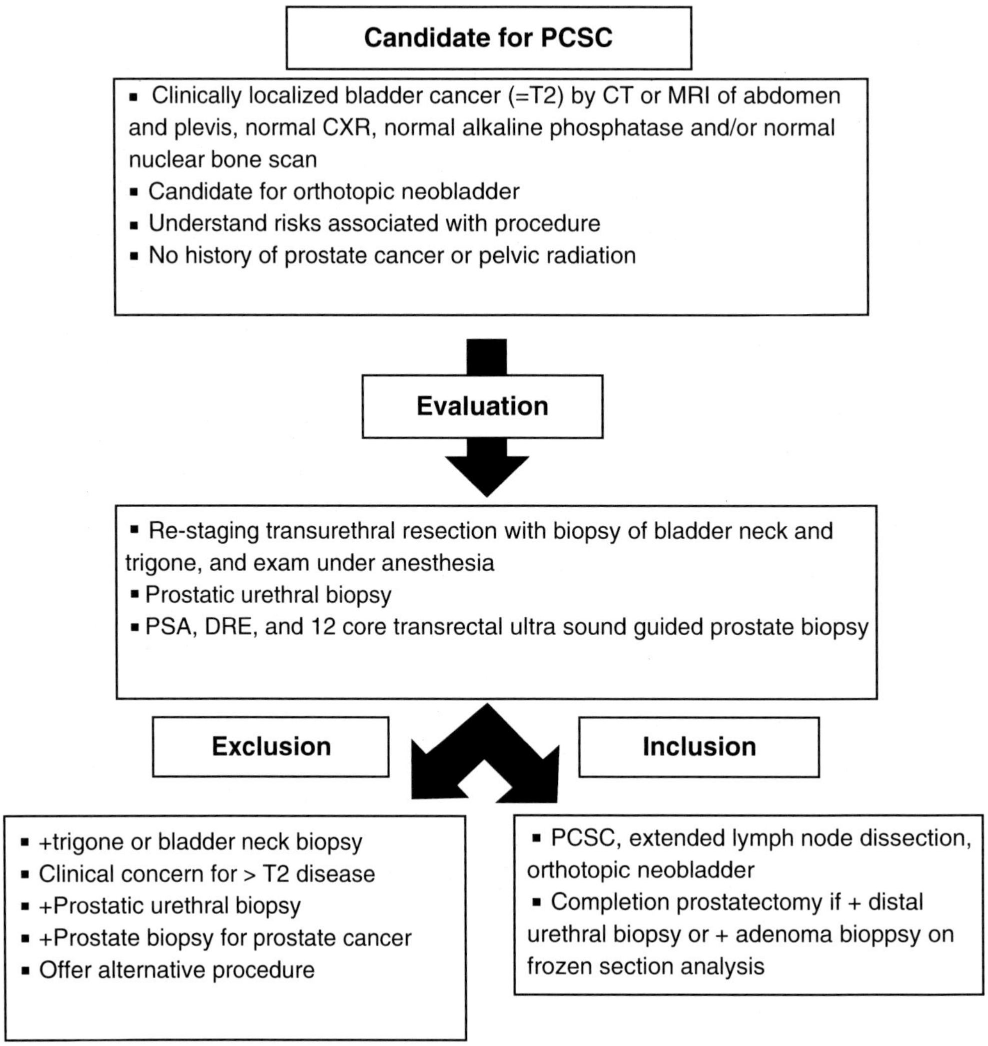

FIG. 15.5. Algorithm for patient selection for prostate capsule sparing cystectomy. *PCSC* prostate capsule sparing cystectomy; *CT* computed tomography; *MRI* magnetic resonance imaging; *CXR* chest radiograph; *PSA* prostate specific antigen; *DRE* digital rectal exam

our institution. As a basis for our selection, we have utilized the results of our retrospective pathologic study as well as algorithms in the literature that have appeared to result in the best oncologic outcomes (Fig.15.5). Our primary endpoint in this study is urinary function at 6 months and 1 year as assessed by the bladder cancer index, a validated health related quality of life instrument for patients with cancer of the bladder . Secondary endpoints will include surgical margins, perioperative complications, sexual function as assessed by the bladder cancer index, and rates of prostate cancer, local recurrence, and metastatic disease as assessed by routine follow-up.

A prostatic urethral biopsy will be used to identify evidence of urothelial carcinoma in the prostatic urethra. Also, patients will undergo an extended core (12 cores) transrectal ultrasound guided biopsy prior to enrollment in the study (20) regardless of prostate specific antigen or digital rectal exam which no studies have identified as predictive of prostate cancer in the bladder cancer population. However, some studies have used digital rectal exam, prostate specific antigen (and percent free prostate specific antigen) as exclusion criteria (6, 16). Those patients found to have prostate cancer will be excluded from the study. Patients will also be excluded from the study if they have had prior radiation to the pelvis or prostate cancer treatment.

Conclusions

While concerns over the risk of prostate cancer, residual urothelial carcinoma, increased local recurrence and metastatic disease appear to call into question the oncologic soundness of prostate capsule sparing cystectomy, the functional outcomes reported in the literature require us to examine this treatment as a potential option for some patients. Concerns have been raised over "less" radical surgeries in the past including partial nephrectomy and time has shown in appropriately selected patients, these procedures can potentially improve quality of life without compromising cancer control. The literature would suggest that patients with T2 disease or less not involving the trigone, bladder neck, or prostatic urethra and with no evidence of prostate cancer as assessed by prostate specific antigen, digital rectal exam, and transrectal ultrasound guided prostate biopsy using a 12 core technique who are suitable candidates for orthotopic neobladder might benefit from this less invasive procedure. In addition, the safe guard of frozen sections of the prostate adenoma and prostatic urethra should add a second opportunity not to leave behind disease. We hope a prospective study with a well defined patient population and validated instrument will determine the value of this procedure.

References

1. Steers WD. Voiding dysfunction in the orthotopic neobladder. World J Urol 2000; 18:330–7.
2. Schoenberg MP, Walsh PC, Breazeale DR, Marshall FF, Mostwin JL, Brendler CB. Local recurrence and survival following nerve sparing radical cystoprostatectomy for bladder cancer: 10-year followup. J Urol 1996; 155: 490–4.
3. Kessler TM, Burkhard FC, Perimenis P, et al. Attempted nerve sparing surgery and age have a significant effect on urinary continence and erectile function after radical cystoprostatectomy and ileal orthotopic bladder substitution. J Urol 2004; 172:1323–7.
4. Zippe CD, Raina R, Massanyi EZ, et al. Sexual function after male radical cystectomy in a sexually active population. Urology 2004; 64:682–5; discussion 685–6.
5. Vallancien G, Abou El Fettouh H, Cathelineau X, Baumert H, Fromont G, Guillonneau B. Cystectomy with prostate sparing for bladder cancer in 100 patients: 10-year experience. J Urol 2002; 168:2413–7.
6. Martis G, D'Elia G, Diana M, Ombres M, Mastrangeli B. Prostatic capsule- and nerve-sparing cystectomy in organ-confined bladder cancer: preliminary results. World J Surg 2005; 29:1277–81.
7. Botto H, Sebe P, Molinie V, Herve JM, Yonneau L, Lebret T. Prostatic capsule- and seminal-sparing cystectomy for bladder carcinoma: initial results for selected patients. BJU Int 2004; 94:1021–5.
8. Hautmann RE, Stein JP. Neobladder with prostatic capsule and seminal-sparing cystectomy for bladder cancer: a step in the wrong direction. Urol Clin North Am 2005; 32:177–85.
9. Millin T. Retropubic prostatectomy: a new extravesical technique report on 20 cases. 1945. J Urol 2002; 167:976–9; discussion 980.
10. Turner WH, Markwalder R, Perrig S, Studer UE. Meticulous pelvic lymphadenectomy in surgical treatment of the invasive bladder cancer: an option or a must? Eur Urol 1998; 33 Suppl 4:21–2.
11. Hautmann RE. Neobladder and bladder replacement. Eur Urol 1998; 33:10 pages following 512.
12. Hautmann RE. Urinary diversion: ileal conduit to neobladder. J Urol 2003; 169:834–42.
13. Arroyo C, Andrews H, Rozet F, Cathelineau X, Vallancien G. Laparoscopic prostate-sparing radical cystectomy: the Montsouris technique and preliminary results. J Endourol 2005; 19:424–8.
14. Wood DP, Jr., Montie JE, Pontes JE, Levin HS. Identification of transitional cell carcinoma of the prostate in bladder cancer patients: a prospective study. J Urol 1989; 142:83–5.
15. Revelo MP, Cookson MS, Chang SS, Shook MF, Smith JA, Jr., Shappell SB. Incidence and location of prostate and urothelial carcinoma in prostates from cystoprostatectomies: implications for possible apical sparing surgery. J Urol 2004; 171:646–51.

16. Pinthus JH, Nam RK, Klotz LH. Prostate sparing radical cystectomy–not for all, but an option for some. Can J Urol 2006; 13 Suppl 1:81–7.
17. Romero FR, de Castro MG, Andriolo Junior A, de Meneses AH, Fernandes RC, Perez MD. Coexistence of prostate neoplasia in patients undergoing radical cystoprostatectomy due to vesical neoplasia. Int Braz J Urol 2004; 30:296–301.
18. Ruffion A, Manel A, Massoud W, et al. Preservation of prostate during radical cystectomy: evaluation of prevalence of prostate cancer associated with bladder cancer. Urology 2005; 65:703–7.
19. Soulie M, Straub M, Game X, et al. A multicenter study of the morbidity of radical cystectomy in select elderly patients with bladder cancer. J Urol 2002; 167:1325–8.
20. Siu W, Dunn RL, Shah RB, Wei JT. Use of extended pattern technique for initial prostate biopsy. J Urol 2005; 174:505–9.
21. Colombo R, Bertini R, Salonia A, et al. Overall clinical outcomes after nerve and seminal sparing radical cystectomy for the treatment of organ confined bladder cancer. J Urol 2004; 171:1819–22; discussion 1822.
22. Muto G, Bardari F, D'Urso L, Giona C. Seminal sparing cystectomy and ileocapsuloplasty: long-term followup results. J Urol 2004; 172:76–80.
23. Nieuwenhuijzen JA, Meinhardt W, Horenblas S. Clinical outcomes after sexuality preserving cystectomy and neobladder (prostate sparing cystectomy) in 44 patients. J Urol 2005; 173:1314–7.
24. Saidi A, Nahon O, Daniel L, Lay F, Lechevallier E, Coulange C. [Prostate-sparing cystectomy: long-term functional and oncological results in a series of 25 cases]. Prog Urol 2004; 14:172–7; discussion 176.
25. Spitz A, Stein JP, Lieskovsky G, Skinner DG. Orthotopic urinary diversion with preservation of erectile and ejaculatory function in men requiring radical cystectomy for nonurothelial malignancy: a new technique. J Urol 1999; 161:1761–4.
26. Gilbert SM, Wood DP, Weizer AZ, et al. Measuring Health-Related Quality of life Outcomes in Bladder Cancer Patients Using the Newly Validated Bladder Cancer Index, American Urological Association, Atlanta, GA, 2006.
27. Terrone C, Cracco C. Scarpa RM et al.: Supra-ampullar cystectomy with preservation of sexual function and ileal orthotopic reservoir for bladder tumor: twenty years of experience. Eur Urol 2004 46:264.
28. Ghanem AN: Experience with 'capsule sparing' cystoprostadenectomy for orthotopic bladder replacement: overcoming the problems of impotence, incontinence and difficuilt urethral anastomosis. BJU Int 2002 90:617.
29. Girgin C, Oder M, Sahin MO et al.: Erection-and ejaculation-preserving cyctectomy with orthotopic urinary diversion: is it feasible? J Androl 2006 27:263.
30. Guazzoni G, Cestari A, Colombo R et al.: Laparoscopic nerve- and seminal-sparing cystectomy with orthotopic ileal neobladder: the first three cases. Eur Urol 2003 44:567.

16 Preservation of Reproductive Organs in Women

Lambda Msezane and Gary D. Steinberg

Contents

Abstract The gold standard therapy for muscle invasive urothelial carcinoma of the bladder in women is radical cystectomy with anterior pelvic exenteration which involves removal of the lymph nodes, uterus, ovaries, fallopian tubes, bladder, anterior vaginal wall and urethra. For all women there is much concern about sexual function and quality of life after cystectomy and urinary diversion. In this chapter we will explore the advances made in preservation of the reproductive organs in females and review the current rates of concomitant involvement of each with urothelial carcinoma.

Keywords Cystectomy, Reproductive organs, Female, Bladder, Female sexual dysfunction, Pelvic exenteration

1. History

Cancer of the bladder is estimated to effect 16,730 American women in 2006 based on the incidence rates over the last 20 years (1). The gold standard therapy for muscle invasive urothelial carcinoma of the bladder in women is radical cystectomy with anterior pelvic exenteration. This procedure involves removal of the lymph nodes, uterus, ovaries, fallopian tubes, bladder, anterior vaginal wall and urethra. The anterior pelvic exenteration allows for greater access to the bladder and removal of the surrounding tissues that may be at risk of involvement with cancer (2). In previous studies, rates of vaginal wall recurrence had been reported as high as 15–28% (3) as well as concomitant urethral involvement in 36% of patients (4). More recent studies however, have demonstrated lower rates of involvement. Often at times the symptoms that women experience with cancer of the bladder, namely hematuria, dysuria, frequency and urgency are misdiagnosed as urinary tract infections or signs of aging and definitive diagnoses of bladder cancer are delayed. This may lead women to presenting themselves with higher stage disease at diagnosis. While the majority of these women are in their seventh decade, 17% of new cases occur in women aged 55–64 and survival rates for all age groups are increasing (1). For all women, and especially those diagnosed in the younger age groups, there is much concern about sexual function and quality of life after

From: *Current Clinical Urology: Bladder Cancer,* Edited by: C.T. Lee and D.P. Wood,
DOI; 10.1007/978-1-59745-417-9_16,

cystectomy and urinary diversion. The efforts put forth by urologists to preserve sexual function in men have far outweighed those directed toward women. Male patients have benefited from the development of nerve sparing prostatectomy and cystoprostectomy by Walsh from Johns Hopkins (5, 6). In addition, the majority of the outcome of these studies is directed toward male sexual potency and satisfaction postoperatively. Little attention was paid to preserving the urethra and reproductive organs, as well as sexual function in females until recently. Eventually, methods of vaginal reconstruction were developed for patients that had been sexually active preoperatively. This involved either tubularization of the remaining posterior vaginal wall or dissecting it anteriorly off of the rectum and advancing the posterior wall forward to recreate a foreshortened cylinder. These procedures, which decrease the diameter and/or the length of the vagina, may lead to significant dyspareunia (7). Additional postoperative complaints include vaginal dryness, loss of climax and clitoral sensation, and the psychological implications of urinary diversion including a change in body image and feelings of sexuality. Loss of ovarian hormones in premenopausal women may lead to excessive dryness and vaginal atrophy as well (7). Alternatively, the vagina may be reconstructed at a later date using rectus myocutaneous flaps or bowel segments. In the mid 1990s urologists began to realize that preservation of sexual function, which had been a goal for men undergoing cystectomy for some time, should be attempted in females as well.

Advances in surgical technique have led to the creation of orthotopic urinary reservoirs anatomically positioned to allow the patient "near normal" micturition. Initially, this technique was offered only to male patients, because of concerns of cancer recurrence if the urethra was left *in situ* as well as a lack of understanding of female pelvic anatomy and continence mechanisms. However, orthotopic urinary tract replacement has been adapted to include females for the past 10–15 years (8). The preservation of the urethra as well as the vagina to maintain neurovascular innervation and pelvic floor support has lead to the evolution of the less radical tissue sparing cystectomy. In addition, the desire to preserve sexual function and quality of life in these patients has motivated urologists into adapting the extirpative radical procedure to allow for preservation of the female reproductive organs when appropriate.

In this chapter we will explore the advances made in preservation of the reproductive organs in females and review the current rates of concomitant involvement of each with urothelial carcinoma. Data on subsequent local recurrence rates is presently limited.

2. Technique

In 1999, Schoenberg et al. described their technique of urethral and vaginal preservation in seven patients undergoing radical cystectomy (9). After staging lymphadenectomy, dissection is performed to mobilize the ovaries and fallopian tubes. One or both ovaries are spared in premenopausal women to avoid hormone deprivation. Dissection down towards the bladder with ligation of the ureters is performed and the bladder is retracted medially to allow visualization of the lateral vascular pedicles from the internal iliac artery and vein. The parasympathetic autonomic innervation of the corpora cavernosa clitoris arises lateral to the cervix and courses along the posterolateral aspect of the vagina (Fig.16.1). Release of these

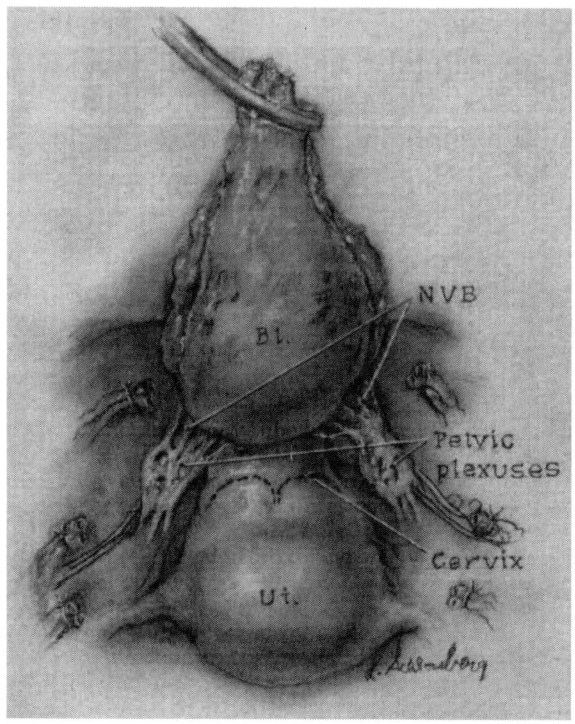

Fig. 16.1. Anatomy of the autonomic innervation of the corpora cavernosa clitoris. The nerves arise lateral to the cervix and course along the lateral aspect of the vagina near the vesicovaginal junction. Bl, Bladder. Ut, Uterus. NVB, Neurovascular bundles. Reproduced with permission from (9)

neurovascular bundles may be done by releasing the fibrovascular pedicles ventral to the vesicovaginal junction. Dissection continues in the usual fashion with ligation of the dorsal venous complex and division of the urethra, sparing the distal two thirds of the urethra without disrupting the endopelvic fascia and the anterior and dorsal supporting ligaments. Dissection then proceeds retrograde along a plane between the bladder and vagina. This vesicovaginal space is developed bluntly and vessels can be ligated as encountered. At the vaginal cervical junction the cardinal ligaments are first divided and then the vagina is dissected from the cervical attachments to allow release of the bladder and uterus (Fig.16.2). The vaginal defect is then closed with a running suture.

The authors admit that preserving the neurovascular bundles has not been shown to alter the return of continence or sexual function in women and the mechanisms involved in these functions have yet to be elucidated. Stenzl et al. performed extensive anatomic studies in order to determine the amount of urethra needed to preserve continence and the innervation required for rhabdoshpincter function (10). They reported that the entire rhabdosphincter, innervated by the pudendal nerve, lies in the distal half of the urethra. The autonomic nervous system controls the smooth muscle along the urethra. Through cadaveric dissection they confirmed the course of these nerves through the pelvis in order to develop a technique to preserve them. By sparing the lateral vaginal walls they found that the majority of the pelvic plexus fibers could be preserved. The urethra is dissected distally to 1 cm from the neck of the bladder and the rest left *in situ*. They reported good results with continence and low residual urinary volumes in their initial studies. Stenzl et al. reviewed their experience in 101 women undergoing radical cystectomy with orthotopic reconstruction (11). Sixty-six women underwent bilateral nerve sparing, six of whom required clean intermittent catheterization (9%). This was compared to 0 out of

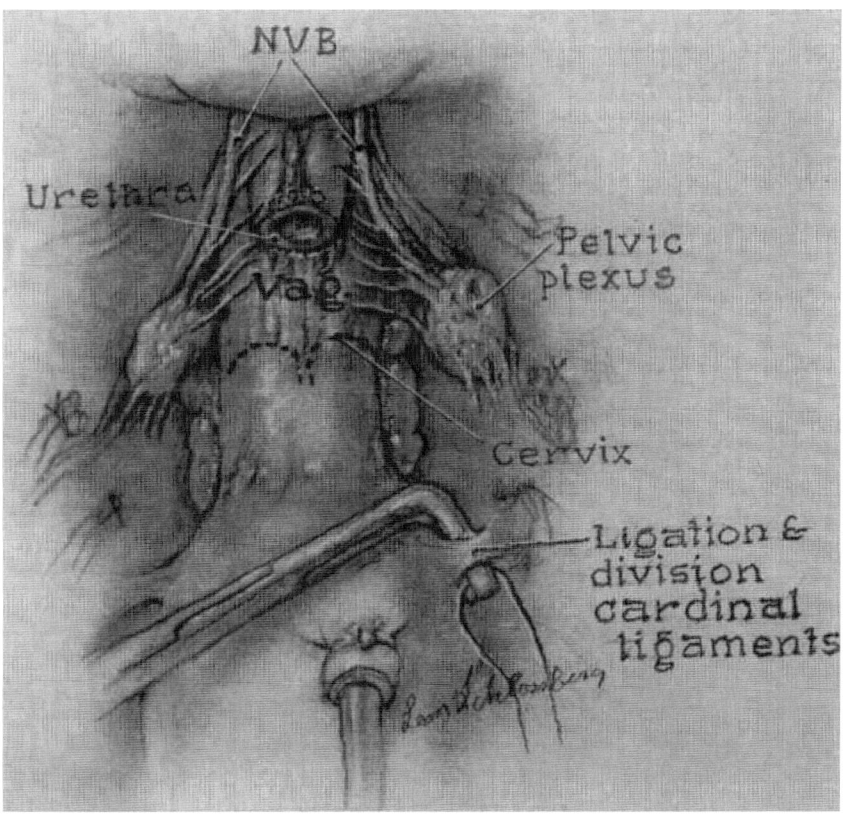

FIG. 16.2. Anatomy of the pelvis showing the pelvic plexus and cardinal ligaments at the vaginocervical junction. *NVB* neurovascular bundles. Reproduced with permission from (9)

28 patients with unilateral nerve sparing (0%) and 5 out of 7 patients with no nerve sparing (72%). The authors concluded that sparing of the autonomic innervation to the smooth muscle of the preserved urethra helped in preventing hypercontinence. Several authors argue that nerve sparing cystectomy leads to improved sexual function as well, although the mechanism of this is unknown.

Our preferred technique of female cystectomy is an antegrade approach. A plane is developed sharply between the posterior bladder wall and anterior vagina. The superior, lateral, and posterior bladder pedicles are ligated using the Ligasure device, pushing the neurovascular bundles posteriorly and laterally. The apex and anterior wall of the vagina are identified with the aid of a sponge stick in the vaginal vault. Antegrade dissection of the posterior wall of the bladder is continued off the anterior vaginal wall to the neck of the bladder. There is minimal dissection along the pelvic floor to spare branches of the pudendal nerve to the striated sphincter. The proximal urethra is then transected at the neck of the bladder, preserving the urethra, using a nerve sparing technique. Minimal dissection of the endopelvic fascia and the area anterior to the urethra is performed, preserving the pubourethral suspensory ligaments, rhabdosphincter region, anterior vaginal support and dorsal venous complex (Fig. 16.3). The specimen is removed, and the vagina is inspected for any injury. A frozen section is obtained from the neck of the bladder.

The most important factor in choosing to preserve organs is that cancer control is not compromised. Proper selection of patient prior to surgery is crucial. It has been shown that diffuse carcinoma in situ (CIS), trigonal involvement, bladder neck tumors, and large bulky tumors are often associated with extension into the urethra and vagina. Preoperative evaluation includes CT or MRI scan of the abdomen and pelvis and bimanual exam under anesthesia to determine any involvement in the gross pelvic sidewall and organ.

3. Orthotopic Neobladder

Orthotopic continent urinary diversion was originally described by Camey et al. in order to allow a patient to void in a more anatomical fashion (12). The majority of these procedures have been performed on men while the urethra has routinely been removed in the female radical cystectomy specimen due to its short

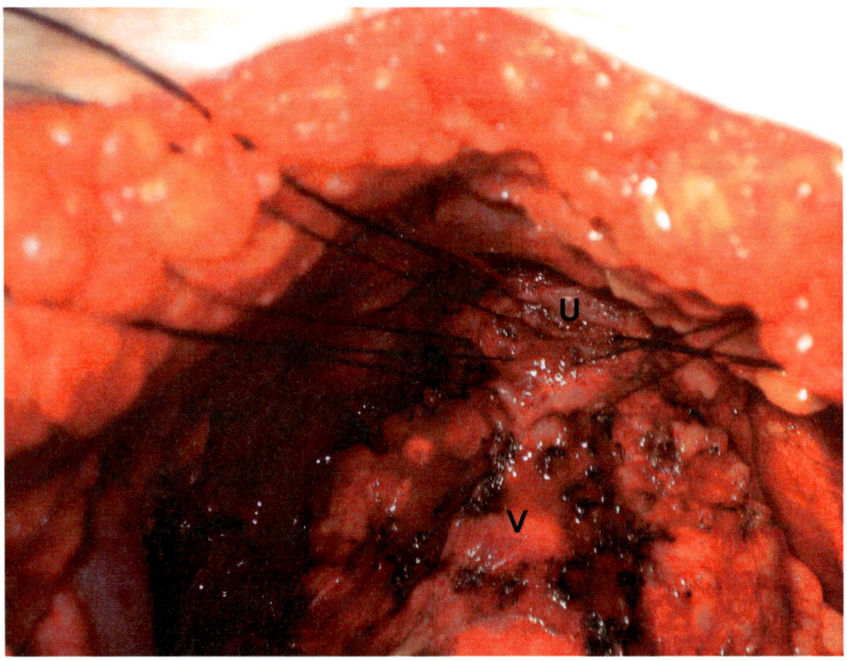

FIG. 16.3. Intraoperative photo showing transected urethra (U) with stay sutures and preserved vagina (V) during a radical cystectomy with orthotopic neobladder reconstruction. The neurovascular bundles course lateral to the vagina

length and concern of risk of concomitant involvement with carcinoma. Stein and Stenzl successfully described the technique in women in 1994 (13–15). These authors reported that to maintain the continence mechanism in women, preservation of the distal two-thirds of the urethra and its innervation is required. A small study on the effect of preservation of the urethra on cancer control after radical cystectomy in females had been performed prior to the 1990s. A concomitant incidence of 36% urethral involvement was found by De Paepe et al. in a study of 22 female cystectomy specimens examined (16). This rate is high in comparison to more contemporary series. Coloby et al. found a rate of 7% in their series of 47 patients and found that bladder neck involvement was an important predictor of urethral involvement (17). This was confirmed in a series of 67 women undergoing surgery for transitional cell carcinoma, where Stein et al. pathologically reviewed bladder and urethral specimens for concomitant cancer involvement (18). They found that 13% of patients (9/67) had proximal and mid urethral involvement with tumor while none had distal urethral involvement. All women with urethral involvement also had bladder neck involvement, and no women without bladder neck tumors had urethral tumor. If the urethra was involved, there was a more common association with high grade and stage disease and metastatic pelvic lymph nodes. Chen et al. reported an incidence of urethral involvement in 8% of women undergoing radical cystectomy for transitional cell carcinoma (19). Stenzl et al. report a rate of 2% urethral tumor recurrence with a mean follow-up of 5.5 years (20). In our series of fifty orthotopic diversions in women performed in the past 9 years only one patient had a urethral recurrence. This patient had pT3 N0 disease. The low incidence of urethral involvement in the current series points to the feasibility of offering women the opportunity to void in a more normal anatomic position while maintaining cancer control. By paying special attention to the bladder neck and obtaining intraoperative frozen sections, the appropriate candidates may be chosen for orthotopic diversion. Evaluation of the bladder neck and urethra should include preoperative bimanual exam with palpation of the urethra and anterior vaginal wall, cystoscopy with bladder neck biopsy, and intraoperative frozen section of the bladder neck prior to reconstruction. The long term rate of urethral recurrence after preservation of the urethra for orthotopic continent urinary diversion is presently unknown but will be important to determine.

4. Anterior Vaginal Wall Preservation

With the advent of orthotopic neobladder creation in females came the modification to allow preservation of the anterior vaginal wall. Some believe that this can improve continence and decrease fistula formation by preventing overlapping suture lines. The technique involves dissecting the plane between the posterior wall of the bladder and the anterior vagina (Fig. 16.4). Placing a sponge stick into the vaginal vault and elevating it cephalad improves identification of the apex and anterior wall of the vagina. A supracervical hysterectomy can be preformed at this time, or the uterus may be spared. The dissection is carried down to the level of the neck of the bladder and then one moves anteriorly to incise the proximal urethra circumferentially. The incision is carried posteriorly to connect the posterior plane of dissection. Inspection of the anterior vaginal wall is made to ensure no vaginotomies were made which should be repaired. One can then proceed with the creation of the diversion (21). Chang et al. reviewed their experience with this technique in 21 females undergoing anterior vaginal wall preservation during radical cystectomy. One patient experienced a neobladder-vagina fistula. Five others had minor complications, mainly ileus. All patients had negative posterior bladder wall and urethral margins with one patient having a positive distal ureteral margin only. Seventy-one percent (15/21) used 0–1 pads per day for stress incontinence. None needed more than two. Nine percent (2/21) required intermittent catheterization for incomplete emptying. These authors argue that preservation of the anterior vaginal wall (1) reduces the risk of fistula formation, (2) maintains pelvic support due to decreased dissection around the vaginal apex and lateral vaginal margins, (3) prevents pelvic prolapse and (4) preserves the vaginal vault length with regards to width and depth. In their 12 month follow-up one patient with T3b disease had a recurrence consistent with traditional series' results. Ali-El-Dein et al. also support the idea that preserving part of or the entire vagina can prevent hypercontinence by providing posterior support (22). In their study of 100 females who underwent cystectomy for organ confined bladder cancer followed by orthotopic reconstruction, they evaluated continence postoperatively. They found through videourodynamics and imaging that the problem of hypercontinence was related to mechanical obstruction. The pouch falls posteriorly into the pelvic cavity which leads to angulation of the posterior pouch-urethral junction. The pouch can also herniate through the prolapsed vaginal stump.

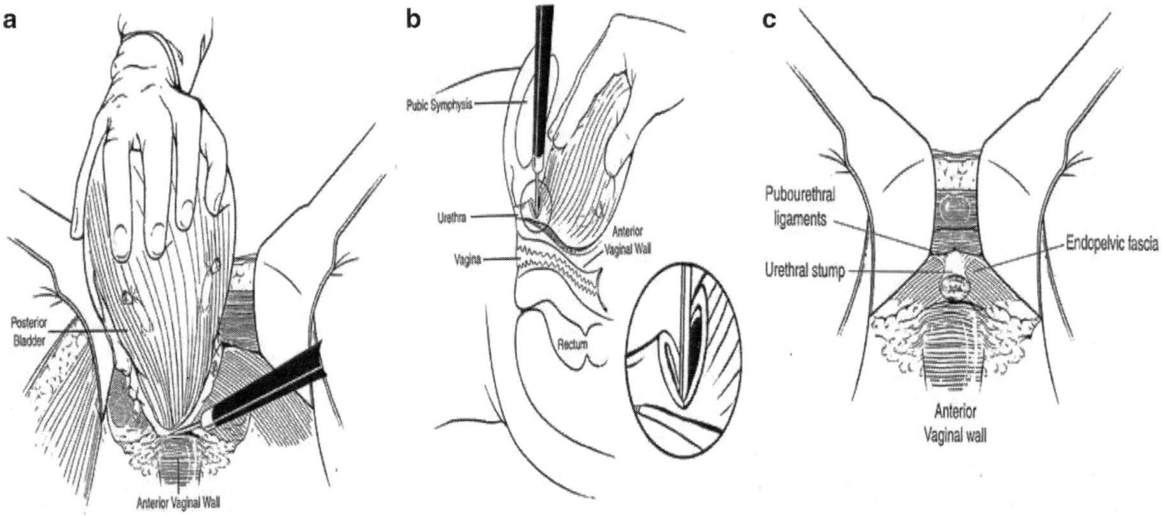

FIG. 16.4. Preservation of the anterior vaginal wall during cystectomy. A, Plane between anterior vaginal wall and posterior bladder. B, Circumferential division of the urethra. C, Resultant preserved surgical bed prior to reconstruction. Reproduced with permission from (21) (4, Part 1 of 2)

Patients in retention were found to have acute pouch-urethral angles (mean of 72°) on imaging as opposed to an obtuse angel (90–160°) found in those who voided well. The authors modified their surgical technique to help prevent this by preserving the medial ends of the round ligament to the vaginal stump to anchor it and by suspending the pouch at its dome to the rectus muscle. Their rates of retention went from 18.7 (14 of 75) to 8% (2 of 25) after this modification. Preservation, in part or in whole, of the vagina could maintain this posterior support and prevent the acute angulation that occurs. Omental interposition and autonomic nerve sparing may prevent urethral-neobladder angulation and decrease voiding dysnergia as well. Presently, we create a peritoneal flap from the posterior wall of the vagina and suture it to the endopelvic fascia (Fig. 16.5), as described by Puppo et al., for posterior support to prevent incomplete neobladder emptying (23).

Neobladder-vaginal fistula (NVF) is a known complication after radical cystectomy. The incidence is reportedly 3–5% in several series (21, 24, 25). In a review of our experience, 4 out of 50 patients who underwent vaginal-sparing cystectomy with orthotopic neobladder creation for invasive urothelial cell carcinoma developed NVF (26). An inadvertent injury to the anterior vaginal wall was identified in 2 of the 4 patients during the dissection of the bladder neck and urethra. The injuries were repaired primarily with a two layer closure and placement of an omental interposition flap. The third patient developed the NVF secondary to cancer recurrence in the pelvis and no obvious cause was identified in the fourth patient. The majority of studies reporting NVF point to vaginal injury as the most common cause of this fistula (21). Care must be taken during the dissection of the vesicovaginal plane, especially in the region of the bladder neck and urethra (Fig. 16.6). We minimize blunt dissection in this area and sharply dissect the posterior urethra to try and prevent NVF. The anterior vaginal wall must be inspected meticulously to identify any tears needing repair.

5. Rates of Gynecologic Organ Involvement

In a study of 68 females undergoing radical cystectomy between 1994 and 2000, Chang et al. reviewed pathologic findings to evaluate the incidence of uterine and adnexal involvement with urothelial or primary malignancy (27). Sixty-four patients had transitional cell carcinoma. Forty patients had gynecologic pathology to review. The mean age was 64 years old. Invasive urothelial carcinoma was identified in two specimens (5%), both of which occurred in the uterus. The authors reported a high suspicion of uterine involvement

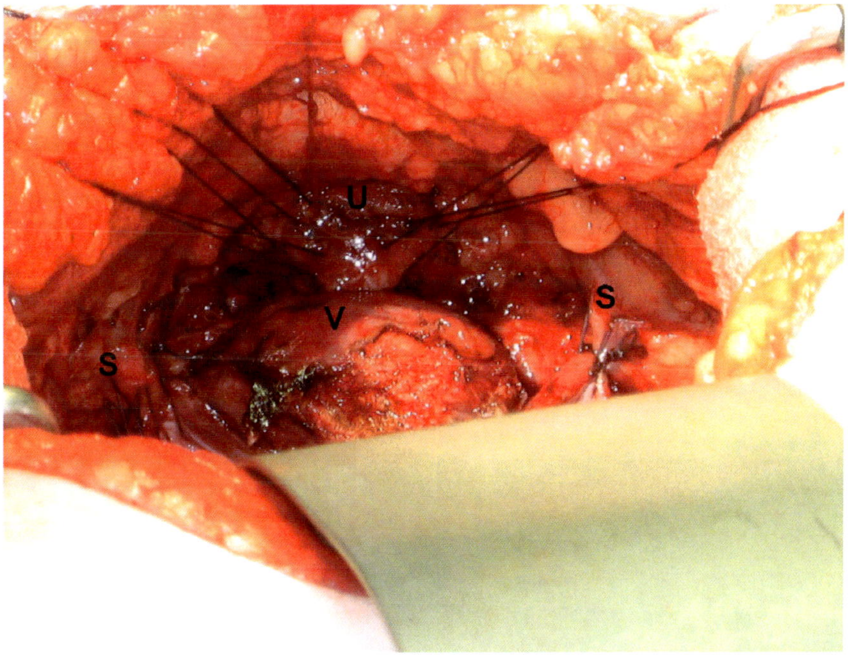

FIG. 16.5. Intraoperative photo demonstration of the preserved vagina (V) and urethra (U) after removal of the bladder. Note the suspension sutures (S) from the posterior vaginal fascia to the obturator internus fascia that lend posterior support to the vagina

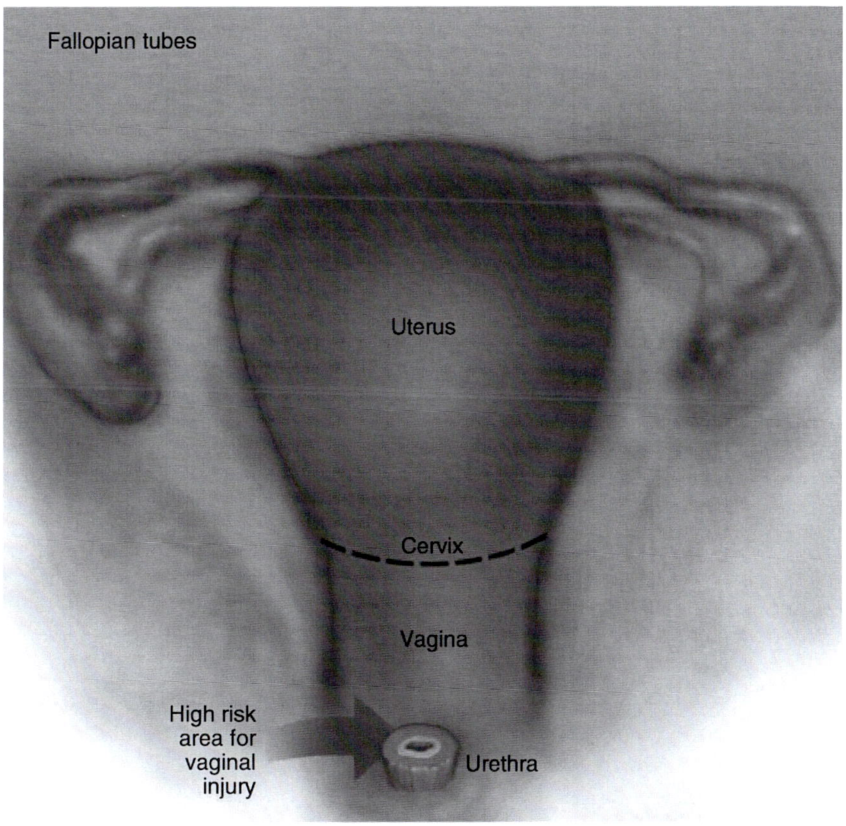

FIG. 16.6. Schematic of area at high risk for vaginal injury during the dissection of the bladder off of the vagina and transection of the urethra. Reproduced with permission from (26)

during surgery. One uterine specimen contained sarcoma which was not suspected intraoperatively. At 2 years follow-up there were no recurrences.

Ali-El-Dein et al. reported on the incidence of gynecologic organ involvement with malignancy in 609 females undergoing cystectomy between 1983 and 2001 (28). They found that 16 of 609 (2.6%) patients had involvement of the uterus, ovaries and/or vagina over a mean follow up of 4.3 years. The majority of these patients had squamous cell carcinoma (64%) and these patients were found to have less incidence of gynecologic organ involvement than patients with transitional cell carcinoma – 1.8 vs. 7.1%, $p = 0.01$. Grade 3 tumors were associated with malignancy in gynecological organs more often the grade 2 and 1 (7.6 vs. 1.7 and 1.5, respectively). Patients with lymph node involvement were more likely to have organ involvement (6.7 vs. 1.5%, $p = 0.01$). Posterior wall tumors were more often associated than other locations, but this was not statistically significant. Notably, they did not find any incidental primary gynecologic malignancy in the specimens although 13% had benign lesions.

With these rates of 2.6–5% it does seem reasonable to preserve the reproductive organs in the female cystectomy patient without compromise of cancer control. Ali-El-Dein et al. recommended exclusion of patients with high grade tumors and positive lymph nodes since these factors were associated with a significantly higher rate of gynecologic organ involvement.

6. Sexual Function After Cystectomy: Quality of Life

The majority of the outcome of these studies after radical cystectomy in females has focused on cancer control and urinary function. In order to assess the impact of radical cystectomy on sexual function Zippe et al. evaluated 27 sexually active females postoperatively (29). Their main concern was the impact of removal of the neurovascular bundles and injury to the blood supply to the clitoris during the dissection around the bladder and urethra. Patients completed a modified Index of Female Sexual Function questionnaire before and after surgery reporting on pain-free intercourse, degree of vaginal lubrication, sexual desire, orgasm, and overall sexual satisfaction. The mean age was 54.79 and mean follow-up was 24 months. Thirteen patients were premenopausal. The mean score preoperatively was 17.4 out of 25 total points. Post cystectomy the score decreased to 10.6 ($p \leq 0.05$) with 45% of patients experiencing decreased or no orgasm, 41% with decreased lubrication, 37% with decreased desire and dyspareunia in 22%. There was no significant difference in the changes that occurred postcystectomy between the premenopausal and postmenopausal women. Overall 52% reported becoming dysfunctional postoperatively, confirming the fact that this is a prevalent problem in all age groups of females undergoing cystectomy. Thirteen patients (48%) were unable to have successful vaginal intercourse at all. It is hard to distinguish the cause of dysfunction as being due to surgically induced changes (i.e., nerve injury or disruption of blood supply) or to the psychological impact of having cancer and undergoing urinary diversion, although it is clear that both play a major role in outcome. The authors found no difference in the change in IFSF score between the Indiana (seven patients), Studor pouch (ten patients), and ileal conduit (ten patients) diversions. Due to this finding they suggest that vaginal sparing procedures may not portend better sexual function outcomes although their numbers were small and surgical technique was not elaborated. Horenblas et al. reported on three females undergoing organ sparing cystectomy who maintained adequate lubrication and orgasm (30).

The Cleveland clinic group that introduced the concept of "quality of life cystectomy" for female patients with cancer of the bladder is a proponent of the preservation of the neurovascular structures to maintain sexual function (31). Bhat et al. recently reported on the retrospective comparison of six women undergoing nerve sparing verses seven women undergoing non-nerve sparing cystectomy (32). Using the Female Sexual Function Index they analyzed vaginal lubrication, desire, arousal, ability to achieve orgasm, and overall sexual satisfaction. The nerve sparing group had a mean age of 55.9 and follow-up for 13 months. There was no significant decline in scores after surgery – 24.5 preoperatively vs. 22.3 postoperatively – and all patients were sexually active at 1 year. This differed from the non-nerve-sparing group. These patients had a mean age of 56.9 and follow-up of 14 months. Their scores declined significantly from 25 preoperatively to 11 postoperatively with the patients experiencing vaginal dryness, lack of arousal, and dyspareunia. Only one patient was sexually active after cystectomy.

Quality of life studies in the gynecologic literature regarding sexual dysfunction after hysterectomy and oophrectomy are scarce. It is known that many women experience sexual dysfunction after these procedures but the exact causes have not been elucidated. As the gynecologists focus more on these issues, improved surgical techniques and preoperative counseling will help the female cystectomy patient as well.

Large scale prospective comparative studies are needed to assess sexual outcomes after organ-sparing radical cystectomy. In addition, a validated questionnaire is needed to assess sexual dysfunction more thoroughly.

7. Conclusion

Historically anterior pelvic exenteration was the standard of care for women with bladder cancer, but preservation of the pelvic organs is now becoming a priority. Properly selected patients with bladder carcinoma can safely undergo organ sparing radical cystectomy and diversion. Initial results are promising with regards to continence, cancer control and preservation of sexual function. Long term follow up is needed to assess the rate of recurrence in the preserved organs as well as the rate of primary malignancy. Prospective studies are still needed to assess the quality of life impact and specifically sexual outcomes after organ sparing radical cystectomy.

References

1. American Cancer Society Surveillance Research, Cancer Facts and Figures 2006. Atlanta: American Cancer Society, 2006.
2. Marshall FF, Treiger FG. Radical cystectomy (anterior exenteration) in the female patient. Urol Clin North Am 18: 765, 1991.
3. Chin JL, Wolf RM, Huben RP, et al. Vaginal recurrence after cystectomy for bladder cancer. J Urol 134: 58, 1985.
4. Paepe ME, Rubin A, Mahadevia P. Urethral involvement in female patients with bladder cancer. Cancer 65: 1237, 1990.
5. Walsh PC, Lepor H, Eggleston JC. Radical prostatectomy with preservation of sexual function: anatomical and pathological considerations. Prostate 4: 473, 1983.
6. Schlegal PH, Walsh PC. Neuroanatomical approach to radical cystoprostatectomy with preservation of sexual function. J Urol 138: 1402, 1987.
7. Schover LR, von Eschenbach AC. Sexual function and female radical cystectomy: A case series. J Urol 134: 465, 1985.
8. Ghoneim MA. Orthotopic bladder substitution in women following cystectomy for bladder cancer. Urol Clin North Am 24: 255, 1997.
9. Schoenberg M, Hortopan S, Schlossberg L, Marshall F. Anatomical anterior exenteration with urethral and vaginal preservation: Illustrated surgical method. J Urol 161: 569, 1999.
10. Stenzl A, Colleselli K, Poisel S, Feichtinger H, Pontasch H, Bartsch G. Rationale and technique of nerve sparing radical cystectomy before an orthotopic neobladder procedure in women. J Urol 154: 2044, 1995.
11. Stenzl A, Ladislav J, Coloby P, Golia S, Bartsch G, Marek B, Tadao K, Robertson C. Urethra-sparing cystectomy and orthotopic urinary diversion in women with malignant pelvic tumors. Cancer 92: 1864, 2001.
12. Camey M, Le Duc A. L'enterocystoplastie avec cystoprostatectomie totale pour cancer de la vessie. Ann Urol 13: 114, 1979.
13. Stein JP, Stenzl A, Esrig D, et al. Lower urinary tract reconstruction following cystectomy in women using the Kock ileal reservoir with bilateral ureteroileal urethrostomy: Initial clinical experience. J Urol 152: 1404, 1994.
14. Stenzl A, Colleselli K, Bartsch G. Continent reservoir to the urethra in the female. J Urol part 2, 151: 204A; videotape V-19, 1994.
15. Colleselli K, Strasser H, Moriggl B, Stenzl A, Poisel S, Bartsch G. Hemi-Kock to the female urethra: anatomical approach to the continence mechanism to the female urethra. J Urol part 2, 151: 500A; abstract 1089, 1994.
16. De Paepe ME, Andre R, Mahadevia P. Urethral involvement in female patients with bladder cancer. A study of 22 cystectomy specimens. Cancer 65: 1237, 1990.
17. Coloby PJ, Kakizoe T, Tobisu K, Sakamoto M. Urethral involvement in female bladder cancer patients: mapping of 47 consecutive cystourethrectomy specimens. J Urol 152: 1438, 1994.
18. Stein J, Cote R, Freeman J, Esrig D, Elmajian D, Groshen S, Skinner E, Boyd S, Lieskovsky G, Skinner D. Indications for lower urinary tract reconstruction in women after cystectomy for bladder cancer: A pathological review of female cystectomy specimens. J Urol 154: 1329, 1995.
19. Chen M, Pisters L, Malpica A, Pettaway C, Dinney C. Risk of urethral, vaginal, and cervical involvement in patients undergoing radical cystectomy for bladder cancer: results of a contemporary cystectomy series from M.D. Anderson Cancer Center. J Urol 157: 2120, 1997.
20. Stenzl A, Draxl H, Posch B, Colleselli K, Falk M, Bartsch G. Bladder cancer: The risk of urethral tumors in female bladder cancer: can the urethra be used for orthotopic reconstruction of the lower urinary tract? J Urol 153: 950, 1995.
21. Chang S, Cole E, Cookson M, Peterson M, Smith J. Preservation of the anterior vaginal wall during female radical cystectomy with orthotopic urinary diversion: technique and results. J Urol 168: 1442, 2002.
22. Ali-El-Dein B, Gohma M, Ghoneim M. Critical evaluation of the problem of chronic urinary retention after orthotopic bladder substitution in women. J Urol 168: 587, 2002.
23. Puppo P, Introini C, Calvi P, Naselli A. Prevention of chronic urinary retention in orthotopic bladder replacement in the female. Eur Urol 47: 674–78, 2005.
24. Ali-El-Dien B, El-Sobky E, Hohenfellner M, Ghoneim MA. Orthotopic bladder substitution in women: functional evaluation. J Urol 161: 1875, 1999.
25. Abol-enein H, Ghoneim M. Functional results of orthotopic ileal neobladder with serous-lined extramural ureteral reimplantation: experience with 450 patients. J Urol 165: 1427, 2001.
26. Rapp D, O'Connor C, Katz E, Steinberg G. Nepbladder-vaginal fistula after cystectomy and orthotopic neobladder construction. BJU Int 94: 1092, 2004.
27. Chang SS, Cole E, Smith JA, Cookson MS. Pathological findings of gynecologic organs obtained at female radical cystectomy. J Urol 168: 147, 2002.

28. Ali-El-Dein B, Abdel-Latif M, Mosbah A, Eraky I, Shaaban A, Taha N, Ghoneim M. Secondary malignant involvement of gynecologic organs in radical cystectomy speciments in women: Is it mandatory to remove these organs routinely? J Urol 172: 885, 2004.
29. Zippe C, Raina R, Shah A, Massanyi E, Agarwal A, Ulchaker J, Jones S, Klein E. Female sexual dysfuction after radical cystectomy: a new outcome measure. Urology 63: 1153, 2003.
30. Horenblas S, Meinhardt W, Ijzerman W, Moonen L. Sexuality preserving cystectomy and neobladder: Initial results. J Urol 166: 837, 2001.
31. Zippe C, Nandipati K, Agarwal A, Rupesh R. Female sexual dysfunction after pelvic surgery: The impact of surgical modifications. BJU 96: 959, 2005.
32. Bhat A, Nandipati K, Nivedita D, Ulchaker J, Jones S, Rackley R, Zippe C. Neurovascular preservation in orthotopic cystectomy: Impact on female sexual function. Urology 67: 185, 2006.

17
Nerve Sparing Radical Cystectomy

Edward M. Schaeffer, Matthew E. Nielsen, Mark L. Gonzalgo, and Mark P. Schoenberg

Contents

Abstract Radical cystectomy is the definitive surgical treatment for a high-risk and invasive bladder and is governed by the general principles of aggressive extirpation. In the modern era, understanding the functional anatomy of the pelvic autonomic plexus and cavernosal nerves has facilitated the development of techniques of radical cystectomy which spare sexual function without compromising on the primary goal of oncological control. This chapter describes the surgical anatomy and approaches and outcomes relevant to the nerve sparing radical cystectomy.

As the definitive surgical treatment for high-risk and invasive bladder cancer, radical cystectomy is governed by the general principles of aggressive extirpation common to all oncological surgical procedures. In the modern era, advances in our understanding of the functional anatomy of the pelvic autonomic plexus and cavernosal nerves have facilitated the development of techniques with enhanced precision that attempt to spare sexual function without compromising the primary goal of oncological control. Anatomic nerve-sparing radical cystectomy for bladder cancer builds upon the foundations of techniques developed in the surgical management of prostate cancer, utilizing precise dissection in the process of tumor extirpation enabling oncologic control and anatomic reconstruction. This chapter describes the surgical anatomy, approaches and outcomes relevant to this approach.

Keywords Cystectomy, Nerve sparing, Sexual function

1. Arterial and Venous Anatomy

The bladder and prostate receive blood supply from the superior and inferior vesical arteries, two branches of the anterior trunk of the hypogastric artery. The prostatic arterial supply can be divided into two main groups of vessels, the capsular and urethral branches. The capsular arteries run along the pelvic sidewall and inferolateral prostate in the lateral pelvic fascia.

From: *Current Clinical Urology: Bladder Cancer,* Edited by: C.T. Lee and D.P. Wood,
DOI; 10.1007/978-1-59745-417-9_17, © Humana Press, a Part of Springer Science + Business Media, LLC 2010

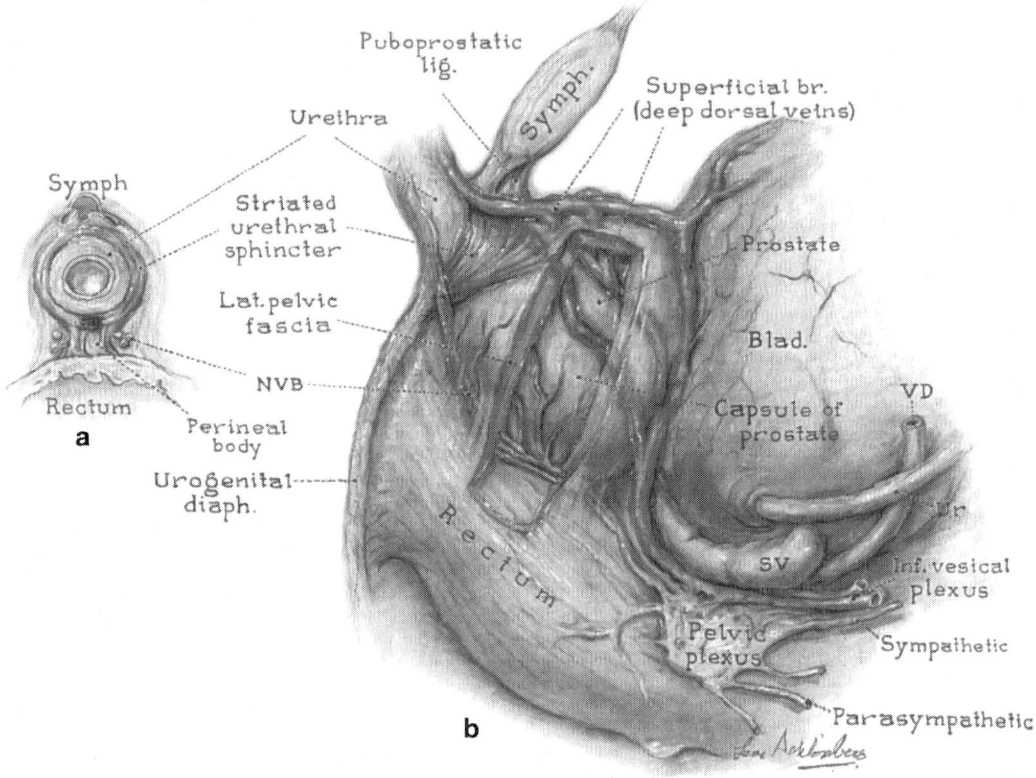

FIG. 17.1. (**a**) Cross section of urethra distal to the apex of the prostate. (**b**) Lateral view of male pelvis depicting relationship of bladder, prostate, pelvic plexus and neurovascular bundle

These branches perforate into the prostate and provide macroscopic anatomic landmarks for the branches of the pelvic plexus that innervate the corpora cavernosa (Fig. 17.1) (1, 2). In females, the inferior and superior vesical arteries supply the bladder, ureters and vagina (3). Perforating vessels from the inferior vesical artery run along the lateral aspect of the vagina and, as in males, act as landmarks for branches of the pelvic plexus supplying the cavernosal bodies of the clitoris (Fig. 17.2) (3).

2. Pelvic Plexus

Dual autonomic innervation of the lower urinary tract is derived from the pelvic plexus and consists of parasympathetic fibers from the sacral center (S2–S4) and sympathetic fibers from the thoracolumbar center (L1–L2) (1, 4–6). This plexus innervates the bladder, ureters, seminal vesicles, prostate, membranous urethra and cavernosal bodies. Somatic nerves also run through this plexus, supplying the levator ani, coccygeus muscles and a portion of the striated urethral sphincter. The plexus lies in a retroperitoneal location beside the rectum, 5–11 cm from the anal verge, and is perforated by the inferior vesicle artery (1). The nerves supplying autonomic innervation to the membranous urethra and cavernosal bodies travel outside the prostatic capsule in the lateral pervic fascia between the rectum and the prostate. Preservation of these nerves, lying in the neurovascular bundle of Walsh (NVB), is essential for preservation of potency (6, 7). Additionally, experimental and clinical outcomes data suggest preservation of the neurovascular bundle may also contribute to return of continence postoperatively, via collateral branches to the striated sphincter (8–10). This observation may have functional relevance to continence outcomes in patients undergoing cystectomy with orthotopic urinary reconstruction. In females, the pelvic plexus also provides dual autonomic innervation to the female urethra. These fibers run in the lateral vaginal walls dorsal to the urethra and also supply the cavernosal bodies of the clitoris controlling its engorgement and contributing to female sexual arousal (11).

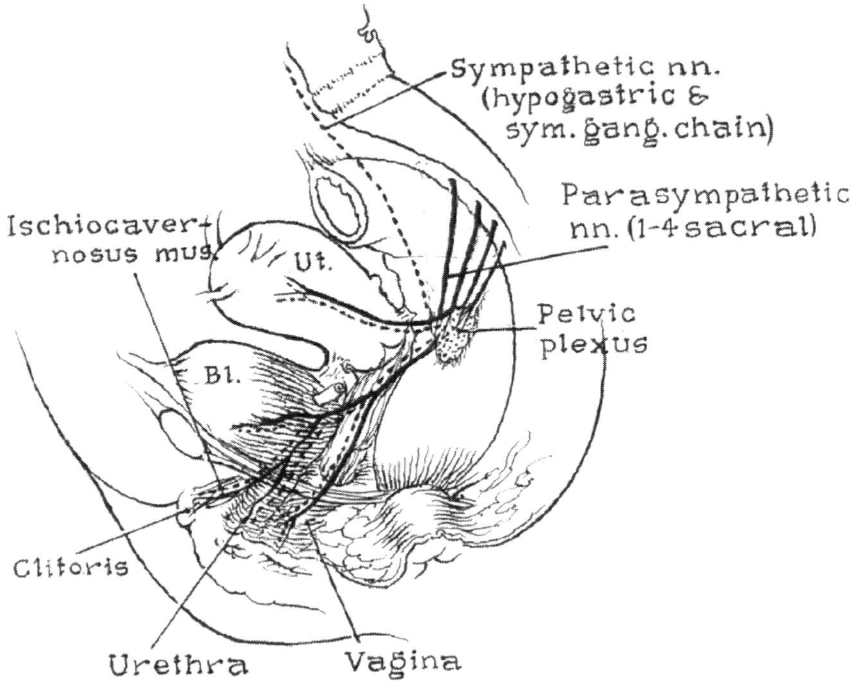

FIG. 17.2. Lateral view of female pelvis demonstrating relationship of bladder, uterus, vagina, pelvic plexus and neurovascular bundle

3. Anatomic Associations

The lower genitourinary organs are extraperitoneal. The bladder is anchored to the anterior abdominal wall by the urachus and the superior portion of the bladder is covered by peritoneum. The ureter is retroperitoneal as it enters the pelvis and crosses anterior to the iliac vessels. Classically it courses over the vessels at the bifurcation of the external iliac and hypogastric arteries and runs lateral to the crossing vas deferens.

The prostate is invested in the prostatic and levator fascia. Between these fascial layers lies the neurovascular bundle of Walsh (12) which provides both autonomic innervation and blood supply to the prostate (1, 2). Distal branches of the NVB facilitate engorgement of the erectile bodies of the corpora cavernosa, resulting in erection. Branches of the pudendal nerve provide the principal somatic innervation of the external striated urethral sphincter, surrounding the membranous urethra distal to the apex of the prostate. This sphincter consists of slow-twitch fibers responsible for passive urinary control (12). Somatic nerve fibers coursing in the neurovascular bundle from the pelvic plexus provide additional efferent supply to the sphincter (3, 14).

In females the urethral sphincter invests the distal two thirds of the urethra and consists of both smooth and striated muscle innervated by autonomic fibers from the pelvic plexus and somatic fibers from the pudendal nerve. It and the bladder lie anterior to the anterior vaginal wall.

4. Preoperative Considerations

We routinely review existing pathology, perform restaging with transurethral resection and update axial imaging as part of our preoperative surgical evaluation. We utilize pelvic MR imaging with dynamic gadolinium enhancement as this readily demonstrates the extent of the tumor and the involvement of adjacent organs (13). This imaging complements the clinical and pathologic staging as these staging modalities are less informative in the detection of extravesical disease. Together this provides an accurate assessment of the tumor type, anatomic location and extent of the disease and is valuable preoperatively when counseling patients on the possibility of a nerve-sparing approach. For example, bulky disease suggesting extravesical extension may result in a modification of the surgical approach (antegrade or retrograde extirpation) with consequences relevant to the feasibility of nerve-sparing (unilateral or bilateral). Location of the disease is also important in evaluating females for a reproductive organ sparing/ nerve sparing procedure as urethral recurrences are associated with primary tumors located at the bladder neck/trigone. Ultimately, however, these decisions are made intraoperatively, including a tactile assessment of the dissection planes between the pelvic organs and the surrounding neural structures.

5. Surgical Technique

5.1. Positioning and Instrumentation

The patient is positioned supine over the break in the table. The patient is not positioned in lithotomy as we do not routinely perform a simultaneous urethrectomy and cystoprostatectomy. If adverse pathology is noted after a final review of the fixed specimen we will perform a staged urethrectomy shortly after recovery from the initial surgical procedure. Nerve sparing in women can also feasibly be performed in a supine position with the legs spread as this will permit access to the vaginal vault during the dissection.

The operation can be performed with standard surgical instruments. A Balfour retractor with narrow and wide malleable blades is sufficient for retraction. The surgeon should be equipped with a fiberoptic headlight and 2.5 power surgical loupes to aid in the visualization of the fine anatomic structures including the neurovascular bundles.

5.2. Surgical Narrative

A low midline incision is made from the pubis to the umbilicus. The extraperitoneal space of Retzius is developed and the Balfour retractor inserted.

Complete bilateral pelvic lymphadenectomy is performed. The dissection begins medial to the genitofemoral nerve and includes lymphatic tissue from the external iliac artery and vein and the obturator fossa. The dissection extends deep to the pelvic sidewall, caudally to the femoral canal and cranially to the bifurcation of the iliac artery.

Dissection then proceeds to the division of the vas deferens laterally at its entrance to the inguinal ring and inferomedially at the ejaculatory duct. The excised portion is removed and dissection continues with medial retraction of the bladder permitting identification and ligation of the obliterated umbilical artery. This embryologically important vessel may remain patent and contribute to vesical blood supply; thus, ligation with hemo-clips prior to transaction is prudent.

One can perform the extirpative portion of the procedure in the extra-peritoneal space in which the lower genitor-urinary organs lie, as this simplifies bowel retraction and lessens evaporative fluid losses during surgery. To continue extra-peritoneally, one develops the plane between the bladder and the peritoneum by gently sweeping the peritoneum cranially at the level of the obliterated umbilical artery. If the planes are well-preserved the edge of peritoneum is readily noted. This plane is started deep and carried anteriorly to the medial and median umbilical ligaments. When these are taken the intraperitoneal intestines are free and easily retracted cranially. This technique also allows for easy delineation of the retrovesical cul-de-sac and subsequently, the vascualar pedicles of the bladder. A more conventional intra/extra-peritoneal approach may also be utilized if the planes between the bladder and peritoneum are fused either by tumor or other preoperative conditions including radiation or chemotherapy. For this approach, the retrovesical cul-de-sac can be exposed through incising the posterior peritoneum.

After exposure of the retrovesical space and delineation of the vascular pedicles to the bladder, nerve sparing is initiated. When attempting nerve-sparing we avoid the use of electocautery and other energy sources in the region of the neurovascular bundle to minimize the possibility of thermal injury. Our standard approach begins in a retrograde manner. The endopelvic fascia and apex of the prostate are exposed with cranial retraction of the bladder and removal of the overlying adipose tissue. Along the midline at the prostatic apex the superficial dorsal vein is isolated and ligated. The lateral endopelvic fascia is then divided sharply to expose the apex of the prostate. Investing levator ani muscles are swept laterally off the apex of the prostate toward the pelvic diaphragm. Next, the puboprostatic ligaments are released sharply, a process aided by gentle downward pressure with a sponge stick. These maneuvers free and expose the apex of the prostate to allow for accurate identification and subsequent control of the dorsal vein complex. A 3-0 Monocryl (poliglecaprone) suture is pre-placed through the dorsal venous complex. While applying downward pressure on the anterior surface of the prostate, the vein is scored with a #15 knife blade and then released with Metzenbaum scissors exposing the urethra. The transected dorsal vein complex is precisely over sewn with the preplaced monocryl suture, approximating the leaflets of the exposed vein anterior and lateral to the urethra. Deep, broad bites across the dorsal vein should be avoided as they may inadvertently damage the adjacent pelvic floor and striated spincter. Closure of the bleeding back (prostatic) side of the dorsal vein with a running 2-0 absorbable suture reduces blood loss and enhances visualization.

The urethra may now be divided. If orthotopic urinary reconstruction is planned, sutures can be preplaced into the urethra. The neurovascular bundle is now approached, first on the side contralateral to the tumor. Identification and release are initiated first with medial retraction of the prostate and dissection and release of the lateral prostatic fascia. The neurovascular bundle is released with a large blunt right angle. When perforating vessels are encountered, they should be isolated, clipped and divided as electocautery can damage the nerves. Complete release of the NVB will allow it to fall away from the lateral pedicle of the prostate. This can then safely be taken with hemoclips exposing Denovillier's fascia and the seminal vesicles laterally just behind the fascia. Disection and release of the seminal vesicles is next performed with a blunt upward retraction. The vascular pedicles to the seminal vesicles enter at their tips and as they are in close proximity to the NVBs, they are carefully controlled with hemo-clips. Dissection can continue in a retrograde manner with ligation of the remainder of the inferior vesical artery and the superior vesical artery.

Alternatively, an antegrade approach may also be utilized for a nerve-sparing radical cystoprostatectomy. After development of the retrovesical cul-de-sac between the bladder and rectum, the vesical pedicles can be ligated. During this approach, special attention is required during ligation of the inferior vesical pedicle as these vessels perforate the pelvic plexus containing the autonomic nerves to the cavernosal bodies. In particular at the prostato-vesical junction, ligation of the pedicle should be performed with medial retraction of the specimen to carefully delineate the pedicle from the seminal vesicle, as the neurovascular bundle runs laterally along the tip of the SV. Precise attention to the anatomic relations of the structures is of particular import in this step in the antegrade dissection, as the distal investment of the NVB in the prostatic fascia pulls the NVB closer to the specimen. Once the pedicles are taken, the lateral pelvic fascia overlying the neurovascular bundle and the endopelvic fascia overlying apex of the prostate are released exposing the neurovascular bundle and the apex of the prostate. The dissection can continue in a completely antegrade fashion or the NVB can be released at the apex of the prostate as described above.

Once the specimen is removed, margins can be assessed and reconstruction can proceed, the topics are discussed in greater detail in the additional chapters.

Ligation of the major vascular pedicles to the bladder can be controlled with hemoclips or an endoGIA reticulating staple device. If rapid ligation with the stapling device is utilized, the stapler should be inserted in an antegrade fashion so as to mitigate the risk of inadvertent injury to the pelvic plexus and its branches. The staples should be placed inferior to the ureteral stump and parallel the rectum. Care should be taken not to incorporate the obturator nerve or accessory vessels to the cavernosal bodies. Although these stapling devices offer the advantages of rapid vascular control one must ensure that the NVBs are completely released and free from the inferior vesical pedicle so that they are not encorporated in stapling device

Nerve sparing in female patients undergoing uretheral sparing cystectomy is also possible. Details of the female reproductive organ preserving cystectomy are outlined in this chapter. In women the nerves contributing to clitoral engorgement and sexual arousal also emanate from the pelvic plexus and move anteriorly with the inferior vesical artery along the fascial investments of the lateral vaginal walls (11). Accordingly, preservation of the lateral and anterior vaginal walls during bladder extirpation ensures optimal nerve preservation.

6. Outcomes

6.1. Oncologic Control

Long term follow-up data demonstrates that nerve sparing radical cystoprostatectomy does not compromise cancer control and can enhance post operative quality of life. The 10 year survival rate, free of local recurrence is 94% in the Johns Hopkins series (14, 15). The Bern group report similarly rates low of local recurrences, in particular, 3% in patients with organ-confined disease (≤pT2 N0) and 11% in nonorgan confined disease (>T2 N0) (16). These results are comparable to other large series that do not routinely employ a nerve sparing approach (17, 18). Modification of the techniques with unilateral nerve sparing can be implemented in patients with large unilateral tumor burdens. In these patients, wide unilateral local excision can be employed to ensure optimal tumor extirpation (16).

Female urethra sparing surgery also does not appear to compromise oncologic outcomes with disease specific and disease free survival comparable to patients with complete pelvic exenterations. Stein and Coloby retrospectively step sectioned the urethra in female patients with bladder cancer who underwent a complete cystourethrectomy and found urethral tumor involvement in, 6 to 10% of the cases (19, 20). In these studies there was a strong correlation between urethral involvement and tumor in the neck of the bladder or trigone. This association is also supported by retrospective analyses by Ashworth and Stenzl who noted a 1.4–2% incidence of urethral tumor recurrences and correlated a risk of urethral recurrence with primary tumor involvement at the bladder neck (21, 22). Accordingly, preoperative cystoscopy and staging can aid in the identification of candidates who can optimally benefit from urethral sparing/nerve sparing cystectomy with minimal oncological risk (23).

6.2. Sexual Function

Nerve sparing increases potency rates after radical cystoprostatectomy (24). Rates of potency vary and are likely dependent on factors including age and medical comorbidities such as diabetes and peripheral vascular disease. The Johns Hopkins series reported 42% potency in men with good preoperative erectile function (15). In men younger than 50, potency was recovered in 62%. Increased rates of potency after nerve sparing approaches have been reported by other institutions (25, 26). Studer and associates have confirmed the initial observations of Schoenberg et al. of age-related return of sexual function (16, 27). In multi-variate analyses of their series, age <65 was significantly associated with recovery of erectile function (16). This association of age and return of erectile function correlates with data from radical prostatectomy series that have reported both earlier and ultimately better return of sexual function (7, 28). The mechanism underlying this recovery is unknown but may stem from improved regenerative/recovery potential of the younger tissues.

The functional outcomes of women undergoing female organ sparing cystectomy has not been thoroughly explored, however, early reports suggest preoperative sexual function can be preserved with a nerve sparing technique (29, 30). Bhatt and collegues demonstrated, in a limited case matched series, near preservation of all domains (desire, arousal, lubrication, orgasm, satisfaction and pain) of the female sexual function index (FSFI) when nerve preservation was utilized (29). This was contrasted in a small matched series of women who did not undergo nerve sparing and experienced declines in FSFI comparable to other reports (31, 32).

7. Summary

Advances in the understanding of the functional anatomy of the male and female pelvis have facilitated the development of techniques that optimize preservation of structures contributing to sexual function while maintaining oncological control. Continued delineation of the precise mechanisms of nerve injury and regeneration will direct further advances in the preservation and return to the baseline function of patients with bladder cancer undergoing extirpation and reconstruction.

References

1. Lepor H, Gregerman M, Crosby R, Mostofi FK, Walsh PC. Precise localization of the autonomic nerves from the pelvic plexus to the corpora cavernosa: a detailed anatomical study of the adult male pelvis. J Urol 1985;133(2):207–12.
2. Walsh PC. Anatomic Radical Retropubic Prostatectomy, 8th ed. Philadelphia, Pennsylvania: Saunders;2002.
3. Jimenez VK, Marshall FF. Surgery of bladder cancer. In: Walsh PC. et al. (eds.). Campbell's Urology, 8th ed. Philadelphia, Pennsylvania: Saunders;2002.
4. Lue TF, Zeineh SJ, Schmidt RA, Tanagho EA. Neuroanatomy of penile erection: its relevance to iatrogenic impotence. J Urol 1984;131(2):273–80.
5. Schlegel PN, Walsh PC. Neuroanatomical approach to radical cystoprostatectomy with preservation of sexual function. J Urol 1987;138(6):1402–6.
6. Walsh PC, Donker PJ. Impotence following radical prostatectomy: insight into etiology and prevention. J Urol 1982; 128(3):492–7.
7. Walsh PC, Marschke P, Ricker D, Burnett AL. Patient-reported urinary continence and sexual function after anatomic radical prostatectomy. Urology 2000;55(1):58–61.
8. Steiner MS, Morton RA, Walsh PC. Impact of anatomical radical prostatectomy on urinary continence. J Urol 1991;145(3):512–4; discussion 4–5.
9. Wei JT, Dunn RL, Marcovich R, Montie JE, Sanda MG. Prospective assessment of patient reported urinary continence after radical prostatectomy. J Urol 2000;164(3 Pt 1):744–8.
10. Nelson CP, Montie JE, McGuire EJ, Wedemeyer G, Wei JT. Intraoperative nerve stimulation with measurement of urethral sphincter pressure changes during radical retropubic prostatectomy: a feasibility study. J Urol 2003;169(6):2225–8.

11. Stenzl A, Colleselli K, Poisel S, Feichtinger H, Pontasch H, Bartsch G. Rationale and technique of nerve sparing radical cystectomy before an orthotopic neobladder procedure in women. J Urol 1995;154(6):2044–9.
12. Stedmann's. Stedmann's Medical Dictionary, 27th ed. Philadelphia, Pennsylvania: Lippincott Williams and Wilkins; 2000.
13. Tekes A, Kamel IR, Imam K, Chan TY, Schoenberg MP, Bluemke DA. MR imaging features of transitional cell carcinoma of the urinary bladder. AJR Am J Roentgenol 2003;180(3):771–7.
14. Brendler CB, Steinberg GD, Marshall FF, Mostwin JL, Walsh PC. Local recurrence and survival following nerve-sparing radical cystoprostatectomy. J Urol 1990;144(5):1137–40; discussion 40–1.
15. Schoenberg MP, Walsh PC, Breazeale DR, Marshall FF, Mostwin JL, Brendler CB. Local recurrence and survival following nerve sparing radical cystoprostatectomy for bladder cancer: 10-year followup. J Urol 1996;155(2):490–4.
16. Kessler TM, Burkhard FC, Studer UE. Clinical indications and outcomes with nerve-sparing cystectomy in patients with bladder cancer. Urol Clin North Am 2005;32(2):165–75.
17. Hautmann RE, de Petriconi R, Gottfried HW, Kleinschmidt K, Mattes R, Paiss T. The ileal neobladder: complications and functional results in 363 patients after 11 years of followup. J Urol 1999;161(2):422–7; discussion 7–8.
18. Stein JP, Lieskovsky G, Cote R, et al. Radical cystectomy in the treatment of invasive bladder cancer: long-term results in 1,054 patients. J Clin Oncol 2001;19(3):666–75.
19. Coloby PJ, Kakizoe T, Tobisu K, Sakamoto M. Urethral involvement in female bladder cancer patients: mapping of 47 consecutive cysto-urethrectomy specimens. J Urol 1994;152(5 Pt 1):1438–42.
20. Stein JP, Cote RJ, Freeman JA, et al. Indications for lower urinary tract reconstruction in women after cystectomy for bladder cancer: a pathological review of female cystectomy specimens. J Urol 1995;154(4):1329–33.
21. Ashworth A. Papillomatosis of the urethra. Br J Urol 1956;28(1):3–13.
22. Stenzl A, Draxl H, Posch B, Colleselli K, Falk M, Bartsch G. The risk of urethral tumors in female bladder cancer: can the urethra be used for orthotopic reconstruction of the lower urinary tract? J Urol 1995;153(3 Pt 2):950–5.
23. Stenzl A, Holtl L. Orthotopic bladder reconstruction in women–what we have learned over the last decade. Crit Rev Oncol Hematol 2003;47(2):147–54.
24. Walsh PC, Mostwin JL. Radical prostatectomy and cystoprostatectomy with preservation of potency. Results using a new nerve-sparing technique. Br J Urol 1984;56(6):694–7.
25. Ramon J, Leandri P, Rossignol G, Gautier JR. Preservation of urinary continence and potency after cystoprostatectomy. Prog Clin Biol Res 1992;378:125–32.
26. Zippe CD, Raina R, Massanyi EZ, et al. Sexual function after male radical cystectomy in a sexually active population. Urology 2004;64(4):682–5; discussion 5–6.
27. Bjerre BD, Johansen C, Steven K. Sexological problems after cystectomy: bladder substitution compared with ileal conduit diversion. A questionnaire study of male patients. Scand J Urol Nephrol 1998;32(3):187–93.
28. Quinlan DM, Epstein JI, Carter BS, Walsh PC. Sexual function following radical prostatectomy: influence of preservation of neurovascular bundles. J Urol 1991;145(5):998–1002.
29. Bhatt A, Nandipati K, Dhar N, et al. Neurovascular preservation in orthotopic cystectomy: impact on female sexual function. Urology 2006;67(4):742–5.
30. Bjerre BD, Johansen C, Steven K. A questionnaire study of sexological problems following urinary diversion in the female patient. Scand J Urol Nephrol 1997;31(2):155–60.
31. Volkmer BG, Gschwend JE, Herkommer K, Simon J, Kufer R, Hautmann RE. Cystectomy and orthotopic ileal neobladder: the impact on female sexuality. J Urol 2004;172(6 Pt 1):2353–7.
32. Zippe CD, Raina R, Shah AD, et al. Female sexual dysfunction after radical cystectomy: a new outcome measure. Urology 2004;63(6):1153–7.

18
Quality of Care Indicators for Radical Cystectomy

Matthew R. Cooperberg and Badrinath R. Konety

Contents

Abstract Radical cystectomy is the gold standard treatment for invasive bladder cancer, and requires high standards for both surgical skill and ancillary support to achieve consistently good outcomes. As is the case elsewhere in the health care system, increasing attention has been paid in recent years to the quality of care delivered before, during, and after surgery. Defining high-quality care in the context of cystectomy, however, is far from straightforward. Multiple outcomes are relevant – perioperative morbidity and mortality, long-term oncologic outcomes, and urinary and sexual health-related quality of life – as there exists as yet no consensus on the best way to measure these outcomes and appropriately risk-adjust them based on patient case mix.

The process of identification and validation of structural aspects of care and processes of care which are likely to predict good outcomes is in an early stage for cystectomy. Several candidate measures have been examined, and each is controversial to some extent with respect to its relevance to cystectomy outcomes. The time from diagnosis to cystectomy, adequacy of lymphadenectomy, and availability of orthotopic diversion are three process measures which are good candidate indicators of quality care. Surgical volume, both surgeon- and hospital-specific, has received a great deal of attention in the media, but results of the studies to date must be interpreted cautiously, and the implications of policies implicitly or explicitly driving regionalization of cystectomy care should be carefully considered. It is critical that clinicians specializing in the care of bladder cancer, rather than regulators or insurers, continue to direct progress in forging consensus on approaches to measurement and reporting of quality outcomes for radical is in an early stage for cystectomy.

Keywords Bladder neoplasms, Radical cystectomy, Quality of health care, Health care quality indicators, Surgical volume, Outcome assessment (health care), Process assessment (health care), Quality of life

1. Introduction: Quality Health Care

Over 9,000 radical cystectomies are performed annually in the United States (1). The pre-, peri-, and postoperative

From: *Current Clinical Urology: Bladder Cancer,* Edited by: C.T. Lee and D.P. Wood,

DOI; 10.1007/978-1-59745-417-9_18,

care of men and women undergoing this procedure is challenging by any measure, and the quality of care delivered to these patients is a subject of increasing interest. However, in evaluating the criteria by which quality cystectomy care may be assessed, we must consider the complexities of the answer to the question of what in fact constitutes quality care. Efforts to measure quality health care focus on one or more aspects of Donabedian's well-cited triad of structure, process, and outcomes (2). *Structural measures* focus on concrete and easily measurable aspects of health care quality such as adequacy of physical plant facilities and nurse-to-patient ratios. Structural measures are usually easy to assess; however, their relationship to the outcomes is not always clear, and adequate structures are generally accepted as necessary but not sufficient to assure high-quality care.

Outcomes represent the true end-points of interest for the assessment of the quality of health care, comprising both beneficial and adverse impacts of interventions on quantity and quality of life, including complications and treatment-related morbidity, modification of disease-specific mortality, and impact on patient health-related quality of life (HRQOL). Improving outcomes is the focus of the large majority of clinical research and the evidence-based medicine movement. However, using outcomes to define quality is invariably problematic. Ultimately, the majority of differences in the outcomes are attributable to factors external to the delivery of health care (3, 4). Complication and mortality outcomes, for example, may be driven at least as much by patient factors such as comorbidity and disease stage as by the clinician's decision-making, and in the absence of a generally accepted risk-adjustment system, outcomes-based quality reporting will drive physicians to turn away higher risk patients. HRQOL outcomes are increasingly recognized as at least as important as mortality outcomes, but are even more problematic: who assesses HRQOL, in what setting, using what methods and criteria, and incorporating what techniques for risk-adjustment will all exert significant impact on outcomes.

Given the difficulties with measuring and interpreting outcomes, most quality measurement efforts focus on *processes* of care. Processes are aspects of health care delivery directly attributable to the health care system which are believed, based on clinical evidence and/or expert opinion, to affect outcomes consistently across a large spectrum of patients. Examples of processes felt to be well-validated as measures of quality care include use of beta-blockade after myocardial infarction and prevalence of regular ophthalmologic examination among diabetics. Two groups over the past few years have made strides towards establishing a criteria for quality care for prostate cancer (5, 6). In contrast, accepted quality of care indicators do not yet exist for radical cystectomy or other aspects of bladder cancer care. Nonetheless, a growing body of literature has emerged which identifies structures and processes of care which may be important and meaningful determinants of patient centered outcomes in bladder cancer (see Fig. 18.1).

2. Structural Measures

Many structural aspects of cystectomy care – adequacy of operating room and patient care unit facilities, certification of surgeons and other providers, etc. – are supported as quality metrics by common sense if not by high-level clinical evidence, and already are used extensively as evaluation criteria by accreditation organizations. Others, such as ready availability of radiation therapy, chemotherapy infusion, and psychological and other supportive care, are also important at an intuitive level. Some of these measures are included in a set of quality of care indicators proposed by an expert panel specifically for early stage prostate cancer care (6), but they have not yet been formally evaluated in the context of bladder cancer.

One structural aspect of cystectomy quality, however, which has been the focus of significant scrutiny in recent years, is both surgeon- and hospital-based surgical volume. Evidence has accumulated over the past quarter-century linking surgical volume with outcomes in other disease conditions, and has engendered significant discussion regarding both the explanations for and the significance of the findings. The volume-outcomes relationship was first noted by Luft et al. in 1979 (7) and since then, has been extensively explored in a number of areas in surgery and medicine. The Institute of Medicine commissioned a systematic review of the United States and European literature, analyzing 135 studies involving 27 different diagnoses and procedures. The authors of the review found that in general a higher volume does associate with better outcomes, but that the magnitude of the relationship varies widely, as does the methodological quality of the studies (8).

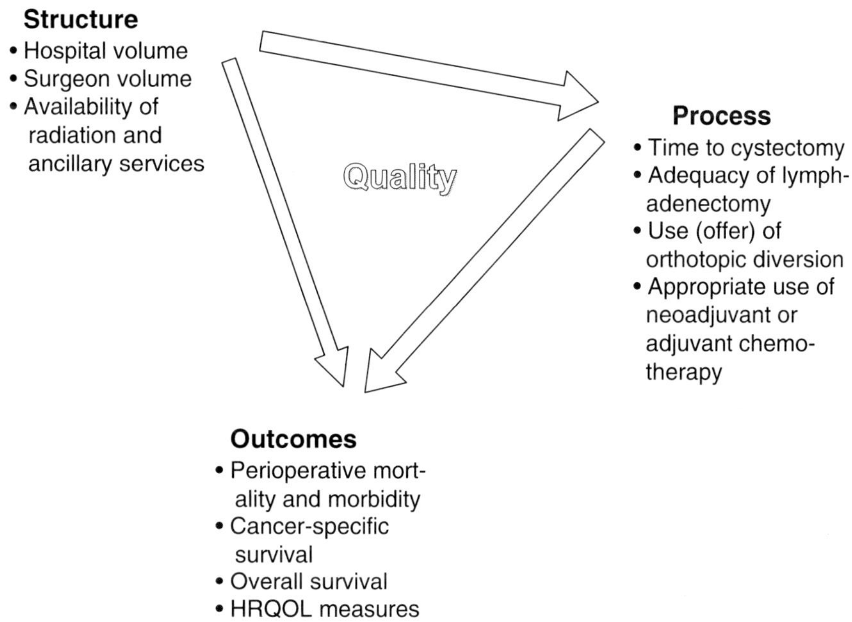

FIG. 18.1. The quality triad: examples of candidate measures specific to cysectomy. Structural aspects of care may be associated directly with outcomes, but in general they help drive clinical processes which in turn are believed to contribute to outcomes. Although the arrows are drawn as one-way, better insights into which outcomes are most important – and how they should be assessed – should be expected to lead to improved measures of structural and process-related quality of care

In the 1990s, the volume-outcome relationship in cardiac surgery was felt to be sufficiently strong that the New York State Department of Health now publishes the annual volume and mortality rates for every cardiac surgeon in the state. Dudley et al. analyzed claims data for admissions in California in 1997, and concluded that of over 58,000 admissions for 11 selected conditions, low volume hospital status could account for 26% (95% CI 13–37%) of the 2,315 deaths observed (9). Begg et al. were the first to focus on cancer care; they analyzed five major cancer operations in the Surveillance, Epidemiology and End Results (SEER) Medicare database and found a significant association between volume and outcomes in four of the five (10). In urologic oncology specifically, most of the focus on volume and outcomes to date has been on radical prostatectomy, with fewer studies on radical cystectomy, radical nephrectomy, and testis cancer management (11).

Surgical volume is gaining importance as a measure of quality at the health policy level. The Leapfrog Group, a coalition of 160 large payors who purchase insurance for over 34 million Americans, have created formal designations for high volume centers for five complex procedures (coronary artery bypass graft, percutaneous coronary intervention, pancreatic resection, esophageal cancer surgery, and abdominal aortic aneurysm repair) and high-risk obstetric care, and explicitly encourages volume-based hospital referral among other initiatives (12). The Centers for Medicare and Medicaid Services (CMS) is likewise piloting programs to provide surgical volume and quality information to patients, and as of 2006 will only provide coverage for bariatric surgery performed at high-volume centers with low mortality data (13).

In cystectomy, as in the other operations to date, most of the insights have been garnered from analysis of large administrative databases. Birkmeyer et al. were the first to report on the impact of both hospital (14) and surgeon (15) volume on radical cystectomy, one of the fourteen major cardiovascular and oncologic operations analyzed using data from Medicare and the Health Care Utilization Project (HCUP)'s Nationwide Inpatient Sample (NIS). They found that hospitals in the highest quintile of volume had lower postoperative mortality than those in the lowest quintile (2.9 vs. 6.4%, adjusted OR 0.46, 95% confidence interval 0.37–0.58). A noteworthy finding was that the highest quintile hospital cystectomy volume was >11 cases per year; the middle quintile was 4–5 cases, and the lowest was fewer than two cases annually (14). The authors found in an analysis of Medicare data that surgeon volume accounted for 39% of the effect of hospital volume on outcomes; tertiles of surgeon volume were <2, 2–3.5, and >3.5 cases annually (15).

A more recent analysis of NIS data focused on radical cystectomies reported on 13,824 cases between 1988 and 1999, examining patients according to the age group and correcting the year of surgery. In this study, overall mortality (2.9%) was lower than that reported by Birkmeyer et al. (14, 15) and hospital volumes were lower (tertiles defined by <1.5, 1.5–2.75, and ≥2.75 annual cases), as were surgeon volumes (tertiles ≤ 1, 1.1–1/.5, >1.5 cases per year). Mortality varied significantly with hospital volume (4.7, 3.3, and 2.7% by tertile, $p < 0.001$). Surgeon volume predicted mortality only among patients between 50–69 years old (2.5, 1.8, and 1.4% mortality by tertile, $p = 0.046$). In multivariate analysis, the significance of hospital volume in predicting mortality was lost in a model which also included surgeon volume along with patient's age, length of stay, and total number of hospital procedures. Low surgeon volume predicted longer length of stay, and high hospital volume was associated with lower average charges (16).

A followup analysis of NIS data from 1998 to 2002 focusing on complication rates reported a slightly lower overall mortality rate (2.57%) and a complication rate of 28.4%; on multivariate analysis, patient factors including age and comorbidity predicted outcomes, as did hospital factors including urban location, size, and teaching status. High volume status per se had less of a protective effect for complications (OR 0.83, 95% CI 0.69–1.01) than did classification as a large bed, urban, teaching hospital (OR 0.71, 95% CI 0.63–0.82) (17). NIS data have also demonstrated markedly lower charges for cystectomy if performed by a high-volume surgeon and/or in a high-volume hospital (18). A final analysis from this data source recently found that hospital high volume status (>3 cases annually) for radical cystectomy predicted reduced mortality (multivariate OR 0.59, 95% CI 0.36–0.97), but neither urologic specialty designation (i.e., high-volume status for multiple urologic procedures) nor meeting volume criteria for the Leapfrog procedures were significantly associated with the outcome (19).

Elting et al. performed an analysis of 1,302 cystectomies at 133 hospitals over a 3 year period using the Texas Hospital Discharge Public Use Data File. They defined three volume groups, not by tertile but rather by requiring that at least 25% of patients and at least five hospitals fall into each group, yielding thresholds of ≤ 3, 4–10, and >10 cases annually to define low, moderate, and high volume centers. Using these much more stringent definitions of high volume compared to the prior studies (only 23 and 5 hospitals met criteria, respectively, for moderate and high volume), they reported mortality rates of 3.1, 2.9, and 0.7% at each tertile ($p = 0.04$) and complication rates of 15.9, 12.1, and 9.0% ($p = 0.01$). Of note all five of the high volume hospitals (accounting for 33% of the cases) were academic medical centers. Teaching status per se was not a predictor of outcome, but for-profit centers had mortality and complication rates of 2.6 and 13.4%, respectively, compared to 0.4 and 6.3% for non-profits. On multivariate analysis, hospital volume, patient's age, patient comorbidity, and nurse-to-bed ratio were all strong predictors of outcomes (20). Studies examining the association between cystectomy volume and outcome are summarized in Table 18.1.

As noted above, a focus on hospital volume for procedures is already starting to drive policy at the

TABLE 18.1. Studies of association between cystectomy volume and outcome.

Study	Data source	Definition of high volume	Major finding
Birkmeyer (14)	NIS	>11 (hospital)	OR 0.46 (95% CI 0.37–0.58) for mortality
Konety (16)	NIS 1988–1999	≥2.75 (hospital)	OR 0.70 and 0.51 vs. moderate- and low-volume for mortality
Konety (19)	NIS 1998–2002	>3 (hospital)	OR 0.59 (95% CI 0.36–0.97) for mortality
Elting (20)	Texas Hospital Discharges 1999–2001	>10 (hospital)	OR 0.35 (95% CI 0.10–1.27) for mortality
Konety (17)	NIS 1998–2002	>3 (hospital)	OR 0.83 (95% CI 0.69–1.01) for complications
Birkmeyer (15)	NIS	>3.5 (surgeon)	OR 0.69 (95% CI 0.49–0.97) for mortality

payor level, if not directly at the accreditation/regulatory level. However, the association is far from definitive. Welke et al. analyzed nearly 950,000 Medicare patients undergoing coronary artery bypass graft surgery at 850 hospitals between 1996 and 2001. They found that the hospital volume predicted mortality at a statistically significant but clinically negligible level of accuracy (concordance index 0.52), and that the ranges in mortality figures for each quintile of hospitals grouped by volume were broader than the difference even between the highest and lowest quintiles (mortality ranges from lowest to highest quintiles: 1–17, 2–12, 2–10, 2–9, 3–11%) (21). Ward et al. likewise analyzed mortality outcomes using the HCUP Iowa State Inpatient Dataset found that hospitals meeting the Leapfrog Group's standards for volume for the five tracked procedures did not have substantially different in-hospital mortality rates than those not meeting the standards, and that applying volume standards would significantly impact revenue for low-volume hospitals and substantially increase patient's travel time (22). Indeed, many rural areas simply lack the referral base to support even a single high-volume center for some procedures (23).

In another recent study, Khuri and Henderson stressed the important observation that most of volume-outcome studies have been performed based on retrospective review of administrative and claims-based datasets, which typically allow for a relatively inaccurate case-mix and/or risk adjustment. By contrast, the Veterans Administration (VA)'s National Surgical Quality Improvement Program (NSQIP) registry reflects clinical data entered prospectively by trained nurses; careful analyses of NSQIP data failed to demonstrate significant association between hospital volumes and outcomes (24). These authors cite previous work comparing the NSQIP to the VA's ICD-9 code-based administrative database, which demonstrated that the administrative database performed poorly in predicting both preoperative risk factors [positive predictive value (PPV) 0.34] and postoperative outcomes (PPV 0.23) confirmed by NSQIP (25).

There is significant public interest in the issue of surgical volume, and there does appear to be a publication bias toward papers showing a positive association between volume and outcomes generally appearing in prominent journals than negative studies. Moreover, the effects of volume-based referrals are already evident in treatment trends. The proportion of United States hospitals performing cystectomy varied showing a rise of 45 to 50% from 1988 to 1996, but between 1996 and 2000 fell to 39% (1). With the greatest attention to surgical volume developing in the last few years, particularly with respect to cystectomy, this trend might be expected to continue and possibly accelerate, as has been demonstrated in a preliminary analysis of the NIS data (26). Another variable which may be accelerating concentration of cystectomy care may be reimbursement, which has either remained stagnant or declined relative to various office and ambulatory surgical procedures in urology.

Nonwhite patients and those with Medicaid or no insurance are already significantly less likely to receive health care in general (27) and radical cystectomy in particular (28) at high volume hospitals, and any policies which potentiate trends toward regionalization must avoid worsening the already profound disparities in the quality of health care across sociodemographic groups. Surgical volume may be a proxy structural measure indicating availability of certain essential resources such as qualified personnel, adequate number of beds etc. to deliver advanced care to people afflicted with bladder cancer and may only be useful in that context.

3. Process Measures

3.1. Time to Cystectomy

Invasive bladder cancer can be an aggressive lesion with a rapid natural history, and multiple studies have now confirmed the importance of minimizing the time interval between diagnosis of invasive disease and radical cystectomy. Chang et al. reported that 81% of patients with a delay of >90 days from diagnosis to surgery had extravesical tumor extension on pathology, vs. 52% of those with a delay ≤90 days ($p = 0.01$); conversely, organ-confined disease on pathology was associated with a mean 48 day delay, compared to 75 days for extravesical disease ($p = 0.02$) (29). However these results assume equivalent clinical stage at the outset and do not necessarily account for understaging at the time of diagnosis. Sanchez-Ortiz et al. found that among 265 cystectomy patients, a delay of >12 vs. ≤ 12 weeks yielded nearly a doubling of risk of both extravesical tumor progression (84 vs. 48%) and 3-year mortality (75 vs. 38%), with a hazard ratio (HR) for mortality of 2.5 (95% CI 1.3–4.8, $p = 0.006$). With the adjustment for tumor and the nodal stage, the HR was 1.9 (95% CI 1.0–3.8, $p = 0.05$) (30).

May et al. found more modest differences of 34 vs. 55% for progression-free survival among those with a

TABLE 18.2. Studies examining impact of delayed time to cystectomy.

Study	N	Time threshold	Major outcome
Chang (29)	303	90 days	81% of delayed patients had extravesical disease vs. 52% of non-delayed
Sanchez-Ortiz (30)	265	12 weeks	OR 1.9 (95% CI 1.0–3.8) for mortality
May (31)	189	3 months	34% progression-free survival for delayed vs. 55% for non-delayed patients
Mahmud (32)	1,592	12 weeks	OR 1.2 (95% CI 1.0–1.5) for mortality

delay >3 vs. ≤ 3 months ($p = 0.04$); with adjustment for stage and grade, the difference in delay was no longer statistically significant (31). In a population-based analysis of cystectomy patients in Quebec, Mahmud et al. found that those with a delay >12 weeks faced an increased risk of death (HR 1.2, 95% CI 1.0–1.5, $p = 0.05$). Of concern is their finding that the median delay increased from 23 to 50 days between 1990 and 2002 (32). Studies examining the impact of time to cystectomy are summarized in Table 18.2. An important source of potential confounding in these series, particularly with respect to mortality outcomes, is that patient factors such as advanced disease and/or comorbidities requiring workup and/or medical optimization prior to surgery may contribute to both delay in surgery and to outcome. However, the preponderance of evidence suggests that time to surgery could be an important process indicator for quality care. Further directed studies will be required to more precisely define the metrics of this process measure.

3.2. Adequacy of Lymphadenectomy

Pelvic lymphadenectomy is an integral part of the procedure of radical cystectomy, important because adequate nodal staging can help guide adjuvant and secondary therapy, and in some cases extirpation of micrometastatic nodal disease can yield long-term cure. Adequacy of lymphadenectomy, therefore, is another potential indicator of quality. Honma et al. reported that among patients with node-positive disease after cystectomy, removal of at least 13 nodes was associated with improved disease-specific survival; moreover those who had fewer than four nodes positive but had removal of fewer than 13 nodes had outcomes comparable to those with a more extended lymphadenectomy and found to have at least four nodes positive (33). Koppie et al. analyzed 1,121 patients undergoing cystectomy over a 15 year period, who had a median of nine nodes removed (range 0–53). They in fact could not identify a threshold above which outcomes reached a plateau; rather, they found a continuous dose-response relationship between more extensive lymphadenectomy and greater probability of survival (34).

Nodal count is admittedly an imperfect proxy for quality of lymphadenectomy, as the yield depends on fixation and analysis by the pathology department as well as the on the surgeon's technique. One analysis, for example, found that submitting lymphatic tissue in multiple anatomic packets rather than as a single specimen increased mean nodal yield from 2.4 to 8.5 for standard template, and from 22.6 to 36.5 for extended template lymphadenectomy (35). However, because accurate staging is an important goal of lymphadenectomy, both surgeon and pathologist contribute to the quality of the nodal analysis.

Secondary analysis of a large cooperative group trial involving 268 patients treated by 106 surgeons found on multivariate analysis that having <10 nodes removed predicted notably worse survival (HR for mortality 1.96, $p = 0.0001$) (36). An even larger analysis from the SEER registry found that among 1,923 cystectomy patients those with a limited lymphadenectomy (<4 nodes examined) had significantly higher disease-specific mortality across all stages than those with more nodes examined. 40.3% of the cohort had no nodes removed and/or analyzed, and 12.7% had 1–3 nodes analyzed. While relatively few patients in most series have fewer than four nodes removed, this study is particularly important because it is based on multi-institutional registry data involving many different surgeons and pathologists, and has still proved the importance of nodal yield (37).

3.3. Use of Orthotopic Diversion

Existing literature does not demonstrate a quality of life benefit for continent rather than incontinent diversion, as will be discussed in further detail below. Nonetheless, many experts in the field consider orthotopic neobladder to be the optimal diversion in terms of functional and cosmetic outcomes for appropriately selected patients (38). While this logic holds merit, particularly for younger patients, the decision on the type of diversion approach should be driven by patient factors: personal preferences and coping ability as well as functional status and biology. It is of particular importance that in the older patient, appropriately tailoring the type of diversion to the patient's desires and physiology may be regarded as an indicator of high quality care.

Gore et al. conducted an analysis of predictive factors for continent diversion in the Medicare population. Of the 3,611 patient treated over an 8 year period, 19.9% received a continent diversion. The authors found that patient factors were strong drivers of outcomes on multivariate analysis, with older age, African–American race, higher comorbidity, female gender, and lower educational level all associated with lower likelihood of continent diversion, as was surgery in the initial three rather than the latter 6 years of the study. However, the single strongest factor predictive of continent diversion was surgery at a designated comprehensive cancer center (OR 5.50, 95% CI 4.20–7.22). Other included treatment at an academic center (OR 1.43, 95% CI 1.14–1.81) and treatment at a high-volume center, defined by 5 cases per year (OR 1.49 compared to <5 cases per year, 95% CI 1.19–1.86) (38).

An ongoing analysis of Medicare patients undergoing cystectomy in 1992, 1995, 1998, and 2001 found on average 370 continent diversions annually, compared to 2,433 incontinent diversions. There was significant regional and year-to-year variation, with no clear trends evident over time (39). Another ongoing study comparing diversion approaches in the United States (NIS data) and Sweden (population-based registry data) found much more prevalent use of continent diversion in Sweden (34% in 2002) than in the United States (7.4% in 2002). Interestingly, while this study found an increase in continent diversion use in the United States from 4.4% in 1997, over the same 5-year interval continent diversion fell from 38% of cases in Sweden in 1997 (Konety et al., unpublished data).

The strong impact of provider factors suggests that some otherwise eligible patients at lower volume or non-cancer center designated hospitals may not be offered continent diversion. Alternatively, it may reflect stronger recommendation for continent diversion by surgeons operating at cancer centers or high volume hospitals, or differences in preferences among patients living near or seeking referral to these centers. While there is no optimal rate of continent diversion indicative of high-quality care, *offering* continent diversion with appropriate counseling to a patient without contraindications is an important process indicator.

4. Outcomes

Outcomes, as discussed above, tend to reflect patient factors as much as quality of care per se, but nonetheless are critical aspects of quality assessment. Perioperative morbidity and mortality certainly are important markers of quality care, assuming incorporation of adequate mechanisms for risk adjustment. In an analysis of 2,538 radical cystectomies included in the NSQIP registry, Hollenbeck et al. reported that 30.5% of the patients had at least one postoperative complication. Surgeon level of training predicted likelihood of complications, as did perioperative factors such as anesthetic agent, operative time, and transfusion requirement. However, equally important were patient factors including age, American Society of Anesthesiologists (ASA) score, functional status, preoperative pulmonary and renal disease (40).

In a followup study, the authors reported 30- and 90-day mortality of 2.9 and 6.8%, respectively, noting that 30-day mortality may inadequately capture late development of perioperative morbidity and/or appropriateness of case selection. On multivariate analysis, they found that patient age, ASA class, functional status, and serum albumin were characteristics which consistently predict both prolonged length of stay and mortality, and could be used in development of case mix adjustment for reporting outcomes (41). Others have found that obesity is an independent predictor of increased blood loss, operative time, and complication rates, with a stronger predictive effect than ASA status (42, 43).

Beyond perioperative morbidity and mortality, cause-specific and overall mortality are both important measures. While the latter is influenced more by nontreatment related patient factors, it will also capture relatively subtle treatment-related morbidity. If a patient undergoes pelvic chemoradiation therapy, for example, and experiences a remission of cancer but dies of sequelae of a hip fracture due to accelerated osteoporosis, the death may not be classified as cancer-specific, but be reflected in overall mortality figures. Here again, care must be taken to adjust mortality outcomes appropriately for cancer stage and grade, use of additional therapy such as radiation and chemotherapy, and relevant patient factors.

As the majority of men and women undergoing radical cystectomy should now expect to survive at least 5 years after surgery, increasing attention is being focused on patient-centered HRQOL as an important outcome to be measured and potentially reported. Experience in the prostate cancer literature has demonstrated definitively that accurate HRQOL measurement requires a direct report by the patient rather an assessment by the physician (44). Toward this end, three bladder cancer-specific patient-reported HRQOL instruments have been developed in recent years. The Functional Assessment of Cancer Therapy-Vanderbilt Cancer Index (FACT-VCI) assesses general and disease-specific HRQOL via a 45-item questionnaire which assesses domains including physical, social/family, emotional, and functional well-being as well as "additional concerns," incorporating questions on urinary, sexual, bowel function (45). The Bladder Cancer Index (BCI) is a 34-item instrument assessing only disease-specific HRQOL in six domains: sexual, urinary, and bowel function and bother (46). The Functional Assessment of Cancer Therapy-Bladder Cancer (FACT-Bl) adds several questions on bladder function to the well-validated FACT (47). These instruments have the potential to standardize HRQOL assessment after cystectomy, but have not yet been externally validated or widely accepted. Two additional instruments for superficial and invasive cancer, the EORTC-QLQ-BLS24 and EORTC-QLQ-BLM30, respectively, have been described but not formally assessed or validated (48). Analytic studies to date have used a variety of different approaches to HRQOL assessment, complicating comparisons among papers.

Several studies have focused on the impact of the type of urinary diversion on HRQOL. It must be stressed that none of these has been a randomized trial, and none fully captures baseline (preoperative) HRQOL, so results must be interpreted with caution, especially with respect to general rather than disease-specific HRQOL. Patients electing incontinent diversion, for example, may have more medical comorbidity, functional limitation, and/or social isolation than those choosing orthotopic diversion, and may therefore have lower HRQOL scores based on issues unrelated to choice of diversion. Results will also vary markedly based on which questions are asked. In a recent review of the field, Gerharz et al. appropriately concluded that the available literature is "rather of extensive but generally of questionable quality," (49) and reiterated the need for prospective, controlled studies of HRQOL outcomes.

Using modifications of four general HRQOL surveys assessing mood, sexual history, body image, urinary problems, and overall quality of life, Hart et al. found no significant differences among patients undergoing ileal conduit, continent cutaneous diversion, or orthotopic diversion (50). Fujisawa et al. surveyed patients using the general HRQOL Short Form-36 (SF-36) and several questions on micturition, finding no significant differences between ileal conduit and orthotopic neobladder patients (51). Hara et al., also using the SF-36, likewise found no differences between ileal conduit and orthotopic neobladder patients (52), as did Mansson et al. in examining differences between continent cutaneous and orthotopic diversion patients (47). Allareddy et al. conducted a long-term (median 100 months since diagnosis) questionnaire study using the FACT-Bl, and found no differences between conduit and continent diversion across any of the general or disease-specific HRQOL domains; for that matter there were no significant differences between radical cystectomy and patients and bladder cancer patients with intact bladders (53).

In contrast, using the European Organisation for Research and Treatment of Cancer (EORTC)'s Quality of Life Questionnaire-Cancer-30 (QLQ-C30) and locally-determined urinary questions, Hobisch et al. found markedly better HRQOL among orthotopic neobladder patients compared to ileal conduit patients in terms of both general and disease-specific domains as well as satisfaction. In this series, however, conduit patients were older, less educated, and less likely to be married (54). Using the SF-36 and Functional Assessment of Cancer Therapy-General (FACT-G) to measure general and cancer-related HRQOL, respectively, Dutta et al. found more modest HRQOL advantages to neobladder over ileal conduit diversion, mostly in terms of emotional well-being, with higher satisfaction among both groups. Their conduit patients again were on an average older than the neobladder patients (55). On the other hand, Gilbert et al. found on using the BCI that urinary function in particular is superior among ileal conduit patients compared to neobladder patients. The BCI has not yet been published in full length form, however, making interpretation of these results difficult (46).

5. Conclusions: Challenges

A recent analysis of the financial impact of surgical complications in the private sector found that the adjusted cost of complications is borne by both the hospital and the payor – hospital reimbursement and costs without complications averaged $14,266 and $10,978, respectively, whereas with complications those values rose to $21,911 and $21,156, respectively. While the hospital profit margin fell from 23.0 to 3.4% with complications, then, the $7,645 increase in cost to the payor markedly exceeded the $2,533 decrease in hospital profit (56). Health care payors – and the businesses and government purchasers who bear the cost of their premiums – clearly have a strong vested interest in reducing complications, and their interest in predictors of poor outcomes can only increase with ongoing increases in health care costs. Certainly a fair assessment of cystectomy quality of care must evaluate a mix of structure, process, and outcome measures, and should focus on the structures and processes most closely and reliably associated with relevant outcomes.

To the extent that surgical volume as a structural measure does predict outcomes, it is clearly a surrogate for pre-, peri-, and postoperative processes, and does not in itself denote a high-quality care. Some of these processes should be measurable with improved accuracy as hospitals gradually move to electronic medical records systems which will facilitate collection of more accurate data than that available in claims-based databases. Others, however, such as intraoperative surgical decision-making, are by nature intangible and will remain difficult to measure reliably. There are of course some low-volume hospitals and low-volume surgeons that provide excellent care and yield excellent outcomes. From a policy standpoint, it would be a disservice both to these providers and the patients they serve to exclude them based on regulation or reimbursement from performing cystectomies or other complex procedures. Rather, a system of required reporting based on volume and outcomes may make more sense, assuming outcomes are appropriately risk-adjusted; high quality providers should be able to stand behind their outcomes data regardless of their volume.

Critical elements of such a reporting system, however, are still lacking. A sufficiently accurate system of case-mix adjustment must be generally accepted by both surgeons and payors. To the growing extent that outcomes of bladder cancer care reflect more than morbidity and mortality of the cancer and treatment, an assessment of patient-reported HRQOL is increasingly important. However, a well-validated HRQOL instrument for bladder cancer has yet to be developed. It is quite possible, in fact, that the absence of consensus regarding the HRQOL impact of continent vs. incontinent diversion reflects lack of sensitivity of bladder cancer HRQOL instruments published to date with respect to outcomes most relevant to patients.

There exist inherent conflicts in the quality of literature in bladder cancer to date which illustrate the overlapping challenges of selecting and implementing quality metrics. If, for example, health care payors or regulatory agencies determine that, based on proven benefits of treatment at high-volume centers, cystectomies should be performed only by high-volume surgeons, patients would almost certainly face longer wait-times between diagnosis and surgery, and it is far from clear with respect to this trade-off whether the benefits of regionalization would outweigh the drawbacks. Furthermore, identifying a measure as a quality indicator will cause providers to focus on it for quality improvement efforts, perhaps at the expense of other (perhaps more important) aspects of quality which are not measured. By analogy, payors focused a great deal of effort on reducing hospital length of stay in the 1990s, and in the example of cystectomy, median length of stay fell from 13 days in 1988–1990 to 9 days in 1997–2000. However, during the same time, the percent of cystectomy patients discharged to subacute care facilities nearly tripled, from 5.3 to 13.2% (1).

In addition to the aspects of care discussed in this chapter, potential quality indicators for cystectomy care may include general aspects of postoperative care such as preoperative assessment of factors such as cardiac risk profile and albumin level, appropriate use of thromboembolism prophylaxis measures and antibiotics, early ambulation and enteral nutrition. Other indicators will be specific to cystectomy, potentially including documentation of adequate staging and upper tract evaluation, intraoperative placement of ureteric stents, and appropriate use of neoadjuvant or adjuvant chemotherapy. Certainly, much work will be needed to be done to define and validate a reliable and meaningful set of quality indicators. A crucial task in the near future will be achieving consensus on which processes and outcomes should be measured, how these data should be collected, with whom they should be shared, and how they should be reported to the public, to payors, and to regulatory agencies. These decisions will be made one way or another in the coming years; it will be incumbent upon the urologic community to assume and retain the leadership of the process of defining quality of radical cystectomy care, and of overall bladder cancer care.

References

1. Taub DA, Dunn RL, Miller DC, Wei JT, Hollenbeck BK. Discharge practice patterns following cystectomy for bladder cancer: evidence for the shifting of the burden of care. J Urol 2006;176(6):2612–8.
2. Donabedian A. Evaluating the quality of medical care. The Milbank Mem Fund Q 1966;44(3S):166–206.
3. Brook RH, McGlynn EA, Cleary PD. Quality of health care, part 2: Measuring quality of care. N Engl J Med 1996;335(13):966–70.
4. Eddy DM. Performance measurement: problems and solutions. Health Aff (Millwood) 1998;17(4):7–25.
5. Gagliardi AR, Fleshner N, Langer B, Stern H, Brown AD. Development of prostate cancer quality indicators: a modified Delphi approach. Can J Urol 2005;12(5):2808–15.
6. Spencer BA, Steinberg M, Malin J, Adams J, Litwin MS. Quality-of-care indicators for early-stage prostate cancer. J Clin Oncol 2003;21(10):1928–36.
7. Luft HS, Bunker JP, Enthoven AC. Should operations be regionalized? The empirical relation between surgical volume and mortality. N Engl J Med 1979;301(25):1364–9.
8. Halm EA, Lee C, Chassin MR. Is volume related to outcome in health care? A systematic review and methodologic critique of the literature. Ann Intern Med 2002;137(6):511–20.
9. Dudley RA, Johansen KL, Brand R, Rennie DJ, Milstein A. Selective referral to high-volume hospitals: estimating potentially avoidable deaths. JAMA 2000;283(9):1159–66.
10. Begg CB, Cramer LD, Hoskins WJ, Brennan MF. Impact of hospital volume on operative mortality for major cancer surgery. JAMA 1998;280(20):1747–51.
11. Joudi FN, Konety BR. The impact of provider volume on outcomes from urological cancer therapy. J Urol 2005;174(2):432–8.
12. Galvin RS, Delbanco S, Milstein A, Belden G. Has the leapfrog group had an impact on the health care market? Health Aff (Millwood) 2005;24(1):228–33.
13. Centers for Medicare & Medicaid Services. Medicare expands national coverage for bariatric surgery procedures. 2006. (Accessed Dec 2, 2006, at http://www.cms.hhs.gov/apps/media/press/release.asp?Counter = 1786.)
14. Birkmeyer JD, Siewers AE, Finlayson EV, et al. Hospital volume and surgical mortality in the United States. N Engl J Med 2002;346(15):1128–37.
15. Birkmeyer JD, Stukel TA, Siewers AE, Goodney PP, Wennberg DE, Lucas FL. Surgeon volume and operative mortality in the United States. N Engl J Med 2003;349(22):2117–27.
16. Konety BR, Dhawan V, Allareddy V, Joslyn SA. Impact of hospital and surgeon volume on in-hospital mortality from radical cystectomy: data from the health care utilization project. J Urol 2005;173(5):1695–700.
17. Konety BR, Allareddy V, Herr H. Complications after radical cystectomy: analysis of population-based data. Urology 2006;68(1):58–64.
18. Konety BR, Dhawan V, Allareddy V, O'Donnell MA. Association between volume and charges for most frequently performed ambulatory and nonambulatory surgery for bladder cancer. Is more cheaper? J Urol 2004;172(3):1056–61.
19. Konety BR, Allareddy V, Modak S, Smith B. Mortality after major surgery for urologic cancers in specialized urology hospitals: are they any better? J Clin Oncol 2006;24(13):2006–12.
20. Elting LS, Pettaway C, Bekele BN, et al. Correlation between annual volume of cystectomy, professional staffing, and outcomes: a statewide, population-based study. Cancer 2005;104(5):975–84.
21. Welke KF, Barnett MJ, Sarrazin MS, Rosenthal GE. Limitations of hospital volume as a measure of quality of care for coronary artery bypass graft surgery. Ann Thorac Surg 2005;80(6):2114–9.
22. Ward MM, Jaana M, Wakefield DS, et al. What would be the effect of referral to high-volume hospitals in a largely rural state? J Rural Health 2004;20(4):344–54.
23. Dimick JB, Finlayson SR, Birkmeyer JD. Regional availability of high-volume hospitals for major surgery. Health Aff (Millwood) 2004:Suppl Web Exclusive: VAR45–53.
24. Khuri SF, Henderson WG. The case against volume as a measure of quality of surgical care. World J Surg 2005;29(10):1222–9.
25. Best WR, Khuri SF, Phelan M, et al. Identifying patient preoperative risk factors and postoperative adverse events in administrative databases: results from the Department of Veterans Affairs National Surgical Quality Improvement Program. J Am Coll Surg 2002;194(3):257–66.
26. Modak S, Konety BR. Where are patients with major urologic cancers undergoing surgery? Changing trends in delivery of surgical and non-surgical care. J Urol 2006:Abstract 174.
27. Liu JH, Zingmond DS, McGory ML, et al. Disparities in the utilization of high-volume hospitals for complex surgery. JAMA 2006;296(16):1973–80.
28. Allareddy V, Konety BR. Race and outcome following radical cystectomy: the effect of hospital volume. J Urol 2006:Abstract 24.
29. Chang SS, Hassan JM, Cookson MS, Wells N, Smith JA, Jr. Delaying radical cystectomy for muscle invasive bladder cancer results in worse pathological stage. J Urol 2003;170(4 Pt 1):1085–7.
30. Sanchez-Ortiz RF, Huang WC, Mick R, Van Arsdalen KN, Wein AJ, Malkowicz SB. An interval longer than 12 weeks between the diagnosis of muscle invasion and cystectomy is associated with worse outcome in bladder carcinoma. J Urol 2003;169(1):110–5; discussion 5.
31. May M, Nitzke T, Helke C, Vogler H, Hoschke B. Significance of the time period between diagnosis of muscle invasion and radical cystectomy with regard to the prognosis of transitional cell carcinoma of the urothelium in the bladder. Scand J Urol Nephrol 2004;38(3):231–5.
32. Mahmud SM, Fong B, Fahmy N, Tanguay S, Aprikian AG. Effect of preoperative delay on survival in patients with bladder cancer undergoing cystectomy in Quebec: a population based study. J Urol 2006;175(1):78–83; discussion.
33. Honma I, Masumori N, Sato E, et al. Removal of more lymph nodes may provide better outcome, as well as more accurate pathologic findings, in patients with bladder cancer–analysis of role of pelvic lymph node dissection. Urology 2006;68(3):543–8.
34. Koppie TM, Vickers AJ, Vora K, Dalbagni G, Bochner BH. Standardization of pelvic lymphadenectomy performed at radical cystectomy: can we establish a minimum number of lymph nodes that should be removed? Cancer 2006;107(10):2368–74.
35. Bochner BH, Herr HW, Reuter VE. Impact of separate versus en bloc pelvic lymph node dissection on the number of lymph nodes retrieved in cystectomy specimens. J Urol 2001;166(6):2295–6.

36. Herr HW, Faulkner JR, Grossman HB, et al. Surgical factors influence bladder cancer outcomes: a cooperative group report. J Clin Oncol 2004;22(14):2781–9.
37. Konety BR, Joslyn SA, O'Donnell MA. Extent of pelvic lymphadenectomy and its impact on outcome in patients diagnosed with bladder cancer: analysis of data from the Surveillance, Epidemiology and End Results Program data base. J Urol 2003;169(3):946–50.
38. Gore JL, Saigal CS, Hanley JM, Schonlau M, Litwin MS. Variations in reconstruction after radical cystectomy. Cancer 2006;107(4):729–37.
39. Konety BR, Joyce GF, Wise M. Urologic Diseases in America: Bladder and upper tract urothelial cancer. J Urol 2007;177:1636–45.
40. Hollenbeck BK, Miller DC, Taub D, et al. Identifying risk factors for potentially avoidable complications following radical cystectomy. J Urol 2005;174(4 Pt 1):1231–7; discussion 7.
41. Hollenbeck BK, Miller DC, Taub DA, et al. The effects of adjusting for case mix on mortality and length of stay following radical cystectomy. J Urol 2006;176(4 Pt 1):1363–8.
42. Chang SS, Jacobs B, Wells N, Smith JA, Jr., Cookson MS. Increased body mass index predicts increased blood loss during radical cystectomy. J Urol 2004;171(3):1077–9.
43. Lee CT, Dunn RL, Chen BT, Joshi DP, Sheffield J, Montie JE. Impact of body mass index on radical cystectomy. J Urol 2004;172(4 Pt 1):1281–5.
44. Litwin MS, Lubeck DP, Henning JM, Carroll PR. Differences in urologist and patient assessments of health related quality of life in men with prostate cancer: results of the CaPSURE database. J Urol 1998;159(6):1988–92.
45. Cookson MS, Dutta SC, Chang SS, Clark T, Smith JA, Jr., Wells N. Health related quality of life in patients treated with radical cystectomy and urinary diversion for urothelial carcinoma of the bladder: development and validation of a new disease specific questionnaire. J Urol 2003;170(5): 1926–30.
46. Gilbert SM, Wood DP, Weizer A, et al. Measuring health-related quality of life outcomes in bladder cancer patients using the newly validated Bladder Cancer Index (BCI). J Urol 2006;176(4 Pt 2):Abstract 36.
47. Mansson A, Davidsson T, Hunt S, Mansson W. The quality of life in men after radical cystectomy with a continent cutaneous diversion or orthotopic bladder substitution: is there a difference? BJU international 2002;90(4):386–90.
48. Botteman MF, Pashos CL, Hauser RS, Laskin BL, Redaelli A. Quality of life aspects of bladder cancer: a review of the literature. Qual Life Res 2003;12(6):675–88.
49. Gerharz EW, Mansson A, Hunt S, Skinner EC, Mansson W. Quality of life after cystectomy and urinary diversion: an evidence based analysis. J Urol 2005;174(5):1729–36.
50. Hart S, Skinner EC, Meyerowitz BE, Boyd S, Lieskovsky G, Skinner DG. Quality of life after radical cystectomy for bladder cancer in patients with an ileal conduit, cutaneous or urethral kock pouch. J Urol 1999;162(1):77–81.
51. Fujisawa M, Isotani S, Gotoh A, Okada H, Arakawa S, Kamidono S. Health-related quality of life with orthotopic neobladder versus ileal conduit according to the SF-36 survey. Urology 2000;55(6):862–5.
52. Hara I, Miyake H, Hara S, et al. Health-related quality of life after radical cystectomy for bladder cancer: a comparison of ileal conduit and orthotopic bladder replacement. BJU international 2002;89(1):10–3.
53. Allareddy V, Kennedy J, West MM, Konety BR. Quality of life in long-term survivors of bladder cancer. Cancer 2006; 106(11):2355–62.
54. Hobisch A, Tosun K, Kinzl J, et al. Quality of life after cystectomy and orthotopic neobladder versus ileal conduit urinary diversion. World J Urol 2000;18(5):338–44.
55. Dutta SC, Chang SC, Coffey CS, Smith JA, Jr., Jack G, Cookson MS. Health related quality of life assessment after radical cystectomy: comparison of ileal conduit with continent orthotopic neobladder. J Urol 2002;168(1):164–7.
56. Dimick JB, Weeks WB, Karia RJ, Das S, Campbell DA, Jr. Who pays for poor surgical quality? Building a business case for quality improvement. J Am Coll Surg 2006;202(6): 933–7.

Section 3
Continent Diversion: Problems and Solutions

19 Continent Diversion: QOL of Orthotopic Diversion vs. Ileal Conduit

Scott M. Gilbert and Cheryl T. Lee

Contents

Abstract The attendant requirement of urinary diversion following radical cystectomy results in several functional consequences that impact health-related quality of life (HRQOL) in bladder cancer patients managed with surgery. While significant developments in urinary reconstruction have increased the availability of several different forms of continent diversion, the majority of cystectomy patients still receive an incontinent urinary reconstruction. Many surgeons argue, that improved techniques have resulted in reduced complications from continent urinary diversion, and that these types of reconstruction offer better functional and health-related quality of life outcomes compared to incontinent diversion. Certainly, this premise holds intuitive validity; however, this has not been demonstrated reliably to date.

While research aimed to address the relative benefit of continent urinary diversion from the perspective of functional outcomes and HRQOL has been an active area of investigation for many years, limitations in methodology and a lack of reliable disease-specific instruments to measure these outcomes have resulted in a lack of progress. To date, high-quality evidence indicating that one type of urinary diversion is superior to another does not exist. Addressing issues related to problematic measurement and improving the quality of research are imperatives to moving the field forward. Currently, there are several disease-specific instruments in various stages of development and testing. A validation of these measures, and systematic assessment of HRQOL will inform the debate regarding the optimal type of urinary diversion.

Keywords Bladder cancer, Urinary diversion, Health-related quality of life, Functional outcomes, Complications

1. Introduction

Although the majority of incidents of bladder cancer cases are non-muscle invasive, approximately 25% of the greater than 60,000 cancers diagnosed in the United States each year are more advanced and require aggressive surgical intervention (1). Currently,

From: *Current Clinical Urology: Bladder Cancer,* Edited by: C.T. Lee and D.P. Wood,
DOI: 10.1007/978-1-59745-417-9_19, © Humana Press, a part of Springer Science+Business Media, LLC 2010

cystectomy is the standard treatment for these more advanced cancers, and offers long-term disease-specific survival rates over 70% in cases with pathological T2 disease (2). Accordingly, greater than 10,000 cystectomies are performed each year in the United States (3). However, radical surgery is not reserved for muscle-invasive disease, and may also be indicated in high-risk noninvasive cases, including those characterized by disease progression, failed response to conservative management (endoscopic- and intravesical-therapies), and presence of rare but aggressive histological features. While improvements in perioperative care have decreased the surgical morbidity following cystectomy (4), the attendant complications associated with urinary diversion continue to present substantial challenges. Cystectomy patients face a multitude of health consequences related to surgical intervention; most are related to the consequent metabolic effects, changes in urinary, bowel and sexual function and altered body image that result from urinary diversion. As a result, the functional and health-related quality of life issues following surgery are extremely important for this group of patients.

The detrimental impact of these important health changes has long been recognized as a major shortcoming of surgery, and has prompted interest in limiting the functional complications associated with urinary diversion. Development of and refinements in various forms of continent urinary diversion have been directed toward addressing this problem, and many surgeons maintain that continent urinary reconstruction is associated with fewer functional impairments compared to incontinent diversion (5, 6). As a result, the options and recommended use of continent diversion have expanded, as evidenced by recent estimates suggesting that 80% of men and greater than 65% of women with invasive bladder cancer are candidates for orthotopic continent urinary diversion (7). The majority of cystectomy patients, however, do not receive continent reconstruction (8). Although the reasons are not entirely clear, significant baseline infirmity and comorbidity, technical complexity, risk of complications (9) and lack of definitive evidence suggesting a health-related quality of life benefit are likely to be contributing factors.

To date, the optimal type of urinary reconstruction has not been firmly established. While previous work has suggested complications may be modifiable and that cancer control and survival are independent of the type of urinary diversion used (5, 10, 11), the slow adoption of continent diversion probably reflects a level of uncertainty regarding the advantages proposed by advocates of continent diversion. Undeniably, the application of continent urinary diversion to restore anatomic and functional voiding, avoid external urinary collection and preserve body image all hold intuitive value. However, this assertion has not yet been supported by high-level evidence. Although an extensive amount of effort has been focused in this area, limitations in the quality of research and methodology have been prevalent, and to date, we still do not know if continent urinary diversion truly offers significant advantages (9, 12, 13). The objectives of this chapter are therefore to outline the perspective of health-related quality of life assessment, review the current state of knowledge regarding urinary diversion outcomes, and introduce several bladder cancer-specific HRQOL instruments currently in development.

2. Health-Related Quality of Life Assessment

Increasingly, health-related quality of life (HRQOL) has become an important outcome measure, particularly in diseases in which treatment is associated with potential functional impairments. Given the significant impact of urinary diversion on several aspects of recovery and function, HRQOL assessment has become an essential component in evaluating the success of invasive bladder cancer treatments. Broadly defined, HRQOL is a patient's evaluation of the impairments, effects and general state of health following the disease and its management (14). Although comprehensive in scope, this definition can be focused on several principal elements (functional status, disease-related and treatment-related symptoms, psychological functioning and social adjustment) that form a multidimensional construct (15). The patient perspective is implied in these definitions, and because physician assessments may be incomplete or inaccurate, patient reported impairments and concerns should be used to ensure that the patient perspective is adequately captured during HRQOL assessment.

In assessing HRQOL, general and disease-specific approaches should be differentiated. General HRQOL instruments, such as the sickness impact profile (SIP) (16) and the Medical Outcomes Study SF-36 (17) are designed to measure the effect of disease and treatment on the physical, emotional, psychological and social well-being for any disease. Accordingly, general HRQOL instruments can be used to assess the impact of disease and therapy across disease states and populations. Disease-specific instruments differ in that the questions used for assessment are detailed and highly relevant for a particular disease and its treatment. The expanded prostate cancer index composite (EPIC) (18), which measures sexual, urinary, bowel and hormonal outcomes in prostate cancer patients, is an example. The advantage of using disease-specific measures is the ability to more accurately assess the effects, complications and impairments that are important for a particular disease. In bladder cancer, questions regarding urinary, sexual and gastrointestinal function, as well as body image, are highly relevant, and impairments in those areas may go unrecognized using more general measures. Intermediate instruments which are cancer-specific but apply to different types of cancer are also available. The two most common are the functional assessment of cancer therapy (FACT) (19) and the European Organization for Research and Treatment of Cancer EORCT-QOL-C30 (20), both of which have been used in several different cancers and settings.

A major limitation in the assessment of bladder cancer-specific HRQOL to date has been the use of nondisease-specific measures. While some groups have recognized this deficit and attempted to capture the urinary and sexual effects following cystectomy and urinary diversion using informally developed questions, the result of this work is of uncertain value given the lack of proper psychometric evaluation. Although such questions may have content validity, the extent to which they measure the impairments they intend to (construct 2 validity) or how well they correlate with other formally developed HRQOL assessment instruments (criterion validity) has not been established. Accordingly, the development and psychometric assessment of most bladder cancer-specific HRQOL questionnaires has been inadequate and incomplete thus far. Formal development and assessment of HRQOL measures is based on evaluating *validity*, *reliability* and *responsiveness*. As previously indicated, validity ensures that questions measure what they purport to measure. Reliability is based on an instrument's ability to provide the same results on several different occasions given stable disease, and responsiveness is a measure of the ability to detect true but clinically meaningful changes in the quality of life (21). In the context of these important and well-developed psychometric properties, the development of previous bladder cancer HRQOL instruments has been limited, even marginal by many standards, raising substantial concern regarding the quality of prior HRQOL research in this area. In the absence of formal development, and proper psychometric evaluation, we cannot be certain the questionnaires used to date measure what they intended to with reliability or with the ability to detect nuanced but clinically important differences. In this setting, important symptoms related to urinary leakage, sexual dysfunction, bowel bother and body image may not have been assessed adequately.

Although significant gains have been advanced in other cancers, few responsive, disease-specific HRQOL measures are available for bladder cancer. This deficiency is an active area of interest, and there are several instruments currently in various phases of development and assessment. Bladder cancer presents several challenges which are likely to have limited the development of HRQOL measures thus far. One challenge has been the ability to develop responsive questions that measure HRQOL impairments equally well in both men and women. As indicated by others (22), the assessment of sexual functions across gender following cystectomy and urinary diversion can be difficult without relying on gender-specific questions. Although different issues may be responsible for sexual dysfunction, measuring erectile dysfunction in men and vaginal shortening and changes in perineal sensation in women with a single instrument facilitates administration, interpretation and comparison. A second problematic issue relates to the use of several standard types of urinary diversion. Measuring urinary function and dysfunction across diversion types within a single HRQOL domain requires an inclusive approach which captures the different sources of urinary dysfunction for each type of diversion. For example, measuring incontinence in patients managed with an incontinent diversion is in-of-itself troublesome. However, urinary leakage, skin excoriation and urine odor resulting from suboptimal stomal placement, stomal retraction or lack of appliance adherence are readily understandable impairments which make the concept of urinary dysfunction following ileal conduit diversion more understandable. This underscores the need to focus on measuring specific impairments and symptoms for each diversion type and then constructing a summary measure to facilitate comparison between diversions. For valid assessment, questions must address different facets of dysfunction, such as issues related to catheterization in those managed with continent nonorthotopic diversion, day-time and night-time urinary incontinence for those with a continent orthotopic diversion, and appliance malfunction and urine leakage for those with an incontinent ileal conduit diversion.

The advanced age of the general bladder cancer population offers an additional challenge in assessing HRQOL following cystectomy, as competing comorbidities and health detriments may overwhelm otherwise detectable differences. Contributing to this problem is the attenuation of sexual function that accompanies aging, making some HRQOL domains potentially less relevant than others. This should not deter clinicians or researchers, as the HRQOL detriments experienced by patients with high presurgical function and expectations, whether young or old, can be substantial. Although research will be more difficult given the clinical characteristics of invasive bladder cancer and the age structure of the bladder cancer population, clinically meaningful impairments and treatment effects should be uncovered so that the quality of cancer survivorship can be optimized following cystectomy and urinary diversion.

3. HRQOL Assessment in Bladder Cancer

Although proponents of orthotopic diversion maintain that the potential advantages of this approach, including preservation of anatomic voiding and avoidance of urinary stoma formation, translate into improved outcomes, this has not been determined reliably. Experienced groups have reported improvement in short- and long-term complications (5), as well as satisfactory urinary continence in up to 95% of patients following continent urinary diversion (23). However, these results are probably not generalizable, and may over-estimate the proposed HRQOL benefit of continent orthotopic urinary diversion. The initial research comparing ileal conduit diversion to continent diversions has produced mixed results (24–30) (Table 19.1). While general HRQOL appears to be similar in both, specific issues concerning body image, problematic urine leakage and decreased sexual functioning have been inconsistent, although more commonly reported for ileal conduit diversion (37). However, given the substantial methodological shortcomings, reliable interpretation is difficult.

Several recent reviews have evaluated existing bladder cancer HRQOL studies (9, 13, 22, 38). Although this previous research has characterized some of the common complications and shared HRQOL impairments associated with urinary diversion, limitations in methodology and a lack of valid disease-specific HRQOL measures has prevented more meaningful comparisons between different types of urinary diversions. While some studies have used validated instruments, up to two-thirds have not (13). In cases in which properly designed and validated HRQOL instruments have been used, HRQOL assessment has been more general, and therefore not responsive to the specific concerns that most researchers and clinicians are interested in capturing in this population. These fundamental problems have hampered the interpretability of bladder cancer related HRQOL research to date. Consequently, there is currently no evidence supporting one type of urinary diversion over another.

Despite these limitations, the work done thus far has elucidated some of the more general aspects of HRQOL following cystectomy and urinary diversion. While general HRQOL appears to return to baseline by 1 year following surgery (39), HRQOL impairments specific to the type of urinary diversion used may persist. Each type of urinary diversion is associated with a different set of well-described treatment-related effects. For patients managed with an ileal conduit, concern centers around the urinary stoma, external urinary appliance and the consequent negative impact on body image. Other factors that appear to be of particular concern to this group include urinary leakage, skin irritation and excoriation, sexual dysfunction, and gastrointestinal problems (31, 40–45). Urinary incontinence, particularly nighttime incontinence, appears to be the principal issue in patients managed with continent orthotopic urinary diversion (neobladder), while catheterization poses its own set of concerns related to frequency, discomfort and inconvenience following continent cutaneous diversion (12). Gastrointestinal complaints, such as diarrhea, has been found more commonly following orthotopic continent urinary diversion, which is consistent with the increased bowel length required for formation of this type of urinary diversion (39). Others have reported that urinary leakage is a greater concern among patients treated with ileal conduit compared to continent diversion (24, 32, 46). However, this was not confirmed in a more recent study which documented significantly greater urine leakage and decreased control in patients managed with orthotopic continent urinary diversion (47).

TABLE 19.1. Summary of previous bladder cancer HRQOL studies.

Study	Year	Instrument	Patients	Design	Population	Findings
Bjerre et al. (23)	1995	Unvalidated author-designed questionnaire	67	Cross-sectional	Denmark	General QOL similar between groups, incontinence more bothersome in IC group
Conde Redondo et al. (31)	2001	Unvalidated author-designed questionnaire	33	Cross-sectional	Spain	Problems with urine leakage and depression more common in IC group
Dutta et al. (28)	2002	SF-36 FACT-G	72	Cross-sectional	United States	Marginally higher HRQOL scores detected in NB group
Fujisawa et al. (25)	2000	SF-36	56	Cross-sectional	Japan	No differences detected between groups
Gilbert et al. (32)	2007	BCI	315	Cross-sectional	United States	Decreased urinary HRQOL among NB patients
Hara et al. (27)	2002	SF-36 Unvalidated author-designed questionnaire	85	Cross-sectional	Japan	No differences detected in general HRQOL
Hart et al. (33)	1999	POMS Sexual history form Body image scale	221	Cross-sectional	United States	Deceased social function among IC group
Hobisch et al. (26)	2000	EORTC-QOL-C30 Unvalidated author-designed questionnaire	102	Cross-sectional	Austria	Higher levels of HRQOL in NB group
Kitamura et al. (34)	1999	EORTC-QOL-C30 Unvalidated author-designed questionnaire	79	Cross-sectional	Japan	Difficulty in social function and travel more common in IC group
Mansson et al. (30)	2002	FACT-BL Hospital anxiety and depression scale	64	Cross-sectional	Sweden	Incontinence more problematic in NB group
McGuire et al. (35)	2000	SF-36	92	Cross-sectional	United States	General HRQOL equivalent between groups
Protogerou et al. (29)	2004	EORTC-QOL-C30 Unvalidated author-designed questionnaire	108			Urinary and sexual function impairments present following cystectomy but no HRQOL differences between groups
Salinas Sanchez et al. (36)	2001	SF-36	49	Cross-sectional	Spain	HRQOL lower than general population

The impact of these various HRQOL outcomes may affect the quality of life beyond the obvious functional impairments documented to date. Several prior studies have found that patients treated with orthotopic continent diversion are more likely to travel and engage in leisure activities and suffer less social deficits than those managed with incontinent diversions (29, 33, 34, 48, 49). While reservations regarding the external urinary appliance, body image and potential urine odor may result in less social behavior, the results from these studies should not be generalized. Limitations in research methodology, including lack of adjustment for case mix and susceptibility to selection basis, probably explain these observations. This underscores one of the difficulties in bladder cancer HRQOL research; patients with continent urinary diversion tend to be more active than their older, more infirm ileal conduit counterparts, and thus, comparison of HRQOL outcomes may not be balanced.

4. Improving HRQOL Assessment and Research

Despite an extensive number of studies, the widely held notion that continent urinary diversion is associated with superior quality of life outcomes has not been supported by high-quality evidence. The majority of studies have suffered from methodological flaws, ranging from cross-sectional assessment and unavailability of reliable disease-specific HRQOL measures. The latter is a major disadvantage, as the measures used to date are not likely to be responsive to changes specific to urinary diversion (13). Consequently, interpreting and synthesizing the results of previous research presents challenges on several levels. Given these limitations and the lack of reliable results, comparing HRQOL outcomes between continent and incontinent urinary diversion based on prior research is a real challenge. The HRQOL benefits and detriments associated with different forms of urinary diversion, however, remain important concerns for both the patients and the physicians alike. In order to move this area forward, the limiting flaws of previous HRQOL research must be addressed systematically. To this end, prospective longitudinal HRQOL assessment using disease-specific, reliable and responsive measures is necessary. Implicit in this strategy is baseline measurement to control for individual and group variation, repeated measures to ensure an adequate understanding of how HRQOL changes with time following treatment, and long-term follow-up to determine the stability of HRQOL scores. Such methodology will limit, although not entirely eliminate, susceptibility to selection bias and provide more reliable and informative results (13).

5. Development of Bladder Cancer-Specific HRQOL Questionnaires

In response to the recognized deficits in bladder cancer-specific HRQOL assessment, several groups have developed disease-specific HRQOL measures (37, 47, 50). The Functional Assessment of Cancer Therapy (FACT) group expanded the more general FACT cancer-specific questionnaire to measure impairments experienced by bladder cancer patients following treatment (12). The resulting FACT-BL contains 12 additional items which assess symptoms related to urinary incontinence, diarrhea, body image, sexual function and stomal issues. Although the FACT-BL has been commonly used in bladder cancer HRQOL assessment, there is limited information regarding its reliability, validity and responsiveness. The EORTC-QOL-BML30 is an adaptation of the C30 questionnaire developed by the European Organization for Research and Treatment of Cancer. The questionnaire contains 30 additional questions specific to bladder cancer and its treatment, and is currently in the final phases of development (12, 22). Additional HRQOL instruments developed for bladder cancer patients include the Vanderbilt Cystectomy Index (FACT-VCI) (50), a cystectomy-specific instrument based on the FACT and developed by researchers at Vanderbilt Medical Center. In addition to the general FACT questions, it contains 17 additional items which measure consequent health effects ranging from functional concerns (gastrointestinal, urinary and sexual dysfunction) to more general HRQOL concerns (body image changes and impact on social activity). More recently, the group at the University of Michigan developed the Bladder Cancer Index (BCI) to measure HRQOL impairments across the continuum of bladder cancer treatments (endoscopic-based, intravesical therapy, and cystectomy with urinary diversion). Unlike the FACT-BL and FACT-VCI, BCI items were based on iterative content development phases consisting of physician, patient and family interviews and group sessions, and repeated factor analysis (47). An early cross-sectional study evaluating the responsiveness of the BCI revealed relatively low urinary scores in patients managed with orthotopic continent urinary diversion compared to those receiving an ileal conduit. Urinary incontinence, leakage and lack of control appeared to be significant contributing factors (Figure 19.1) (47). However, additional studies accounting for baseline status, and optimally, adjusting for patient preference, are needed to effectively compare HRQOL outcomes in different types of urinary diversion. As with the EORTC-QOL instruments and the FACT-VCI, the BCI is currently being assessed in prospective longitudinal studies.

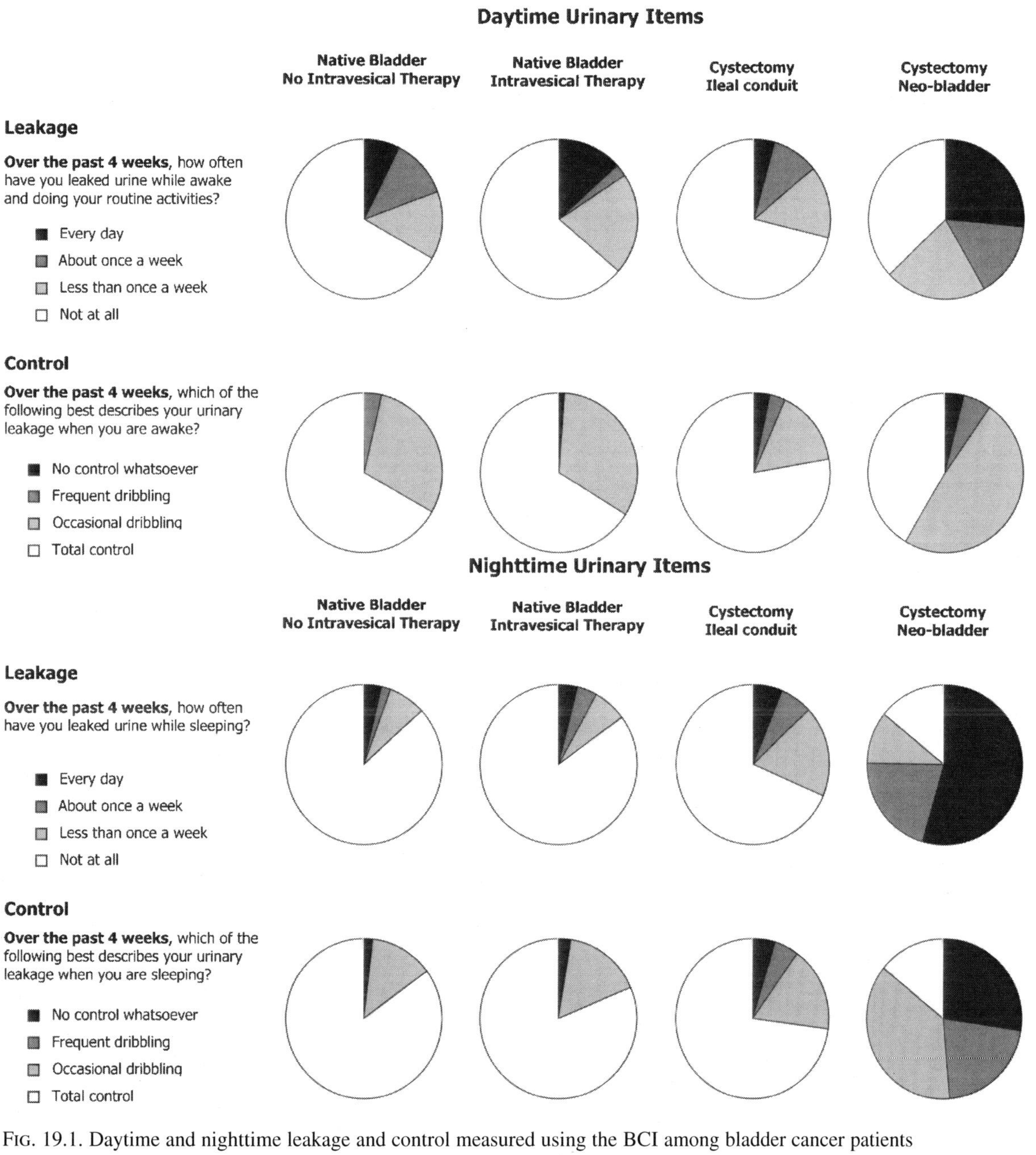

FIG. 19.1. Daytime and nighttime leakage and control measured using the BCI among bladder cancer patients

6. Conclusions

While all surgeons involved in treating bladder cancer undoubtedly strive to limit the adverse impact of cystectomy, the necessity of urinary diversion results in associated attendant complications and HRQOL impairments. Although avoiding an external stoma and appliance and restoring anatomic voiding have been proposed as ways to improve outcomes, a HRQOL benefit favoring orthotopic continent urinary diversion has not been readily detectable thus far. This is certainly related to limitations in the research performed to date, but may also be related to underappreciated but important functional impairments specific to continent diversion. The impact of urinary incontinence, hyper-continence, sexual dysfunction and gastrointestinal complaints have not been adequately assessed following continent diversion, and these functional detriments may be further exacerbated by patient expectations that are unmet by post diversion outcomes. Additional research using reliable and responsive HRQOL measures specific for the HRQOL concerns and complications associated with urinary diversion will contribute substantially to the understanding of these complex issues and help to move the field forward.

References

1. Jemal A, Siegel R, Ward E, Murray T, Xu J, Thun MJ. Cancer statistics, 2007. CA Cancer J Clin 2007;57(1):43–66.
2. Stein JP, Lieskovsky G, Cote R, Groshen S, Feng AC, Boyd S, et al. Radical cystectomy in the treatment of invasive bladder cancer: ling-term results in 1054 patients. J Clin Oncol 2001;19:666–675.
3. Hollenbeck BK, Dunn RL, Miller DC, Daignault S, Taub DA, Wei JT. Volume-based referral for cancer surgery: informing the debate. J Clin Oncol 2007;25:91–96.
4. Taub DA, Dunn RL, Miller DC, Wei JT, Hollenbeck BK. Discharge practice patterns following cystectomy for bladder cancer: evidence for the shifting of the burden of care. J Urol 2006;176:2612–2617.
5. Madersbacher S, Studer UE. Contemporary cystectomy and urinary diversion. World J Urol 2002;20:151–157.
6. Hautmann RE, Volkmer BG, Schumacher MC, Gschwend JE, Studer UE. Long-term results of standard procedures in urology: the ileal neobladder. World J Urol 2006;24:305–314.
7. Hautmann RE. Which patients with transitional cell carcinoma of the baldder or prostatic urethra are candidates for an orthotopic neobladder? Curr Urol Rep 2000;1(3):173–179.
8. Gore JL, Saigal CS, Hanley JM, Schonlau M, Litwin MS. Urologic disease in America project: variations in reconstruction after radical cystectomy. Cancer 2006;107(4):729–737.
9. Gerharz EW, Mansson A, Hunt S, Skinner EC, Mansson W. Quality of life after cystectomy and urinary diversion: an evidence-based analysis. J Urol 2005:1729–1736.
10. Clark PE. Urinary diversion after radical cystectomy. Curr Treat Options Oncol 2002;3(5):389–402
11. Krupski T, Theodorescu D. Orthotopic neobladder following cystectomy: indications, management, and outcomes. J Wound Ostomy Continence Nurs 2001;28(1):37–46
12. Botteman MF, Pashos CL, Hauser RS, Laskin BL, Redaelli A. Quality of life aspects of bladder cancer: a review of the literature. Qual Life Res 2003;12:675–688.
13. Porter MP, Penson DF. Health related quality of life after radical cystectomy and urinary diversion for bladder cancer: a systematic review and critical analysis of the literature. J Urol 2005;173:1318–1322.
14. Cella DF, Tulsky DS. Quality of life in cancer: definition, purpose and methods of measurement. Cancer Invest 1993; 11:327–336.
15. Aaronson NK. Quality of life: what is it? How should it be measured? Oncology (Huntingt) 1988;2:69
16. Bergner M, Bobbitt RA, Carter WB, et al. The sickness impact profile: development and final revision of a health status measure. Med Care 1981;23(3 Suppl):S27–S43.
17. Ware JE Jr, Sherbourne CD. The MOS 36-item short-form health survey (SF-36). I. Conceptual framework and item selection. Med Care 1992;30(6):473–483.
18. Wei JT, Dunn RL, Litwin MS, Sandler HM, Sanda MG. Development and validation of the expanded prostate cancer index composite (EPIC) for comprehensive assessment of health-related quality of life in men with prostate cancer. Urology 2000;56:899–905.
19. Cella DF, Tulsky DS, Gray G, et al. The Functional Assessment of cancer therapy scale: development and validation of the general measure. J Clin Oncol 1993;11(3):570–579.
20. Aaronson NK, Ahmedzai S, Bergman B, et al. The European Organization for Research and Treatment of Cancer QOL-C30: a quality-of-life instrument for use in international clinical trials in oncology. J Natl Cancer Inst 1993;85(5):365–376.
21. Hays RD, Hadorn D. Responsiveness to change: an aspect of validity, not a separate dimension. Qual Life Res 1992; 1(1):73–75.
22. Porter MP, Wei JT, Penson DF. Quality of life issues in bladder cancer patients following cystectomy and urinary diversion. Urol Clin N Am 2005;32:207–216.
23. Hautmann RE, De Petriconi R, Gottfried HW, Kleinschmidt K, Mattes R, Paiss T. The ileal neobladder: complications and functional results in 363 patients after 11 years of followup. J Urol 1999;161:422–428.
24. Bjerre BD, Johansen C, Steven K. Helath-related quality of life after cystectomy: bladder substitution compared with ileal conduit diversion. A questionnaire survey. Br J Urol 1995;75:200.
25. Bjerre BD, Johansen C, Steven K. Sexological problems after cystectomy: bladder substitution compared to ileal conduit diversion. A questionnaire survey of male patients. Scand J Urol Nephrol 1998;32:187
26. Fujisawa M, Isotani S, Gototh A, Okada H, Arakawa A, Kamidono S. Health-related quality of life with orthotopic neobladder versus ileal conduit according to SF-36 survey. Urology 2000;55:862.

27. Hobisch A, Tosun K, Kinzl J, Kemmler G, Bartsch G, Holtl L, et al. Quality of life after cystectomy and orthotopic neobladder versus ileal conduit urinary diversion. World J Urol 2000;18:338.
28. Hara I, Miyake H, Hara S, Gotoh A, Nakamura I, Okada H, et al. Health-related quality of life after radical cystectomy for bladder cancer: a comparison of ileal conduit and orthotopic bladder replacement. BJU Int 2002;89:10.
29. Dutta SC, Chang SS, Coffey CS, Smith JA Jr., Jack G, Cookson MS. Health related quality of life assessment after radical cystectomy: comparison of ileal conduit with continent orthotopic neobladder. J Urol 2002;168:164.
30. Promogerou V, Moschou M, Antoniou N, Varkarakis J, Bamias A, Deliveliotis C. Modified S-pouch neobladder vs ileal conduit and a matched controlled population: a quality of life survey. BJU Int 2004;94:350.
31. Henningsohn L, Wijkstrom H, Dickman PW, Bergmark K, Steineck G. Distressful symptoms after radical cystectomy with urinary diversion for urinary bladder cancer: a Swedish population-based study. Eur Urol 2001;40:151.
32. Mansson A, Johnson G, Mansson W. Quality of life after cystectomy: comparison between patients with conduit and those with continent caecal reservoir urinary diversion. Br J Urol 1988;62(3):240–245.
33. Okada Y, Oishi K, Schichiri Y, et al. Quality of life survey or urinary diversion patients: comparison of continent urinary diversion versus ileal conduit. Int J Urol 1997;4(1)26–41.
34. Hobisch A, Tosun K, Kinzl J, et al. Life after radical cystectomy and orthotopic neobladder versus ileal conduit urinary diversion. Semin Urol Oncol 2001;19(1):18–23.
35. McGuire MS, Grimaldi G, Grotas J, Russo P: The type of urinary diversion after radical cystectomy significantly impacts on the patient's quality of life. Ann Surg Oncol 2000;7:4
36. Salinas Sanchez AS, Segura Martin M, Lorenzo Romero JG, Hernandez Millan I, Fernandez Olano C, Virseda Rodriguez JA: [Quality of life of patients after radical surgery of bladder cancer]. Arch Esp Urol 2001;54:787–795.
37. Mansson A, Davidsson T, Hunt S, Mansson W. The quality of life in men after radical cystectomy with a continent cutaneous diversion or orthotopic bladder substitution: is there a difference? BJU Int 2002;90:386.
38. Nabi G, Yong SM, Ong E, McPherson G, Grant A, N'Dow J. Is orthotopic bladder replacement the new gold standard? Evidence from a systematic review. J Urol 2005;174:21–28.
39. Hardt J, Filipas D, Hohenfellner R, Egle UT. Quality of life in patients with bladder carcinoma after cystectomy: first results of a prospective study. Qual Life Res 2000;9(1):1–12.
40. Jones MA, Breckman B, Hendry WK. Life with an ileal conduit: results of questionnaire surveys of patients with urological surgeons. Br J Urol 1980;52:21.
41. Fossa SD, Reitan JB, Ous S, Kaalhus O. Life with an ileal conduit in cystectomized bladder cancer patients: expectations and experiences. Scand J Urol Nephrol 1987;21:97.
42. Mommsen S, Jakobsen A, Sell A. Quality of life in patients with advanced bladder cancer. A randomized study comparing cystectomy and irradiation – the Danish Bladder Cancer Study Group (DAVECA protocol 8201). Scand J Urol Nephrol Suppl 1989;125:115
43. Chadwick DJ, Stower MJ. Life with urostomy. Br J urol 1990;65:189.
44. Nordstrom GM, Nyman CR. Male and female sexual function and activity following ileal conduit urinary diversion. Br J Urol 1992;70:33.
45. Nordstrom G, Nyman CR, Theorell T. Psychosocial adjustment and general state of health in patients with ileal conduit urinary diversion. Scand J Urol Nephrol 1992;26:139.
46. Conde Redondo C, Estebanez Zarranz J, Rodriguez Tovez A, et al. [Quality of life in patients treated with orthotopic bladder substitution versus cutaneous ileostomy.] Actas Urol Esp 2001;25(6):435–444.
47. Gilbert SM, Wood DP, Dunn RL et al. Measuging health-related quality of life outcomes in bladder cancer patients using the bladder cancer index (BCI). Cancer 2007;109: 1756–1762.
48. Kitamura H, Miyao N, Yanase M et al. Quality of life in patients having ileal conduit, continent reservoir or orthotopic neobladder after cystectomy for bladder carcinoma. Int J Urol 1999;6(8):393–399.
49. Hart S, Skinner EC, Meyerowitz BE, et al. Quality of life after radical cystectomy for bladder cancer in patients with an ileal conduit, cutaneous or urethral Kock pouch. J Urol 1999;162(1):77–81.
50. Cookson MS, Dutta SC, Chang SS, Clark T, Smith JA Jr, Wells N: Health related quality of life in patients treated with radical cystectomy and urinary diversion for urothelial carcinoma of the bladder: development and validation of a new disease specific questionnaire. J Urol 2003; 170:1926

20 Voiding Dysfunction After Orthotopic Diversion

Jerilyn M. Latini

Contents

Abstract Orthotopic urinary diversion is a major advancement in the surgical management of patients requiring cystectomy for benign and malignant causes. Prevention of voiding dysfunction and incontinence after orthotopic urinary diversion is a focus of the comprehensive preoperative and postoperative algorithm. Preoperatively patients must be counseled about the benefits of and potential difficulties with orthotopic diversions, carefully instructed in the importance of timed voiding and what we currently believe are the best techniques to void effectively and efficiently, and they must be presented with realistic expectations in terms of the potential need for intermittent self-catheterization and treatment for incontinence depending on patient specific factors. Just as with any reconstructive surgical endeavor, outcomes should be realistically presented and discussed with the patient because voiding dysfunction and incontinence following orthotopic urinary diversion can cause significant reduction in the quality of life. A combination of educational, pharmacological, surgical, or catheterization strategies are available for the management of voiding dysfunction and incontinence after orthotopic urinary diversion. Education and counseling preoperatively, meticulous technique at the time of surgery, and ongoing instructions with long-term follow up can help prevent future issues with voiding dysfunction and incontinence after orthotopic urinary diversion to maximize quality of life and long term functional outcomes.

Keywords Neobladder, Urinary reservoirs, Continent, Urination/voiding disorders, Urodynamics

From: *Current Clinical Urology: Bladder Cancer,* Edited by: C.T. Lee and D.P. Wood,
DOI: 10.1007/978-1-59745-417-9_20,

1. Introduction

Following the description of the original surgical technique for internal urinary diversion in 1852 by Simon (1), numerous procedures have been developed to divert or reconstruct the urinary tract. Historically, three main categories of urinary diversions have been described: formation of a fistulous tract between the ureters and intact intestine, implantation of the ureters into a partially excluded segment of the gastrointestinal tract, and implantation of the ureters into a surgically created bladder fashioned from an excluded segment of the gastrointestinal tract (2). The first two types of diversions include continent diversions with the anal sphincter (elimination of urine by evacuation) and have declined in popularity with time. The third type has come to the forefront and continues to be modified internationally. Subdivided into appliance-dependent urinary diversions (conduits), continent catheterizable reservoirs and orthotopic bladder replacements or urinary diversions (neobladders), this chapter will focus on neobladders.

Ortho ("correct") topic ("of a place") urinary diversions or neobladders are anastomosed to the urethra, relying on the intact rhabdosphincter continence mechanism, rather than other continent urinary diversions that utilize the anal sphincter or an intestinal valve for continence. The goals of orthotopic diversion are: volitional residual-free voiding through the urethra, continence, avoidance of intermittent catheterization and maintenance of potentially sterile urine. Orthotopic urinary diversion after cystectomy affords patients the natural desire to void through the urethra. However, this desired outcome must be balanced with alterations in voiding and continence that occur with surgical creation of a new bladder from a segment of intestine. In recent years, our knowledge of the potential manifestations of voiding dysfunction that can occur after orthotopic urinary diversion has increased considerably. This knowledge has provided us with the opportunity to counsel our patients so that they can make a well-informed decision about their choices for urinary diversion after cystectomy. This chapter will discuss the potential dysfunction that may occur and the mechanisms underlying that dysfunction with regard to voiding and continence. Knowledge of the underlying pathogenesis and identification of risk factors will enable the development of strategies to prevent voiding dysfunction from occurring after orthotopic urinary diversion. Principal issues include patient selection, the design of orthotopic diversions, meticulous surgical technique, and when voiding dysfunction and/or incontinence do occur, how to evaluate and manage them appropriately.

Orthotopic urinary diversion encompasses a number of different surgical procedures and makes comparison of techniques and functional outcomes which are difficult at best. Measures of the prevalence, severity and character of functional outcomes in the contemporary literature are confounded by variability in endpoints, definitions, patient age and sex, choice of surgical technique, prior surgery or radiation therapy, quality and duration of follow up, and may contain bias depending on the entity reporting the data. Only recently have validated outcome instruments and voiding logs been used in the assessment of voiding dysfunction and continence after orthotopic diversion.

2. Physiology and Biomechanics of Orthotopic Urinary Diversions

Various gastric, ileal, ileocolonic, and colonic orthotopic diversions have been described. Voiding dysfunction and incontinence has been reported for all intestinal segments used in orthotopic diversion. The prevalence of voiding dysfunction appears to vary with the surgical technique used. The type, length and configuration of the intestinal segment used to create the orthotopic diversion directly impacts voiding pressures and patterns, and the risk of voiding dysfunction and incontinence. Urodynamic findings depend on the type, length and configuration of the intestinal segment use for orthotopic diversion.

The storage characteristics of orthotopic diversions depend on the type of intestinal segment, its length, and its surgical configuration. In addition to these factors, continence is dependent on timed voiding, adequate storage of urine in a low-pressure storage system, and a functional continence mechanism. Efficient voiding is dependent on the generation of an adequate abdominal contraction of sufficient duration and amplitude, coordinated with appropriate relaxation of the pelvic floor and sphincter mechanisms. Sphincteric mechanics and function are related to patient sex and age, effects of prior abdominopelvic surgery and/or radiation, vascular and neurological comorbidities, and parity in women. The relationships between native bladder contraction for voiding and sphincteric control of continence are dramatically altered with surgical creation of an orthotopic diversion.

The clinical and urodynamic goals of any orthotopic diversion should be to reproduce normal voiding habits. Continent diversions should: provide adequate capacity of approximately 500 cc at low storage pressures <15–40 cm H_2O (3), empty completely with <100 cc residual urine four to six times daily, allow the patient to sleep without awakening at night, ensure preservation of upper tract function in the long-term, provide voluntary reliable control of continence and evacuation, and allow for maintenance of a normal body image.

2.1. Rationale for Detubularization and Reconfiguration of the Intestinal Segment

The efficacy of an orthotopic diversion to store urine depends on detubularization of the intestinal segment, sufficient capacity, proper configuration and positioning of the neobladder in the pelvis (4). Refashioning the intestine into a pouch rather than a conduit is based on Goodwin's (5) work with augmentation cystoplasty. The shortest possible length of intestine should be used to create a low-pressure reservoir of adequate volume, minimizing gastrointestinal and metabolic sequelae. This is accomplished by detubularization and reconfiguration of a sufficient length of intact intestine (4, 6). Detubularization (incising the intestine along its antimesenteric border) and reconfiguration (folding and sewing the edges together) into spherical or ellipsoid configurations greatly increases the capacity/volume and decreases pressure.

Coordinated intestinal muscular/nerve activity propels intestinal contents in the normal aboral direction. These spontaneous intestinal contractions are physiological, whereas in the neobladder they are considered pathological. Detubularization interrupts rhythmic intestinal peristaltic contractions and elevated intraluminal pressures by preventing complete transmission of myogenic activity from longitudinal muscle to the inner circular muscle. Detubularization delays the onset and reduces the amplitude of pressures due to these spontaneous contractions.

An important clinical correlation is that neobladder over-distension is counterproductive because it destroys the added pressure generated by intestinal contractions that can help with emptying. With over distention, the pressure rise produced with spontaneous intestinal contractions at a given volume is further reduced, decreasing the efficiency of voiding. This implies that the voiding characteristics may very well change with time and could contribute to the development of retention. Therefore patients should be instructed to void at volumes less than capacity starting immediately postoperatively once their catheter is removed. The loss of myogenic activity from detubularization may lead to a higher incidence of retention, but all things considered, it is a more significant factor in terms of protecting the urinary tract from high pressures, decreasing susceptibility for reflux and pyelonephritis, and improving continence. Detubularization is more vital to promoting continence than the configuration of the orthotopic diversion. The concern is that if the spontaneous intestinal contractions are of large enough amplitude they can overwhelm the pelvic floor and sphincter mechanisms, thereby promoting incontinence.

Reconfiguration is also important. For a given length of intestine, reservoir volume and intraluminal pressure depends on the geometric configuration (4). The goal of reconfiguration is to obtain a spherical or ellipsoid reservoir. Spheres have the greatest volume for the smallest surface area and shortest initial length of intestine. Spherical reservoirs with larger radius (r) and volume (v) have lower filling pressures (p) without coordinated contractions (4, 5). According to the Laws of Laplace and Pascal: for a given wall tension (t), a larger radius results in decreased pressure. Geometric pouch capacity is determined by the configuration ($v = r2 \times h$), accommodation ($t = p \times r3$), and compliance or viscoelastic properties of the intestine (5). Clinical observations corroborate these mechanical principles: spherical configurations have the lowest luminal pressures while tubular configurations have the highest. In neobladders constructed from 40 cm of ileum with a diameter of 3.2 cm, when the pressure volume relationships for a tubular reservoir were compared with that of a detubularized spherical reservoir, the tubular reservoir had substantially smaller capacity and larger pressures for a given volume than the detubularized intestine. The volume of a U-shaped configuration has been shown to be less than those of the S, W or Koch pouches (7).

Colonic segments tend to have higher intraluminal pressures even when detubularized compared with the small intestine (8–11). When the colon is used, spontaneous myogenic contractions are more common and may be triggered by ingestion of food, other physiological reflexes, or humoral factors that may still exist despite detubularization. The presence of these contractions may not lead to incontinence per se (12) but increasing the amplitude of the contractions may (11, 13).

3. Urodynamic Characteristics of Orthotopic Urinary Diversions

Urodynamic characteristics are related to the type of intestinal segment, its length and surgical configuration, as well as the time since surgical creation of the orthotopic diversion. With filling and emptying over time (cycling), reservoir capacity increases, especially over the first 9–12 months. Maximal capacity varies with the intestinal segment used and its configuration (4, 7, 11). Generally, neobladder capacities are greater and pressures are lower for the Studer and Hautmann ileal orthotopic diversions than for Mainz ileocecal and some Camey II ileal neobladders. The most capacious appears to be the Kock orthotopic diversion (14). An extensive review of over 2,000 patients reported in the literature by Steers (14) shows that the capacity of ileal orthotopic diversions ranges from 270 to 770 mL at 3–54 months after surgery. The author notes that capacity increases with time and the length of follow up may explain some of the differences in reported capacities.

Reservoir capacity, rate of diuresis, efficacy of emptying and urethral resistance determines the reservoir's functional stability. If emptying is incomplete or chronically delayed, neobladders can become over distended and decompensated. Steers' (14) review of over 2,000 orthotopic diversion patients reported in the literature showed residual urine volumes from 1 to 170 mL for patients voiding spontaneously. No mention is made of catheterized volumes for those patients who catheterized for incomplete emptying or due to urinary retention. Conversely, defunctionalized orthotopic diversions lose capacity over time, as would be expected (15).

Emphasis has been placed on attaching the orthotopic diversion directly to the urethra with the neobladder neck positioned in the most dependent position within the pelvis to maximize complete emptying (16–19). After orthotopic urinary diversion, patients are typically instructed to abdominally strain to void and to consciously learn to relax the pelvic floor to allow for complete emptying. The relative voiding efficiency of abdominal straining was compared with the orthotopic diversion's intrinsic contractions (20). Voiding pressures with colonic orthotopic diversions are generally higher and the more colon that is used, the less the abdominal straining needed, whereas ileal orthotopic diversions required the most abdominal straining.

The compliance of and pressures within an orthotopic diversion are very important key concepts to optimal neobladder function. Intraluminal pressures should be kept low during filling and storage to preserve neobladder function, urinary continence, and upper tract function. It has been well established that if reservoir pressure exceeds 40 cm water at functional capacity, then deterioration of renal function can occur (3). There should be no spontaneous, intrinsic neobladder contractions causing increases in neobladder intraluminal storage pressures. The concern is that if neobladder compliance is poor or spontaneous intestinal contractions are of large enough amplitude, that elevated pressures can overwhelm ureteral peristalsis and lead to transmission of the elevated pressures to the pelvicaliceal system with deterioration of the upper tracts. Additionally, if neobladder compliance is poor or spontaneous intestinal contractions are of large enough amplitude, then elevated pressures can overwhelm the pelvic floor and sphincter mechanisms, thereby promoting incontinence.

4. Voiding and Continence with an Orthotopic Urinary Diversion

Beginning from the time that the postoperative catheter is removed from the orthotopic urinary diversion, it is imperative to avoid over distension of the neobladder with careful and specific patient instruction in timed voiding. The patient should be instructed to always void before the neobladder capacity is reached and before any sensation of fullness is perceived. Timed voiding every 3–4 h around the clock with volumes less than about 500 cc is required and not negotiable. Intermittent self-catheterization may be needed to assist with complete emptying and may be required to keep neobladder volumes low.

During timed voiding, the neobladder pressure generated by abdominal straining should be of sufficient amplitude to overcome pelvic muscle and sphincter mechanisms and of sufficient duration to allow for efficient and complete emptying. The use of abdominal straining to void falls into two patterns. Some patients strain throughout voiding whereas others strain only at the end of voiding (21). Urine flow rates of 12–19 mL/s are reported. Maximal voiding pressures necessary for neobladder emptying range from 40 to 80 cm water. Excessive abdominal straining has been postulated to predispose women to pelvic floor prolapse and subsequent obstruction or incontinence. However, a correlation between the amount of abdominal straining and the development of prolapse or incontinence has not been shown. Notably, a significant number of both male and female patients develop abdominal or inguinal hernias, which decrease the voiding efficiency by virtue of impaired abdominal straining. Hernias should be screened for, recognized and repaired.

Patients must be instructed to void routinely by the clock (timed voiding) rather than waiting for the sensation of neobladder fullness. It was hypothesized that sensation from the intestinal orthotopic diversion was transmitted to the spinal cord, resulting in the conscious perception of fullness. However this was tested in sigmoid neobladders and found to be false. Urodynamic studies showed that the sigmoid does not transmit sensation of reservoir fullness (20). Rather, neobladder sensation and a vague sensation of fullness appear to be conveyed via either peritoneal or pelvic floor striated muscle afferents. Given this information, patients must not wait for the conscious perception of reservoir fullness to void or wait until maximal capacity is reached. Instead patients must void by the clock at an interval that prevents neobladder volume from reaching maximal capacity, in an effort to prevent decompensation of the orthotopic diversion with time – usually every 3–4 h around the clock.

5. Evaluation of Voiding Dysfunction After Orthotopic Diversion

Any patient with sepsis, hydronephrosis, urinary retention, or suspicion of a fistula (vesicovaginal or vesicorectal) should be evaluated early. During the first 6–12 months after orthotopic diversion, lower urinary tract symptoms and incontinence typically improve. After 6–12 months, patients with persistent or worsening lower urinary tract symptoms, incomplete emptying, or incontinence warrant evaluation. Careful history and physical examination should include abdominal and inguinal examination for hernia, determination of intestinal function to assess for constipation and fecal impaction, pelvic examination for pelvic floor prolapse, and a focused neurourological examination. In women with incontinence, it is crucial to determine if leakage occurs from the urethra and/or the vagina. Careful pelvic examination with the use of methylene blue in the neobladder or fluoroscopic techniques are required to rule out a fistula. Computed tomography cystogram is very useful to evaluate for a fistula, in addition to charcoal studies, cystoscopy, voiding cystourethrography and fluoroscopic urodynamics.

Cystourethroscopy is indicated to rule out a urethral or neobladder neck stricture in all patients with voiding dysfunction and incontinence because a stricture can lead to difficulty in voiding and/or urinary retention with overflow incontinence. Cystourethroscopy should also be performed for recurrent urine infections, hematuria, to rule out the presence of a calculus or other pathology. Retroperitoneal and transabdominal ultrasound is useful in evaluating hydronephrosis and upper tract changes that may be associated with poor neobladder compliance and high neobladder pressures, obstruction or reflux.

Video fluoroscopic urodynamics are invaluable in evaluating patients with voiding dysfunction or incontinence after orthotopic diversion to help determine a cause and guide management. Urodynamics evaluates neobladder capacity, compliance, stability (presence or absence of intrinsic neobladder contractions), and sensation. Steers (14) presents a review of reported urodynamic parameters for many types of small intestine and colonic neobladders. A general review will be presented here and the reader is directed to this comprehensive report (14) for further details. Fluoroscopy allows for evaluation of the neobladder neck, neobladder shape and position, neobladder stability, presence or absence of spontaneous neobladder contractions, presence or absence of reflux, both at rest and with voiding. Fluoroscopically, the neobladder neck should be in the most dependent position compared with the rest of the neobladder, and a lateral view will help determine if there is any angulation of the urethra.

Residual urine volumes can be measured via catheterization or by transabdominal ultrasound. Fluoroscopic pressure-flow studies with residual urine measurement are used to evaluate voiding in terms of incomplete emptying and retention. Although there are no pressure-flow nomograms for neobladders, the presence of extremely high voiding pressures with an inability to empty implies obstruction (16, 17). Measurement of abdominal pressures during urodynamics assesses the strength and coordination of abdominal efforts for voiding with pelvic floor relaxation. Pelvic muscle electromyography is useful to evaluate pelvic muscle and urethral sphincter recruitment, synergy/dyssynergy, and whether the patient is able to relax the pelvic floor during voiding. Sometimes, as patients Valsalva and raise abdominal pressure to void, they simultaneously contract their pelvic floor causing pseudodyssynergia. Leak point pressure testing with Valsalva and cough efforts should be measured in varying positions with the use of fluoroscopy to characterize continence mechanisms and incontinence. Abdominal leak point pressure evaluation is valuable in assessing bladder outlet resistance, whereas urethral closure pressures and urethral functional length measurements are not typically useful due to a lack of normative data.

6. Voiding Dysfunction

Conceptually and clinically, voiding dysfunction after orthotopic diversion can be categorized into failure to empty the neobladder or failure to store urine in the neobladder. Table 20.1 lists the reported rates of voiding dysfunction, specifically urinary incontinence, enuresis and intermittent self-catheterization, for some of the contemporary series of orthotopic urinary diversions available presently in the literature. Gilbert, et al. used a validated health-related quality of life instrument to measure the outcomes in patients with bladder cancer (51). 122 patients underwent an orthotopic diversion. As assessed in a self-reported questionnaire, 8% of patients had no urinary control or had frequent dribbling and 40% of patients had urinary leakage at least once per week. Nighttime incontinence was a considerable problem with 49% having no urinary control or frequent dribbling and 75% of patients had urinary leakage at least once per week. Despite the day and nighttime incontinence, patients were happy with the orthotopic diversion registering 85 on a scale from 0 (terrible) to 100 (perfect). A control group with nonmuscle invasive bladder cancer treated by transurethral resection alone had a 'bother' score of 91.

6.1. Failure to Empty

It is reported that approximately less than 5–25% of patients must self catheterize for incomplete neobladder emptying (14), although some studies have reported catheterization rates over 80% (67). Urinary retention may be more common in women than men with orthotopic diversions. The cause of incomplete emptying and retention are unclear. Obstruction may be due to inferior displacement of the neobladder neck causing angulation of the urethra. Lengthening the urethra in an attempt to preserve continence or creation of a nipple or elongated neobladder neck anastomosed to the urethra is believed to contribute to obstruction. Patients who are able to void effectively have wide funneling of the neobladder neck with straining, consistent with the idea that adequate pelvic floor relaxation is necessary for effective voiding after orthotopic diversion. In some men and women, ability to maintain abdominal straining and high abdominal pressures may be lacking. For certain female patients, obstruction of their orthotopic diversion is similar to a prolapsed bladder or cystocele in some ways. Attention to preservation of vaginal tissues, levator muscles, and pelvic floor fascia in women may prevent prolapse, and retropubic support to secure proper neobladder orientation may be indicated (68).

A misleading term has been used in the literature – hypercontinence. This is a misnomer and really describes retention of residual urine and not continence per se. Importantly, the fact that with time, an orthotopic diversion increases its capacity does not imply that this is always desirable and advantageous in terms of voiding and continence. The term hypercontinence should not be used or advocated as a concept. Incomplete neobladder emptying and retention of residual urine should be recognized for what it is and managed appropriately.

Management of incomplete emptying involves timed voiding, physical therapy of the pelvic muscle to promote relaxation of the pelvic floor with voiding efforts, and intermittent self-catheterization to empty post-void residual urine. Intermittent self-catheterization may be recommended twice daily (once after the first morning void and once after the last void before bedtime) or as often as after every volitional void. Some patients empty their neobladder exclusively via intermittent self-catheterization and do not attempt to void at all due to the ease and relative efficiency of intermittent self-catheterization and the futility of efforts to volitionally void. Management of retention relies primarily with intermittent self-catheterization every 4–6 h around the clock based on neobladder capacity, compliance, presence or absence of intrinsic neobladder contractions, presence or absence of reflux, and associated lower urinary tract symptoms (41, 69).

Physical therapy techniques for the pelvic muscle are primarily concerned with the mechanics and coordination of the pelvic floor: locating, contract-

TABLE 20.1. Voiding dysfunction with orthotopic urinary diversions (14).

Type	Follow-up (month)	Number of patients	Age (years)	Sex	% UI	% Enuresis	% ISC	References
Camey	11	13	62	Male	7	38		(22)
	12	44	60	Male	0	33	0	(23)
		10		Male	20	10		
		18	60	Male		62	17	(24)
	30	27	57	Male	11	44	0	(25)
	46	32	58	Male	13	47	19	(25)
Mainz	42	108	57	Male	12	11	11	(26)
		8	60	Male	25	25		(11)
		14		Male	14	21		(27)
R Colon	12	38		36M/2F	0	8	8	(28)
Sigmoid		4	60	Male	50	50		(11)
	38	24		Male	6	44	24	(29)
	12	27		Male	0	33		(30)
	38	50	64	Male	11	90	0	(31)
	18	50	65	Male	15	91	24	(32)
		14		Male	21	57	0	(33)
		9		Female	0	33	11	(33)
Koch		87		Male	6	16		(34)
		155	66	Male	13	14	5	(35)
	48	35		Male	29			
		34	67	Female	12	18	15	(36)
		17		Female	7	13		(37)
	24	225		Male	8	25		(38)
	35	29	62	Female	4	14	10	(39)
Hautmann	36	200	61	Male	10	7	4	(40)
	55	13		Male	11	7		(41)
	6	12	59	Female	0	8		(16)
	54	363		Male	3	33	4	(42)
	50			M/F	7	14	4	(43)
	19	61		Male	5	33	5	(44)
		5	60	Male	20	20		(11)
	33	12		Female	17	50	25	(44)
	12	60	48	Female	26	14	14	(45)
	6	10		Female	30		10	(46)
	20	19	58	15M/4F		85	10	(47)
	16	37		Male	6	20		(48)
		16	60	Male	0	18	6	(24)
	19	67	56	9F/58M	5	27	15	(49)
	37	655	63	Male			12	(50)
	35	122	69	93M/29F	8	47	8	(51)

(continued)

TABLE 20.1. (continued)

Type	Follow-up (month)	Number of patients	Age (years)	Sex	% UI	% Enuresis	% ISC	References
Studer	34	33	63	Male	9	18	0	(21)
	9	167	64	Male	10	15		(52)
	18	22	48	Male	0	55	27	(18)
	74	40		Male	10	20		(53)
	17	66		Male	12	43	21	(54)
		40			0	18	8	(47)
	18	100	60	Male	10	40		(55)
	6	44		Male	3	70		(56, 57)
	12	25		Male	10	26		(58)
	12	24		Male	0	25	0	(59)
	42	21	64	Male	0	5		(60)
	37	62	58	Male	10	40	25	(32)
	57	57	60	53M/4F	4	11	9	(61)
	12	482		442M/40F	8	21	7	(62)
N-Shaped Ileal	38	52	60	Male	5	34	0	(63)
	38	6	47	Female	5	34	83	(63)
Goodman	37	95	65	75M/20F	9	18	2	(64)
Stanford	28	96		89M/7F	22	17		(65, 66)
Gastric	18	28	60	Male	7	39	3	(12)
	21	4	65	6M, 7F	15	7	70	(14)
		6	62.5	Male	67	67		(11)
Mean	26.7	4,072 (sum)	60		11.2	30.8	13.4	

UI urinary incontinence; *ISC* intermittent self-catheterization

ing and especially relaxing the pelvic floor. Specific techniques are used to help patients with contraction and bracing of the abdomen to assist with emptying. Various sitting positions and hand pressure are used to facilitate evacuation. Manual therapy techniques on the viscera and musculature of the pelvis are used because myofascial restrictions in these areas also contribute to voiding dysfunction. There may be a place for the use of alpha-adrenergic medications to decrease activity in sympathetic adrenergic nerves to the pelvic floor during voiding. For patients with incontinence, the focus is on pelvic muscle strengthening and coordination with activities, and timed voiding.

For some women with neobladder prolapse, a properly fitted pessary may be useful for symptoms of pelvic pressure. Unfortunately, in our experience, the pessary does little to assist with incomplete emptying or retention by the time the prolapse is recognized because over distention of the neobladder has often already taken its toll. Patients are relegated to chronic intermittent self-catheterization by that time and placement of the pessary does nothing for the neobladder dysfunction. If the neobladder neck is not in the most dependent position in the pelvis, some have recommended surgical repositioning of the neobladder neck (18). However, if the neobladder has been over distended and retention is based more on that issue, then surgery to reposition the bladder neck will do little to help. For inadequate or excessive neobladder capacity, surgical reconstruction may be an option but is not commonly performed.

6.2. Failure to Store

Failure to store urine can occur during the daytime, night-time or both. A history of preoperative stress incontinence in women appears to be an important predictive factor for incontinence after orthotopic diversion (45). In both women and men, daytime incontinence due to reduced urethral outlet resistance can be accentuated by low neobladder capacity, reduced neobladder compliance, elevated neobladder pressures, or intrinsic contractions of the neobladder (neobladder overactivity). In a review of over 2,200 patients with follow up of 26 ± 18 months, daytime incontinence occurred in 13.3 ± 13.6% patients (14). The Cochrane Collaboration has reported outcomes for use of intestinal segments for intractable incontinence or after cystectomy. The reported relative risk for both daytime and night-time incontinence was 1.0 suggesting no difference between varieties of orthotopic techniques, however a clinical difference may exist but could not be demonstrated statistically given that the confidence intervals were wide (70, 71).

Incontinence may improve or resolve in the 6–12 months after surgical diversion, as neobladder capacity increases with time. Evaluation should typically be delayed until a year after orthotopic diversion for this reason. A trend towards lower maximal urethral closure pressures has been reported in patients with stress incontinence, although no normative data exists for patients with orthotopic diversions (27). Functional urethral length does not appear to correlate with daytime incontinence (72). Risk factors for daytime incontinence include patient age older than 65 years (15% in patients older than 65 years vs. 5% in those younger than 65 years) (52), the use of colonic intestinal segments for orthotopic diversion, and possibly a lack of nerve sparing technique (47).

Continence may decrease 5–10 years after orthotopic diversion due to effects of aging on the sphincter mechanism and changes in the neobladder itself (73). Preservation of autonomic innervation at the time of diversion is intended to facilitate continence (74), however a significant percentage of patients develop retention with time. The highest rates of urinary retention have occurred in those patients where nerve-sparing techniques were utilized (14), whereas nerve sparing surgery reduces both daytime and night-time incontinence (52). They reported a 15% incidence of daytime incontinence and 25% incidence of night-time incontinence with nonnerve sparing surgery compared with 5% for both daytime and night-time incontinence in those undergoing nerve sparing techniques.

Night-time incontinence is one of the most common and frustrating issues after orthotopic urinary diversion. Night-time incontinence is a consequence of reduced or absent neobladder sensation that allows excessive night-time urine volumes to overcome urethral closure mechanisms. This is compounded by any impairment of the continence mechanisms at the neobladder outlet and decreased urethral strength following surgical dissection, relative decrease in urethral tone during sleep, and by the physiological diuresis that occurs with aging. It is further exacerbated by the loss of the physiological bladder storage reflexes and lack of neobladder sensation of fullness. Night-time incontinence improves to varying degrees within the first 12 months after surgery, as neobladder capacity increases. Just as with daytime incontinence, the main risk factor for night-time incontinence appears to be age greater than 65 years.

6.3. Management Strategies

Often daytime and night-time incontinence improves with time as the orthotopic diversion's capacity increases, especially during the first 12 months following surgery. Persistent stress incontinence is managed with physical therapy for the pelvic muscle for strengthening and coordination, endoscopic injection of periurethral bulking agents (75–77), surgical placement of a perineal (78) or pubovaginal sling (79), or surgical placement of an artificial urinary sphincter (80, 81). An alpha-adrenergic medication may be of use in some patients. Incontinence related to intrinsic contractions of the neobladder must be recognized and treated. This can be managed with loperamide alone or in combination with an anticholinergic medication that exerts an effect on intestinal motility, to, in essence, inhibit the neobladder overactivity. Overflow incontinence is managed with routine intermittent self-catheterization.

Night-time incontinence is managed by limiting fluid intake after dinnertime, elevation of the lower extremities in the evenings to help fluid mobilization, adjustment of medications and maximization of treatment for other medical issues such as congestive heart disease and peripheral edema, and primarily with the use of an alarm clock to awaken the patient several times per night to void (19). If there is also an element of incomplete neobladder emptying, intermittent self-catheterization before bedtime is a necessary adjunct (82). The efficacy and safety of 1-deamino-D-Arg-8 vasopressin (DDAVP) is not known in patients with orthotopic urinary diversions. Given the risk of hyponatremia, and the unknown effects of DDAVP on fluid absorption in patients with orthotopic diversions, it cannot be recommended at this time. The use of anticholinergics or tricyclic antidepressants at bedtime may be considered but are often ineffective.

7. Conclusions

Prevention of voiding dysfunction and incontinence after orthotopic urinary diversion is paramount. Preoperatively patients must be counseled about the benefits of and potential difficulties with orthotopic diversions, be carefully instructed in the importance of timed voiding and what we currently believe are the best techniques to void effectively and efficiently, and be presented with realistic expectations in terms of the potential need for intermittent self-catheterization and treatment for incontinence depending on patient specific factors. At the time of surgical diversion, one should aim to use an adequate length of ileum with a spherical or ellipsoid configuration, avoid creation of an oversized neobladder, carefully prevent injury to the pelvic floor musculature and innervation, avoid the use of excessive urethral length, not create a nipple or elongated neobladder neck for anastomosis to the native urethra, position the neobladder neck in the most dependent position, and create retropubic support of the neobladder to secure proper orientation where appropriate.

Postoperatively it is imperative to avoid over distension of the neobladder with careful and specific patient instruction in timed voiding, and to always void before neobladder capacity is reached and before any sensation of fullness is perceived. Timed voiding every 3–4 h around the clock with volumes less than about 500 cc is required and not negotiable. Intermittent self-catheterization may be needed to assist with complete emptying and may be required to keep neobladder volumes low.

Orthotopic urinary diversion is a major advancement in the surgical management of patients requiring cystectomy. However outcomes should be realistically presented and discussed with the patient considering orthotopic diversion because voiding dysfunction and incontinence cause significant reduction in quality of life. It cannot be overemphasized that regular urological follow up in terms of voiding outcomes is crucial regardless of how far out a patient is from surgical creation of the orthotopic diversion. A combination of educational, pharmacological, surgical, or catheterization strategies are necessary in the management of voiding dysfunction after orthotopic urinary diversion. Education and counseling pre operatively, meticulous technique at the time of surgery, and ongoing instruction with long-term follow up after surgery can help prevent future issues with voiding dysfunction and incontinence after orthotopic urinary diversion to maximize quality of life and long term functional outcomes.

References

1. Simon J. Ectropia vesica (absence of the anterior walls of the bladder and pubic abdominal parieties); operation for directing the orifices of the ureters into the rectum; temporary success; subsequent death; autopsy. Lancet 1852;2:568.
2. Hinman F, Weyrauch HM. A critical study of the different principles of surgery which have been used in ureterointestinal implantation. Trans Am Assoc Genitourin Surg 1936;29:15–16.

3. McGuire EJ, Woodside JR, Borden TA et al. Prognostic value of urodynamic testing in myelodysplastic patients. J Urol 1981;126:205.
4. Hinman F Jr. Selection of intestinal segments for bladder substitution: physical and physiological characteristics. J Urol 1988;139:519–523.
5. Goodwin WE, Turner RD, Winter CC. Results of ileocystoplasty. J Urol 1958;80:461–466.
6. Ekman 1965 Ekman H, Jacobsson B, Kock N, et al. The functional behavior of different types of intestinal bladder urinary substitutes. In: Proceedings of the XIII Congres de la Societe Internationale d'Urologie, vol II, discussions and free communications; 1965. London: E and S Livingstone.
7. Colding-Jorgensen M, Poulsen AL, Steven K. Mechanical characteristics of tubular and detubularized bowel for bladder substitution; theory, urodynamics and clinical results. Br J Urol 1993;72:586–593.
8. Chen KK, Chang LS, Chen MT. Neobladder construction using completely detubularized sigmoid colon after radical cystoprostatectomy. J Urol 1991;146:311–315.
9. Lobel B, Guille F, Olivo JF, et al. Variations of intestinal motor activity in bladder replacements and in the intestine. Arch Ital Urol Androl 1993a;65:615–623.
10. Lobel B, Guille F, Cipolla B, et al. Does detubularization improve continence in bladder replacement?. Arch Ital Urol Androl 1993b;65:625–628.
11. Santucci RA, Park CH, Mayo ME, et al. Continence and urodynamics parameters of continent urinary reservoirs: comparison of gastric, ileal, ileocolic, right colon, and sigmoid segments. Urol 1999;54:252–257.
12. Iwakiri J, Gill H, Anderson R, et al. Functional and urodynamic characteristics of an ileal neobladder. J Urol 1993;149: 1072–1076.
13. Bachor R, Frohneberg D, Miller K, et al. Continence after total bladder replacement: urodynamic analysis of the ileal neobladder. Br J Urol 1990;65:462–466.
14. Steers WD. Voiding dysfunction in the orthotopic neobladder. W J Urol 2000;18:330–337.
15. Kock NG, Nilson AE, Norlen L, et al. Changes in renal parenchyma and the upper urinary tract following urinary diversion via a continent ileum reservoir: an experimental study in dogs. Scand J Urol Nephrol 1978 49 (Suppl) 11–22.
16. Jarolim L, Babjuk M, Hanus T, et al. Female urethra-sparing cystectomy and orthotopic bladder replacement. Eur Urol 1997;31:173–177.
17. Mikuma N, Hirose T, Yokoo A, et al. Voiding dysfunction in ileal neobladder. J Urol 1997;158:1365–1368.
18. Porru D, Madeddu G, Campus G, et al. Urodynamic analysis of voiding dysfunction in orthotopic neobladder. W J Urol 1999;17:285–289.
19. Studer UE, Zingg EJ. Ileal orthotopic bladder substitute. What have we learned from 12 years experience with 200 patients. Urol Clin North Am 1997;24:781–800.
20. Koraitim MM, Atta MA, Foda MK. Desire to void and force of micturition in patients with intestinal neobladders. J Urol 1996;155:1214–1216.
21. Casanova GA, Springer JP, Gerber E, et al. Urodynamic and clinical aspects of ileal low pressure bladder substitutes. Br J Urol 1993;72:728–735.
22. Wu TT, Lee YH, Hauang JK, Jiaan BP, Yu CC. Functional and urodynamic characteristics of Camey II ileal neobladder. Urol Inter 1996;57(4):213–217.
23. Melchior H, Spehr C, Ingeborg K-W, Persson MC, Juenemann KP. The continent ileal bladder for urinary tract reconstruction after cystectomy: a survey of 44 patients. J Urol 1987;139:714–718.
24. Villanueva BA, Rioja SC, Sanz VJI, Rioja SLA. Urodynamic basis and findings in detubularised intestine neobladder: bladder substitutions and continent urinary reservoirs. Arc Esp Urol 1992;45(9):937–948.
25. Nesrallah LJ, Srougi M, Dall'Oglio MF. Orthotopic ileal neobladder: the influence of reservoir volume and configuration on urinary continence and emptying properties. BJU Int 2004;94(1):194.
26. Leissner J, Stein R, Hohenfellner R, Koho U, Riedmiller H, Schroder A, Lampel A et al. Radical cystoprostatectomy combined with Mainz pouch bladder substitution to the urethra: long-term. Br J Urol Int 1999;83(9):964–970.
27. Kakizaki H, Shibata T, Ameda K, et al. Continence mechanism of the orthotopic neobladder: urodynamic analysis of ileocolic neobladder and external urethral sphincter functions. Int J Urol 1995;2:267–272.
28. D'Orazio OR, Lambert OL, Vallati JC. Total and immediate daytime and nighttime continence with a right colonic neobladder – What makes it possible? AN 11-year followup. J Urol 2005;174(5):1882–1886.
29. Da Pozzo LF, Colombo R, Pompa P, Montorsi F, Di Girolamo V, Rigatti P. Detubularized sigmoid colon for bladder replacement after radical cystectomy. J Urol 1994;152(5 Pt 1):1409–1412.
30. Reddy PK, Lange PH, Fraley EE. Total bladder replacement using detubularized sigmoid colon: Technique and results. J Urol 1991;145(1):51–55.
31. Laguna MP, Brenninkmeier M, Belon JA. Long-term functional and urodynamic results of 50 patients receiving a modified sigmoid neobladder created with a short distal segment. J Urol 2005;174(3):963–967.
32. Schrier BP, Laguna MP, Van Der Pal F. Comparison of orthotopic sigmoid and ileal neobladders: continence and urodynamic parameters. European Urol 2005;47(5):679–685.
33. Fujisawa M, Isotani S, Gotoh A. Voiding dysfunction of sigmoid neobladder in women: a comparative study with men. Eur Urol 2001;40(2):191–195.
34. Skinner DG, Boyd SD, Lieskovsky G, Bennett C, Hopwood B. Lower urinary tract reconstruction following cystectomy: experience and results in 126 patients using the Kick ileal reservoir with bilateral ureteroileal urethrostomy. J Urol 1999;146:756.
35. Elmajian DA, Stein JP, Esrig D, Freeman JA, Skinner EC, Boyd SD, Lieskovsky G et al. The Kock ileal neobladder: updated experience in 295 male patients. J Urol 1996;156(3):920–925.
36. Stein JP, Grossfeld GD, Freeman JA, Esrig D, Ginsberg DA, Cote RJ, Skinner EC et al. Orthotopic lower urinary tract reconstruction in women using the Kock ileal neobladder: updated experience in 34 patients. J Urol 1997;158(2):400–405.
37. Grossfeld GD, Stein JP, Bennett CJ, Ginsberg DA, Boyd SD, Lieskovsky G, Skinner DG. Lower urinary tract reconstruction in the female using the Kock ileal reservoir with bilateral ureteroileal urethrostomy: update of continence results and fluorourodynamic findings. Urol 1996;48(3):383–388.
38. Kurzrock EA, Tomasic NA, Razi SS, Skinner DG, Bennett CJ. Flurourodynamic and clinical evaluation in males following construction of a Kock ileal-urethral reservoir. Urol 1995;46(6):801–803.

39. Nesrallah LJ, Almeida FG, Dall'oglio MF. Experience with the orthotopic ileal neobladder in women: a mid-term follow-up. BJU Int 2005;95(7):1045–1047.
40. Hautmann RE, Miller K, Steiner U, Wenderoth U. The ileal neobladder: 6 Years of experience with more than 200 patients. J Urol 1993;150(1):40–45.
41. Hautmann RE, Paiss T, De Petriconi R. The ileal neobladder in women: 9 years experience in 18 women. J Urol 1996;155: 76–81.
42. Hautmann RE, de Petriconi R, Gottfried HW, Kleinschmidt K, Mattes R, Paiss T. The ileal neobladder: complications and functional results in 363 patients after 11 years of follow-up. J Urol 1999;161(2):422–428.
43. Hollowell CM, Christiano AP, Steinberg GD. Technique of Hautmann ileal neobladder with chimney modification: interim results in 50 patients. J Urol 2000;163(1):47–50.
44. Arai Y, Taki Y, Kawase N, Terachi T, Kakehi Y, Okada T, Okabe T et al. Orthotopic ileal neobladder in male patients: functional outcomes of 66 cases. Int J Urol 1999;6(8):388–392.
45. Aboseif SR, Borirakchanyavat S, Lue TF, et al. Continence mechanism of the ileal neobladder in women: a urodynamics study. W J Urol 1998;16:400–404.
46. Ali-el-Dein B, el-Sobky E, Hohenfellner M, Ghoneim MA. Orthotopic bladder substitution in women: functional evaluation. J Urol 1999;161(6):1875–1880.
47. Park JM, Montie JE. Mechanisms of incontinence and retention after orthotopic neobladder diversion. Urol 1998;51: 601–609.
48. Jensen JB, Lundbeck F, Jensen KM. Complications and neobladder function of the Hautmann orthotopic ileal neobladder. BJU Int 2006;98(6):1289–1294.
49. Katoh N, Ono Y, Sahashi M, Kinukawa T, Matsuura O, Oshima S. Hautmann's Ileal neobladder: experience of 37 cases. Hinyokika Kiyo 1996;42(6):417–421.
50. Simon J, Bartsch G Jr, Kufer R. Neobladder emptying failure in males: incidence, etiology and therapeutic options. J Urol 2006;176(4 Pt 1):1468–1472; discussion 1472.
51. Gilbert SM, Wood DP, Dunn RL, Weizer AZ, Lee CT, Montie JE, Wei JT. Measuring health-related quality of life outcomes in bladder cancer patients using the Bladder Cancer Index (BCI). Cancer 2007;109(9):1756–1762.
52. Turner WH, Danuser H, Moehrle K, et al. The effect of nerve sparing cystectomy technique on postoperative continence after orthotopic bladder substitution. J Urol 1997;158:2118–2122.
53. Studer UE, Danuser H, Thalmann GN, Springer JP, Turner WH. Antireflux nipples or afferent segments in 70 patients with ileal low pressure bladder substitutes: longterm results of a prospective randomized trial. J Urol 1996;156(6): 1913–1917.
54. Gburek BM, Lieber MM, Blute ML. Comparison of Studer ileal neobladder and ileal conduit urinary diversion with respect to perioperative outcome and late complications. J Urol 1998;160(Pt 1):721–723.
55. Regalado PR, Huguet PJ, Errando SC, Lima BX, Chechile TG, Villavicencio MH. Orthotopic bladder replacement: II Functional results and complications in patients with Studer-type ileal neobladder. Arc Esp Urol 1997;50(3):234–241.
56. GutierrezBanos JL, Martin Garcia B, Hernandez Rodriguez R, Portillo Martin JA, Correas MA, Del Valle Schaan JI et al. Studer's type ileal neobladder. Study of complications and continence. Actas Urol Esp 1998;22(10):828–834 (erratum in Actas Urol Esp 1999;23(1):82).
57. Gutierrez Banos JL, Martin Garcia B, Hernandez Rodriguez R, Portillo Martin JA. Correas Gomez MA, del Valle Schaan JI, Monge Mirallas JM et al. Substitutive orthotopic ileocystoplasty. The Studer's technique. Arch Esp Urol 1995;48(8): 783–790.
58. Yokoo A, Hirose T, Mikuma N, Tskamoto T. Ileal neobladder for bladder substitution after radical cystectomy. Int J Urol 1998;5(3):219–224.
59. Rawal S, Kumar P, Kaul R. The "pitcher pot" ileal neobladder: early experiences. Jpn J Clin Oncol 2006;36(11):717–722.
60. Obara W, Isurugi K, Kudo D. Eight year experience with Studer ileal neobladder. Jpn J Clin Oncol 2006;36(7):418–424.
61. Tanaka T, Kitamura H, Takahashi A. Long-term functional outcome and late complications of Studer's ileal neobladder. Jpn J Clin Oncol 2005;35(7):391–394.
62. Studer UE, Burkhard FC, Schumacher M. Twenty years experience with an ileal orthotopic low pressure bladder substitute-lessons to be learned. J Urol 2006;176(1): 161–166.
63. Joniau S, Benijts J, Van Kampen M. Clinical experience with the N-shaped ileal neobladder: assessment of complications, voiding patterns, and quality of life in ore series of 58 patients. European Urol 2005;47(5):666–672; discussion 672–673.
64. Koie T, Hatakeyama S, Yoneyama T. Experience and functional outcome of modified ileal neobladder in 95 patients. J Urol 2006;13(9):1175–1179.
65. Cancrini A, DeCarli P, Fattahi H, Pompeo V, Cantiani R, Von Heland M. Orthotopic Ileal neobladder in female patients after radical cystectomy: Two-year experience. J Urol 1995;153(3 Pt 2):956–958.
66. Cancrini A, De Carl P, Pompeo V, Fattahi H, Lamanna L, Giuseppe C, Cantiani R et al. Lower urinary tract reconstruction following cystectomy: experience and results in 96 patients using the orthotopic ileal bladder substitution of Studer et al. Eur Urol 1996;29(2):204–209.
67. Joniau S, Benijts J, Van Kampen M Clinical experience with the N-shaped ileal neobladder: assessment of complications, voiding patterns, and quality of life in ore series of 58 patients. European Urol. 2005 47(5):666–672; discussion 672–673
68. Puppo P, Introini C, Calvi P, et al. Prevention of chronic urinary retention in orthotopic bladder replacement in the female. Eur Urol 2005;47:674–678; discussion 678.
69. Mills RD, Studer UE. Female orthotopic bladder substitution: a good operation in the right circumstances. J Urol 2000;163:1501–1504.
70. Yong SM, Dublin N, Pickard R, et al. Urinary diversion and bladder reconstruction/replacement using intestinal segments for intractable incontinence or following cystectomy. Cochrane Library, Issue 1, Oxford 2003.
71. Nabi G, Cody J, Dublin N, et al. Urinary diversion and bladder reconstruction/replacement using intestinal segments for intractable incontinence or following cystectomy. Cochrane Library, Issue 1, Oxford 2006.
72. Gasparini ME, Hinman F, Presti C, et al. Continence after radical cystoprostatectomy and total bladder replacement: a urodynamics analysis. J Urol 1992;148:1861–1864.

73. Madersbacher S, Mohrloe K, Burkhard F, et al. Long term voiding pattern of patients with ileal orthotopic neobladder substitutes. J Urol 2002;157:2052–2057.
74. El-Bahnasawy MS, Gomha MA, Shaaban AA. Urethral pressure profile following orthotopic neobladder: differences between nerve sparing and standard radical cystectomy techniques. J Urol 2006;175:1759–1763; discussion 1763.
75. Tchetgen MB, Sanda MG, Montie JE, et al. Collagen injection for the treatment of incontinence after cystectomy and orthotopic neobladder reconstruction in women. J Urol 2000;163:212–214.
76. Pruthi RS, Petrus CD, Bundrick WS. New onset vesicovaginal fistula after transurethral collagen injection in women who underwent cystectomy and orthotopic neobladder creation: presentation and definitive treatment. J Urol 2000; 164:1638–1639.
77. Wilson S, Quek ML, Ginsberg DA. Transurethral injection of bulking agents for stress urinary incontinence following orthotopic neobladder reconstruction in women. J Urol 2004;172:244–246.
78. Minowada S, Sasaki Y, Kano M, et al. Sling operation for male urinary incontinence after ileal neobladder reconstruction: a case report. Int J Urol 1995;2:132–133; discussion 134.
79. Quek ML, Ginsberg DA, Wilson S, et al. Pubovaginal slings for stress urinary incontinence following radical cystectomy and orthotopic neobladder reconstruction in women. J Urol 2004;172:219–221.
80. Schettini M, Diana M, Gallucci M. Treatment of urinary incontinence with AMS 800 artificial urinary sphincter. Int Surg 1998;83:257–261.
81. O'Connor RC, Kuznetsov DD, Patel RV, et al. Artificial urinary sphincter placement in men after cystectomy with orthotopic ileal neobladder: continence, complications, and quality of life. Urol 2002;59:542–545.
82. El-Bahnasawy MS, Magdy SO, Gomha MA, et al. Persistent and occasional nocturnal enuresis in orthotopic urinary diversion: is there a urodynamics difference? BJU Int 2005;96:1373–1377.

21
Overcoming the Stigma of Complications of Continent Cutaneous Diversion

Niels-Erik B. Jacobsen

Contents

Abstract The introduction of continent cutaneous diversions have increased the acceptability and decreased the stigmata associated with bladder cancer therapy. The understanding of the complications associated with continent cutaneous diversions is of vital importance for individuals caring for bladder cancer patients. The utilization of such techniques requires significant understanding of the immediate and long-term complications to allow for appropriate patient selection for individuals undergoing radical cystectomy. The appropriate selection criteria, immediate and late complications are reviewed. The chapter is organized by patient aspects such as capabilities, selection criteria, and QOL concerns. The complications are described by those associated with the reservoir, the continence mechanism or the stoma. This review serves as a valuable reference for the care of bladder cancer patients prior to and after receiving a continent cutaneous diversion.

Keywords Diversion, Continent, Cutaneous, Neobladder, Incontinence, Perforation, Infection, Hernia, Stenosis, Stricture, Metabolic

From: *Current Clinical Urology: Bladder Cancer,* Edited by: C.T. Lee and D.P. Wood,
DOI: 10.1007/978-1-59745-417-9_21,

1. Introduction

The field of lower urinary tract reconstruction and urinary diversion has undergone considerable change over the past three decades. Although conduit diversion remains the most common form of urinary diversion performed worldwide, continent diversion has become popular in recent years (1). Two general forms of continent urinary diversion are available: continent cutaneous diversion (CCD) and orthotopic neobladder replacement (ONB), each of which comprises the numerous individual techniques. Relative to ONB, CCD is performed much less commonly. In fact, ONB accounts for 50–90% of all urinary diversions performed at some centers (2–5). Multiple explanations exist, not the least of which is the capability to void per urethra rather than catheterize via an abdominal wall stoma. The perception that CCD is associated with a higher complication rate and a lower quality of life relative to ONB also plays a role. Regardless, CCD remains a valid alternative to ONB and may represent the most appropriate option in a subset of patients considering continent urinary diversion.

The purpose of this chapter is to review the incidence, presentation, and evaluation of the salient complications of CCD and to outline available treatment options and important preventive measures. Discussion will also be given on the patient selection process for CCD and its role in minimizing the potential complications thereof.

2. Patient Selection

Patient selection is the single most important determinant of outcome following urinary diversion. The selection process is individualized and must take into account the medical, physical, and psychological needs and capabilities of the patient (6). Foremost among the medical considerations is the indication for urinary diversion which includes bladder cancer, neurogenic bladder dysfunction, disabling urinary incontinence, interstitial cystitis, radiation cystitis, and hemorrhagic cystitis. Amongst bladder cancer patients it is of the utmost importance that the selected urinary diversion does not compromise the oncologic principles of radical cystectomy. Patients who require urethrectomy based on tumor involvement of the bladder neck (women) or urethral margin (men and women) are inappropriate candidates for ONB replacement. Likewise, patients with stress urinary incontinence secondary to sphincteric dysfunction should not undergo orthotopic diversion since continued voiding dysfunction is virtually guaranteed and will have significant impact on the quality of life (QOL). In both circumstances, patients who wish to remain continent post-operatively are better served by CCD. Additional medical considerations include renal function, hepatic function, prior abdominal radiotherapy and the presence of gastrointestinal disease (7). Renal dysfunction (serum creatinine >2 ng/mL) and moderate to severe hepatic dysfunction represent absolute contraindications to continent diversion of any type since the risk of developing metabolic complications is unreasonably high (8). Relatively long segments of ileum, colon or both are used in the construction of continent urinary diversion. The presence of gastrointestinal disease or radiation change may impact the type and length of bowel available for reconstruction. Accordingly, patients in whom a segment of colon will be used for diversion require preoperative colonoscopy or a barium enema study to rule out significant pathology. Advanced age (>75 years), medical comorbidity and neoplastic pelvic lymphadenopathy are not considered contraindications to continent urinary diversion (1, 9, 10).

The primary physical consideration when selecting a urinary diversion is the manual dexterity of the patient. Successful continent cutaneous diversion requires that clean intermittent catheterization (CIC) be performed on a regular basis. Patients who do not possess the manual dexterity to perform CIC are inappropriate candidates for CCD. Likewise, patients who are deemed incapable of adhering to a strict catheterization schedule, by way of mental defect or not, should not be offered CCD. Patient compliance with regular long-term follow-up is important with any form of urinary diversion but it is mandatory when considering CCD or ONB.

In addition to patient compliance, psychological considerations include the perception of body image as well as coping ability. Patients in whom the thought of an abdominal wall stoma provokes extreme anxiety are better served by orthotopic replacement, unless otherwise contraindicated. Conversely, patients who are unwilling to accept the higher risk of diurnal (13%) and nocturnal (28%) incontinence that comes with ONB, should be offered CCD wherein the risk of incontinence is less than 5% (11, 12).

3. Quality of Life

The perception of many urologists and patients, in turn, is that orthotopic diversion provides a QOL advantage over CCD and conduit diversion (13). Unfortunately, this opinion has been drawn from the findings of poorly designed studies many of which used unvalidated QOL instruments. Not a single randomized, controlled study has examined this question. As such, the current body of evidence is insufficient to conclude that one form of urinary diversion is superior to another in terms of health-related QOL (14, 15). In fact, many studies have found that QOL is similar among the three available options for diversion as well as in comparison to age-matched controls (15–17). Most patients report good QOL overall and general satisfaction irrespective of the type of urinary diversion performed (18). The role of proper patient selection in this regard cannot be overstated.

4. Overview of Complications

The performance of continent urinary diversion is technically demanding and carries with it a higher complication rate than does conduit diversion. However, with improvements in surgical technique, perioperative care and postsurgical follow up, the incidence of complications following continent diversion, including CCD, have fallen to an acceptable level (19). Large series with appropriately long follow-up demonstrate an early (within 30 days of surgery) complication rate of 15% (0–24%) (19–23). The majority of early complications are unrelated to the diversion and consist of wound infection/abscess (2.5%) and prolonged ileus (>7 days)/ small bowel obstruction (3.5%) primarily. Only 3–4% of patients require reoperation within the early postoperative period indicating that most early complications resolve with conservative management. Late complications occur in 40% (25–48%) of patients who undergo CCD. In contrast to early complications, the majority of late complications involve the CCD and a greater proportion of patients require surgical or endourologic intervention for resolution (14–33%). The most common late complications include ureteral obstruction (8.3%), difficult catheterization (7.9%) and reservoir calculi. The incidence of early and late complications in our Indiana pouch series is 20 (4% reoperation) and 32% (14% re-operation), respectively (23). Although at least one intrainstitutional review has found a higher rate of complications and reoperation with CCD compared to ONB in the long-term, most large ONB series report early (19–30%) and late (14–34%) complication rates similar to those of CCD (7, 24–26).

The complications associated with CCD can be divided into two groups according to whether they are related or unrelated to the diversion (Table 21.1).

TABLE 21.1. Overview of complications of continent urinary diversion.

General	Specific
Metabolic	Reservoir
Bowel	Leak
Prolonged ileus (>7 days)	Spontaneous perforation
Bowel obstruction	Stones
Anastomotic leak	Urinary tract infection
Enteric fistula	Malignancy
Uretero-intestinal anastomosis	Efferent limb
Leak	Stomal stenosis
Stricture	Difficult catheterization
	Parastomal hernia
	Incontinence
	Reservoir-related
	Continence mechanism-related

Complications unrelated to CCD include those germane to the performance of a laparotomy and bowel resection. Diversion-related complications arise directly from the CCD itself and can be categorized according to the specific component involved: reservoir, continence mechanism, stoma/efferent limb and ureterointestinal anastomosis. Only complications specific to CCD will be discussed in this chapter.

5. Complications Related to the Reservoir

5.1. Prolonged Urinary Leakage

Up to 10% of patients will have prolonged urinary leakage in the early postoperative period (6, 19). The relative incidence may be higher amongst ONB patients versus CCD patients based on the potential for leakage from the urethrovesical anastomosis (19). The usual manner of presentation is high-volume output from the intraabdominal drain, however, some patients may develop generalized peritonitis secondary to the irritative effects of urine. The diagnosis is confirmed by the finding of an elevated fluid creatinine level relative to serum. It is imperative that catheter patency is confirmed at the bedside. Mucous production by interposed bowel can impair emptying and propagate leakage, therefore it is important to institute scheduled catheter irrigations of the reservoir on postoperative day one prophylactically. While radiologic investigation is not necessary initially, prolonged leakage warrants further evaluation. A retrograde contrast study of the reservoir using fluoroscopy or computed tomography (CT) is useful to rule out the development of a chronic fistula, which is rare.

The majority of urine leaks emanate from a non-watertight suture line and will close spontaneously with appropriate drainage of both the diversion and abdomen (19). The reservoir catheter may be removed when leakage has resolved and the patient is competent to begin CIC via the efferent limb. Following this, the intra-abdominal drain can be removed if output remains low. On occasion, closed suction drains lying directly adjacent to a suture line may perpetuate leakage. Options in this circumstance include conversion to gravity drainage (i.e. take drain-off suction) as well as incremental advancement of the drain away from the suture line.

5.2. Spontaneous Rupture

Spontaneous intraperitoneal rupture of the urinary reservoir is a rare event among patients with continent cutaneous diversions, however, the incidence is known to be as high as 10% in high risk groups such as spinal-cord-injured patients (27). In combination with data extrapolated from the bladder augmentation literature, wherein the incidence of spontaneous perforation is up to 13%, factors associated with rupture include bowel segment, reservoir configuration, catheterization schedule, catheterization injury, chronic infection, reservoir ischemia, trauma, and neurologic dysfunction (28). The common end-product of all such risk factors is the generation of excessively high intraluminal pressure within the reservoir. Most commonly, this is due to incomplete or infrequent emptying secondary to impaired sensation, poor patient compliance or difficult catheterization. Although the normal sensation of bladder fullness is lost following cystectomy and urinary diversion, most patients with CCD or ONB describe a general awareness of reservoir distention, albeit reduced (29). Sensory impairment is even more pronounced among patients with baseline neurologic dysfunction. In these patients not only is the risk of perforation elevated, but so too are the consequences and potential morbidity since clinical presentation can be atypical and the diagnosis delayed. While some authors speculate that the segment of bowel used for urinary reconstruction may predispose toward spontaneous rupture, others have found no such association (28, 30). Theoretically, colonic reservoirs generate higher intraluminal pressures than ileal or ileocecal segments due to greater myogenic activity as demonstrated in urodynamic studies (31–34). More important than bowel type, however, is reservoir configuration. Detubularization and folding of bowel into a sphere minimizes the propagation of peristaltic activity and achieves the lowest intraluminal pressure possible according to Laplace's law (12). Spontaneous rupture secondary to reservoir ischemia is also a concern. Factors associated with ischemic injury include poor surgical technique, chronic overdistention and also transmural infection (28, 35–37).

Spontaneous rupture of a continent urinary reservoir is a true urologic emergency. Most patients present with an acute onset of generalized peritonitis, however, small contained leaks may cause localized pain only. It is not uncommon for patients to describe difficulty with catheterization of the efferent limb. In this context, abdominal pain should raise suspicion for perforation especially in patients with neurologic impairment in whom the presentation may be atypical. The diagnosis is confirmed by the intraperitoneal extravasation of contrast on retrograde fluoroscopic or CT imaging. Immediate treatment involves indwelling catheter decompression of the reservoir as well as the empiric administration of broad spectrum antibiotics. Chronic bacteriuria is common to all forms of CCD due to non-sterile intermittent catheterization, therefore, it must be assumed that extravasated urine is infected (38). Antibiotic treatment can be tailored according to the results of urine culture. Case reports demonstrate that small perforations with minimal extravasation may heal with conservative management, however, this circumstance is uncommon (39). The majority of perforations, including those that are large, remote from the time or surgery, or associated with significant peritonitis require open exploration, drainage, and repair (29).

Obviously, the key treatment for spontaneous perforation is prevention. All patients should be advised on the importance of maintaining a strict catheterization schedule in order to ensure complete emptying of urine and evacuation of mucus and debris. Patients who cannot adhere to such a regimen, due to either poor manual dexterity or mental defect, are inappropriate candidates for continent urinary diversion and should undergo incontinent diversion instead.

5.3. Reservoir Calculi

The formation of reservoir calculi is relatively common following continent urinary diversion with an overall incidence of 10% (40–42). Among continent diversions, calculi appear to be more common in cutaneous diversions (0–43%) than in orthotopic diversions (0.5–30%). The wide range in reported incidence reflects a difference in predisposing factors as determined by reservoir design and function. Recognized risk factors for calculi formation include foreign bodies, chronic bacteriuria, mucus production, urine stasis and diversion-related metabolic changes (43–46). Foreign bodies, such as metallic staples, act as a nidus for calculi formation and represent the single most important etiologic factor in this setting. Not surprisingly, diversions with an intussuscepted nipple valve constructed using metallic staples, such as the Kock pouch or Kock ileal neobladder, have the highest incidence at 26–43% and 10–30%, respectively (19, 42, 43, 47). Diversions which reduce staple exposure or negate their use altogether, such as the Indiana pouch or Studer ileal neobladder, have the lowest incidence at 5% or less (19, 42, 48, 49).

Most reservoir calculi are composed of struvite indicating that chronic bacteriuria is an important etiologic factor (43). Up to 80% of CCD are chronically colonized by bacteria secondary to nonsterile catheterization (50). By comparison, the majority of ONB patients who void spontaneously will have sterile urine for 4 months from the time of surgery (51). This difference in the rate of bacteriuria likely accounts for the higher incidence of calculi observed in CCD patients (29, 45, 50). Reservoir calculi are also composed of variable amounts of calcium oxalate indicating that metabolic factors are also involved. Hypercalciuria, secondary to metabolic acidosis-induced bone demineralization, is common in this population. Enteric hyperoxaluria may develop whenever large segments of ileum are used for urinary reconstruction (8). The urinary excretion of calcium, phosphate, and magnesium has been shown to be higher in continent diversions than in ileal conduits (52). Urinary stasis is a well-known risk factor for calculi formation regardless of the presence or type of urinary diversion. Interestingly, although lower tract calculi are more common among continent diversions versus incontinent diversions, there appears to be no difference in the incidence of upper tract calculi (29).

Typically patients with reservoir calculi are asymptomatic and most cases are diagnosed incidentally during routine radiologic follow up. Additional manners of presentation include gross hematuria, the sensation of pressure, incontinence, difficulty with catheterization, and symptomatic urinary tract infection (29, 46). If reservoir calculi are suspected on plain film, a noncontrast CT of the abdomen and pelvis should be performed in order to accurately evaluate stone burden, adjacent anatomy, and the presence of upper-tract calculi.

The treatment of reservoir calculi presents somewhat a challenge. First, the risk of treatment-related perforation of a thin-walled reservoir exceeds that for the native bladder. Second, endoscopic access through the efferent limb risks damage the continence mechanism which places an obvious upper limit on instrument size. In this regard it is important to discern the type of continence mechanism and the bowel segment used in the creation of the efferent limb (i.e. appendix vs. tapered ileum). Third, the spontaneous passage of residual fragments is often impeded by the continence mechanism. As such, secondary procedures are frequently necessary to achieve stone-free status. Fortunately, a number of treatment options are available for reservoir calculi. These include shock wave lithotripsy, open stone removal, and endoscopic or percutaneous techniques (53). Shock wave lithotripsy is rarely appropriate for reservoir calculi because of the difficulty with fragment passage. It is reserved for small calculi in the reservoir or upper tracts or for patients with extensive comorbidity and large stone burden requiring combination therapy. Most small stones are amenable to endoscopic lithotripsy and extraction through the efferent limb (53). Available flexible cystoscopes are of sufficiently small diameter (15 Fr) that the risk of damage to any component of the diversion is low. Large stone burdens are more appropriately treated percutaneously using the same techniques and instruments as used for percutaneous nephrolithotripsy (53–58). Percutaneous access, via one or more Amplatz sheaths or laparoscopic trocars, allows the expeditious fragmentation and removal of large calculi and avoids damage to the efferent limb and continence mechanism. The proximity of the reservoir to adjacent bowel and mesentery must be determined on preoperative CT to avoid injury when establishing percutaneous access. An alternative is to gain access under CT guidance directly. Electrohydraulic, ultrasound, and laser lithotripsy devices are all suitable for use in continent diversions (29). Intraoperative fluoroscopy is often essential since stone fragments are easily hidden by mucosal folds (53). Perforation of the reservoir intraoperatively can be avoided by periodic decompression or through the use of an open rather than closed percutaneous system. Open cystolithotomy is rarely indicated for the treatment of reservoir calculi. The few circumstances in which open surgery may be appropriate include the need for additional open procedure or an extremely large stone burden whereby percutaneous lithotripsy cannot be performed safely or expeditiously.

As is the case for most diversion-related complications, the best management strategy for reservoir calculi is prevention. Although the treatment of asymptomatic bacteriuria is not recommended, urease-producing bacteria are an exception and warrant antibiotic therapy even in the absence of symptoms. Certainly all symptomatic urinary tract infections deserve appropriate treatment. Pouch irrigations with hemiacidrin, which acidifies the urine, or acetohydroxamic acid, which inhibits bacterial urease, represent additional measures which may prevent the formation of struvite stones (59). Daily irrigations with sterile water is a simple maneuver which has been shown to reduce the incidence of reservoir calculi from 43 to 7% in some series (45). Reason for this involves the evacuation of mucous, crystals, and bacteria from the reservoir, all of which are known to propagate stone formation. Dietary strategies, including oral hydration (2–3 L/day) and the avoidance of foods high in oxalate, are also important. Patients with hypercalciuria secondary to chronic metabolic acidosis warrant oral alkalinization therapy with bicarbonate or citrate.

5.4. Metabolic Complications

Metabolic abnormalities are common to all forms of urinary diversion in which bowel mucosa is exposed to urine. The type and severity of metabolic change depends upon the length and segment of bowel used, contact time with urine and baseline renal function. Ileum and colon, the bowel segments used most commonly in urinary diversion, possess similar transport properties. When exposed to urine these segments tend to secrete sodium and bicarbonate and absorb hydrogen, chloride, and ammonium resulting in the development of hyperchloremic metabolic acidosis (60). Due to a larger absorptive surface area and longer contact time with urine, continent diversions have a higher rate of hyperchloremic metabolic acidosis than do ileal or colon conduits, estimated at 50 and 15%, respectively (61–63). Fortunately, most patients do not develop clinically significant metabolic change if renal and hepatic function is normal (64). Metabolic acidosis is minimized through the upregulation of acid excretion by the kidneys, while ammoniagenic encephalopathy is avoided through the hepatic metabolism of ammonium to urea (8). As such, it is essential that any patient in whom continent urinary diversion is considered have normal renal and hepatic function at baseline. Patient compliance is important since regular and complete emptying of the reservoir further reduces the risk of metabolic complications.

Patients with significant electrolyte or acid–base disturbance may have fatigue, weight loss, anorexia, and polydipsia. A history of urinary retention or difficult/infrequent catheterization may be provided. Serum chemistries reveal a nonanion gap acidosis, as well as hyperchloremia and azotemia. Initial management involves prompt drainage of urinary reservoir with an indwelling catheter and empiric antibiotic therapy if urinary tract infection is suspected. Alkalinization with bicarbonate or citrate is indicated in symptomatic patients as well as in those with mild chronic metabolic acidosis. Typically, ammoniagenic encephalopathy occurs in the setting of liver dysfunction. Encephalopathic patients in whom liver function was known to be normal previously should be suspected of harboring systemic infection since bacterial endotoxins may induce transient hepatic dysfunction and, in turn, the accumulation of ammonium (65). Acute management in this setting includes urinary drainage and systemic antibiotics. Oral neomycin and lactulose, which reduce the production and absorption of ammonia from the intestinal tract, are also appropriate (66).

5.5. Urinary Tract Infection

Asymptomatic bacteriuria is common to all forms of cutaneous urinary diversion. The incidence is as high as 80–90% amongst CCD patients, presumably due to clean, yet not sterile, intermittent catheterization (50, 67). Conversely, bacteriuria is uncommon after ONB replacement since most patients void spontaneously without the need for catheterization. About 4 months following surgery, most patients with Kock ileal neobladders have sterile urine (51). Interestingly, one study of ONB patients found that the incidence of symptomatic urinary tract infection (UTI) was not associated with the need for intermittent catheterization (68). Nonetheless, risk factors for bacteriuria following CCD include intermittent catheterization and high postvoid residual urine volume (38). There is also suggestion that bacterial colonization is more common among ileal diversions than in colonic diversions (68). *Escherichia coli* is the most frequently isolated microorganism, although other gram-negative Enterobacteriaceae and gram-positive cocci are also identified (38).

Urosepsis in the early postoperative period occurs in up to 2% of patients, usually because of ureteral stent occlusion (29, 69, 70). In the long-term, 0.9–5.8% of CCD patients develop acute pyelonephritis (19). Traditionally, CCD has been performed with a nonrefluxing ureterointestinal anastomosis based on the rationale that this minimizes the risk of pyelonephritis in the face of prevalent bacteriuria (71). However, one series examining this issue in the Indiana pouch found no difference in the rate of pyelonephritis between refluxing and nonrefluxing anastomoses (71). Furthermore, numerous studies have shown that nonrefluxing ureterointestinal anastomoses significantly increase the risk of anastomotic stricture over direct refluxing techniques (71, 1).

While the significance of bacteriuria in the setting of urinary diversion is not entirely clear, most authorities agree that in the absence of symptoms, antibiotic therapy is not warranted (6, 48, 72). Urea-splitting organisms, such as Proteus, represent an exception to this rule. Documentation of such organisms requires treatment, even if asymptomatic, based on the potential for struvite stone formation (6, 43). Established indications for antibiotic treatment include symptomatic UTI and pyelonephritis. While the treatment of CCD patients with recurrent symptomatic UTI or recurrent pyelonephritis is controversial, prophylactic antibiotics may be appropriate. At a minimum, patients with recurrent UTI warrant radiologic investigation to rule out the presence of stones or ureterointestinal stricture.

6. Complications Related to the Continence Mechanism

6.1. Incontinence

The incidence of incontinence following continent cutaneous diversion varies widely among reports. This is due not only to differences in continence mechanism design, but also, and perhaps more importantly, to differences in the timing and method of assessment. The lack of a uniform definition of postoperative continence is central to this problem. Nonetheless, reports exist of incontinence rates as high as 20% (73). Fortunately, with growing experience and improvements in surgical technique, the rate of postoperative incontinence amongst contemporary CCD series has fallen to 3.2%, overall (19). In comparison, daytime and nighttime incontinence remains a problem in 13 and 28% of orthotopic neobladder patients, respectively (12, 74). This is an important point since urinary control is a major determinant of quality of life following continent urinary diversion (12).

Broadly speaking, incontinence following continent cutaneous diversion is caused by either low outlet resistance (i.e. incompetent continence mechanism) or high intraluminal pressure (i.e. hypercontractile or poorly compliant reservoir). Lack of formal comparison makes it difficult to assess the relative efficacy of available continence mechanisms, however, it appears that incontinence is more frequent with the intussuscepted nipple valve (5.8%) than with the tunneled appendix (3.0%) or plicated ileocecal valve (0.6%) (19). In regard to bowel type, the incidence of incontinence appears to be similar in ileal, colonic, and ileocecal reservoirs. Interestingly, urodynamic studies have shown that colonic segments maintain greater myogenic activity and, in turn, generate higher intraluminal pressure (12).

The evaluation of urinary incontinence in CCD patients follows the same principles as that designed for patients with an intact bladder. Key points to focus on during history taking include timing of incontinence, precipitating factors, frequency, and ease of catheterization, "voided" volumes, abdominal pain, and sensation of fullness. Incontinence with stress points towards an incompetent continence mechanism, while infrequent or difficult catheterization of small volumes may suggest overflow incontinence. Abdominal pain associated with sudden onset of explosive incontinence should raise suspicion of pouchitis, a rare transmural infection of the reservoir that necessitates temporary catheter drainage and broad spectrum antibiotics for resolution. Physical examination includes evaluation of the stoma for signs of stenosis, prolapse, or parastomal hernia as well as of the reservoir for evidence of distension. Catheterization should be performed to confirm patency of the efferent limb and continence mechanism as well as to obtain urine for cytology and microbiologic analysis. While catheterization may provide an estimate of postvoid residual urine volume, abdominal ultrasonography may be more accurate. Additional radiologic investigation includes a retrograde contrast study to determine the anatomy and patency of the efferent limb as well as the integrity of the continence mechanism. If incontinence is suspected to be related to the reservoir, urodynamic testing will provide valuable insight into its capacity, compliance, contractility and intraluminal pressure.

The etiology of reservoir-related incontinence (high intraluminal pressure) includes hypercontractile peristaltic activity, low reservoir compliance and low reservoir capacity. Each can be prevented or minimized by following three established surgical principles of reservoir construction. First, the bowel segment must be adequately detubularized. This inhibits effective propagation of myogenic activity and prevents the development of high intraluminal pressure. Second, the reservoir configuration should be spherical. According to Laplace's law, wall tension is lower and compliance is higher in spheres compared to cylinders of the same radius (12). Third, the reservoir should be constructed from a sufficient length of bowel to ensure adequate capacity. By following these simple rules, a reservoir of suitable capacity (500 mL) and compliance (intraluminal pressure <15 cm water at capacity) will be constructed and the risk of incontinence minimized. The treatment of established reservoir-related incontinence usually involves open revision and ileal patch augmentation (23, 29). The frequency and severity of incontinence may be reduced with anticholinergic therapy, however, most reports indicate that the result of such treatment is unsatisfactory (12, 75–77).

Incontinence due to low outlet resistance usually requires open revision of the continence mechanism. Similar to reservoir-related incontinence, the key to managing outlet failure is through prevention. Valvular incompetence appears to be least common with the plicated ileocecal valve and, as such, it is the preferred continence technique for CCD diversion at our institution (19). Technical points which improve the long-term integrity of this valve include tapering the efferent limb over a small 12 Fr catheter and reinforcing the ileocecal valve along the antimesenteric border of the cecum and terminal ileum with a series of interrupted silk Lembert sutures. Surgical options in the uncommon event of valvular incompetence vary from repeat plication to complete disassembly and tunneled implantation of a tapered ileal segment (78, 79).

Reasons for failure of an intussuscepted nipple include fistula formation, nipple fibrosis or nipple dessusception. A fistula may arise secondary to injury caused by the alignment pin of modern staplers or as a result of catheter trauma. Preventive measures include closure of the pinhole defect and confirmation of facile catheterization at the time of diversion. Small fistulas can be repaired primarily while larger fistulas usually require construction of a new efferent limb (29). Nipple fibrosis is caused by ischemia and usually presents incontinence or difficult catheterization. Definitive treatment requires the complete reconstruction of a new continence mechanism and efferent limb. Nipple dessusception, or prolapse, results from inadequate fixation of the nipple to the reservoir (80). Fixation of the nipple to the wall of the reservoir using staples or an absorbable mesh collar seems to reduce the incidence of prolapse (80, 81). Treatment options include repeat stapling of the valve or construction of a new limb.

7. Complications Related to the Stoma and Efferent Limb

7.1. Parastomal Hernia

The incidence of parastomal hernia following continent cutaneous diversion is less than 5% (19, 82, 83). Most cases present within 6–12 months of surgery. Predisposing factors include obesity, multiple previous abdominal operations, parastomal wound infection, and stomal position lateral to the rectus muscle (84). Most patients are symptomatic and present with such complaints as abdominal wall deformity, parastomal pain, difficult catheterization and urinary incontinence. Few patients present with bowel obstruction. Diagnostic clues include parastomal pain which resolves in the supine position as well as the development of delayed urinary incontinence after an initial period of dryness (82). Physical examination in the supine and upright position, with and without performance of the Valsalva maneuver usually confirms the diagnosis. Equivocal cases, particularly obese patients, require CT imaging.

Anatomically, there exist two forms of parastomal herniation (84). The first is an extraperitoneal sliding hernia in which the continence mechanism and reservoir themselves herniate through the fascial defect. The second, and more common type, is an eccentric hernia in which intra-abdominal viscera herniate alongside the stoma and the continence mechanism remains intraperitoneal.

While numerous surgical treatments for parastomal hernia have been described, the most effective involves transabdominal repair of the fascial defect and repositioning of the stoma (29, 84). Fascial defects smaller than 6 cm may be closed primarily while those larger than 6 cm require external reinforcement with Marlex mesh (80, 84). Repositioning of the efferent limb allows its placement through the rectus muscle via an appropriately small hiatus. Revision or reinforcement of the continence mechanism should also be performed if simultaneous urinary incontinence exists.

7.2 Stomal Stenosis and Difficult Catheterization

Historically complications related to the efferent limb and stoma affected as many as 20–50% of CCD patients, the most common being difficult catheterization and stomal stenosis (85–87). With improvements in surgical technique the overall incidence of such complications has fallen to 8% (19). There appears to be different levels of risk among the various types of continence mechanisms. The incidence is highest with the tunneled appendix (18%), intermediate with the intussuscepted nipple valve (9%) and lowest with the tapered/plicated ileocecal valve (3%) (19). In our experience with the Indiana pouch using a tapered ileal efferent limb and plicated ileocecal valve, the incidence of difficult catheterization and stomal stenosis are 2% each (23). Established risk factors for stomal stenosis include ischemia and anastomotic tension, both of which are to be avoided (19, 29). Although the risk of stomal stenosis also appears to be higher in appendiceal limbs, incorporation of a V-plasty, which creates a wide distal funnel, has minimized this complication (85). Treatment of established stenosis usually begins with progressive stomal dilation in combination with strict adherence to an intermittent catheterization schedule. Should this fail, treatment options include endoscopic incision of the scar or creation of a V-plasty. The most definitive treatment involves complete mobilization of the efferent limb down to fascia, excision of the strictured segment and formation of a new stoma.

Reasons for difficult catheterization include false passage formation, stomal stenosis, redundancy of the efferent limb, and poor fixation or stenosis of the continence mechanism. False passages within the efferent limb are not uncommon and largely arise from improper catheterization technique. In this circumstance catheter drainage can almost always be established endoscopically. After a brief period of catheterization (3–7 days), the false passage will heal and the patient can resume intermittent catheterization provided that repeat instruction has been given in the interim. Persistent difficulty with catheterization warrants endoscopic and radiographic investigation of the efferent limb to determine both the cause and location of blockage. Redundancy or kinking of the efferent limb usually requires surgical correction and is best avoided at the time of original surgery. The ideal efferent limb closely approximates the diameter of the catheter, provides just enough length to avoid anastomotic tension, and maintains a straight course into the continence mechanism and reservoir. Fixation of the continence mechanism to the abdominal wall avoids kinking of the efferent limb as the reservoir fills. The treatment of stomal stenosis and stenosis of the continence mechanism has already been discussed.

8. Complications Related to the Uretero-Intestinal Anastomosis

What constitutes the gold-standard ureterointestinal anastomosis is a matter of some controversy. Refluxing and nonrefluxing anastomoses represent the two general types, each comprising numerous individual techniques. Traditionally, nonrefluxing anastomoses have been recommended for continent cutaneous diversions based on the high incidence of bacteriuria within the reservoir (50, 67). It is felt by some that a nonrefluxing anastomosis prevents the development of pyelonephritis and, potentially, renal dysfunction. While some studies have documented a lower incidence of pyelonephritis with nonrefluxing anastomoses, others have found no difference (71, 88). Furthermore, the implications of reflux and pyelonephritis in the adult kidney are unknown at this time. Presumably, they are of less clinical importance than in children (29, 89, 90). Less contentious is the association of anastomotic technique and stricture formation. Most series have found a higher incidence of stricture formation with nonrefluxing anastomoses (3.6–13%) vs. refluxing anastomoses (1.7–4.2%) (6, 29, 71, 91). Weighing the genuine risk of anastomotic stricture against the theoretic benefit of preventing reflux, it is our practice to perform direct refluxing ureterointestinal anastomoses on all continent cutaneous diversions. Until well-designed prospective randomized trials with adequate follow up are conducted, the ideal anastomotic technique will remain controversial.

Regardless of the type of anastomosis performed, it is of the utmost importance to follow basic surgical tenets in order to prevent or minimize the development of anastomotic complications. First, the blood supply to the distal ureter must be maintained. Preservation of the vascularized peri-adventitial tissue along the entire length of the ureter will accomplish this goal.

Second, the anastomosis should be free of tension. This is achieved by ensuring that adequate ureteral length and mobility is available. Third, the ureter should be free of kinks or twists, especially the left ureter where it is transposed beneath the sigmoid mesentery. Fourth, the anastomosis must be made water tight and created over an indwelling ureteral stent to ensure patency.

8.1. Uretero-Intestinal Anastomotic Leak

Leakage from the ureterointestinal anastomosis is uncommon today due to the routine use of ureteral stents which bridge the anastomosis in the early postoperative period (91). Amongst contemporary series, the incidence of anastomotic leak is only 2% (6). Indwelling and exdwelling ureteral stents appear to be equally effective in this regard, however, indwelling stents may increase the rate of UTI (57). While practice patterns vary, stents are usually removed prior to discharge providing that a retrograde stentogram has confirmed anastomotic patency and absence of leakage.

The drainage of high volumes of fluid with an elevated creatinine level should raise suspicion for an anastomotic leak. The diagnosis is confirmed by a retrograde pouchogram or a stentogram if the stent is still in place. The vast majority of leaks can be treated conservatively with high success (6). Rarely is open surgical management necessary. If the stent has already been removed, initial management involves the placement of a percutaneous nephrostomy catheter and continued closed suction intraabdominal drainage. Should leakage persist, an antegrade ureteral stent is advised. Anastomotic leaks which occur in the presence of the original ureteral stent may be observed since most will resolve within a few days. If early resolution does not occur, a retrograde stentogram should be performed to assess the severity of leakage followed by the placement of a percutaneous nephrostomy drain to divert the urinary stream. Persistent leakage beyond the early postoperative period is a recognized risk factor for anastomotic stricture (6).

8.2. Uretero-Intestinal Anastomotic Stricture

Similar to anastomotic leak, the incidence of anastomotic stricture has fallen since ureteral stents were incorporated into the construction of urinary diversions on a routine basis. Overall, stricture formation occurs in less than 5% of anastomoses as documented by large contemporary series (19). Risk factors for anastomotic stricture include anastomotic leak, infection, prior pelvic radiotherapy, nonrefluxing anastomoses and poor surgical technique (6, 19, 78). The pathophysiology of stricture formation involves periureteral fibrosis, progressive scarring, and consequent obstruction. This is to be differentiated from obstruction secondary to ureteral edema following stent removal which occurs in approximately 3% of patients in the early postoperative period (6). Provided that anastomotic leakage is not present, ureteral edema is of no long-term consequence and treatment need only involve temporary decompression via percutaneous nephrostomy. Recurrence of urothelial carcinoma is included in the differential diagnosis of anastomotic stricture and must be ruled out prior to assigning treatment in those patients with a history of bladder cancer.

Due to the slow progressive nature of stricture formation, most patients remain asymptomatic and the diagnosis is usually made incidentally during routine postsurgical evaluation. Although most anastomotic strictures present within 2 years of surgery, some may not become apparent until 6 years or beyond underscoring the importance of long-term follow up (71, 92). The demonstration of hydroureteronephrosis raises suspicion for obstruction while the diagnosis is confirmed by diuretic renal scan or intravenous pyelography. Alternatively, a retrograde pouchogram may be used to rule out obstruction if a direct refluxing anastomosis was performed. In cases of high grade obstruction, an antegrade nephrostogram may better define the length, site, and severity of stricture. The minimum diagnostic algorithm to rule out tumor recurrence at the anastomosis includes contrast-enhanced CT of the abdomen and pelvis as well as urinary cytology. Endoscopic visualization and biopsy of the anastomotic site is recommended if preliminary studies are suspicious for neoplastic regrowth. A baseline determination of renal function is appropriate in all patients since it may guide subsequent treatment recommendations.

The first step in the management of anastomotic stricture usually consists of percutaneous nephrostomy drainage. Indications for its use include symptomatic renal colic, suspicion of upper urinary tract infection and compromised renal function. If the function of the ipsilateral renal unit is poor at baseline, functional studies can be repeated following a short period of decompression. Percutaneous access also allows the performance of antegrade contrast studies to further define stricture anatomy as well as the aspiration of urine for diagnostic cytology.

Following initial decompression, management of anastomotic stricture is individualized and depends on a number of factors: (1) ipsilateral renal function, (2) number, length, and location of the stricture(s), (3) history of radiation to the abdomen or pelvis, and (4) benign or malignant etiology. If renal function is poor (< 10% split renal function), treatment of the stricture is inappropriate and nephrectomy should be considered. Patients with recurrent urothelial tumor must undergo a complete metastatic reevaluation. If tumor is limited to the ureter, the primary treatment options include open excision and reimplantation as well as nephroureterectomy. Poor surgical candidates, those with a solitary kidney, and those with small, solitary low grade tumors may be candidates for endoscopic ablative therapy. The treatment of patients with advanced or metastatic disease is primarily medical. In advance of chemotherapy, these patients may be considered for antegrade stent insertion.

The primary treatment options for benign anastomotic stricture include balloon dilation, endoscopic incision and open surgical revision. Endoscopic balloon dilation, performed under fluoroscopic guidance, is the least invasive modality and also the least effective. Although reported success rates vary among studies, long-term patency rates rarely exceed 30% (72). Stricture recurrence typically occurs within 1–2 years of dilation, however, long-term radiologic follow up is advised. Endoscopic incision, the most commonly employed treatment for anastomotic stricture, is more effective than balloon dilation with short and long-term patency rates of 66–88% and 32–75%, respectively (72, 93, 71, 94). Predictors of treatment success following balloon dilation or endoscopic incision include stricture length less than 2 cm, stricture onset within 7 months of urinary diversion, and ipsilateral split renal function greater than 25% (6, 95–100). The incision should extend through the full thickness of the scar and may be performed using a cold knife, cutting current electrocautery or Holmium:YAG laser. Similar to endopyelotomy, most authorities recommend leaving a large caliber ureteral stent (≥12 Fr) for a period of 4–6 weeks following incision (6). It has also been suggested that endoscopic incision in combination with either balloon dilation or the injection of corticosteroids into the stricture may improve long-term patency rates (101, 102).

Open surgical revision is the definitive treatment option for anastomotic stricture with long-term patency rates as high as 90% (78, 101). However, since it is the most invasive of the available treatment options, and portends the highest risk of morbidity, it is used primarily after endourologic management has failed. Most strictures are amenable to excision and primary reanastomosis, however, long strictures may necessitate ileal interposition or transureteroureterostomy. If reconstruction is not possible, nephrectomy may be indicated. It is important that all excised segments undergo pathologic review in order to exclude the presence of malignancy.

9. Conclusion

The complications of continent cutaneous diversion as they relate to the reservoir, continence mechanism, stoma/efferent limb, and ureterointestinal anastomosis are not infrequent. However, with improvements in surgical technique and postoperative care, the incidence of CCD-related complications has fallen to an acceptable level. Most large series with appropriate follow up demonstrate similar complication and reoperation rates following CCD and ONB. Furthermore, quality of life data indicate that no single urinary diversion technique demonstrates clear superiority over another. Most patients report good overall QOL and general satisfaction regardless of the type of urinary diversion performed. In this regard, the importance of proper patient selection and meticulous surgical technique cannot be overstated. Continent cutaneous diversion remains a viable alternative to orthotopic reconstruction, especially for patients who wish to maintain urinary control but are not willing to accept the higher risk of nocturnal incontinence associated with ONB. Likewise, patients with intrinsic sphincter dysfunction and those with neoplastic involvement of the urethral margin who require urethrectomy are inappropriate candidates for ONB and are better served by CCD if postoperative continence is a goal.

References

1. Hautmann RE. 15 years experience with the ileal neobladder. What have we learned?. Urologe A 2001; 40(5):360–7.
2. Studer UE, Zingg EJ. Ileal orthotopic bladder substitutes. What we have learned from 12 years' experience with 200 patients. Urol Clin North Am 1997; 24(4):781–93.
3. Hautmann RE, de Petriconi R, Gottfried HW, Kleinschmidt K, Mattes R et al. The ileal neobladder: complications and functional results in 363 patients after 11 years of follow-up. J Urol 1999; 161(2):422–7.

4. Stein JP, Skinner DG. Application of the T-mechanism to an orthotopic (T-pouch) neobladder: a new era of urinary diversion. World J Urol 2000; 18(5):315–23.
5. Montie JE, Wei JT. Formation of an orthotopic neobladder following radical cystectomy: historical perspective, patient selection and contemporary outcomes. J Pelvic Surg 2002; 8:141.
6. Farnham SB, Cookson MS. Surgical complications of urinary diversion. World J Urol 2004; 22(3):157–167.
7. Hautmann RE, Schumacher M, Gscgwend JE, Studer UE, Volkmer BG. Long-term results of standard procedures in urology: the ileal neobladder. World J Urol 2006; 24(3): 305–14.
8. DeMarco RT, Koch MO. Metabolic complications of continent urinary diversion. AUA Update Series 2003; 22(15):114–9.
9. Parekh DJ, Clark T, O'connor J, Jung C, Chang SS et al. Orthotopic neobladder following radical cystectomy in patients with high perioperative risk and co-morbid medical conditions. J Urol 2002; 168(6):2454–6.
10. Tefilli MV, Gheiler EL, Tiguert R, Grignon DJ, Forman JD et al. Urinary diversion-related outcome in patients with pelvic recurrence after radical cystectomy for bladder cancer. Urology 1999; 53(5):999–1004.
11. Rowland RG. The long-term study of continent cutaneous urinary reservoirs and neobladders. J Urol 1996; 155:1217.
12. Steers WD. Voiding dysfunction in the orthotopic neobladder. World J Urol 2000; 18(5):330–337.
13. Dutta SC, Chang SC, Coffey CS, Smith JA Jr, Jack G et al. Health related quality of life assessment after radical cystectomy: comparison of ileal conduit with continent orthotopic neobladder. J Urol 2002; 168(1):164–7.
14. Porter MP, Penson DF. Health related quality of life after radical cystetomy and urinary diversion for bladder cancer: a systematic review and critical analysis of the literature. J Urol 2005; 173(4):1318–22.
15. Gerharz EW, Mansson A, Hunt S, Skinner EC, Mansson W. Quality of life after cystectomy and urinary diversion: an evidence based analysis. J Urol 2005; 174(5):1729–36.
16. Ohrstrom M, Davidsson T, Mansson W, Wohlfart B, Ekelund M. Working capacity and well-being after radical cystectomy with continent cutaneous diversion. Eur Urol 2006; 49(4):691–7.
17. Pazooki D, Edlund C, Dahlstrand C, Lindholm E, Tornqvist H et al. Continent cutaneous urinary diversion is still a valid alternative after cystectomy for bladder carcinoma. Scan J Urol Nephrol 2005; 39(6):468–73.
18. Hart S, Skinner EC, Meyerowitz BE, Boyd S, Lieskovsky G et al. Quality of life after radical cystectomy for bladder cancer in patients with an ileal conduit, cutaneous or urethral Kock pouch. J Urol 1999; 162(1):77–81.
19. Rowland RG. Complications of continent cutaneous reservoirs and neobladders-series using contemporary techniques. AUA Update Ser 1995; 14(25):202–207.
20. Thuroff JW, Alken P, Riedmiller H, Jacobi GH, Hohenfellner R. 100 cases of Mainz pouch: continuing experience and evolution. J Urol 1988; 140(2):283–8.
21. Riedmiller H, Thuroff J, Hohenfellner R. Continent urinary diversion: The Mainz pouch procedure. Prob in Urol 1991; 5:283–91.
22. Mansson W, Davidsson T, Colleen S. The detubularized right colonic segment as urinary reservoir: evolution of technique for continent diversion. J Urol 1990; 144(6): 1359–61.
23. Bihrle R. The Indiana pouch continent urinary reservoir. Urol Clin North Am 1997; 24(4):773–9.
24. Crivellaro S, Michaels MJ, Kocjancic E, Libertino JA. The Lahey clinic experience with continent urinary diversion. BJU Int 2004; 94:1087–1091.
25. Stein JP, Dunn MD, Queck ML, Miranda G, Skinner DG. The orthotopic T pouch ileal neobladder: experience with 209 patients. J Urol 2004; 172(2):584–7.
26. Meyer JP, Drake B, Boorer J, Gillat D, Persad R et al. A three-centre experience of orthotopic neobladder reconstruction after radical cystectomy: intial results. BU Int 2004; 94(9):1317–21.
27. Pazooki D, Edlund C, Karlsson AK, Dahlstrand C, Lindholm E et al. Continent cutaneous urinary diversion in patients with spinal cord injury. Spinal Cord 2006; 44(1):19–23.
28. Defoor W, Tackett L, Minevich E, Wacksman J, Sheldon C. Risk factors for spontaneous bladder perforation after augmentation cystoplasty. Urology 62(4):737–741.
29. Ginsberg DA, Rovner ES, Raz S. Complications of continent urinary diversion. In: Taneja SS, Smith RB, Ehrlich RM, eds. Complications of Urologic Surgery: Prevention and management, 3rd ed. Philadelphia: WB Saunders, 2001: 454–467.
30. Shekarriz B, Upadhyay J, Demirbilek S, Barthold JS, Gonzalez R. Surgical complications of bladder augmentation: comparison between various enterocystoplasties in 133 patients. Urology 2000; 55(1):123–8.
31. Chen KK, Chang LS, Chen MT. Neobladder construction using completely detubularized sigmoid colon after radical cystoprostatectomy. J Urol 1991; 146(2):311–5.
32. Lobel B, Guille F, Olivo JF, Gosselin A, Goldwasser B. Variations of intestinal motor activity in bladder replacements and in the intestine. Arch Ital Urol Androl 1993; 65(6):615–23.
33. Lobel B, Guille F, Cipolla B, Roth S, Shalev M et al. Does detubularization improve continence in bladder replacement?. Arch Ital Urol Androl 1993; 65(6):625–8.
34. Santucci RA, Park CH, Mayo ME, Lange PH. Continence and urodynamic parameters of continent urinary reservoirs: comparison of gastric, ileal, ileocolic, right colon, and sigmoid segments. Urology 1999; 54(2):252–7.
35. Bauer SB, Hendren WH, Kozakewich H et al. Perforation of the augmented bladder. J Urol 1992; 148:699–703.
36. Crane JM, Scherz HS, Billman GF et al. Ischemic necrosis: a hypothesis to explain the pathogenesis of spontaneously ruptured enterocystoplasty. J Urol 1991; 146:141–144.
37. Essig KA, Sheldon CA, Brandt MT et al. Elevated intravesical pressure causes arterial hypoperfusion in canine colocystoplasty: a fluorometric assessment. J Urol 1991; 146: 551–553.
38. Wullt B, Agace W, Mansson W. Bladder, bowel and bugs: bacteriuria in patients with intestinal urinary diversion. World J Urol 2004; 22(3):186–95.
39. Gupta NP, Nabi G, Ansari MS. Conservative management of spontaneous rupture of a sigmoid colon neobladder. Urol Int 2002; 69(4):325–6.
40. Holmes DG, Thrasher JB, Park GY, Kueker DC, Weigel JW. Long-term complications related to the modified Indiana pouch. Urology 2002; 60:603–06.

41. Skinner DG, Lieskovsky G, Boyd SD. Continuing experience with the continent ileal reservoir (Kock pouch) as an alternative to cutaneous urinary diversion: an update after 250 cases. J Urol 1987; 137:1140–145.
42. Terai A, Ueda T, Kakehi Y, Terachi T, Arai Y, Okada Y, Yoshida O. Urinary calculi as a late complication of the Indiana continent urinary diversion: comparison with the Kock pouch procedure. J Urol 1996; 155:66–68.
43. Ginsberg D, Huffman JL, Lieskovsky G, Boyd S, Skinner DG. Urinary tract stones: a complication of the Kock pouch continent urinary diversion. J Urol 1991; 145(5):956–9.
44. Steven K, Poulsen AL. The orthotopic Kock ileal neobladder: functional results, urodynamic features, complications and survival in 166 men. J Urol 2000; 164:288–295.
45. Hensle TW, Bingham J, Lam J, Shabsigh A. Preventing reservoir calculi after augmentation cystoplasty and continent urinary diversion; the influence of an irrigation protocol. BJU Int 2004; 93(4):585–7.
46. Edin-Liljegren A, Grenabo L, Hedelin H, Jonsson O, Akerlund S et al. Concrement formation and urease-induced crystallization in urine from patients with continent ileal reservoirs. Br J Urol 1996; 78(1):57–63.
47. Arai Y, Kawakita M, Terachi T, Oishi K, Okada Y, Takeuchi H, Yoshida O. Long-term followup of the Kock and Indiana pouch procedures. J Urol 1993; 150(1):51–5.
48. Hautmann RE. Neobladder and bladder replacement. Eur Urol 1998; 33(5):512–22.
49. Abol-Enein H, Ghoneim MA. Functional results of orthotopic ileal neobladder with serous-lined extramural ureteral reimplantation: experience with 450 patients. J Urol 2001; 165:1427–432.
50. Akerlund S, Berglund B, Kock NG, Philipson BM. Voiding pattern, urinary volume, composition and bacterial contamination in patients with urinary diversion via a continent ileal reservoir. Br J Urol 1989; 63(6):619–23.
51. Skinner DG, Boyd SD, Lieskovsky G, Bennett C, Hopwood B. Lower urinary tract reconstruction following cystectomy: experience and results in 126 patients using the Kock ileal reservoir with bilateral ureteroileal urethrostomy. J Urol 1991; 146(3):756–60.
52. Terai A, Arai Y, Kawakita M, Okada Y, Yoshida O. Effect of urinary intestinal diversion on urinary risk factors for urolithiasis. J Urol 1995; 153(1):37–41
53. L'Esperance JO, Sung J, Marguet C, L'Esperance A, Albala DM. The surgical management of stones in patients with urinary diversions. Curr Opin Urol 2004; 14:129–134.
54. Hollensbe DW, Foster RS, Brito CG, Kopecky K. Percutaneous access to a continent urinary reservoir for removal of intravesical calculi: a case report. J Urol 1993; 149(6):1546–547.
55. Thomas R, Lee S, Salvatore F, Blank B, Harmon E. Direct percutaneous pouch cystostomy with endoscopic lithotripsy for calculus in a continent urinary reservoir. J Urol 1993; 150(4):1235–237.
56. Seaman EK, Benson MC, Shabsigh R. Percutaneous approach to treatment of Indiana pouch stones. J Urol 1994; 151(3):690–2.
57. Roth S, Van Ahlen H, Semjonow A, Von Heyden B, Hertle L. Percutaneous pouch lithotripsy in continent urinary diversions with narrowed Mitrofanoff conduit. Br J Urol 1994; 73(3):316–8.
58. Beiko DT, Razvi H. Stones in urinary diversions: update on medical and surgical issues. Curr Opin Urol 2002; 12:297–303
59. Williams JJ, Rodman JS, Peterson CM. A randomized double-blind study of acetohydroxamic acid in struvite nephrolithiasis. N Engl J Med 1984; 311(12):760–4.
60. Koch MO, McDougal WS, Thomson CO. Mechanisms of solute transport following urinary diversion through intestinal segments: An experimental study with rats. J Urol 1991; 146:1390–7.
61. Bowels WT, Tall BA. Urinary diversion in children. J Urol 1967; 78:597–605.
62. McDougal WS. Metabolic complications of urinary intestinal diversion. J Urol 1992; 147:1199–1207.
63. Poulsen AL, Steven K. Acid-base metabolism following bladder substitution with the ileal urethral Kock reservoir. BJU Int 1996; 78:47–53.
64. Kock MO, McDougal WS, Reddy PK et al. Metabolic alterations following continent urinary diversion through colonic segments. J Urol 1991; 145:270–2.
65. McDougal WS, Wilmore DW, Pruitt BA. Glucose-dependent hepatic membrane transport in non-bacteremic and bacteremic thermally injured patients. J Surg Res 1977; 22:697–708.
66. Edwards RH. Hyperammonemic encephalopathy related to ureterosigmoidostomy. Arch Neurol 1984; 41:1211–2.
67. Terai A, Arai Y, Okada Y, Yoshida O. Urinary bacteriology of contient urinary reservoirs and calculus formation. Int J Urol 1994; 1(4):332–6.
68. Wood DP Jr, Bianco FJ Jr, Pontes JE, Heath MA, DaJusta D. Incidence and significance of positive urine cultures in patients with an orthotopic neobladder. J Urol 2003; 169(6):2169–9.
69. Elmajian DA, Stein JP, Esrig D, Freeman JA, Skinner ED et al. The Kock ileal neobladder: updated experience in 295 male patients. J Urol 1996; 156(3):920–5.
70. Cancrini A, De Carli P, Pompeo V, Fattahi H, Lamanna L et al. Lower urinary tract reconstruction following cystectomy: experience and results in 96 patients using the orthotopic ileal bladder substitution of Studer et al. Eur Urol 1996; 29(2):204–9.
71. Pantuck AJ, Han KR, Perrotti M, Weiss RE, Cummings KB. Ureteroenteric anastomosis in continent urinary diversion: long-term results and complications of direct versus nonrefluxing techniques. J Urol 2000; 163:450–55.
72. Hafez KS, Wolf JS Jr. Update on minimally invasive management of ureteral strictures. J Endourol 2003; 17:453–464
73. Bachor R, Hautmann R. Options in urinary diversion: a review and critical assessment. Semin Urol 1993; 11(4):235–50.
74. Balbay MD, Slaton JW, Trane N, Skibber J, Dinney CP. Avoiding urinary diversion in patients with locally advanced rectal cancer: the rationale for bladder sparing. J Urol 1999; 161:90A.
75. Christmas TJ, Smith GL, Rickards D. Diagnosis and management of high-pressure peristaltic contractions in cystoplasties. Br J Urol 1997; 79(6):879–82.
76. Fowler JE, Clayton M, Mouli K, et al. Effect of liquid diphenoxylate hydrochlorid and atropine sulfate (Lomotil) instillations on dynamics and function of continent cecal urinary reservoirs. J Urol 1987; 183:735–8.
77. Jakobsen H, Steven K. Lack of effect of cholinergic blocking and alpha-adrenergic stimulation on nocturnal incontinence after ileocecal bladder replacement. A controlled randomized study. Br J Urol 1989; 63:379–83.

78. Wilson TG, Moreno JG, Weinberg A et al. Late complications of the modified Indiana pouch. J Urol 1994; 151:331–4.
79. de Kernion JB, Trapasso JG. Urinary diversion and continent reservoir. In: Gillenwater JY, Grayhack JT, Howards SS, eds. Adult and Pediatric Urology. 3rd ed. St. Louis, Mo: Mosby-Year Book, 1996:1465–1500.
80. Lieskovsky G, Boyd SD, Skinner DG. Management of late complications of the Kock pouch form of urinary diversion. J Urol 1987; 137(6):1146–50.
81. Skinner DG, Lieskovsky G, Boyd S. Continent urinary diversion. J Urol 1989; 141:1323–1327.
82. Mastrandrea FD, Helal MA, Kahn P, Pow-Sang JM, Sanford EF et al. The Florida pouch procedure: six year follow-up. J Urol 1995; 53:241A.
83. Lieskovsky G, Skinner DG, Boyd SD. Complications of the Kock pouch. Urol Clin North Am. 1988; 15:195–205.
84. Helal M, Austin P, Spyropoulos E, Pow-Sang J, Persky L et al. Evaluation and management of parastomal hernia in association with continent urinary diversion. J Urol 1997; 157:1630–1632.
85. Woodhouse CRJ, Malone PR, Cumming J et al. The Mitrofanoff principle for continent urinary diversion. Br J Urol 1989; 63:53–7.
86. Leonard MP, Gearhart JP, Jeffs RD. Continent urinary reservoirs in pediatric urologic practice. J Urol 1990; 144:330–3.
87. Dykes EH, Duffy PG, Ransley PG. The use of Mitrofanoff principle in achieving clean intermittent catheterization and urinary continence in children. J Pediatr Surg 1991; 26:535–8.
88. Richie JP, Skinner DG. Urinary diversion: the physiologic rationale for non-refluxing colon conduit. Br J Urol 1975; 47:269–75.
89. McDougal W. Use of intestinal segments and urinary diversion. In: Walsh PC, Vaughan ED Jr, Wein AJ, eds. Campbell's Urology, 8th ed., vol. 4. Philadelphia: WB Saunders, 2002:3745–88.
90. Studer UE, Danuser H, Thalmann GN et al. Antireflux nipples or afferent tubular segments in 70 patients with ileal low pressure bladder substitutes; the long term results of a prospective randomized trial. J Urol 1996; 156: 1913–7.
91. Regan JB, Barrett DM. Stented versus nonstented ureteroileal anastomoses: is there a difference with regard to leak and stricture?. J Urol 1985; 134:1101–3.
92. Malgieri JL, Persky L. Ileal loop in the treatment of radiation-treated pelvic malignancies: a comparative review. J Urol 1978; 120:32–4.
93. Wolf JS Jr, Elashry OM, Clayman RV. Long-term results of endoureterotomy for benign ureteral and ureteroenteric strictures. J Urol 1997; 158:759–764.
94. Scheider AW, Conrad S, Busch R. The cold-knife technique for endourological management of stenosis in the upper urinary tract. J Urol 1991; 146:961–5.
95. Martin EC, Fankuchen EL, Casarella WJ. Percutaneous dilation of ureteroenteric strictures or occlusions in ileal conduits. Urol Radiol 1982; 4:19–21.
96. Banner MP, Pollack HM. Dilation of ureteral stenosis: techniques and experiences in 44 patients. Am J radiol 1984; 143:789.
97. Shapiro MJ, Banner MP, Amendola MA et al. Balloon catheter dilation of ureteroenteric strictures: long-term results. Radiology 1988; 168:385–7.
98. Beckmann CF, Roth RA, Bihrle W. Dilation of benign ureteral strictures. Radiology 1989; 172:437–41.
99. Netto NR Jr, Ferreira U, Lemos GC et al. Endourological management of ureteral strictures. J Urol 1990; 144:631–4.
100. Johnson CD, Oke EJ, Dunnick NR. Percutaneous balloon dilatation of ureteral strictures. Am J Radiol 1987; 148:181–4.
101. Kramolowsky EV, Clayman RV, Weyman PJ. Endourological management of ureteroileal anastomotic strictures: is it effective?. J Urol 1987; 137:390–4.
102. Meretyk S, Albala DM, Clayman RV et al. Endoureterotomy for treatment of ureteral strictures. J Urol 1992; 147:1502–6.

Part III
Locally Advanced / Distant Disease: Multi-Modality Treatement

22
Neoadjuvant Chemotherapy: The New Standard

Karen Giselle Chee and Primo N. Lara

Contents

Abstract Bladder cancer, most often of the transitional cell type (TCC), is the fourth most commonly diagnosed malignancy in the United States (1). About 75% of patients are diagnosed with localized disease at initial presentation, with about 20% having loco-regionally advanced (stage II/III) disease (2). Following radical cystectomy or definitive radiation therapy, recurrence risk in these patients exceeds 50% (3). Table 22.1 summarizes the data of the recent outcome for patients with locally advanced bladder cancer treated with cystectomy alone.

The high incidence of distant recurrence in patients with presumed early stage disease is principally due to the presence of distant micrometastases at the time of local therapy. Because of this, recent research has revolved around peri-operative systemic therapy, either as neoadjuvant or adjuvant treatment, aimed at eradicating micrometastatic deposits. Alternative (non-cystectomy) approaches for localized disease have also been investigated, particularly radiation therapy with or without chemotherapy. This review summarizes current data on therapeutic strategies for locally advanced bladder cancer.

Keywords Bladder carcinoma, Neoadjuvant chemotherapy, Adjuvant chemotherapy

1. Definitive Local Therapy: Radiation Therapy Alone vs. Combined Modality Chemoradiation

In the United States, radical cystectomy has been considered the standard local treatment for patients with locally advanced bladder cancer for the past thirty years. However, in Europe and Canada, radiation therapy is often considered a reasonable alternative to cystectomy. The contribution of chemotherapy in the context of radiation therapy (either as a radiosensitizer and/or as systemic therapy for occult micrometastases) has not yet been definitively established in

From: *Current Clinical Urology: Bladder Cancer,* Edited by: C.T. Lee and D.P. Wood,
DOI: 10.1007/978-1-59745-417-9_22,

TABLE 22.1. A summary of the data of the recent outcome for patients with locally advanced bladder cancer treated with cystectomy alone (Stein et al. (4)).

Stage of disease (N = 1,054)	10-year relapse-free survival (RFS; %)
T2	78
T3a	76
T3b	50
T4	45
Overall recurrence rate	30
Distant recurrence	22
Madersbacher et al. (5)	
Stage of disease	5-year relapse-free survival (RFS; %)
Organ-confined	73
Extravesical disease (no lymph node involvement)	56
Distant relapse among patients with organ-confined disease	25

this disease. Furthermore, patients receiving primary radiation therapy often are not completely surgically staged, precluding direct comparisons with surgical cohorts. Patients selected for primary radiation therapy are therefore likely to have a high rate of occult, undocumented regional or distant micrometastases, reducing the likelihood of cure with local therapy alone. In at least one trial of patients receiving radiation alone as principal therapy, a 5-year survival rate of 31% and a 5-year local control rate of 35% were observed (6).

Concurrent chemoradiation has also been tested formally in this setting. Coppin et al. conducted a small randomized phase II trial of radiation alone vs. radiation plus concurrent cisplatin for locally advanced bladder cancer (7). At study completion, the trial accrued 50 patients in each arm. Local recurrence was significantly lower in patients receiving combined modality therapy (52% vs. 29%, $p < 0.05$). While there was an encouraging trend favoring the chemoradiation arm with respect to an overall 3-year survival, the results did not reach statistical significance, most likely due to the small sample size.

Hussain et al. also performed a phase II trial in 56 patients who were unresectable or medically unfit for a cystectomy (8). Patients received combined chemoradiation therapy with cisplatin 75 mg/m^2 on day 1 and 5-FU 1 g/m^2/d on days 1–4, on a 28-day cycle. Two cycles of chemotherapy were given during radiation with another two cycles given as consolidation after completion of radiation therapy. In this poor-risk population, planned therapy was completed in only 57% of the patients. The overall response rate was 51% and the 5-year survival rate was a dismal 32%.

In light of these and other data, one can summarise that radiation therapy (either alone or in combination with chemotherapy) for locally advanced disease has resulted in relatively disappointing outcomes, due, in large part, to the substantial understaging of patients treated with this strategy. Nevertheless, radiation remains an option for a subset of patients who are either not candidates for cystectomy, or are interested in bladder preservation.

1.1. Neoadjuvant Chemotherapy

In an attempt to improve overall survival, studies have been done to evaluate the role of neoadjuvant and adjuvant chemotherapy in patients with locally advanced bladder cancer. Neoadjuvant therapy has the advantage of providing the earliest systemic therapy to the primary tumor and to the micrometastatic sites. Other possible advantages for the neoadjuvant approach include (1) chemotherapy delivery through intact vasculature (which is often affected by surgery or radiation therapy); (2) downstaging of tumor size prior to a cystectomy; (3) the potential for delaying cystectomy if an observed pathological complete response (pCR) is achieved; (4) the potential to increase complete resection rates; and (5) better tolerability compared to the adjuvant therapy approach. To date, the results of randomized clinical trials appear to favor neoadjuvant systemic therapy in muscle invasive bladder cancer.

The earliest trials in neoadjuvant chemotherapy utilized single-agent platinum as the base regimen. Wallace et al. performed a combined analysis of two small randomized trials that were initially designed to test the survival benefit of neoadjuvant single-agent cisplatin prior to radiation in patients with T2–T4 bladder cancer (9). Both trials failed to reach their individual accrual goals. The combined analysis included 255 patients with the two treatment groups each compared to its corresponding control group. Data were pooled and analyzed. No difference in overall survival was found between single-agent cisplatin-treated patients and those who did not receive neoadjuvant therapy.

Another trial of 122 patients evaluating the role of neoadjuvant single agent cisplatin has also been reported (10). In this trial, the observed time to relapse was different between the two arms (30.3 months vs. 13.1 months favoring the chemotherapy arm with a $p = 0.0501$). However, the time to death did not differ significantly between the two groups ($p = 0.139$).

A meta-analysis of the studies evaluating the potential role of single-agent platinum therapy revealed a hazard ratio (HR) of 1.15 (95% CI: 0.90–1.47) for survival and of 1.14 (95% CI: 0.83–1.55) for disease-free survival (11). The confidence intervals clearly cross 1, demonstrating no benefit to single agent neoadjuvant cisplatin in this setting. Given the results of these trials, the use of single-agent platinum as neoadjuvant therapy cannot be recommended.

The pursuit of combination platinum-based neoadjuvant chemotherapy regimens is logical since response and survival rates for metastatic bladder cancer are higher with combination chemotherapy regimens compared to single agent therapy (12). This culminated in two large phase III trials, summarized below, that established neoadjuvant platinum-based chemotherapy as the standard of care in locally advanced bladder cancer.

The first definitive trial to define the role of multiagent neoadjuvant therapy was conducted by the Medical Research Council's Advanced Bladder Cancer Group. This group tested the combination of CMV (cisplatin, methotrexate and vinblastine) (13). A total of 976 patients were randomized to cystectomy or definitive radiation therapy with or without neoadjuvant CMV. With a median follow-up of 7 years, the observed median survivals were 44 months and 37.5 months for the CMV arm vs. the no CMV arm, respectively. The HR for survival was 0.85 with a $p = 0.048$ in favor of the neo-adjuvant chemotherapy, corresponding to a 15% reduction in the risk of death during the course of the study.

The United States Intergroup led by the Southwest Oncology Group performed a similar trial employing neoadjuvant MVAC (methotrexate, vinblastine, adriamycin and cisplatin) followed by cystectomy vs. cystectomy alone (14). In this trial, 307 patients were followed for a median of 8.4 years. At the study's conclusion, the HR for survival was 0.74 ($p < 0.05$, one-sided) in favor of the neoadjuvant MVAC approach. This represented a 26% reduction, in the risk of death, which was due to MVAC. Median survival time for patients in the MVAC arm was 77 months vs. just 46 months for patients who did not receive MVAC. Interestingly, a complete pathological response of 38% was observed in patients receiving neoadjuvant chemotherapy.

Of note, there were smaller trials that had previously failed to show benefit for the neoadjuvant approach. Bassi et al. reported the results of a phase III trial utilizing neoadjuvant MVAC (15). With a total of 206 patients (much smaller than the Intergroup trial), no survival advantage was found in patients who received neoadjuvant therapy.

The Italian Bladder Tumor Study Group performed a multicenter randomized phase III study comparing neoadjuvant chemotherapy followed by cystectomy vs. cystectomy alone (16). The chemotherapy regimen was MVEC (methotrexate, vinblastine, epidoxorubicin and cisplatin), where the anthracycline doxorubicin was substituted for its analogue epidoxorubicin. With a median follow-up of 33 months, no differences were found in either disease free or overall survival between the study arms.

Two Nordic studies, each with different neoadjuvant cisplatin-based chemotherapy regimens, also reported a lack of statistical power to detect a difference in overall survival (17–18). The first study by the Nordic Cooperative Bladder Cancer Study Group randomized 325 patients to receive neoadjuvant cisplatin and doxorubicin followed by short-term radiotherapy and cystectomy vs. short-term radiotherapy and cystectomy. In that trial, the overall survival rate was 59% in the chemotherapy group and 51% in the control group. A second Nordic cystectomy trial randomized patients to receive neoadjuvant cisplatin and methotrexate followed by cystectomy vs. proceeding directly to cystectomy. 317 patients were recruited to the trial. With a median follow-up of 5.3 years, the estimated 5-year overall survival was 53% in the chemotherapy arm vs. 46% in the control arm. When the two Nordic studies were combined, however, an observed HR for survival of 0.80 (95% CI: 0.64–0.99) favoring the chemotherapy arm was reported (19). A common theme among these "negative" trials is that they were all statistically underpowered to detect a clinically meaningful difference in outcome between the treatment arms.

Subsequently, a meta-analysis of all published randomized trials of neoadjuvant chemotherapy demonstrated a HR of 0.86 (95% CI: 0.77–0.095, $p = 0.003$) in favor of a neoadjuvant platinum-based combination chemotherapy approach. This was calculated to be equivalent to a 5% absolute improvement in survival at 5 years (11). There was also a disease-free survival benefit found with chemotherapy (HR = 0.78 with 95% CI: 0.71–0.86, $p < 0.0001$). Given the overall benefit seen in this meta-analysis, the use of neoadjuvant platinum-based chemotherapy is considered the standard of care in the management of locally advanced/muscle-invasive bladder cancer.

2. Adjuvant Chemotherapy

Another approach at delivering systemic therapy for patients with locally advanced disease is in the postoperative (or adjuvant) setting. As an example of this approach, Skinner et al. performed a randomized trial of adjuvant cisplatin, adriamycin, and cytoxan (CAP) vs. observation in patients with completely surgically-resected bladder cancer (20). With only 91 patients evaluated, the 5-year disease-free survival (DFS) was 51% vs. 34% ($p < 0.011$) favoring the use of CAP. The 5-year overall survival was 44% vs. 39% ($p = 0.0062$) for the CAP and observation arms, respectively. However, the DFS curves of the two groups did cross after 7 years. In addition, there were noted deviations from the pre-defined treatment protocol, including an unplanned interim analysis.

Another trial by Stockle et al. suggested benefit of the addition of adjuvant chemotherapy in this setting (21). However, this particular trial was plagued by methodological problems which placed its conclusions in doubt.

In another study, Freiha et al. randomized patients to receive adjuvant CMV after radical cystectomy vs. observation. The freedom from disease progression in the adjuvant chemotherapy arm was superior to the observed group (median 37 vs. 12 months, respectively with $p = 0.01$) (22). There was also a trend favoring the chemotherapy arm in terms of overall survival (median 63 vs. 36 months, $p = 0.32$). Unfortunately, this trial was closed prematurely before accruing the intended number of patients, thereby preventing the possibility of full assessment of the benefits of adjuvant therapy.

A recent meta-analysis of a series of adjuvant chemotherapy trials did yield a HR of 0.75 in favor of chemotherapy ($P = 0.019$), but problems with the individual trials included in the analysis obviously confound the results. (11)

There is currently an ongoing NCI-sponsored phase III clinical trial evaluating immediate and delayed adjuvant chemotherapy in patients who have undergone a radical cystectomy for stage III or stage IV transitional cell carcinoma of the bladder urothelium (23). Within 3 months after surgery, patients are randomized to receive one of three different combination chemotherapy regimens vs. no treatment until the cancer returns. The results of this trial may help better define the role of adjuvant therapy in the treatment of bladder carcinoma.

3. Neoadjuvant vs. Adjuvant Therapy

In other solid tumors such as breast cancer, neoadjuvant and adjuvant chemotherapy can be given interchangeably with relatively equivalent benefit in disease-free and overall survival. The theoretical advantages of adjuvant therapy include better patient selection for those who can tolerate therapy and the opportunity for more accurate pathological staging via surgical specimens. However, as noted above, the results of adjuvant trials in bladder cancer are inconclusive. Many of these clinical trials have shown either the lack of statistical power due to the size of the trials and early termination, used ineffective chemotherapy regimens, or had protocol deviations which have made generalizable interpretations difficult.

To date, there is ample evidence supporting the use of neoadjuvant therapy. The potential benefit of adding adjuvant chemotherapy to patients who received prior chemotherapy and definitive local therapy has not been satisfactorily answered. To address this issue, Millikan and colleagues performed a perioperative trial incorporating MVAC in patients with locally advanced bladder cancer (24). The trial was designed to compare an adjuvant treatment arm to a neoadjuvant arm. Patients were randomized to receive either cystectomy followed by MVAC for five cycles vs. MVAC for two cycles followed by cystectomy and another with three cycles of MVAC. This trial, closed early due to dwindling accrual, reported no difference in the overall 5-year survival between the two arms. The authors concluded that there was no preferred sequence to therapy. Interestingly, the complete pathological response rate in the neoadjuvant arm approached 40%, consistent with the findings of the US Intergroup MVAC study. Patients achieving a complete pathological response, documented in the resected specimen, had an encouraging survival of 88% at a median follow-up of 6.8 years.

The actual role and benefit of adjuvant chemotherapy therefore remains unknown. Given the inadequate supportive data for adjuvant treatment, neoadjuvant chemotherapy should still be considered the standard of care while adjuvant therapy still remains investigational.

4. Recent Trials and Developments

While there has been general consensus on the benefits attained with neoadjuvant chemotherapy in addition to definitive surgical or radiation therapy, there are ongoing studies evaluating novel combinations of chemotherapy that aim to increase efficacy while decreasing the toxicities associated with older regimens. MVAC has long been studied in patients with bladder cancer – principally in the metastatic and perioperative settings. When used in the neoadjuvant clinical trials, toxicities associated with this particular regimen included 57% grade III-IV granulocytopenia, 10% grade III stomatitis, and 7% grade III-IV anemia (14). However, neoadjuvant MVAC did not result in increased death or surgical complication rates.

Newer chemotherapy regimens have been tested in the metastatic setting that suggest improved efficacy and display better toxicity profiles resulting in a shift of the treatment paradigm for patients with advanced bladder carcinoma. Von Der Masse et al. performed a trial evaluating the activity of gemcitabine and cisplatin (GC) vs. MVAC in patients with metastatic disease (25). Although survival was similar between the arms, the group of patients who received GC did show less grade III/IV toxicities. Current trials are underway evaluating the efficacy of GC in the neoadjuvant setting (26).

Cisplatin-based chemotherapy cannot easily be given in every patient with bladder carcinoma where many patients have renal dysfunction precluding cisplatin therapy.

Given the clinical activity of a platinum agent in bladder cancer lines, carboplatin has been studied as a viable alternative to cisplatin. There have been multiple phase II trials evaluating carboplatin combinations which report RR varying from 38 to 60%, CR rates from 12 to 25%, and manageable toxicities (27–28). Smith et al. recently reported the final results of a neoadjuvant paclitaxel, carboplatin, and gemcitabine (PCaG) trial in patients with locally advanced disease (29). 68 patients were enrolled in one of two arms: PCaG for three cycles followed by cystectomy or PCaG for 6 cycles with an endpoint of resectability. While this combination of agents did demonstrate activity, there were some notable toxicities including four deaths during chemotherapy (with only one death apparently clearly chemotherapy related). Currently, there is an ongoing SWOG phase II clinical trial evaluating these same three cytotoxic agents given on an alternative (i.e., better tolerated) day 1 and 8 every 21 days to patients with stage II or III bladder cancer.

The integration of taxanes in recent trials, such as those mentioned above, has been done to investigate the potential of increasing the efficacy of the known neo-adjuvant chemotherapy regimens while minimizing toxicities. Burch et al. performed a phase II study of paclitaxel and cisplatin in patients with advanced urothelial cancer and reported a response rate of 70% with 32% complete responses (CR) (30). Another phase II multi-center trial enrolled patients with advanced urothelial cancer and used docetaxel and cisplatin as the chemotherapeutic regimen (31). An overall response rate of 58% was seen among 38 patients with 2 CR at 3–4 years follow-up. Given these results, both paclitaxel and docetaxel have been assessed in neoadjuvant regimens.

A phase II trial utilizing paclitaxel and cisplatin in a neoadjuvant approach of 42 patients reported a 76% major response rate with 22% complete responses (32). Three patients with T4 disease experienced a pathological CR. While the expected hematologic toxicities occurred, no grade IV neutropenia was observed. Another neoadjuvant phase II trial using docetaxel in lieu of paclitaxel was tested with cisplatin in 50 patients (33). The reported 5-year survival rate was 52% with 37% pathological CR, equivalent to what is seen in some earlier neoadjuvant trials.

While some of these other non-cisplatin-based regimens are encouraging, they have yet not displayed results that are better than cisplatin-based regimens. Thus, cisplatin-based combination therapy is preferred in this curative setting outside of a clinical trial. However, non-cisplatin regimens are a viable alternative to patients who have contra-indications to cisplatin.

5. Neoadjuvant Therapy: Is There a Role for Bladder Conservation?

Given the sensitivity of bladder cancer to chemotherapy agents, primary tumors can regress such that no primary tumor is found at cystoscopy following administration of neoadjuvant chemotherapy (pT0). The current management of these patients is unclear.

Patients who achieve this particular response and proceed to a cystectomy are found to have durable disease free periods. Millikan et al. followed 63 patients who received neoadjuvant therapy and proceeded to a cystectomy (24). Among those patients, 40% were found to be pT0 at the time of resection. With a median follow-up of 7 years, the disease free survival was 88% among patients with pT0 disease vs. 12% among patients who had any remaining primary tumor present at cystoscopy following neoadjuvant therapy.

Similar results were reported by Grossman et al. (14) In that series of patients, 38% of the patients who received neoadjuvant chemotherapy were found to have no detectable primary tumor at the time of resection. Among those patients, 85% were still alive at 5 years.

With the morbidity and potential mortality associated a cystectomy, there are investigations underway evaluating whether a cystectomy in pT0 patients can be delayed until the tumor recurs in the bladder if the chemotherapy in combination with a trans-urethral resection of the bladder tumor (TURBT) can eradicate local disease. The 10-year outcome of a series of 151 patients was reported by Herr from Memorial Sloan Kettering (34). Patients were treated locally by standard radical cystectomy or by definitive transurethral resection (TUR). There was a subgroup of patients with <pT2 disease at resection following neo-adjuvant MVAC therapy. In this group, 55 patients proceeded to cystectomy and 99 patients were followed with cystoscopic surveillance every 3–6 months for a minimum of 10 years. The 10-year survival rate was 71% vs. 76% ($p = 0.3$) in the cystectomy vs. the cystoscopic surveillance patients, respectively. Of the 99 patients who were followed by surveillance, 34% relapsed in the bladder with a new muscle-invasive tumor. Among those patients with relapsed disease, 53% were successfully treated with salvage therapy via cystectomy. When taken as a whole, 29% of patient in the cystectomy arm and 24% of patients in the surveillance arm died of bladder cancer with 57% of patients in the surveillance arm being able to retain their bladder.

The SWOG (S0219) trial evaluating the role of neoadjuvant gemcitabine, paclitaxel, and carboplatin tests a sequential approach to the treatment of locally advanced bladder cancer. Patients with confirmed residual transitional cell carcinoma are given three cycles of neoadjuvant gemcitabine, paclitaxel, and carboplatin. The chemotherapy is then followed by a repeat TURBT. Patients achieving a complete pathological response have an option, after a balanced discussion with their urologist, of either an immediate cystectomy or cystoscopic surveillance. Patients with any disease (pT1 or greater) at the end of the neoadjuvant chemotherapy will proceed with immediate cystectomy. It may be conceivable that future patients with muscle invasive bladder cancer can delay cystectomy if the primary tumor regresses following chemotherapy.

6. Conclusion

Given the body of clinical evidence, peri-operative chemotherapy, particularly neoadjuvant therapy, should be considered the standard of care for patients with locally advanced urothelial cancer. There are, however, multiple questions that still linger in the care of these patients. The optimal chemotherapy regimen – one with maximum efficacy and minimal toxicity – is still far from reach. For patients who can tolerate it, cisplatin-based combination chemotherapy should be administered. The precise role, if any, for further post-operative chemotherapy has yet to be defined. Certainly, the management of patients who have an excellent response to neoadjuvant therapy with complete resolution of their primary disease is still under investigation. Support for ongoing and planned trials employing peri-operative chemotherapy is essential.

References

1. Jamel A, Siegel R, Ward E, et al. Cancer Statistics, 2006. CA Cancer J Clin. 2006, 56(2): 106–130.
2. SEER Cancer Statistics Review, 1975–2003. National Cancer Institute. www.cancer.gov.
3. Ghoneim, MA, El-Mekresh MM, Mokhtar AA, et al. A predictive model of survival after radical cystectomy for carcinoma of the bladder. BJU Int. 2000, 85: 811–816.
4. Stein JP, Cai J, Groshen S, et al. Radical cystectomy in the treatment of invasive bladder cancer: long-term results in 1054 patients. J Clin Oncol. 2001, 19(3): 666–675.
5. Madersbacher S, Hochreiter W, Burkhard F, et al. Radical cystectomy for bladder cancer today – a homogeneous series without neoadjuvant therapy. J Clin Oncol. 2003, 21(4): 690–696.
6. Scholten AN, Leer JW, Collins CD, et al. Hypofractionated radiotherapy for invasive bladder cancer. Radiother Oncol. 1997, 43(2): 163–169.
7. Coppin CM, Gospodarowicz MK, James K, et al. Improved local control of invasive bladder cancer by concurrent cisplatin and preoperative or definitive radiation. The National Cancer Institute of Canada Clinical Trials Group. J Clin Oncol. 1996, 14(11): 2901–2907.
8. Hussain MH, Glass TR, Forman J, et al. Combination cisplatin, 5-fluorouracil and radiation therapy for locally advan-ced unresectable or medically unfit bladder cancer cases:

A Southwest Oncology Group Study. J Urol. 2001, 165(1): 56–60.
9. Wallace DM, Raghavan D, Kelly KA, et al. Neo-adjuvant (pre-emptive) cisplatin therapy in invasive transitional cell carcinoma of the bladder. Br J Urol. 1991, 67(6): 608–615.
10. Martinez-Pineiro JA, Gonzalez-Martin M, Arocena F, et al. Neoadjuvant cisplatin chemotherapy before radical cystectomy in invasive transitional cell carcinoma of the bladder: a prospective randomized phase III study. J Urol. 1995, 153(3 Pt 2): 964–973.
11. Advanced Bladder Cancer (ABC) Meta-analysis Collaboration. Neoadjuvant chemotherapy in invasive bladder cancer: update of a systematic review and meta-analysis of individual patient data advanced bladder cancer (ABC) meta-analysis collaboration. Eur Urol. 2005, 48(2): 202–205.
12. Brinkley WM, Torti FM. Systemic chemotherapy of transitional cell carcinoma of the urothelium. Semin Surg Oncol. 1997, 13(5): 365–375.
13. Hall RR. Updated results of a randomized controlled trial of neoadjuvant cisplain (C), methotrexate (M) and vinblastine (V) chemotherapy for muscle-invasive bladder cancer. Proc Am Soc Clin Oncol. 2002, 21: 178A: abstr 710.
14. Grossman HB, Natale, RB, Tangen CM, et al. Neoadjuvant chemotherapy plus cystectomy compared with cystectomy along for locally advanced bladder cancer. N Engl J Med. 2003, 349(9): 859–866.
15. Bassi P, Pappagallo GL, Sperandio P, et al. Neoadjuvant M-VAC chemotherapy for invasive bladder cancer: results of a multicenter phase III trial. J Urol. 1996; 155(suppl): 264: abstr 1021.
16. Cortesi E. Neoadjuvant treatment for locally advanced bladder cancer: a randomized prospective clinical trial (meeting abstract). Proc Am Soc Clin Oncol. 1995, Abstr 623.
17. Malmstrom PU, Rintala E, Wahlqvist R, et al. Five year follow-up of a prospective trial of radical cystectomy and neoadjuvant chemotherapy: Nordic Cystectomy Trial I. The Nordic Cooperative Bladder Cancer Study Group. J Urol. 1996, 155: 1903–1906.
18. Sherif A, Rintala E, Mestad O, et al. Neoadjuvant cisplatin-methotrexate chemotherapy for invasive bladder cancer – Nordic cystectomy trial 2. Scand J Urol Nephol. 2002, 36: 419–425.
19. Sherif A, Holmberg L, Rintala E, et al. Neoadjuvant cisplatinum based combination chemotherapy in patients with invasive bladder cancer: a combined analysis of two Nordic Studies. Eur Urol. 2004, 45: 297–303.
20. Skinner DG, Daniels JR, Russell CA, et al. The role of adjuvant chemotherapy following cystectomy for invasive bladder cancer: a prospective comparative trial. J Urol. 1991, 145(3): 459–464.
21. Stockle M, Meyenburg W, Wellek S, et al. Adjuvant polychemotherapy of nonorgan-confined bladder cancer after radical cystectomy revisited: long-term results of a controlled prospective study and further clinical experience. J Urol. 1995, 153(1): 47–52.
22. Freiha F, Reese J, Torti FM. A randomized trial of radical cystectomy versus radical cystectomy plus cisplatin, vinblatine, and methotrexate chemotherapy for muscle invasive bladder cancer. U Urol. 1996, 155(2): 495–499.
23. Phase III Randomized Study of Immediate versus Deferred Adjuvant chemotherapy after Radical Cystectomy in Patients with Stage III or IV Transitional Cell Carcinoma of the Bladder Urothelium. www.cancer.gov
24. Millikan R, Dinney C, Swanson D, et al. Integraded therapy for locally advanced bladder cancer: final report of a randomized trial of cystectomy plus adjuvant M-VAC versus cystectomy with both preoperative and postoperative M-VAC. J Clin Oncol. 2001, 19(20): 4005–4013.
25. Von der Maase H, Sengelov L, Roberts JT, et al. Long-term survival results of a randomized trial comparing gemcitabine plus cisplatin, with methotrexate, vinblastine, doxorubicin, plus cisplatin in patients with bladder cancer. J Clin Oncol. 2005, 23(21): 4602–4608.
26. Cohen SM, Goel A, Phillips J, et al. The role of perioperative chmeotherapy in the treatment of urothelial cancer. Oncologist. 2006, 11: 630–640.
27. Tsavaris N, Kosmas C, Skopelitis H, et al. Methotrexate-paclitaxel-epirubicin-carboplatin (M-TEC) combination chemotherapy in patients with advanced bladder cancer: an open label phase II study. J Chemother. 2005, 17(4): 441–448.
28. Bamias A, Moulopoulos LA, Koutras A, et al. The combination of gemcitabine and carboplatin as first-line treatment in patients with advanced urothelial carcinoma. A Phase II study of the Hellenic Cooperative Oncology Group. Cancer. 2006, 106(2): 297–303.
29. Smith DC, Mackler NJ, Hussain MH, et al. Neoadjuvant paclitaxel (P), carboplatin (Ca), and gemcitabine (G) in patients with locally advanced transitional cell carcinoma (TCC) of the bladder: A final report. Proc Am Soc Oncol. 2006, 24(18s): 226s: Abstr 4541.
30. Burch PA, Richardson RL, Cha SS, et al. Phase II study of paclitaxel and cisplatin for advanced urothelial cancer. J Urol. 2000, 164(5): 1538–1542.
31. Garcia del Muro X, Marcuello E, Guma J, et al. Phase II multicentre study of docetaxel plus cisplatin in patients with advanced urothelial cancer. Br J Cancer. 2002, 86(3): 326–330.
32. Sousa-Escandon A, Vazquez S, Quintero-Aldana G, et al. Neo-adjuvant treatment of infiltrating transitional-cell carcinoma of the bladder with paclitaxel and cisplatin: a phase II trial. Int J Urol. 2002, 9(3): 162–166.
33. Barmias A, Delveliotis C, Karayiannis A, et al. Neoadjuvant chemotherapy with docetaxel and cisplatin in patients with high-risk resectable bladder carcinoma: long term results. Eur Urol. 2004, 46: 344–350.
34. Herr HW. Transurethral resection of muscle-invasive bladder cancer: 10-year outcome. J Clin Oncol. 2001, 19(1): 89–93.

23
Adjuvant Chemotherapy in Bladder Cancer: A Good Concept But Where's the Proof?

Stephen Smith and Timothy Gilligan

Contents

Abstract Cystectomy and pelvic lymphadenectomy for locally advanced (T3/T4, N+) bladder cancer is associated with high rates of disease recurrence and death. In an effort to improve the outlook for patients with this disease, postoperative chemotherapy has been investigated. Using cisplatin-based combinations which are shown to be safe and effective in the metastatic setting, this strategy permits selection and treatment of patients at highest risk for disease recurrence and death, based on findings at the time of surgery. But despite the high prevalence of bladder cancer, studies of adjuvant chemotherapy to date incorporate fewer than 500 patients altogether, and provide insufficient statistical power to show a survival benefit. Furthermore, the clinical significance of a demonstrated improvement in disease-free survival is uncertain given the ability of chemotherapy to salvage some patients at relapse. Although adjuvant chemotherapy is conceptually attractive, enrollment in ongoing clinical trials is needed to identify whether adjuvant chemotherapy cures more patients than surgery alone for locally advanced bladder cancer.

Keywords Bladder cancer, Chemotherapy, Adjuvant, Urothelial carcinoma, Postoperative

1. Eationale for Perioperative Chemotherapy

Survival following radical cystectomy for bladder cancer is unsatisfactory. Five-year survival by pathologic stage is 63–72% for T2, 30–58% for T3, 19–33% for T4 and 4–31% for those with pelvic lymph node metastases (1–5). Systemic chemotherapy increases survival and even results in some long-term complete remissions in the setting of metastatic urothelial carcinoma but the vast majority of patients with metastatic disease die from their cancer. Postoperative chemotherapy has led to increased survival for other apparently less chemosensitive tumors such as breast, lung, and colon cancer patients. It is thus a reasonable hypothesis that administering chemotherapy following radical cystectomy for bladder cancer would decrease the relapse rate and increase survival. Post-operative chemotherapy targets micrometastases that have spread from the cancer prior to resection. Chemotherapy represents a more logical adjuvant treatment than radiation because three quarters of postoperative relapses manifest with distant metastases; local control does not appear to be the main problem with transitional cell carcinoma (TCC).

From: *Current Clinical Urology: Bladder Cancer*, Edited by: C.T. Lee and D.P. Wood,
DOI: 10.1007/978-1-59745-417-9_23,

The demonstration that chemotherapy in metastatic TCC is reasonably safe and effective provided the basis for testing similar agents in the perioperative setting. Historically, single agent chemotherapy in metastatic TCC has produced response rates ranging from 12 to 30% (reviewed in Bamias (6) and Yagoda (7); see also Loehrer (8)), a finding which led to trials of combination chemotherapy to further improve upon these results. Sternberg et al. treated patients with metastatic or unresectable urothelial cancer with MVAC (methotrexate, vinblastine, doxorubicin, and cisplatin), and found a 71% overall response rate (9). More modest but still impressive response rates were seen in later trials, ranging from 39 to 65% (8, 10). Subsequently, randomized, prospective trials showed superiority of MVAC compared to single-agent cisplatin (8) and to the CISCA regimen (cisplatin, cyclophosphamide, and doxorubicin) (10). Other randomized trials showed that MVAC produced longer survival than either docetaxel plus cisplatin[or methotrexate, vinblastine, and carboplatin (11). Similarly, CMV (cisplatin, methotrexate, vinblastine) was shown to result in longer survival than methotrexate plus vinblastine (12). These findings led to the use of MVAC or similar cisplatin-based combinations in all major completed adjuvant trials to date. More recent data has shown similar efficacy and less toxicity with gemcitabine and cisplatin when compared to MVAC (13) in the metastatic setting, leading to the ongoing adjuvant trials using this two-drug combination.

Given poor surgical cure rates and the availability of safe and effective chemotherapies in TCC, the basis for perioperative chemotherapy is clear—although the optimal timing of such therapy is not. Giving chemotherapy after surgery allows the oncologist to risk-stratify patients based on pathological staging and ensures that resection is not delayed by chemotherapy. The major advantage of postoperative chemotherapy is that patients with a low risk of tumor recurrence may thus be spared chemotherapy, with its attendant immediate and long-term morbidities, unless they subsequently relapse. Furthermore, given that a proportion of patients will not respond to chemotherapy, postoperative chemotherapy avoids the risk that outcomes will be compromised by delaying potentially curative resection in patients with chemoresistant tumors. On the other hand, preoperative chemotherapy delivers systemic treatment to any micrometastases sooner without the delay of waiting for cystectomy and recovery therefrom. While some have cited as an advantage the ability of preoperative chemotherapy to identify which patients have chemosensitive tumors, it is unclear how such identification aids the patient. In the end, the question of when and whether to administer perioperative chemotherapy can only be resolved through randomized controlled trials.

2. Evidence Supporting Adjuvant Chemotherapy

After early retrospective data suggested a disease-free survival benefit to adjuvant chemotherapy in high-risk disease (14), several prospective randomized trials were completed. Unfortunately, they accrued insufficient patient umbers and have suffered from flaws in design, execution, and analysis. Four major trials using cisplatin-based combination chemotherapy, along with one meta-analysis, have shown convincing evidence of improved relapse-free but not overall survival with adjuvant treatment of locally advanced bladder cancer (see Table 23.1). Of modest use in clinical decision-making, the available prospective trials have not yet proved that adjuvant chemotherapy leads to longer survival or improved quality of life compared to chemotherapy at time of relapse.

In the largest trial of adjuvant multiagent chemotherapy, Skinner et al. performed radical cystectomy and lymph node dissection on 498 patients with invasive bladder cancer, then randomized those with deeply invasive (pT3/4) or node-positive transitional cell carcinoma to undergo chemotherapy or observation (15). The treatment group of 44 patients was to receive four cycles of post-cystectomy CISCA and their relapse and survival was compared to 47 patients randomized to cystectomy alone. Overall, 36% of the 91 patients in this study had pathological involvement of lymph nodes. Follow-up consisted of routine physical examination, laboratory studies, intravenous pyelogram, and chest radiograph carried out every four months for the first year, then biannually for 3years, and thereafter on a yearly basis.

On the basis of an intent-to-treat analysis, the group receiving chemotherapy had a significantly delayed time to progression at three years (70% were free of disease compared to 46% in the observation group, $p=0.01$, unstratified Wilcoxon test), and their median survival was prolonged at 4.3 years compared to 2.4 years in the observation arm. Although the benefit in median survival was found to be significant ($p=0.0062$, stratified Wilcoxon test), overall survival

TABLE 23.1. Summary of randomized trials of multi-agent adjuvant chemotherapy in transitional cell cancer of the bladder.

				Relapse-free survival	Overall survival	Comment		
References	*N*	*LN*+	Chemotherapy	Chemotherapy	Observation	Chemotherapy	Observation	
Skinner (15)	91	36%	CISCA, CISCA-like regimen for 4 cycles	70% at 3years	46% at 3years (p=0.01, Wilcoxon)	39% at 5years	44% at 5years (p=0.1, Wilcoxon)	Heterogenous chemotherapy Early benefits did not persist Stopped early
Stockle (16, 17); Lehmann (18)	49	60%	MVAC/MVEC for 3 cycles	63% at 3years	13% at 3years (p=0.0005)	39% at 5years, 27% at 10years	17% at 5years, same at 10years (p=0.069)	Borderline survival benefit at 10-years follow-up Stopped early
Freiha (20)	50	70%	CMV for 3 cycles	48% at 5years	20% at 5years (p=0.01)	52% at 5years	36% at 5years (p=0.32)	Salvage therapy given to relapsed controls stopped early
Bono (22)	83	0	Cis+MTX for 3 cycles	49% at nearly 6years (69months)	44% at nearly 6years (p value not given)	49% at nearly 6years	37% at nearly 6years (no p value given)	No benefit to this two-drug combination

p values based on intent-to-treat analysis and log-rank analysis of Kaplan-Meier data, unless otherwise indicated

at 3years was not significantly different between the two arms. (Overall survival at three years was 66% in the group receiving chemotherapy and 50% for those observed ($p=0.1$, stratified Wilcoxon test). Finally, relapse-free and overall survival curves by the Kaplan-Meier method eventually intersect, casting doubt on the durability of the improvements seen in early follow up. It is thus relevant that this study used a statistical test that emphasizes early rather than later events and it has been criticized for this analytic methodology.

In addition, this study was limited by low patient numbers, potential sources of bias, and methodological problems. The small group sizes limited the power of the trial to detect differences, especially in survival. Of 160 patients considered eligible, only 91 were eventually randomized to one of the two groups, raising the possibility of selection bias. Further attrition in patient numbers occurred as the trial progressed, with 11 of 44 patients assigned to receive chemotherapy refusing it (although the results were analyzed on an intent-to-treat basis). Finally, the type and duration of chemotherapy given bore little resemblance to that which was originally intended. Only 21 of 44 patients completed a 4-month course of chemotherapy, and only 48% received the CISCA regimen specified in the protocol; others received combinations of cisplatin with a variety of other agents such as bleomycin, 5-fluorouracil, and vinblastine. The Skinner trial was thus severely underpowered, suffered from numerous protocol violations, and failed to demonstrate a survival advantage with adjuvant chemotherapy but it did generate provocative evidence that adjuvant chemotherapy might be beneficial.

A subsequent prospective trial of postcystectomy chemotherapy was conducted at two German centers by Stockle et al. and began enrollment in 1987 (17). Patients with extravesical (pT3/4) and/or node-positive transitional cell carcinoma were randomized to either three cycles of MVAC (methotrexate, vinblastine, doxorubicin, and cisplatin) or observation. (In one center, epirubicin was substituted for doxorubicin.) Initially designed to detect a 35% benefit in disease-free survival among 100 patients, only 49 were ultimately included in the trial. Twenty-six patients were assigned to receive chemotherapy, of whom seven refused treatment, and 23 were assigned to observation. Follow up consisted of biochemical evaluation, chest radiography, computerized tomography of the abdomen, and sonographic studies of the upper urinary tract. Overall, 60% of the participants had regional lymph node metastases, with a similar proportion in each arm. The primary endpoint was disease relapse, analyzed on an intent-to-treat basis. Patients on the observation arm were not routinely treated with chemotherapy in the event of relapse.

In January 1991, patient recruitment was stopped prematurely due to the interim finding of significantly improved relapse-free survival in the group receiving chemotherapy. This benefit, derived from a higher-than-expected relapse rate in the observation group, persisted at analysis in August 1991: 19/26 (73%) patients in the chemotherapy group were without relapse compared with only 5/23 (22%) in the observation group ($p=0.0012$, log-rank test). As recently published, the benefit in progression-free survival was durable: 44% of patients in the initial chemotherapy arm vs. 13% of controls were alive and without relapse at 10years ($p=0.002$) (18).

At the time of the initial trial, the early benefit in progression-free survival for those in the chemotherapy group prompted the authors to conclude that chemotherapy was beneficial, cease enrollment in the trial, and begin to routinely treat patients with pT3/4 or node-positive TCC with adjuvant chemotherapy. A report of their experience in treating patients with adjuvant chemotherapy was published in 1995 (17). Combining data from the initial randomized trial with that culled from their later off-protocol treatment experience, the updated report confirmed the improvement in relapse-free survival found in the initial group. However, pooling data from a randomized trial and a subsequent nonrandomized case series is not generally considered valid because a case series cannot adequately control for selection bias.

Despite the gain in relapse-free survival seen in the original Stockle trial, data on overall survival was only presented in 2006 (18). Overall survival at 10years for the 26 patients in the chemotherapy group was 27% compared to 17% for controls with a hazard ratio of 1.75 ($p=0.07$). Survival curves diverge early but the extremely small number of subjects left the study massively underpowered and we are left with a provocative but statistically non-significant trend toward a survival benefit. Moreover, the failure to administer chemotherapy to many of the relapsing patients on the observation arm means that any survival benefit is a benefit of postoperative chemotherapy compared to no chemotherapy ever. A more meaningful study would compare postoperative chemotherapy to that at the time of relapse.

Freiha et al. published a third trial of combination adjuvant chemotherapy in 1996 (19). The study began enrollment in April 1986, randomizing postcystectomy patients with extravesical (pT3b/pT4) TCC with or without lymph node involvement to one of two arms. The authors intended to enroll 40 patients per arm, but only 55 patients were enrolled, of whom 50 were available for analysis with a full two years of followup. In this trial, patients undergoing observation were treated with chemotherapy at the time of relapse. The chemotherapy group of 25 patients was to be treated with four cycles of CMV (cisplatin, methotrexate, and vinblastine) starting 6weeks after surgery. Physical examination, laboratory studies, computerized tomography of the abdomen, and chest radiography were carried out every 3 months for the first year, every 4months for the next year, and biannually thereafter. The two groups were similar at baseline, and 70% had lymph node involvement.

At an overall median follow up of 62 months, 12/25 patients (48%) receiving chemotherapy were alive without relapse compared with only 5/25 (20%) of patients in the cystectomy only group. Median time to relapse was 37 months for the chemotherapy group as a whole compared with 12months for the observation group, and a significant benefit in relapse-free survival was found favoring chemotherapy ($p=0.01$, log-rank test with Kaplan-Meier analysis). Like the other two, this trial was closed early because a benefit in freedom from progression was achieved with fewer patients than anticipated. However, the trial was not able to document an overall survival benefit even though median survival was 75% longer in the chemotherapy arm (63 vs. 36 months, $p=0.32$). As noted, patients in the observation arm who relapsed ($n=19$) were offered chemotherapy. Four refused and 15 underwent salvage chemotherapy, resulting in complete remission in three patients. Of 12 patients in the chemotherapy group who relapsed, 11 received additional treatment but died; one underwent chemotherapy followed by surgery and was still alive at the time of analysis. The end result was that 13 of 25 (52%) patients on the adjuvant chemotherapy arm were alive without evidence of disease compared to 8 of 25 (32%) on the observation arm. Although the authors of the study concluded that the failure to demonstrate a survival benefit resulted from the unexpected ability to salvage a few observation patients with chemotherapy at the time of relapse, a more logical conclusion is that the trial was severely underpowered. In this study, the chemotherapy arm lived longer and the absolute difference in survival was 20% while the relative difference in survival was 62%. If a survival benefit of that magnitude were to be confirmed in an adequately powered study, then adjuvant chemotherapy would become the standard of care. The problem with the Freiha study was not that the difference between the two arms was not great enough to be clinically meaningful but rather that there weren't enough patients to conclude that the difference was due to chemotherapy rather than to chance.

The final major trial of combination chemotherapy, an Italian multicenter trial by Bono et al. began accruing in December 1984. Results were published in 1989 (20) and in a follow-up report in 1997 (21). In this trial, postcystectomy patients with muscle-invasive (T2) or extravesical (T3/T4) transitional cell carcinoma without lymph node involvement were randomized to one of two arms. The chemotherapy arm was treated with cisplatin and methotrexate for four cycles, and compared with an observation group in terms of relapse and overall survival. (Patients with lymph node involvement after cystectomy were all treated with chemotherapy as above, and formed an additional, nonrandomized group.) Surveillance with blood chemistries, chest radiography, abdominal ultrasound, physical examination, computerized tomography of the abdomen, and bone scan every 6 months for 2 years then yearly for 5 years is carried out.

In total, 83 patients were randomized into one of two groups: 35 received chemotherapy and 48 were observed. Thirty-one nonrandomized lymph node positive patients were also treated with chemotherapy. Mean follow up for all patients, as published in 1997, was 69 months. Survival and relapse rates were equivalent for the two groups, although the authors do not include p values or basic analysis of differences between the groups. Eighteen out of 35 patients (51%) randomized to chemotherapy progressed during the follow-up period, and the same number of patients died, whereas 27/48 (56%) of observed patients progressed and 30/48 (63%) died. The authors confirmed the ineffectiveness of this two-drug combination in the adjuvant setting and recommended that different combinations (such as MVAC) be used in future adjuvant trials.

3. Meta-Analysis: Is There Consensus?

In an attempt to draw firmer conclusions from the various underpowered studies of adjuvant chemotherapy, a pooled analysis and a meta-analysis were performed. The pooled analysis of five published trials (including the four discussed above, and one trial of single-agent cisplatin (22)) found a significant reduction in risk of death with adjuvant chemotherapy (RR 0.74, CI 0.62–0.88), but did not use individual patient data or data from unpublished sources, and included only 350 patients (23). On the other hand, a meta-analysis conducted by the Advanced Bladder Cancer (ABC) Meta-analysis Collaboration included data on 108 patients from one unpublished trial and reinstated a number of patients from five published randomized trials, so that relapse and survival data were available for 491 patients (24). Four hundred of these were randomized to receive adjuvant multiagent chemotherapy (200 patients) or were observed (200 patients) after cystectomy for TCC; the other 91 patients were randomized between observation ($n = 45$) and adjuvant single-agent cisplatin ($n = 46$). Overall survival data, available for all 400 patients from the multiagent chemotherapy trials, showed that chemotherapy was associated with a 29% relative decrease in the risk of death (HR 0.71; $p = 0.01$). This would translate into an 11% improvement in absolute survival at 3 years, though more patients would be required to show that difference to be statistically significant. In addition, progression-free survival data on 292 evaluable patients showed a 38% relative decrease in the risk of recurrence or death for those on chemotherapy compared to controls (HR 0.62; $p = 0.001$). Subgroup analysis found no difference in outcomes related to patient factors such as age, sex, tumor stage, or nodal status. Adjuvant chemotherapy using single-agent cisplatin was not associated with any survival benefit (HR = 1.01, $p = 0.95$).

As the authors of this meta-analysis point out, the quality of a meta-analysis is ultimately limited by the quality of the included studies. Selection bias, the impact of small group sizes, the irregular delivery of salvage chemotherapy, and the effects of early trial termination are limitations of included studies that impact the meta-analysis as well. Due to these considerations and the low statistical power of the meta-analysis, the authors of the ABC collaboration conclude that there is insufficient evidence upon which to base treatment decisions in patients with invasive bladder cancer after cystectomy. The findings of this meta-analysis serve primarily to confirm findings of improved freedom of recurrence with adjuvant chemotherapy, and to add urgency to efforts to include patients on randomized controlled clinical trials.

4. Conclusion: Evolving Validation of the Adjuvant Concept

The utility of adjuvant chemotherapy for locally advanced TCC remains unproven. Although improved relapse-free survival has been demonstrated by several trials and confirmed in a meta-analysis, it remains unclear whether adjuvant chemotherapy increases overall survival. If postoperative observation, with chemotherapy administered in the event of relapse, leads to the same long-term survival as postoperative chemotherapy, then it may be preferable to observe patients and spare the nonrelapsing patients from the side effects of chemotherapy. The main reason adjuvant chemotherapy remains a contentious issue decades after the first trials began accruing patients is that the published trials suffered from extremely small patient numbers, limitations in methodology and protocol design, and premature trial termination. The history of adjuvant chemotherapy trials is a lesson in the importance of good trial design and careful adherence to research protocols. It is hoped that further studies in adjuvant chemotherapy, including the ongoing randomized controlled trial by the European Organization for the Research and Treatment of Cancer (EORTC), will succeed in these respects. This multicenter study (EORTC 30994, www.cancer.gov/clinicaltrials) will randomize high-risk patients (pathological stage T3–T4 and/or N+ disease) to either adjuvant chemotherapy or observation (and treatment upon relapse) and aims to accrue 660 patients. Cisplatin-based combination chemotherapy consisting of either MVAC, a high-dose version of MVAC, or gemcitabine with cisplatin is to be used with each participating center free to choose which of these three regimens it uses. A second current trial (ITNRC-CU02.00447ST/97, www.cancer.gov/clinicaltrials) will randomize postcystectomy patients to receive gemcitabine and cisplatin or undergo observation after surgery. Both trials are currently enrolling patients. A US trial (CALGB 90104) has closed due to lack of accrual, which had intended to compare sequential doxorubicin and gemcitabine followed by paclitaxel and cisplatin with gemcitabine/cisplatin alone in the adjuvant setting. Given the shortcomings of available data, increased participation in ongoing trials is required to prove whether adjuvant chemotherapy can cure more patients with locally advanced bladder cancer than surgery alone. At this point in time, there is substantially more data supporting the use of preoperative chemotherapy than postoperative chemotherapy.

References

1. Bassi P, Ferrante GD, Piazza N, et al. Prognostic factors of outcome after radical cystectomy for bladder cancer: A retrospective study of a homogeneous patient cohort. J Urol. 1999; 161(5):1494–1497.
2. Ghoneim MA, el-Mekresh MM, el-Baz MA, el-Attar IA, Ashamallah A. Radical cystectomy for carcinoma of the bladder: critical evaluation of the results in 1,026 cases. J Urol. 1997; 158(2):393–399.
3. Madersbacher S, Hochreiter W, Burkhard F, et al. Radical cystectomy for bladder cancer today–a homogeneous series without neoadjuvant therapy. J Clin Oncol. 2003; 21(4):690–696.
4. Pagano F, Bassi P, Galetti TP, et al. Results of contemporary radical cystectomy for invasive bladder cancer: A clinicopathological study with an emphasis on the inadequacy of the tumor, nodes and metastases classification. J Urol. 1991; 145(1):45–50.
5. Stein JP, Lieskovsky G, Cote R, et al. Radical cystectomy in the treatment of invasive bladder cancer: Long-term results in 1,054 patients. J Clin Oncol. 2001; 19(3):666–675.
6. Bamias A, Tiliakos I, Karali MD, Dimopoulos MA. Systemic chemotherapy in inoperable or metastatic bladder cancer. Ann Oncol. 2006; 17(4):553–561.
7. Yagoda A. Chemotherapy for advanced urothelial cancer. Semin Urol. 1983; 1(1):60–74.
8. Loehrer PJ S, Einhorn LH, Elson PJ, et al. A randomized comparison of cisplatin alone or in combination with methotrexate, vinblastine, and doxorubicin in patients with metastatic urothelial carcinoma: A cooperative group study. J Clin Oncol. 1992; 10(7):1066–1073.
9. Sternberg CN, Yagoda A, Scher HI, et al. Preliminary results of M-VAC (methotrexate, vinblastine, doxorubicin and cisplatin) for transitional cell carcinoma of the urothelium. J Urol. 1985; 133(3):403–407.
10. Logothetis CJ, Dexeus FH, Finn L, et al. A prospective randomized trial comparing MVAC and CISCA chemotherapy for patients with metastatic urothelial tumors. J Clin Oncol. 1990; 8(6):1050–1055.
11. Bamias A, Aravantinos G, Deliveliotis C, et al. Docetaxel and cisplatin with granulocyte colony-stimulating factor (G-CSF) versus MVAC with G-CSF in advanced urothelial carcinoma: a multicenter, randomized, phase III study from the Hellenic Cooperative Oncology Group. J Clin Oncol. 2004; 22(2):220–228.
12. Mead GM, Russell M, Clark P, et al. A randomized trial comparing methotrexate and vinblastine (MV) with cisplatin, methotrexate and vinblastine (CMV) in advanced transitional cell carcinoma: results and a report on prognostic factors in a Medical Research Council study. MRC Advanced Bladder Cancer Working Party. British Journal of Cancer, 1998; 78(8):1067–1075.
13. von der Maase H, Hansen SW, Roberts JT, et al. Gemcitabine and cisplatin versus methotrexate, vinblastine, doxorubicin, and cisplatin in advanced or metastatic bladder cancer: Results of a large, randomized, multinational, multicenter, phase III study. J Clin Oncol. 2000; 18(17):3068–3077.
14. Logothetis CJ, Johnson DE, Chong C, et al. Adjuvant cyclophosphamide, doxorubicin, and cisplatin chemotherapy for bladder cancer: An update. J Clin Oncol. 1988; 6(10): 1590–1596.
15. Skinner DG, Daniels JR, Russell CA, et al. The role of adjuvant chemotherapy following cystectomy for invasive bladder cancer: A prospective comparative trial. J Urol. 1991; 145(3):459–64; discussion 464–467.
16. Stockle M, Meyenburg W, Wellek S, et al. Advanced bladder cancer (stages pT3b, pT4a, pN1 and pN2): Improved survival after radical cystectomy and 3 adjuvant cycles of chemotherapy. results of a controlled prospective study. J Urol. 1992; 148(2 Pt 1):302–306; discussion 306–307.
17. Stockle M, Meyenburg W, Wellek S, et al. Adjuvant polychemotherapy of nonorgan-confined bladder cancer after radical cystectomy revisited: Long-term results of a controlled prospective study and further clinical experience. J Urol. 1995; 153(1):47–52.
18. Lehmann J, Franzaring L, Thuroff J, Wellek S, Stockle M. Complete long-term survival data from a trial of adjuvant chemotherapy vs. control after radical cystectomy for locally advanced bladder cancer. BJU Int. 2006; 97(1): 42–47.
19. Freiha F, Reese J, Torti FM. A randomized trial of radical cystectomy versus radical cystectomy plus cisplatin, vinblastine and methotrexate chemotherapy for muscle invasive bladder cancer. J Urol. 1996; 155(2):495–499; discussion 499–500.
20. Bono AV, Benvenuti C, Reali L, et al. Adjuvant chemotherapy in advanced bladder cancer. italian uro-oncologic cooperative group. Prog Clin Biol Res. 1989; 303:533–540.
21. Bono AV, Benvenuti C, Guazzer S, et al. Adjuvant chemotherapy in locally advanced bladder cancer. final analysis of a controlled multicenter study. Acta Urol Ital. 1997; 11(1):5–8.
22. Studer UE, Bacchi M, Biedermann C, et al. Adjuvant cisplatin chemotherapy following cystectomy for bladder cancer: Results of a prospective randomized trial. J Urol. 1994; 152(1):81–84.
23. Ruggeri EM, Giannarelli D, Bria E, et al. Adjuvant chemotherapy in muscle-invasive bladder carcinoma: a pooled analysis from phase III studies. Cancer 2006; 106(4):783–788.
24. Advanced Bladder Cancer (ABC) Meta-analysis Collaboration. Adjuvant chemotherapy in invasive bladder cancer: A systematic review and meta-analysis of individual patient data advanced bladder cancer (ABC) meta-analysis collaboration. Eur Urol. 2005; 48(2):189–199; discussion 199–201.

24
Beyond MVAC: New and Improved Chemotherapeutics

Deborah Bradley and Maha Hussain

Contents

Abstract With the introduction of cisplatin based combination chemotherapy, survival for patients with advanced bladder cancer has doubled from approximately 3–6 months with supportive care alone to over one year. The lack of curative potential coupled with significant potential toxicity fueled the search for more efficacious and less toxic regimens. Although median survivals have marginally improved since the original reports on MVAC, this likely is a result of stage migration and better supportive care. However, several alternative regimens have shown promising activity with less toxicity and applicability to a broader population of patients. Significant steps have also been made in the last several years in understanding the pathobiology of bladder cancer. These advances have led to trials investigating a variety of cytotoxic agents and biologically targeted agents as monotherapy or in combination with chemotherapy in hopes of increasing response rate and overall survival.

Keywords: bladder cancer, urothelial cancer, transitional cell carcinoma, metastatic, cytoxic therapy, targeted agents

1 Introduction: Systemic Chemotherapy for Advanced Bladder Cancer

13,060 patients are expected to die from bladder cancer in 2006.[1] The vast majority of these patients will die from metastatic disease. Systemic chemotherapy is the primary treatment modality for these patients with an expected median survival of 14 months.[2] and a 5-year survival rate of only13%.[2]

Bladder cancer has long been recognized to be a chemo-sensitive disease. Historically, cisplatin was considered the most active single agent. Its activity led

From: *Current Clinical Urology: Bladder Cancer*, Edited by: C.T. Lee and D.P. Wood,
DOI: 10.1007/978-1-59745-417-9_24,

to trials of cisplatin based combination chemotherapy in the 1980's which for the first time in advanced bladder cancer showed an appreciable improvement in overall survival.[3] Of the cisplatin based combination therapies, MVAC (methotrexate, vinblastine, adriamycin and cisplatin) has been established as standard of care based on superior efficacy and survival in two randomized phase III trials conducted over a decade ago (Table 1.).[3–5] MVAC resulted in overall and complete response (CR) rates of 36–59% and 9–35% respectively in the early randomized trials. [3, 5–8] However, it was associated with substantial toxicities, particularly, toxic death rates of 3% to 4% [3, 6] and has doubtful curative potential as reflected by a 3.7% survival at 6 years. [4] To Improve the overall efficacy of MVAC, dose intensification (high-dose (HD-MVAC)) supported by growth factors was investigated in a randomized phase III study and compared to standard MVAC.[7, 9] HD-MVAC resulted in a higher overall response rate (62% compared to 50% (p = 0.06)), a significantly higher CR rate (21% versus 9%) and less toxicity (p = 0.009) as compared with standard dose MVAC and longer progression free survival (9.1 months versus 8.2 months, p = .037). However, the primary endpoint of increased survival was not achieved (15.5 months with HD-MVAC versus 14.1 months with standard MVAC, p =0.122).

Over the last decade, many newer chemotherapeutic agents have been introduced into clinical practice. Two agents with appreciable activity in bladder cancer, gemcitabine and paclitaxel have been of particular interest. Single agent gemcitabine is associated with overall response rates of 24–28%,[10, 11] while paclitaxel resulted in response rates of 42% in the first line setting.[12] In this multicenter trial reported by Roth et al., [12] a response rate of 42% was observed with a CR rate of 27%. Unlike the current schedule, its important to note in this trial paclitaxel was administered as a 24 hour infusion. Based on the promising single agent activity these agents became the backbone of several chemotherapy combinations. Table 2. summarizes results of gemcitabine and paclitaxel-based phase II trials. Overall the data from these trials show an overall response rate of 24–70%, CR rates of 7–32% and median survivals ranging from 7.1–16 months with doublet combinations.

The favorable results observed in phase II studies using combination gemcitabine/cisplatin (GC) led to a phase III trial comparing GC directly with MVAC. [2, 6] Although the study failed to achieve its primary endpoint of superiority, it demonstrated comparable efficacy with regard to overall survival (GC, 13.8 months; MVAC, 14.8 months), time to progressive disease (GC, 7.4 months; MVAC, 7.4 months), and response rate (GC, 49.4%; MVAC, 45.7%), with significantly less febrile neutropenia, neutropenic sepsis, and mucositis. As a result, GC has largely replaced MVAC.

Similarly, the promising activity and favorable toxicity profile of paclitaxel based combinations led to an ECOG phase III trial comparing carboplatin/paclitaxel (CP) to MVAC.[8] The trial was designed to show a 50% improvement in survival over MVAC. Secondary endpoints included comparison of response rate, duration of response, toxicity, and quality of life between the two arms. The accrual target was 330 patients. However, this trial was prematurely closed after 2.5 years due to slow accrual. Based on 80 eligible

TABLE 1. Phase III Trials of MVAC.

Trial	Regimen	Patient number	RR/CR (%)	P value Response rate	Overall survival (months)	P value Overall survival
Logothetis 1990 [5]	MVAC CISCA	110 patients**	65 / 35 46 / 25	<.05	62.6 weeks 40.4 weeks	0.000315
Loehrer 1992 [3, 4]	MVAC Cisplatin	126 120	39 / 13 12 / 3	0.0001	12.5 8.2	<0.0002
von der Maase 2000 [2, 6]	MVAC Gemcitabine/ cisplatin	202 203	46 / 11.9 49 / 12.2	NS	15.2 14	NS
Sternberg 2001 [7, 9]	MVAC HD-MVAC/ G-CSF	129 134	50 / 9 62 / 21	0.06	14.1 15.5	NS
Siefker-Radtke 2002 [64]	MVAC FAP	83 86	59 / 24 42 / 10	NS	12.5 12.5	NS
*Dreicer 2004 [8]	MVAC Carboplatin/ paclitaxel	44 41	36 / 12.8 28 / 2.6	NS	15.4 13.8	NS

MVAC: methotrexate, vinblastine, doxorubicin, cisplatin; CISCA: cisplatin, cyclophosphamide, doxorubicin; FAP: interferon alfa-2b, 5-fluorouracil, cisplatin; HD-MVAC: high-dose MVAC; * trial did not reach accrual, RR: response rate, CR: complete response rate, NS: not significant **number treated in each arm not reported.

patients, the overall survival at a mean follow-up of 32.5 months was 15.4 months for the MVAC arm and 13.8 months for the CP arm (p = 0.65). An overall response rate of 35.9% was observed in the MVAC arm and 28.2% in the CP arm (p = 0.63). Toxicities were greater in the MVAC arm (p = 0.0001) but quality of life assessment was similar in both arms (p = 0.33). Although there was not a significant difference in overall response or survival between patients treated with MVAC or CP, results of this trial must be interpreted with caution as it failed to reach target accrual thus is underpowered.

Three drug combinations mostly based on gemcitabine and paclitaxel have also been investigated in phase II trials with overall response rates of 43–77%, CR rates of 12–32% and median survivals of 11–20 months (Table 3). Overall, they appeared to have a higher response rates than cisplatin based doublets, particularly in patients with visceral disease. Based on the phase II data (response and survival) of paclitaxel + GC combination.[13] , the EORTC conducted a phase III trial, in which 627 patients with previously untreated metastatic urothelial carcinoma were randomly assigned to GC or to triplet GC plus paclitaxel (PCG)[14]. The overall response rates and complete responses were higher with PCG (57% and 15%), than with GC (46% and 10%), but the overall survival with PCG (15.7 months) was not significantly better than with GC (12.8 months).

2. Second Line Chemotherapy

The vast majority of patients treated for metastatic bladder cancer ultimately develop progression of disease. However, there is no currently accepted standard second line chemotherapy regimen. Various agents have been studied in second line phase II (with

TABLE 2. Phase II Trials of Combination Therapy in Advanced Bladder Cancer*.

Trial	Regimen	Patient number	RR / CR (%)	Median survival (months)	TTP (months)
Moore 1999 [127]	Gemcitabine/cisplatin	31	57 / 19	13.2	NR
Kaufman 2000 [128]	Gemcitabine/cisplatin	46	41 / 21.7	14.3	5.5
Hussain 2004 [129]	Gemcitabine/cisplatin	32	65 / 12.5	16.0	NR
Nogue-Aliguer 2003 [19]	Gemcitabine/carboplatin	41	56 / 14.6	10.1	7.2 (PFS)
Redman 1998 [130]	Carboplatin/paclitaxel	35	52 / 20	9.5	NR
Vaughn 2002 [131]	Carboplatin/paclitaxel	37	24 / 8.1	7.1	3 (PFS)
Johannsen 2005 [132]	Carboplatin/paclitaxel	33	57 / 18.2	12	6.5 (PFS)
Dreicer 2000 [133]	Cisplatin/paclitaxel	52	50 / 8	10.6	NR
Burch 2000 [134]	Cisplatin/paclitaxel	34	70 / 32	12.7	7.2
Dimopoulos 1999 [135]	Cisplatin/docetaxel	66	52 / 12	8	5
Garcia del Muro 2002 [136]	Cisplatin/docetaxel	38	58 / 18.4	10.4	6.9
Meluch 2001 [20]	Gemcitabine/paclitaxel	54	54 / 7	14.4	9 (PFS)
Kaufman 2004 [137]	Gemcitabine/paclitaxel	55	40 / 9	11.8	
Theodore 2006 [138]	Gemcitabine/oxaliplatin	30	47 / 10	15	7.0 (PFS)

*Only published trials including 30 or more patients are included. RR: response rate, CR: complete response rate, TTP: time to progression. PFS: progression free survival. NR: not reported.

TABLE 3. Phase II Trials of Multi-Agent Therapy in Advanced Bladder Cancer*.

Trial	Regimen	Patient number	RR / CR (%)	Median survival (months)	TTP (months)
Bajorin 2000 [139]	Paclitaxel/cisplatin/ifosfamide	44	68 / 23	20	NR
Edelman 2000 [140]	Carboplatin/paclitaxel/methotrexate	33	56 /28	15.5	NR
Bellmunt 2000 [13]	Paclitaxel/gemcitabine/cisplatin	58	77.6 / 28	16	NR
Hussain 2001 [91]	Paclitaxel/gemcitabine/carboplatin	49	68 / 32	14.7	NR
Hainsworth 2005[90]	Paclitaxel/gemctiabine/carboplatin	60	43 / 12	11	7.4 (PFS)
Ardavanis 2005 [141]	Gemcitabine/docetaxel	31	51 / 12.9	15	8
Tsavaris 2005 [142]	Methotrexate/paclitaxel/ Epirubicin/carboplatin	40	60 / 35	14	8

*Only published trials including 30 or more patients are included. RR: response rate, CR: complete response rate, TTP: time to progression. PFS: progression free survival. NR: not reported.

vinflunine also in a phase III trial; see below) trials with response rates ranging from 5 to 22%, overall survival of 5–9 months and time to progression of 2.2 to 4.9 months (Table 4).[24–31] Even some of the most active agents in the front line setting, such as paclitaxel, appear to lose activity in cisplatin treated patients.[12, 30]

With modestly active agents, combination chemotherapy has also been investigated in the second line setting. [32–35] However, results of these studies should be interpreted with caution because patients who have shown progression after neoadjuvant or adjuvant chemotherapy are also included in most of these trials. In addition, prior treatment of patients in these trials is mostly limited to older cisplatin based combination regimens that have largely fallen out of favor in the United States.

3. New Cytotoxics

3.1. Anti-Microtubule Agents

Anti-mictrotubule agents are an important class of anti-neoplastics with broad activity in both solid and hematologic neoplasms. Microtubules are critical in mitosis playing a key role in the mitotic spindle apparatus. They are also essential for maintenance of cell shape, cellular motility and attachment, and intracellular transport. Microtubules are highly dynamic structures. [36, 37] Anti-microtubule agents exert their effects by interfering with microtubule dynamics. [36, 37] Main classes of anti-microtubules include vinca alkaloids which act as microtubule depolymerizing agents and taxanes which enhance tubulin polymerization inhibiting the normal dynamic process of the microtubule network leading to inhibition of mitosis and cell division.

Antimicrotubule agents have been widely utilized in the treatment of bladder cancer. Vinblastine was among one of the earliest anti-neoplastics investigated in bladder cancer. Although single agent activity was only ~15%,[38] vinblastine has been an integral component of the original cisplatin based combination regimens (MVAC, MVEC, CMV). The taxanes have been amongst the most active single agents in utothelial cancers. In phase II studies, paclitaxel and docetaxel have resulted in overall response rates of 42%[12] and 31% [39] respectively. Therefore novel agents targeting microtubules are of significant interest.

3.1.1. Epothilones

Epothilones induce microtubule bundling, formation of mitotic spindles and subsequent mitotic arrest in a taxol-like mechanism of action.[40] Four epothilone analogues are currently in clinical trials: BMS-310705, a water soluble semi-synthetic analogue of epothilone B; BMS-247550, aza-epothilone B [Ixabepilone]; EPO906; and epothilone D, KOS-862. Preclinical studies have demonstrated that epothilones competitively bind to microtubules with paclitaxel and inhibit microtubule dynamics in a similar manner. [41] However, epothilones differ from taxanes in several important ways that may result in activity in patients who have shown taxane resistance. Although resistance to epothilones may result from β tubulin mutations, specific mutations associated with paclitaxel resistance may not confer epothilone resistance. [41, 42] In addition, epothilones may also be less susceptible to overexpression of p-glycoprotein, the multidrug efflux pump known to confer resistance to paclitaxel.[36, 43, 44]

TABLE 4. Single Agent Second Line Chemotherapy for Advanced Bladder Cancer*.

Trial	Regimen	Patient number	Response rate	Median survival (months)	TTP (months)
Lorusso[24]	Gemcitabine	31	22.5%	5	3.8
Albers[25]	Gemcitabine	28	11%	8.7	4.9
Pollera[26]	Gemcitabine	14	21%	NR	NR
Witte[27]	Ifosfamide	56	20%	22 **weeks**	9.6 **weeks**
Pronzato[28]	Ifosfamide	20	5%	NR	NR
McCaffrey[29]	Docetaxel	30	13%	9	NR
Vaughn[30]	Paclitaxel	31	10%	7.2	2.2
Culine[31]	Vinflunine	51	18%	6.6	3.0 (**PFS**)
Bellmunt[49]	Vinflunine	370	9%	6.9	3.0 (**PFS**)

*Includes only published trials of 20 or more patients. NR: not reported TTP: Time to progression PFS: Progression free survival

The first epothilone to be tested in bladder cancer is BMS-247550. ECOG reported a study of BMS-247550 in the second line setting. [45] Patients who had failed one previous platinum containing regimen were eligible. Patients were treated with 40 mg/m2 IV over 3 hours on day 1 every 21 days. Activity was only modest with a response rate of 12.2% (0% CR) and overall and progression free survival of 7.5 months and 2.8 months, respectively. Toxicity was significant. Twelve patients (28%) experienced grade 4 toxicity, including leukopenia, neutropenia, ventricular arrhythmia, hypotension, DIC, stomatitis, elevated bilirubin, dyspnea, febrile neutropenia, hypoxia, acidosis, and elevated creatinine. There was one treatment related death. While the data is disappointing, it clearly is not out of line with what is seen with paclitaxel and therefore evaluating this or other epothilones in the front line setting is a legitimate question for future clinical trials.

3.1.2. Vinflunine

Vinflunine is a novel vinca alkaloid that blocks cells at the G2/M phase and induces cell death via apoptosis. In comparison to older vinca alkaloids, vinflunine has shown superior anti-tumor activity against a variety of cell lines and tumor models. [46] Because of cytotoxic activity observed in a murine bladder cancer cell line, [47] vinflunine became attractive for further study in bladder cancer. Another property of vinflunine is that it is thought to be associated with less neurotoxcity, [48] a dose limiting side-effect seen with other vinca alkaloids.

A Phase II study of vinflunine in patients with advanced bladder cancer progressing after a first-line platinum-containing regimen has been reported in Europe.[31] The primary end point of this trial was response rate. Secondary objectives included duration of response, progression free survival, overall survival, and evaluation of treatment related toxicity. Objective responses were observed in 3 of 22 patients (14%) who had received prior vinca alkaloids as a component of MVAC or CMV regimens. The median duration of response was 9.1 months (95% CI: 42–15.0) with a progression free survival of 3.0 months (95% CI: 2.4–3.8) and a median survival of 6.6 months (95% CI: 4.8–7.6).

More recently, preliminary results of a randomized phase III trial of 370 patients with previously treated advanced urothelial carcinoma, comparing vinflunine plus best supportive care (n=253), with best supportive care alone (n=117) was reported.[49] Treatment with vinflunine was associated with an overall response rate of 9% and a statistically nonsignificant increase in survival (6.9 months versus 4.6 months; hazard ratio 0.88, 95% CI, 0.69–1.12). However, a planned multivariate analysis adjusting for prognostic factors, showed a statistically significant effect of vinflunine on overall survival (6.9 months versus 4.3 months, p=0.036).

3.1.3. Halichondrin B Analog: E7389

E7389 is synthetic analog of halichondrin which inhibits microtubule polymerization by suppressing the rate and extent of microtubule growth rather than causing microtubule shortening, a mechanism that is distinct from other anti-microtubules.[50] Preclinical data show that nanomolar levels of E7389 inhibit cancer cell proliferation via induction of dose- and time-dependent cell cycle block at G_2/M, disruption of mitotic spindle formation, and initiation of apoptosis. [51] A multi-center phase I/II trial utilizing this agent in patients with metastatic urothelial cancer with renal dysfunction is ongoing.

3.1.4. ABI-007 (Abraxane)

Although paclitaxel is the most active single agent in bladder cancer and has been used successfully in combination therapy it does have limitations. Due to its poor water solubility, paclitaxel is currently formulated with Cremophor EL (CrEL) (castor oil) and dehydrated ethanol (1:1, vol/vol). [37] The solvent is thought to alter the pharmacokinetics of paclitaxel.[52,53] CrEL micelles can entrap paclitaxel in the plasma compartment limiting tumor uptake. [52,53] Additionally, the solvent is responsible for causing rare hypersensitivity reactions necessitating steroid premedication and long infusion times.

ABI-007 is a nanoparticle albumin bound paclitaxel that exploits a receptor-mediated (gp60) albumin transcytosis pathway to achieve high intracellular tumor concentrations of the active ingredient, paclitaxel. [37,54] SPARC and Caveolin-1 are two albumin binding proteins overexpressed in many cancers thought to aid in preferential drug delivery to tumors. [55–57] In tumor xenografts, at equitoxic dose, treatment with ABI-007 compared to cremophor-based paclitaxel resulted in more complete regressions, longer time to recurrence, longer doubling time, and prolonged survival. [58] In addition, a higher intratumoral accumulation of ABI-007 was seen.

The clinical efficacy of this agent was established by a phase III study of ABI-007 versus standard paclitaxel in patients with metastatic breast cancer. [59] In this trial, ABI-007 demonstrated significantly higher response rates compared with standard paclitaxel (33% v 19%, respectively; P = .001) and significantly longer time to tumor progression (23.0 v 16.9 weeks, respectively; hazard ratio = 0.75; P = .006). The incidence of grade 4 neutropenia was significantly lower for ABI-007 compared with standard paclitaxel (9% v 22%, respectively; P < .001) but grade 3 sensory neuropathy was more common in the ABI-007 arm than in the standard paclitaxel arm (10% vs. 2%, respectively; P < .001) but improved rapidly (median, 22 days). Given the efficacy of paclitaxel in bladder cancer, ABI-007 is being evaluated in the neoadjuvant and metastatic settings. .

3.2. Antimetabolites

Methotrexate and 5-fluorouracil are two of the original cytoxics used to treat bladder cancer. Before the introduction of gemcitabine and taxanes, methotrexate was integral in the treatment of advanced bladder cancer. As a single agent, response rates of 26–44% have been reported. [60–62] Methotrexate is better known as part of earlier cisplatin based combination regimens (MVAC, MVEC, CMV). Historically, activity of 5-fluorouracil was less impressive with response rates of only 15%. [63] Combination regimens including 5-fluorouracil have been investigated but have fallen out of favor based on inferiority when compared to MVAC. [64]

3.2.2. Pemetrexed

Pemetrexed is a novel antimetabolite with multiple enzyme targets involved in both purine and pyrimidine synthesis. Preclinical studies demonstrated appreciable activity in multiple cell lines and xenografts including those resistant to methotrexate and 5-fluorouracil.[65] Its single agent activity was confirmed in multiple solid tumors in early phase II studies.[65] However, a pooled toxicity analysis of 872 patients entered on phase II trials demonstrated a high level of myelosuppression (grade 3–4 neutropenia was observed in 50% of patients).[65] A correlation between folic acid status and incidence of toxicity was shown by several investigators leading to the recommendation that patients undergoing therapy with pemetrexed also be supplemented with folic acid and vitamin B12. [65, 66] A comparative toxicity analysis of patients treated in several trials with (78 patients) or without (246 patients) vitamin supplementation showed that the addition of folic acid and vitamin B12 substantially reduced the incidence of adverse events (grade 4 neutropenia 2.6% vs. 32%, grade 4 thrombocytopenia 0% vs. 8%, grade 3–4 mucositis 1.3% vs. 5%, grade 3–4 diarrhea 2.6% vs. 6%, and toxic death 0% vs. 5%). [65]

Activity in transitional cell carncinoma was demonstrated in a phase II trial. [65] In 31 chemotherapy-naïve patients with advanced bladder cancer a response rate of 32% was observed with a medial survival of 9.4 months. This trial was done before the addition of vitamin supplementation so hematologic toxicity was significant (grade 3–4 neutropenia 71%, febrile neutropenia 26%).

A phase II trial of pemetrexed in combination with gemcitabine as front line therapy for patients with advanced transitional cell carcinoma has also been reported. [67] The overall response rate for the intention-to-treat population was 20% (95% CI 11% to 32%). Median progression free survival in protocol-qualified patients was 3.1 months (95% CI 2.8–4.3 months, 19% censoring). The estimated median overall survival time was 8.1 months (95% CI 4.7–10.3 months, 25% censoring) Based on historic single agent activity with gemcitabine in bladder cancer of 23% and 29% [10, 11, 24, 68] it was felt that the addition of pemetrexed did not provide increased efficacy but did add significant toxicity. A second phase II trial of combination pemetrexed / gemcitabine with vitamin supplementation was conducted by the ECOG. Results showed modest activity but at the cost of significant toxicity.[69]

Pemetrexed has also been evaluated in the second line setting. Sweeney et al [70] reported a phase II trial of pemetrexed as second line therapy in patients with metastatic disease or for first line treatment in patients with disease recurrence within 12 months of completing neoadjuvant or adjuvant therapy. The primary end point of this trial was response rate. 47 patients were analyzed based on intention-to-treat analysis. The overall response rate was 27.7% (95% CI, 15.6% to 42.6%) (6.4% CR, 21.3% PR, and 21.3% had stable disease. The median time to progression was 2.9 months (95% CI, 1.7 months to 4.6 months,) median survival was 9.6 months (95% CI, 5.1 months to 14.6 months) and the 1-year survival was 41.8% (95% CI, 27.5% to 56.0%).

4. Targeted Therapy

4.1. Molecular Changes in Bladder Cancer

Molecularly, bladder cancer can be divided into two distinct groups of disease with different clinical behaviors and prognosis; low grade superficial disease and high grade disease. Low-grade non-invasive papillary tumors are characterized by activating mutations in the *HRAS* gene and fibroblast growth factor receptor 3 gene leading to activation of the mitogen activated protein kinase pathway.[71–73] High-grade tumors are characterized by structural and functional defects in the p53 and retinoblastoma protein (RB) tumor-suppressor pathways leading to genetic instability and development of many other molecular changes.[71–73] The order of these molecular events and signaling pathways involved have not been well defined. However, like in many other tumor types, advanced bladder cancer has been associated with multiple disturbances including mutations and upregulation of oncogenes, tumor suppressor genes, and gene products, disturbances in regulation of the cell cycle, and alterations in DNA methylation (table 5.). [71, 72] Examining the role of specific molecular changes individually and as part of molecular pathways of tumorigenesis provides a framework for devising rational, targeted therapies.

4.2. Targeting molecular changes

The first malignancy identified to have a specific causal chromosomal abnormality was chronic myeloid leukemia (CML) in which a translocation t(9:22) results in a constitutively active BCR-ABL tyrosine kinase leading to the activation of multiple pathways and ultimately the malignant expansion of myeloid cells. Imatinib was designed to block the binding site for ATP in the ABL kinase thereby preventing the phosphorylation of tyrosine residues and therefore activation of signal transduction.[74] In a phase II study, imatinib induced durable complete hematologic responses in 95 percent of patients treated.[75] With the success of imatinib in CML, the process of identifying a target → inhibiting the target → response has became a reality.

However, the molecular changes in other tumor types including bladder cancer remain more elusive. One reason is that unlike CML, in which one molecular event can be identified as causal, there is substantial

TABLE 5. Molecular Changes in Advanced Bladder Cancer.

Alteration	Function	Change	Clinical Association	Frequency
p53	Tumor suppressor gene	Mutation / Deletion	Increased risk of disease progression and recurrence, decreased survival [143-147] in some studies but not all [148, 149]	29 52% [144, 145, 148]
Rb gene	Tumor suppressor gene	Mutation / Deletion	More aggressive disease, progression of disease, decreased survival [146, 147, 150-153]	34–37%[151, 153]
EGFR	Oncogene	Overexpression	Tumor grade, stage, progression and survival [77, 78, 80, 154, 155]	35–86%[81, 155, 156]
Her2/neu	Oncogene	Overexpression	Higher stage, tumor progression, greater incidence metastasis[88, 157-159]. Effect on survival is mixed. [88, 157-159]	26–74%[82, 88, 155-159]
VEGF	Angiogenic factor	Overexpression	Grade, stage, recurrence [105, 106, 160]	unknown
PDGF	Angiogenic factor	Overexpression	Invasion, grade, progression, recurrence[107, 108, 109]	unknown
Cox-2	Angiogenic factor	Overexpression	Invasion [161]	31% [161]
p21	Cell cycle regulator	Decreased expression	Decreased survival[162, 163]	unknown
p27	Cell cycle regulator	Decreased expression	Grade, progression, decreased survival [164-166]	unknown
E-cadherin	Cell adhesion	Decreased expression	Invasion, progression, grade, stage, metastasis, survival [167-171]	unknown
CD 44	Cell adhesion	Decreased expression	Stage, survival[172]	unknown
Urokinase type plasminogen activator	Cell adhesion	Elevated expression	Invasion, metastasis, progression, survival [173, 174]	unknown

Rb = retinoblastoma, EGFR = epidermal growth factor receptor, VEGF = vascular endothelial growth factor, PDGF = platelet derived growth factor, Cox-2 = cyclooxygenase-2,

molecular heterogeneity and complexity in solid tumors. In solid tumors progress is being made. Specifically, significant advances have occurred in understanding the role of tyrosine kinase signaling and angiogenesis, identification of mutations in oncogenes, tumor suppressor genes, and gene products, and identification of the role of cell cycle dysregulation. These advances have led to the development of rational targeted therapies that are currently under investigation in multiple tumor types.

4.3. Blockade of the Epidermal Growth Factor Receptor Family

Many tumor types, including urothelial cancer, express high levels of growth factors and their receptors. Two commonly overexpressed in bladder cancer are the epidermal growth factor receptor (EFGR) and Her-2/neu. Therefore when anti-EGFR therapy became available, trials in urothelial cancer were logical. EGFR is over-expressed in 50% of bladder cancers. [76] Level of expression of EGFR has been correlated with tumor grade, stage, and survival and therefore is a potential prognostic and predictive factor in advanced bladder cancer.[76–81] The role of Her-2/neu is less clear. Reports of Her-2/neu overexpression in urothelial carcinoma range widely (2–74%) and the prognostic significance of Her-2/neu in bladder cancer remains controversial. [82]

4.3.1. Gefitinib

Gefitinib is an orally bioavailable inhibitor of the EGFR. Preclinical work by Dominguez-Escrig et al in EGFR-expressing human bladder cancer cell lines showed promise for gefitinib.[83] However, a SWOG trial investigating the use of gefitinib as a single agent study in patients with advanced transitional cell carcinoma refractory to one prior chemotherapy demonstrated minimal antitumor activity leading to closure of the trial after the first phase of accrual.[84] The CALGB investigated cisplatin, fixed-dose rate gemcitabine, and gefitinib in locally advanced urothelial carcinoma. A total of 27 patients were enrolled before the study was stopped because dose-limiting toxicity exceeded pre-established stopping rules.[85] Of 24 evaluable patients, there were 12 responses. Median time to progression was 6.9 months. Because toxicity was felt to be secondary to fixed dose gemcitabine, a second cohort was accrued using standard gemcitabine dosing.[86] The combination of GC and gefitinib using standard gemcitabine dosing had acceptable toxicity. However, the relative contribution of gefitinib to the efficacy of this regimen remains uncertain given no substantial improvement in response rates or overall survival in comparison to historical results of GC alone.

4.3.2. Lapatinib

Lapatinib, an oral reversible inhibitor of EGFR and HER-2/*neu* receptor tyrosine kinases has also been been evaluated in bladder cancer.[87] However, results have been disappointing with a response rate of 2%, median time to progression of 9 weeks and a median overall survival of 18 weeks in a multicenter phase II trial [87]

4.3.3. Trastuzumab

Trastuzumab is a recombinant humanized monoclonal antibody against Her-2/neu. Based on earlier work of Her-2/neu overexpression in 28% of primary bladder tumors[88] with preclinical data demonstrating synergy between paclitaxel, cisplatin and trastuzumab, a multi-institutional phase II study evaluating the combination of trastuzumab, paclitaxel, carboplatin, and gemcitabine in patients with metastatic urothelial carcinoma and over-expression of Her-2/neu was completed.[89] Of 109 registered patients, 57 (52.3%) demonstrated over-expression of Her-2/neu as determined by immunohistochemistry (93%), gene amplification (26%) and/or elevated serum HER2 levels (23%). HER-2/neu–positive patients demonstrated an increased number of metastases compared with HER-2/neu–negative patients (two *v* one; $P = .014$); a greater probability of having two or more metastatic sites (51% *v* 31%; $P = .051$), and a trend toward more liver and bone metastases. Of the patients with Her-2/neu over-expression, 44 received therapy with the combination. The overall response rate was 70% (95% CI, 55–83%). Five patients had a CR (11%), 26 (59%) a PR. The median time to progression was 9.3 months (95% CI: 6.7–10.2 months) and median survival was 14.1 months (95% CI: 11.5–17.1 months). This compares to an expected overall response rate with paclitaxel/carboplatin/gemcitabine of 43–68% [90, 91] Although, the response rate and median survival were similar to those treated with PCG[91], patients treated with TPCG had higher visceral sites of metastases (liver, lung, or bone), a known independent poor prognostic factor in urothelial carcinoma.[92] While the response rates in this study are promising, defining the role of targeting Her-2/neu in the treatment of bladder cancer requires investigation in a randomized trial.

4.3.4. Cetuximab

Cetuximab is a recombinant, human/murine chimeric monoclonal antibody, that binds specifically to the extracellular domain of the human EGFR, which has been approved by the Food and Drug Administration (FDA) for the treatment of colorectal and head and neck cancer.[93–100] Treatment with cetuximab results in EGF receptor inhibition and down-regulation, resulting in inhibition of the downstream signaling pathways of the EGFR. Based on the preclinical and clinical data that demonstrate the importance of the EGF pathway in urothelial carcinoma, cetuximab efficacy in preclinical urothelial cancer models, and the enhanced clinical efficacy of combining cetuximab with chemotherapy in advanced colorectal and head and neck cancers, a randomized open label phase II trial is currently evaluating the efficacy and safety of the addition of cetuximab to gemcitabine and cisplatin in patients with locally advanced and metastatic urothelial carcinoma.

4.4. Angiogenesis

Angiogenesis appears to be important in the development and progression of bladder cancer. The development of new vasculature has been associated with tumor grade and stage as well as disease progression and presence of metastases.[101–103] Of the angiogenic factors, VEGF has been identified as a crucial regulator of both normal and pathologic angiogenesis. Increased VEGF expression has been measured in most human tumors including those of the bladder. [104–106] Another angiogenic factor shown to be important in the pathobiology of urothelial cancer is platelet-derived endothelial cell growth factor (PDGF). Higher PDGF levels have also been associated with more invasive and higher grade urothelial carcinoma [107, 108] and appear to predict for recurrence and progression. [109] Three agents known to effect angiogenesis have been approved for treatment of other solid tumors in which angiogenesis in known to play a role; sunitinib, sorafenib, and bevacizumab and therefore are of interest in treatment of bladder cancer. Additionally, other anti-angiogenesis agents still in clinical trials are also being investigated in bladder cancer.

4.4.1. SU11248 (Sunitinib)

SU11248 is a novel, multi-targeted, small molecule inhibitor of receptor tyrosine kinases (RTKs), including vascular endothelial growth factor receptor-1 (VEGFR-1), -2, and -3, PDGFR-α and -β, stem cell receptor factor (KIT), and fms-like tyrosine kinase 3 (Flt3) known to inhibit angiogenesis. Sunitinib also exerts direct anti-tumor activity on cells that express target RTKs associated with tumor cell proliferation, such as KIT, PDGFR and RET. This agent has recently been FDA approved for the treatment of metastatic renal cell carcinoma and gastrointestinal stromal tumor on the basis of objective anti-cancer activity observed in clinical trials.[110–112]

Because angiogenesis is thought to play a crucial role in bladder cancer, our group is pioneering a new approach to advanced urothelial cancer, maintenance therapy, with the goal of prolonging progression free survival. The role of sunitinib as maintenance therapy in patients with advanced bladder cancer who have achieved at least stable disease after standard cytotoxic chemotherapy is currently being evaluated as part of a multi-center, randomized phase II trial. Sunitinib in combination with GC is also being studied neoadjvuantly.

4.4.2. BAY 43–9006 (Sorafenib)

Sorafenib is an orally available Raf kinase inhibitor that also directly inhibits VEGFR-2, VEGFR-3, and PDGFR-B affecting both tumor proliferation as well as angiogenesis. Sorafenib was recently approved by the FDA for use in metastatic renal cell carcinoma based on prolongation of progression free survival in a phase II and a phase III trial.[113–115]

Trials are ongoing investigating the role of this drug in patients with advanced urothelial carcinoma.

4.4.3. Bevacizumab

Bevacizumab is an anti-VEGF monoclonal antibody that has been approved for treatment of metastatic colon cancer on the basis of improvement in disease-free and overall survival when combined with chemotherapy.[116] Given the synergistic activity in colon cancer along with promising clinical studies in other solid tumors, bevacuzumab is being investigated in the treatment of advanced bladder cancer. The Hoosier Oncology has completeda single arm phase II study of gemcitabine, cisplatin and bevacizumab in patients with previously untreated locally advanced or metastatic transitional cell carcinoma. The primary outcome of this study is progression free survival. CALGB has planned a phase III randomized study also investigating this combination.

4.4.4. *ZD6474 (Zactima)*

ZD6474 is an orally bioavailable, potent and selective inhibitor of VEGFR-2, EGFR and RET receptor kinases.[117, 118] ZD6474 has shown dose-dependent inhibition of growth in several human cell lines and a dose-dependent supra-additive effect in growth inhibition and in apoptosis when combined with paclitaxel or docetaxel.[119]

In a phase II study involving 168 patients with locally advanced or metastatic non- small cell lung cancer who had failed either first-line and/or second-line platinum- based chemotherapy, ZD6474 was compared to gefitinib. ZD6474 demonstrated a statistically significant improvement in progression free survival over gefitinib HR=0.632 (95% CI 0.44 – 0.90, p<0.011).[120] Another phase II study in the same population of patients compared ZD6474 (100mg or 300mg daily) versus placebo in combination with docetaxel (75mg/m2 every 21 days). Combined use of ZD6474 (100mg or 300mg) and docetaxel prolonged progression free survival, but only ZD6474 100mg plus docetaxel achieved the primary end-point of a 50% prolongation of progression free survival compared with docetaxel alone HR=0.64 (95% CI 0.38 – 1.05, p=0.074) using a preset significance level of 0.2 as opposed to 0.05.[121] The efficacy demonstrated in lung cancer combined with preclinical evidence of synergistic action with paclitaxel has led to a phase II study of docetaxel +/- ZD6474 in metastatic transitional cell carcinoma which is ongoing.

4.5. HDAC Inhibitors

4.5.1. *Suberoylanilide hydroxamic acid (SAHA)/ Depsipeptide*

SAHA and depsipeptide are small molecule inhibitors of histone deacetylase (HDAC). HDACs play a critical role in the equilibrium between histone acetylation and deacetylation necessary for the regulation of gene expression including genes required for the regulation of cell survival, proliferation, differentiation, and apoptosis.[122,123] HDACs also act as members of a protein complex to recruit transcription factors to the promoter region of genes, including those of tumor suppressors, and they affect the acetylation status of specific cell cycle regulatory proteins.[123,124] In addition, HDACs have been shown to be important in regulation of non-histone proteins such as Hsp90 which plays a key role in modulation of cell signaling and degradation of proteins key for continued cell growth. [124] Preclinical trials using bladder xenografts showed suppression of tumor growth by HDACs.[125] In a phase I trial of SAHA administered intravenously, objective tumor regression and clinical improvement in tumor related symptoms has been observed including in patients with bladder cancer.[126] Promising results from preclinical and phase I studies has led to the phase II study of HDAC inhibitors in multiple tumor types including bladder cancer.

5. Conclusion

The therapeutic armamentarium for urothelial cancer is expanding with the development of active new single agents and combination chemotherapy. However, these therapies continue to be palliative with doubtful curative potential in metastatic urothelial cancer. Hence more effective therapy is needed.

With improvements in the understanding of the biology of bladder cancer, new trials utilizing novel and targeted therapeutics as single agents and in combination with chemotherapy are currently underway. To allow accurate interpretation of results, careful attention to study design, patient selection and end-points are particularly important considering that several of the agents being evaluated are non-cytotoxic targeted agents.

References

1 Jemal A, Siegel R, Ward E, et al. Cancer statistics, 2006. CA Cancer J Clin 2006;56:106–130.
2 von der Maase H, Sengelov L, Roberts J460T, et al. Long-term survival results of a randomized trial comparing gemcitabine plus cisplatin, with methotrexate, vinblastine, doxorubicin, plus cisplatin in patients with bladder cancer. J Clin Oncol 2005;23:4602–4608.
3 Loehrer PJ, Sr., Einhorn LH, Elson PJ, et al. A randomized comparison of cisplatin alone or in combination with methotrexate, vinblastine, and doxorubicin in patients with metastatic urothelial carcinoma: a cooperative group study. J Clin Oncol 1992;10:1066–1073.
4 Saxman SB, Propert KJ, Einhorn LH, et al. Long-term follow-up of a phase III intergroup study of cisplatin alone or in combination with methotrexate, vinblastine, and doxorubicin in patients with metastatic urothelial carcinoma: a cooperative group study. J Clin Oncol 1997;15:2564–2569.
5 Logothetis CJ, Dexeus FH, Finn L, et al. A prospective randomized trial comparing MVAC and CISCA chemotherapy for patients with metastatic urothelial tumors. J Clin Oncol 1990;8:1050–1055.

6 von der Maase H, Hansen SW, Roberts JT, et al. Gemcitabine and cisplatin versus methotrexate, vinblastine, doxorubicin, and cisplatin in advanced or metastatic bladder cancer: results of a large, randomized, multinational, multicenter, phase III study. J Clin Oncol 2000;18:3068–3077.
7 Sternberg CN, de Mulder PH, Schornagel JH, et al. Randomized phase III trial of high-dose-intensity methotrexate, vinblastine, doxorubicin, and cisplatin (MVAC) chemotherapy and recombinant human granulocyte colony-stimulating factor versus classic MVAC in advanced urothelial tract tumors: European Organization for Research and Treatment of Cancer Protocol no. 30924. J Clin Oncol 2001;19:2638–2646.
8 Dreicer R, Manola J, Roth BJ, et al. Phase III trial of methotrexate, vinblastine, doxorubicin, and cisplatin versus carboplatin and paclitaxel in patients with advanced carcinoma of the urothelium. Cancer 2004;100:1639–1645.
9 Sternberg CN, de Mulder P, Schornagel JH, et al. Seven year update of an EORTC phase III trial of high-dose intensity M-VAC chemotherapy and G-CSF versus classic M-VAC in advanced urothelial tract tumours. Eur J Cancer 2006;42: 50–54.
10 Moore MJ, Tannock IF, Ernst DS, Huan S, Murray N. Gemcitabine: a promising new agent in the treatment of advanced urothelial cancer. J Clin Oncol 1997;15: 3441–3445.
11 Stadler WM, Kuzel T, Roth B, Raghavan D, Dorr FA. Phase II study of single-agent gemcitabine in previously untreated patients with metastatic urothelial cancer. J Clin Oncol 1997;15:3394–3398.
12 Roth BJ, Dreicer R, Einhorn LH, et al. Significant activity of paclitaxel in advanced transitional-cell carcinoma of the urothelium: a phase II trial of the Eastern Cooperative Oncology Group. J Clin Oncol 1994;12:2264–2270.
13 Bellmunt J, Guillem V, Paz-Ares L, et al. Phase I-II study of paclitaxel, cisplatin, and gemcitabine in advanced transitional-cell carcinoma of the urothelium. Spanish Oncology Genitourinary Group. J Clin Oncol 2000;18:3247–3255.
14 Bellmunt J, von der Maase H, Mead G, et al. Randomized phase III study comparing paclitaxel/cisplatin/gemcitabine and gemcitabine/cisplatin in patients with locally advanced or metastatic urothelial cancer without prior systemic therapy; EORTC30987/Intergroup Study. Journal of Clinical Oncology, ASCO Annual Meeting Proceedings Part I Vol 25, 2007;25:No. 18S (June 20 Supplement): LBA5030.
15 Raghavan D, Shipley WU, Garnick MB, Russell PJ, Richie JP. Biology and management of bladder cancer. N Engl J Med 1990;322:1129–1138.
16 Llado ABJ, Kaiser G, et al. A dose finding study of carboplatin with fixed doses of gemcitabine in "unfit" patients with advanced bladder cancer. Proc Am Soc Clin Oncol 2000;19:344a.
17 Carles J, Nogue M, Domenech M, et al. Carboplatin-gemcitabine treatment of patients with transitional cell carcinoma of the bladder and impaired renal function. Oncology 2000;59:24–27.
18 Shannon C, Crombie C, Brooks A, Lau H, Drummond M, Gurney H. Carboplatin and gemcitabine in metastatic transitional cell carcinoma of the urothelium: effective treatment of patients with poor prognostic features. Ann Oncol 2001;12:947–952.
19 Nogue-Aliguer M, Carles J, Arrivi A, et al. Gemcitabine and carboplatin in advanced transitional cell carcinoma of the urinary tract: an alternative therapy. Cancer 2003;97: 2180–2186.
20 Meluch AA, Greco FA, Burris HA, 3rd, et al. Paclitaxel and gemcitabine chemotherapy for advanced transitional-cell carcinoma of the urothelial tract: a phase II trial of the Minnie pearl cancer research network. J Clin Oncol 2001;19:3018–3024.
21 Sternberg CN, Calabro F, Pizzocaro G, Marini L, Schnetzer S, Sella A. Chemotherapy with an every-2-week regimen of gemcitabine and paclitaxel in patients with transitional cell carcinoma who have received prior cisplatin-based therapy. Cancer 2001;92:2993–2998.
22 Parameswaran RFM, Ansari F, et al. A Hoosier Oncology Group phase II study of weekly paclitaxel and gemcitabine in advanced transitional cell (TCC) carcinoma of the bladder. Proc Am Soc Clin Oncol 2001;20:200a.
23 MacVicar G, Hussain M. Special Considerations on the Management of Elderly Bladder Cancer Patients. In: SP L, M S, C S, eds. Textbook of Bladder Cancer. London: T&F-Informa; 2006.
24 Lorusso V, Pollera CF, Antimi M, et al. A phase II study of gemcitabine in patients with transitional cell carcinoma of the urinary tract previously treated with platinum. Italian Co-operative Group on Bladder Cancer. Eur J Cancer 1998;34:1208–1212.
25 Albers P, Siener R, Hartlein M, et al. Gemcitabine monotherapy as second-line treatment in cisplatin-refractory transitional cell carcinoma - prognostic factors for response and improvement of quality of life. Onkologie 2002;25:47–52.
26 Pollera CF, Ceribelli A, Crecco M, Calabresi F. Weekly gemcitabine in advanced bladder cancer: a preliminary report from a phase I study. Ann Oncol 1994;5:182–184.
27 Witte RS, Elson P, Bono B, et al. Eastern Cooperative Oncology Group phase II trial of ifosfamide in the treatment of previously treated advanced urothelial carcinoma. J Clin Oncol 1997;15:589–593.
28 Pronzato P, Vigani A, Pensa F, Vanoli M, Tani F, Vaira F. Second line chemotherapy with ifosfamide as outpatient treatment for advanced bladder cancer. Am J Clin Oncol 1997;20:519–521.
29 McCaffrey JA, Hilton S, Mazumdar M, et al. Phase II trial of docetaxel in patients with advanced or metastatic transitional-cell carcinoma. J Clin Oncol 1997;15:1853–1857.
30 Vaughn DJ, Broome CM, Hussain M, Gutheil JC, Markowitz AB. Phase II trial of weekly paclitaxel in patients with previously treated advanced urothelial cancer. J Clin Oncol 2002;20:937–940.
31 Culine S, Theodore C, De Santis M, et al. A phase II study of vinflunine in bladder cancer patients progressing after first-line platinum-containing regimen. Br J Cancer 2006;94:1395–1401.
32 Fechner G, Siener R, Reimann M, Kobalz L, Albers P. Randomised phase II trial of gemcitabine and paclitaxel second-line chemotherapy in patients with transitional cell carcinoma (AUO Trial AB 20/99). Int J Clin Pract 2006;60:27–31.
33 Krege S, Rembrink V, Borgermann C, Otto T, Rubben H. Docetaxel and ifosfamide as second line treatment for patients with advanced or metastatic urothelial cancer after

failure of platinum chemotherapy: a phase 2 study. J Urol 2001;165:67–71.
34 Tu SM, Hossan E, Amato R, Kilbourn R, Logothetis CJ. Paclitaxel, cisplatin and methotrexate combination chemotherapy is active in the treatment of refractory urothelial malignancies. J Urol 1995;154:1719–1722.
35 Pagliaro LC, Millikan RE, Tu SM, et al. Cisplatin, gemcitabine, and ifosfamide as weekly therapy: a feasibility and phase II study of salvage treatment for advanced transitional-cell carcinoma. J Clin Oncol 2002;20:2965–2970.
36 Dumontet C, Sikic BI. Mechanisms of action of and resistance to antitubulin agents: microtubule dynamics, drug transport, and cell death. J Clin Oncol 1999;17:1061–1070.
37 Attard G, Greystoke A, Kaye S, De Bono J. Update on tubulin-binding agents. Pathol Biol (Paris) 2006;54:72–84.
38 Blumenreich MS, Yagoda A, Natale RB, Watson RC. Phase II trial of vinblastine sulfate for metastatic urothelial tract tumors. Cancer 1982;50:435–438.
39 de Wit R, Kruit WH, Stoter G, de Boer M, Kerger J, Verweij J. Docetaxel (Taxotere): an active agent in metastatic urothelial cancer; results of a phase II study in non-chemotherapy-pretreated patients. Br J Cancer 1998;78:1342–1345.
40 Bollag DM, McQueney PA, Zhu J, et al. Epothilones, a new class of microtubule-stabilizing agents with a taxol-like mechanism of action. Cancer Res 1995;55:2325–2333.
41 Kowalski RJ, Giannakakou P, Hamel E. Activities of the microtubule-stabilizing agents epothilones A and B with purified tubulin and in cells resistant to paclitaxel (Taxol(R)). J Biol Chem 1997;272:2534–2541.
42 Nettles JH, Li H, Cornett B, Krahn JM, Snyder JP, Downing KH. The binding mode of epothilone A on alpha,beta-tubulin by electron crystallography. Science 2004;305: 866–869.
43 Goodin S, Kane MP, Rubin EH. Epothilones: mechanism of action and biologic activity. J Clin Oncol 2004;22:2015–2025.
44 Lee FY, Borzilleri R, Fairchild CR, et al. BMS-247550: a novel epothilone analog with a mode of action similar to paclitaxel but possessing superior antitumor efficacy. Clin Cancer Res 2001;7:1429–1437.
45 Dreicer R, Li S, Manola J, Haas N, Roth B, Wilding G. Phase II trial of epothilone B analogue BMS-247550 in advanced carcinoma of the urothelium (E3800): A trial of the Eastern Cooperative Oncology Group. J Clin Oncol 2006;24:Abstract 4543.
46 Hill BT, Fiebig HH, Waud WR, Poupon MF, Colpaert F, Kruczynski A. Superior in vivo experimental antitumour activity of vinflunine, relative to vinorelbine, in a panel of human tumour xenografts. Eur J Cancer 1999;35:512–520.
47 Bonfil RD, Russo DM, Binda MM, Delgado FM, Vincenti M. Higher antitumor activity of vinflunine than vinorelbine against an orthotopic murine model of transitional cell carcinoma of the bladder. Urol Oncol 2002;7:159–166.
48 Lobert S, Ingram JW, Hill BT, Correia JJ. A comparison of thermodynamic parameters for vinorelbine- and vinflunine-induced tubulin self-association by sedimentation velocity. Mol Pharmacol 1998;53:908–915.
49 Bellmunt J, von der Maase H, Theodore C, et al. Randomised phase III trial of vinflunine (V) plus best supportive care (B) vs B alone as 2nd line therapy after a platinum-containing regimen in advanced transitional cell carcinoma of the urothelium (TCCU). Sub-category: Bladder Cancer J Clin Oncol 2008;26:abstract 5028.
50 Jordan MA, Kamath K, Manna T, et al. The primary antimitotic mechanism of action of the synthetic halichondrin E7389 is suppression of microtubule growth. Mol Cancer Ther 2005;4:1086–1095.
51 Towle MJ, Salvato KA, Budrow J, et al. In vitro and in vivo anticancer activities of synthetic macrocyclic ketone analogues of halichondrin B. Cancer Res 2001;61:1013–1021.
52 van Zuylen L, Verweij J, Sparreboom A. Role of formulation vehicles in taxane pharmacology. Invest New Drugs 2001;19:125–141.
53 Sparreboom A, van Zuylen L, Brouwer E, et al. Cremophor EL-mediated alteration of paclitaxel distribution in human blood: clinical pharmacokinetic implications. Cancer Res 1999;59:1454–1457.
54 John TA, Vogel SM, Tiruppathi C, Malik AB, Minshall RD. Quantitative analysis of albumin uptake and transport in the rat microvessel endothelial monolayer. Am J Physiol Lung Cell Mol Physiol 2003;284:L187–196.
55 Ho CC, Huang PH, Huang HY, Chen YH, Yang PC, Hsu SM. Up-regulated caveolin-1 accentuates the metastasis capability of lung adenocarcinoma by inducing filopodia formation. Am J Pathol 2002;161:1647–1656.
56 Kato K, Hida Y, Miyamoto M, et al. Overexpression of caveolin-1 in esophageal squamous cell carcinoma correlates with lymph node metastasis and pathologic stage. Cancer 2002;94:929–933.
57 Tahir SA, Yang G, Ebara S, et al. Secreted caveolin-1 stimulates cell survival/clonal growth and contributes to metastasis in androgen-insensitive prostate cancer. Cancer Res 2001;61:3882–3885.
58 Desai N, Trieu V, Yao Z, et al. Increased antitumor activity, intratumor paclitaxel concentrations, and endothelial cell transport of cremophor-free, albumin-bound paclitaxel, ABI-007, compared with cremophor-based paclitaxel. Clin Cancer Res 2006;12:1317–1324.
59 Gradishar WJ, Tjulandin S, Davidson N, et al. Phase III trial of nanoparticle albumin-bound paclitaxel compared with polyethylated castor oil-based paclitaxel in women with breast cancer. J Clin Oncol 2005;23:7794–7803.
60 Turner AG. Methotrexate in advanced bladder cancer. Cancer Treat Rep 1981;65 Suppl 1:183–186.
61 Natale RB, Yagoda A, Watson RC, Whitmore WF, Blumenreich M, Braun DW, Jr. Methotrexate: an active drug in bladder cancer. Cancer 1981;47:1246–1250.
62 Oliver RT, England HR, Risdon RA, Blandy JP. Methotrexate in the treatment of metastatic and recurrent primary transitional cell carcinoma. J Urol 1984;131:483–485.
63 Knight EW, Pagand M, Hahn RG, Horton J. Comparison of 5-FU and doxorubicin in the treatment of carcinoma of the bladder. Cancer Treat Rep 1983;67:514–515.
64 Siefker-Radtke AO, Millikan RE, Tu SM, et al. Phase III trial of fluorouracil, interferon alpha-2b, and cisplatin versus methotrexate, vinblastine, doxorubicin, and cisplatin in metastatic or unresectable urothelial cancer. J Clin Oncol 2002;20:1361–1367.
65 Paz-Ares L, Bezares S, Tabernero JM, Castellanos D, Cortes-Funes H. Review of a promising new agent--pemetrexed disodium. Cancer 2003;97:2056–2063.

66 Worzalla JF, Shih C, Schultz RM. Role of folic acid in modulating the toxicity and efficacy of the multitargeted antifolate, LY231514. Anticancer Res 1998;18:3235–3239.
67 von der Maase H, Lehmann J, Gravis G, et al. A phase II trial of pemetrexed plus gemcitabine in locally advanced and/or metastatic transitional cell carcinoma of the urothelium. Ann Oncol 2006.
68 von der Maase H. Gemcitabine in transitional cell carcinoma of the urothelium. Expert Rev Anticancer Ther 2003;3:11–19.
69 Li S, Dreicer R, Roth B, Manoloa J, Cooney M, Wilding G. Phase II trial of pemetrexed disodium and gemcitabine in advanced carcinoma of the urothelium (E4802): A trial of the Eastern Cooperative Oncology Group. J Clin Oncol 2007;25:abstract 5079.
70 Sweeney CJ, Roth BJ, Kabbinavar FF, et al. Phase II study of pemetrexed for second-line treatment of transitional cell cancer of the urothelium. J Clin Oncol 2006;24: 3451–3457.
71 Knowles MA. Molecular subtypes of bladder cancer: Jekyll and Hyde or chalk and cheese? Carcinogenesis 2006;27: 361–373.
72 Schulz W. Understanding urothelial carcinoma through cancer pathways. Int J Cancer 2006;Mar 23; [Epub ahead of print].
73 Wu XR. Urothelial tumorigenesis: a tale of divergent pathways. Nat Rev Cancer 2005;5:713–725.
74 Druker BJ, Tamura S, Buchdunger E, et al. Effects of a selective inhibitor of the Abl tyrosine kinase on the growth of Bcr-Abl positive cells. Nat Med 1996;2:561–566.
75 Kantarjian H, Sawyers C, Hochhaus A, et al. Hematologic and cytogenetic responses to imatinib mesylate in chronic myelogenous leukemia. N Engl J Med 2002;346:645–652.
76 Chow NH, Liu HS, Lee EI, et al. Significance of urinary epidermal growth factor and its receptor expression in human bladder cancer. Anticancer Res 1997;17: 1293–1296.
77 Nguyen PL, Swanson PE, Jaszcz W, et al. Expression of epidermal growth factor receptor in invasive transitional cell carcinoma of the urinary bladder. A multivariate survival analysis. Am J Clin Pathol 1994;101:166–176.
78 Neal DE, Marsh C, Bennett MK, et al. Epidermal-growth-factor receptors in human bladder cancer: comparison of invasive and superficial tumours. Lancet 1985;1:366–368.
79 Neal DE, Sharples L, Smith K, Fennelly J, Hall RR, Harris AL. The epidermal growth factor receptor and the prognosis of bladder cancer. Cancer 1990;65:1619–1625.
80 Messing EM. Clinical implications of the expression of epidermal growth factor receptors in human transitional cell carcinoma. Cancer Res 1990;50:2530–2537.
81 Bue P, Wester K, Sjostrom A, et al. Expression of epidermal growth factor receptor in urinary bladder cancer metastases. Int J Cancer 1998;76:189–193.
82 Bellmunt J, Hussain M, Dinney CP. Novel approaches with targeted therapies in bladder cancer. Therapy of bladder cancer by blockade of the epidermal growth factor receptor family. Crit Rev Oncol Hematol 2003;46 Suppl:S85–104.
83 Dominguez-Escrig JL, Kelly JD, Neal DE, King SM, Davies BR. Evaluation of the therapeutic potential of the epidermal growth factor receptor tyrosine kinase inhibitor gefitinib in preclinical models of bladder cancer. Clin Cancer Res 2004;10:4874–4884.
84 Petrylak D, Faulkner J, Van Veldhuizen P, Mansukhani M. Evaluation of ZD1839 for advanced transitional cell carcinoma (TCC) of the urothelium: A Southwest Oncology Group Trial. Proc Am Soc Clin Oncol 2003;22:Abstract 1619.
85 Phillips G, Halabi S, Sanford D, et al. Phase II trial of cisplatin, fixed-dose gemcitabine and gefitinib for advanced transitional cell carninoma of the urothelial tract: Preliminary results from CALGB 90102. Journal of Clinical Oncology 2004;22:4540.
86 Philips G, Sanford B, Halabi S, Bajorin D, Small EJ. Phase II study of cisplatin (C), gemcitabine (G) and gefitinib for advanced urothelial carcinoma (UC): Analysis of the second cohort of CALGB 90102. J Clin Oncol 2006;24:abstract 4578.
87 Wülfing C, Machiels J, Richel D, Grimm M. A single arm, multicenter, open label, ph II study of lapatinib as 2L treatment of pts with locally advanced/metastatic transitional cell carcinoma (TCC) of the urothelial tract. J Clin Oncol 2005;23:Abstract 4594.
88 Jimenez RE, Hussain M, Bianco FJ, Jr., et al. Her-2/neu overexpression in muscle-invasive urothelial carcinoma of the bladder: prognostic significance and comparative analysis in primary and metastatic tumors. Clin Cancer Res 2001;7:2440–2447.
89 Hussain MH, MacVicar GR, Petrylak DP, et al. Trastuzumab, paclitaxel, carboplatin, and gemcitabine in advanced human epidermal growth factor receptor-2/neu-positive urothelial carcinoma: results of a multicenter phase II National Cancer Institute trial. J Clin Oncol 2007;25:2218–2224.
90 Hainsworth JD, Meluch AA, Litchy S, et al. Paclitaxel, carboplatin, and gemcitabine in the treatment of patients with advanced transitional cell carcinoma of the urothelium. Cancer 2005;103:2298–2303.
91 Hussain M, Vaishampayan U, Du W, Redman B, Smith DC. Combination paclitaxel, carboplatin, and gemcitabine is an active treatment for advanced urothelial cancer. J Clin Oncol 2001;19:2527–2533.
92 Bajorin DF, Dodd PM, Mazumdar M, et al. Long-term survival in metastatic transitional-cell carcinoma and prognostic factors predicting outcome of therapy. J Clin Oncol 1999;17:3173–3181.
93 Cunningham D, Humblet Y, Siena S, et al. Cetuximab monotherapy and cetuximab plus irinotecan in irinotecan-refractory metastatic colorectal cancer. N Engl J Med 2004;351:337–345.
94 Van Cutsem E, Nowacki M, Lang I, et al. Randomized phase III study of irinotecan and 5-FU/FA with or without cetuximab in the first-line treatment of patients with metastatic colorectal cancer (mCRC): The CRYSTAL trial. J Clin Oncol 2007;25:abstract 4000.
95 Jonker DJ, O'Callaghan CJ, Karapetis CS, et al. Cetuximab for the treatment of colorectal cancer. N Engl J Med 2007;357:2040–2048.
96 Bonner JA, Harari PM, Giralt J, et al. Radiotherapy plus cetuximab for squamous-cell carcinoma of the head and neck. N Engl J Med 2006;354:567–578.
97 Trigo J, Hitt R, Koralewski P, et al. Cetuximab monotherapy is active in patients (pts) with platinum-refractory recurrent/ metastatic squamous cell carcinoma of the head and neck

(SCCHN): Results of a phase II study. Journal of Clinical Oncology 2004;22:abstract 5502.

98 Vermorken JB, Trigo J, Hitt R, et al. Open-label, uncontrolled, multicenter phase II study to evaluate the efficacy and toxicity of cetuximab as a single agent in patients with recurrent and/or metastatic squamous cell carcinoma of the head and neck who failed to respond to platinum-based therapy. J Clin Oncol 2007;25:2171–2177.

99 Vermorken J, Mesia R, Vega V, et al. Cetuximab extends survival of patients with recurrent or metastatic SCCHN when added to first line platinum based therapy - Results of a randomized phase III (Extreme) study. Journal of Clinical Oncology 2007;25:abstract 6091.

100 Saltz LB, Meropol NJ, Loehrer PJ, Sr., Needle MN, Kopit J, Mayer RJ. Phase II trial of cetuximab in patients with refractory colorectal cancer that expresses the epidermal growth factor receptor. J Clin Oncol 2004;22:1201–1208.

101 Jaeger TM, Weidner N, Chew K, et al. Tumor angiogenesis correlates with lymph node metastases in invasive bladder cancer. J Urol 1995;154:69–71.

102 Goddard JC, Sutton CD, Furness PN, O'Byrne KJ, Kockelbergh RC. Microvessel density at presentation predicts subsequent muscle invasion in superficial bladder cancer. Clin Cancer Res 2003;9:2583–2586.

103 Canoglu A, Gogus C, Beduk Y, Orhan D, Tulunay O, Baltaci S. Microvessel density as a prognostic marker in bladder carcinoma: correlation with tumor grade, stage and prognosis. Int Urol Nephrol 2004;36:401–405.

104 Ferrara N, Davis-Smyth T. The biology of vascular endothelial growth factor. Endocr Rev 1997;18:4–25.

105 Yang CC, Chu KC, Yeh WM. The expression of vascular endothelial growth factor in transitional cell carcinoma of urinary bladder is correlated with cancer progression. Urol Oncol 2004;22:1–6.

106 Izawa JI, Slaton JW, Kedar D, et al. Differential expression of progression-related genes in the evolution of superficial to invasive transitional cell carcinoma of the bladder. Oncol Rep 2001;8:9–15.

107 Mizutani Y, Okada Y, Yoshida O. Expression of platelet-derived endothelial cell growth factor in bladder carcinoma. Cancer 1997;79:1190–1194.

108 Li N, Kanda K, Fukumori T, et al. Expression of vascular endothelial growth factor isoforms and platelet-derived endothelial cell growth factor in bladder cancer. Urol Oncol 2000;6:10–15.

109 Li S, Nomata K, Sawase K, Noguchi M, Kanda S, Kanetake H. Prognostic significance of platelet-derived endothelial cell growth factor/thymidine phosphorylase expression in stage pT1 G3 bladder cancer. Int J Urol 2001;8:478–482.

110 Motzer RJ, Rini BI, Bukowski RM, et al. Sunitinib in patients with metastatic renal cell carcinoma. Jama 2006;295:2516–2524.

111 Motzer RJ, Michaelson MD, Redman BG, et al. Activity of SU11248, a multitargeted inhibitor of vascular endothelial growth factor receptor and platelet-derived growth factor receptor, in patients with metastatic renal cell carcinoma. J Clin Oncol 2006;24:16–24.

112 Demetri G, van Oosterom T, Blackstein M, et al. Phase 3, mulitcenter, randomized, double-blind, placebo-controlled trial of SU11248 in patients following failure of imatinib for metastatic GIST. Proc Am Soc Clin Oncol 2005:Abstract 4000.

113 Ratain M, Eisen T, Stadler W, et al. Final findings from a Phase II, placebo-controlled, randomized discontinuation trial (RDT) of sorafenib (BAY 43–9006) in patients with advanced renal cell carcinoma (RCC). Proc Am Soc Clin Oncol 2005:abstract 4544.

114 Ratain MJ, Eisen T, Stadler WM, et al. Phase II placebo-controlled randomized discontinuation trial of sorafenib in patients with metastatic renal cell carcinoma. J Clin Oncol 2006;24:2505–2512.

115 Escudier B, Szczylik C, Eisen T, et al. Randomized Phase III trial of the Raf kinase and VEGFR inhibitor sorafenib (BAY 43–9006) in patients with advanced renal cell carcinoma. Proc Am Soc Clin Oncol 2005:abstract 4510.

116 Hurwitz H, Fehrenbacher L, Novotny W, et al. Bevacizumab plus irinotecan, fluorouracil, and leucovorin for metastatic colorectal cancer. N Engl J Med 2004; 350:2335–2342.

117 Wedge SR, Ogilvie DJ, Dukes M, et al. ZD6474 inhibits vascular endothelial growth factor signaling, angiogenesis, and tumor growth following oral administration. Cancer Res 2002;62:4645–4655.

118 Carlomagno F, Vitagliano D, Guida T, et al. ZD6474, an orally available inhibitor of KDR tyrosine kinase activity, efficiently blocks oncogenic RET kinases. Cancer Res 2002;62:7284–7290.

119 Ciardiello F, Caputo R, Damiano V, et al. Antitumor effects of ZD6474, a small molecule vascular endothelial growth factor receptor tyrosine kinase inhibitor, with additional activity against epidermal growth factor receptor tyrosine kinase. Clin Cancer Res 2003;9:1546–1556.

120 Natale RBD, Govindan R et al. A comparison of the antitumour efficacy of ZD6474 and gefitinib (Iressa) in patients with NSCLC: results of a randomized, double-blind Phase II study. Lung Cancer 2005;49:S37.

121 Herbst RJB, Rowbottom J et al. ZD6474 plus docetaxel in patients with previously treated NSCLC: results of a randomized placebo-controlled Phase II trial. Lung Cancer 2005;49:S35.

122 Wade PA, Gegonne A, Jones PL, Ballestar E, Aubry F, Wolffe AP. Mi-2 complex couples DNA methylation to chromatin remodelling and histone deacetylation. Nat Genet 1999;23:62–66.

123 Arts J, de Schepper S, Van Emelen K. Histone deacetylase inhibitors: from chromatin remodeling to experimental cancer therapeutics. Curr Med Chem 2003;10:2343–2350.

124 Drummond DC, Noble CO, Kirpotin DB, Guo Z, Scott GK, Benz CC. Clinical development of histone deacetylase inhibitors as anticancer agents. Annu Rev Pharmacol Toxicol 2005;45:495–528.

125 Canes D, Chiang GJ, Billmeyer BR, et al. Histone deacetylase inhibitors upregulate plakoglobin expression in bladder carcinoma cells and display antineoplastic activity in vitro and in vivo. Int J Cancer 2005;113:841–848.

126 Kelly WK, Richon VM, O'Connor O, et al. Phase I clinical trial of histone deacetylase inhibitor: suberoylanilide hydroxamic acid administered intravenously. Clin Cancer Res 2003;9:3578–3588.

127 Moore MJ, Winquist EW, Murray N, et al. Gemcitabine plus cisplatin, an active regimen in advanced urothelial

cancer: a phase II trial of the National Cancer Institute of Canada Clinical Trials Group. J Clin Oncol 1999;17: 2876–2881.
128 Kaufman D, Raghavan D, Carducci M, et al. Phase II trial of gemcitabine plus cisplatin in patients with metastatic urothelial cancer. J Clin Oncol 2000;18:1921–1927.
129 Hussain SA, Stocken DD, Riley P, et al. A phase I/II study of gemcitabine and fractionated cisplatin in an outpatient setting using a 21-day schedule in patients with advanced and metastatic bladder cancer. Br J Cancer 2004;91: 844–849.
130 Redman BG, Smith DC, Flaherty L, Du W, Hussain M. Phase II trial of paclitaxel and carboplatin in the treatment of advanced urothelial carcinoma. J Clin Oncol 1998;16:1844–1848.
131 Vaughn DJ, Manola J, Dreicer R, See W, Levitt R, Wilding G. Phase II study of paclitaxel plus carboplatin in patients with advanced carcinoma of the urothelium and renal dysfunction (E2896): a trial of the Eastern Cooperative Oncology Group. Cancer 2002;95:1022–1027.
132 Johannsen M, Sachs M, Roigas J, et al. Phase II trial of weekly paclitaxel and carboplatin chemotherapy in patients with advanced transitional cell cancer. Eur Urol 2005;48:246–251.
133 Dreicer R, Manola J, Roth BJ, Cohen MB, Hatfield AK, Wilding G. Phase II study of cisplatin and paclitaxel in advanced carcinoma of the urothelium: an Eastern Cooperative Oncology Group Study. J Clin Oncol 2000;18:1058–1061.
134 Burch PA, Richardson RL, Cha SS, et al. Phase II study of paclitaxel and cisplatin for advanced urothelial cancer. J Urol 2000;164:1538–1542.
135 Dimopoulos MA, Bakoyannis C, Georgoulias V, et al. Docetaxel and cisplatin combination chemotherapy in advanced carcinoma of the urothelium: a multicenter phase II study of the Hellenic Cooperative Oncology Group. Ann Oncol 1999;10:1385–1388.
136 Garcia del Muro X, Marcuello E, Guma J, et al. Phase II multicentre study of docetaxel plus cisplatin in patients with advanced urothelial cancer. Br J Cancer 2002;86:326–330.
137 Kaufman DS, Carducci MA, Kuzel TM, et al. A multi-institutional phase II trial of gemcitabine plus paclitaxel in patients with locally advanced or metastatic urothelial cancer. Urol Oncol 2004;22:393–397.
138 Theodore C, Bidault F, Bouvet-Forteau N, et al. A phase II monocentric study of oxaliplatin in combination with gemcitabine (GEMOX) in patients with advanced/metastatic transitional cell carcinoma (TCC) of the urothelial tract. Ann Oncol 2006;17:990–994.
139 Bajorin DF, McCaffrey JA, Dodd PM, et al. Ifosfamide, paclitaxel, and cisplatin for patients with advanced transitional cell carcinoma of the urothelial tract: final report of a phase II trial evaluating two dosing schedules. Cancer 2000;88:1671–1678.
140 Edelman MJ, Meyers FJ, Miller TR, Williams SG, Gandour-Edwards R, deVere White RW. Phase I/II study of paclitaxel, carboplatin, and methotrexate in advanced transitional cell carcinoma: a well-tolerated regimen with activity independent of p53 mutation. Urology 2000;55: 521–525.
141 Ardavanis A, Tryfonopoulos D, Alexopoulos A, Kandylis C, Lainakis G, Rigatos G. Gemcitabine and docetaxel as first-line treatment for advanced urothelial carcinoma: a phase II study. Br J Cancer 2005;92:645–650.
142 Tsavaris N, Kosmas C, Skopelitis H, et al. Methotrexate-paclitaxel-epirubicin-carboplatin (M-TEC) combination chemotherapy in patients with advanced bladder cancer: an open label phase II study. J Chemother 2005;17: 441–448.
143 Esrig D, Elmajian D, Groshen S, et al. Accumulation of nuclear p53 and tumor progression in bladder cancer. N Engl J Med 1994;331:1259–1264.
144 Lipponen PK. Over-expression of p53 nuclear oncoprotein in transitional-cell bladder cancer and its prognostic value. Int J Cancer 1993;53:365–370.
145 Sarkis AS, Bajorin DF, Reuter VE, et al. Prognostic value of p53 nuclear overexpression in patients with invasive bladder cancer treated with neoadjuvant MVAC. J Clin Oncol 1995;13:1384–1390.
146 Cordon-Cardo C, Zhang ZF, Dalbagni G, et al. Cooperative effects of p53 and pRB alterations in primary superficial bladder tumors. Cancer Res 1997;57:1217–1221.
147 Chatterjee SJ, Datar R, Youssefzadeh D, et al. Combined effects of p53, p21, and pRb expression in the progression of bladder transitional cell carcinoma. J Clin Oncol 2004;22:1007–1013.
148 Fleshner N, Kapusta L, Ezer D, Herschorn S, Klotz L. p53 nuclear accumulation is not associated with decreased disease-free survival in patients with node positive transitional cell carcinoma of the bladder. J Urol 2000;164: 1177–1182.
149 Schmitz-Drager BJ, Goebell PJ, Ebert T, Fradet Y. p53 immunohistochemistry as a prognostic marker in bladder cancer. Playground for urology scientists? Eur Urol 2000;38:691–699;discussion 700.
150 Cote RJ, Dunn MD, Chatterjee SJ, et al. Elevated and absent pRb expression is associated with bladder cancer progression and has cooperative effects with p53. Cancer Res 1998;58:1090–1094.
151 Cordon-Cardo C, Wartinger D, Petrylak D, et al. Altered expression of the retinoblastoma gene product: prognostic indicator in bladder cancer. J Natl Cancer Inst 1992;84: 1251–1256.
152 Quentin T, Henke C, Korabiowska M, Schlott T, Zimmerman B, Kunze E. Altered mRNA expression of the Rb and p16 tumor suppressor genes and of CDK4 in transitional cell carcinomas of the urinary bladder associated with tumor progression. Anticancer Res 2004;24: 1011–1023.
153 Logothetis CJ, Xu HJ, Ro JY, et al. Altered expression of retinoblastoma protein and known prognostic variables in locally advanced bladder cancer. J Natl Cancer Inst 1992;84:1256–1261.
154 Mellon K, Wright C, Kelly P, Horne CH, Neal DE. Long-term outcome related to epidermal growth factor receptor status in bladder cancer. J Urol 1995;153:919–925.
155 Lipponen P, Eskelinen M. Expression of epidermal growth factor receptor in bladder cancer as related to established prognostic factors, oncoprotein (c-erbB-2, p53) expression and long-term prognosis. Br J Cancer 1994;69: 1120–1125.

156 Ravery V, Grignon D, Angulo J, et al. Evaluation of epidermal growth factor receptor, transforming growth factor alpha, epidermal growth factor and c-erbB2 in the progression of invasive bladder cancer. Urol Res 1997; 25:9–17.
157 Miyamoto H, Kubota Y, Noguchi S, et al. C-ERBB-2 gene amplification as a prognostic marker in human bladder cancer. Urology 2000;55:679–683.
158 Hussain M, Trastuzumab T, Paclitaxel P, Carboplatin C, and Gemcitabine G in Advanced HER2-positive Urothelial Carcinoma: Results of a Multi-Center Phase II NCI Trial. Proc Am Soc Clin Oncol 2005;23:abstract 4507.
159 Sato K, Moriyama M, Mori S, et al. An immunohistologic evaluation of C-erbB-2 gene product in patients with urinary bladder carcinoma. Cancer 1992;70:2493–2498.
160 Inoue K, Slaton JW, Karashima T, et al. The prognostic value of angiogenesis factor expression for predicting recurrence and metastasis of bladder cancer after neoadjuvant chemotherapy and radical cystectomy. Clin Cancer Res 2000;6:4866–4873.
161 Shirahama T, Arima J, Akiba S, Sakakura C. Relation between cyclooxygenase-2 expression and tumor invasiveness and patient survival in transitional cell carcinoma of the urinary bladder. Cancer 2001;92:188–193.
162 Stein JP, Ginsberg DA, Grossfeld GD, et al. Effect of p21WAF1/CIP1 expression on tumor progression in bladder cancer. J Natl Cancer Inst 1998;90:1072–1079.
163 Migaldi M, Sgambato A, Garagnani L, et al. Loss of p21Waf1 expression is a strong predictor of reduced survival in primary superficial bladder cancers. Clin Cancer Res 2000;6:3131–3138.
164 Korkolopoulou P, Christodoulou P, Konstantinidou AE, Thomas-Tsagli E, Kapralos P, Davaris P. Cell cycle regulators in bladder cancer: a multivariate survival study with emphasis on p27Kip1. Hum Pathol 2000;31:751–760.
165 Kamai T, Takagi K, Asami H, Ito Y, Oshima H, Yoshida KI. Decreasing of p27(Kip1)and cyclin E protein levels is associated with progression from superficial into invasive bladder cancer. Br J Cancer 2001;84:1242–1251.
166 Del Pizzo JJ, Borkowski A, Jacobs SC, Kyprianou N. Loss of cell cycle regulators p27(Kip1) and cyclin E in transitional cell carcinoma of the bladder correlates with tumor grade and patient survival. Am J Pathol 1999;155: 1129–1136.
167 Bringuier PP, Umbas R, Schaafsma HE, Karthaus HF, Debruyne FM, Schalken JA. Decreased E-cadherin immunoreactivity correlates with poor survival in patients with bladder tumors. Cancer Res 1993;53:3241–3245.
168 Otto T, Birchmeier W, Schmidt U, et al. Inverse relation of E-cadherin and autocrine motility factor receptor expression as a prognostic factor in patients with bladder carcinomas. Cancer Res 1994;54:3120–3123.
169 Lipponen PK, Eskelinen MJ. Reduced expression of E-cadherin is related to invasive disease and frequent recurrence in bladder cancer. J Cancer Res Clin Oncol 1995;121:303–308.
170 Syrigos KN, Harrington K, Waxman J, Krausz T, Pignatelli M. Altered gamma-catenin expression correlates with poor survival in patients with bladder cancer. J Urol 1998;160:1889–1893.
171 Byrne RR, Shariat SF, Brown R, et al. E-cadherin immunostaining of bladder transitional cell carcinoma, carcinoma in situ and lymph node metastases with long-term followup. J Urol 2001;165:1473–1479.
172 Miyake H, Eto H, Arakawa S, Kamidono S, Hara I. Over expression of CD44V8-10 in urinary exfoliated cells as an independent prognostic predictor in patients with urothelial cancer. J Urol 2002;167:1282–1287.
173 Hasui Y, Marutsuka K, Asada Y, Osada Y. Prognostic value of urokinase-type plasminogen activator in patients with superficial bladder cancer. Urology 1996;47: 34–37.
174 Shariat SF, Monoski MA, Andrews B, Wheeler TM, Lerner SP, Slawin KM. Association of plasma urokinase-type plasminogen activator and its receptor with clinical outcome in patients undergoing radical cystectomy for transitional cell carcinoma of the bladder. Urology 2003;61:1053–1058.

Part IV
Next Steps: Translational Research

25
The Role of Microarray Technologies in Bladder Cancer Management

Marta Sánchez-Carbayo and Carlos Cordón-Cardo

Contents

Abstract The advent of high-throughput methods of molecular analysis has allowed the comprehensive survey of the epigenetic, genetic and protein profiles characteristic of distinct tumor types, and the identification of targets and pathways that may underlie particular clinical behavior. Microarray technologies represent a means for targets and biomarkers identification in bladder cancer. Several groups have used molecular comprehensive profiling by means of microarray technologies of bladder cancer cell lines and bladder tissues to identify signature candidates that robustly distinguish bladder cancer subclasses, and pathways underlying bladder cancer progression. However, further research is warranted in the field to translate the identification of these molecular targets into potential predictive biomarkers of bladder cancer behavior to be applied into routine clinical practice. The challenge remains to optimize the measurement of these targets on noninvasive specimens and to improve outcome stratification, and finally, the clinical management of bladder cancer patients. This chapter summarizes the targets and role of microarray technologies as discovery and validation platforms of targets and biomarkers for the clinical assessment of patients affected with bladder cancer.

Keywords Bladder cancer, DNA microarrays, Transcript microarrays, Protein arrays, Molecular profiling, Tissue arrays

1. Introduction

The use of high-throughput technologies as a means of discovering specific targets and biomarkers should address the specific clinical needs of the spectrum of diseases that comprise uroepithelial neoplasms. Bladder tumors have been traditionally classified into three main groups with distinct clinical behavior, prognosis, and primary managements: nonmuscle invasive (stages Ta-Tis-T1), deep muscle invasive (stages T2–T4), and metastatic disease (N+/M+) (1). Most of the nonmuscle invasive cases are treated conservatively by transurethral removal of the tumor, with or without adjuvant intravesical chemo- or immuno-therapy. Approximately 20% of the nonmuscle invasive tumors are cured by surgical removal of the presenting lesion (five years, no evidence of disease); 50–70% recurs one or more times, but never progresses into invasive disease; and 10–30%

From: *Current Clinical Urology: Bladder Cancer*, Edited by: C.T. Lee and D.P. Wood,
DOI: 10.1007/978-1-59745-417-9_25, © Humana Press, a part of Springer Science+Business Media, LLC 2010

progresses to invasive and potentially lethal disease. Intravesical bacille Calmette-Guerin (BCG) represents the main treatment of carcinoma in situ or high-grade noninvasive bladder carcinoma (2). Muscle infiltrating tumors are generally treated by cystectomy with or without adjuvant chemotherapy. Patients with invasive disease have a 50% chance of relapse within 2 years of surgery and the shortest overall survival (3). There is a major decision dilemma in identifying patients in whom bladder preservation is possible without compromising overall survival, compared with those who require a more aggressive approach to achieve cure. Approximately 50% of patients with muscle infiltrating tumors already harbor or will develop metastatic disease. For patients with locally advanced and/or distant metastases, chemotherapy is the standard of care; yet, despite responses seen in 50% of the cases, their overall cure is less than 10% (3). Although chemotherapy improves the prognosis for patients with distant metastasis, the vast majority die from their disease. It is expected that the comprehensive amount of information provided by microarrays would support and assess the risk stratification of each of these tumor subtypes to recur, progress, respond to intravesical and chemotherapy treatments and ultimately to survive.

The diagnosis and follow-up of patients with bladder cancer is based on the information provided by cystoscopy, the gold standard, in combination with urinary cytology. Many urinary tumor markers have been evaluated for the detection and surveillance of the disease, providing promising results as adjacent tests to cytology. However, they are neither fully validated nor introduced in clinical practice yet (4). In serum, none of the tumor biomarkers evaluated to date has provided sufficient sensitivity and specificity for the early detection of noninvasive bladder cancer, nor favorable efficacy for predicting relapses, response to chemotherapy, and overall survival in patients with advanced disease. Bladder cancer prognostication is based on pathological stage and grade, tumor size, presence of concomitant carcinoma *in situ*, and multicentricity. The presence of lymphovascular and/or perineural invasion, as well as squamous differentiation is considered a poor prognosticator in bladder cancer (1). Numerous individual molecular markers have been identified in the tissue specimens that correlate to some extent with tumor stage, and possibly with prognosis in bladder cancer. However, these molecular prognosticators do not play a role in the clinical routine management of patients with bladder tumors yet. Thus, the need for development of specific tissue and serum tumor markers for prognostic stratification remains. The advent of high-throughput microarrays technologies allowing comprehensive discovery of targets relevant in bladder cancer progression will accelerate the development of novel approaches for specific drug therapies. Although great achievement has been obtained in the identification of critical targets, further investigation is warranted to translate and validate novel biomarkers specific for bladder cancer patients based on the molecular alterations of tumor progression, and multiplexed strategies for their clinical management.

2. High-Throughput Profiling Using Array Technologies

The initial development of array technologies focused on transcript comprehensive platforms. The versatility of the array design has allowed improvement in the printing and labelling strategies to adapt multiplexing measurement to other nucleic acids and even to proteins and specific peptides. This section summarizes the experimental designs and achievements obtained by each of these technologies in the discovery and validation of targets and biomarkers proven to be potentially useful clinically, along the progression of the bladder cancer. The initial transcript profiling studies using cDNA and oligonucleotide arrays is being complemented by profiling analyses at the DNA level (either using CGH or SNP arrays), and furthermore by means of protein profiling using antibody and protein arrays (Fig. 25.1).

(a) Transcript based arrays

(1) *Using in vitro models.* Expression profiling using bladder cancer cell lines has been used to gain insight into the molecular events associated with the disease. Targets identified differentially expressed in the cells have been shown to be of clinical relevance when validated on human specimens of patients with bladder cancer. It has been possible to assign potential functional roles to novel genes in both the signalling pathways controlling bladder cancer development and the phenotypic changes associated with the same.. The technology can be applied to *gene and pathway discovery* in bladder cancer associated with exposure of bladder cancer cell lines to several anti-neoplastic drugs. Tumor cell growth inhibition mediated by genistein was induced in the susceptible bladder tumor line

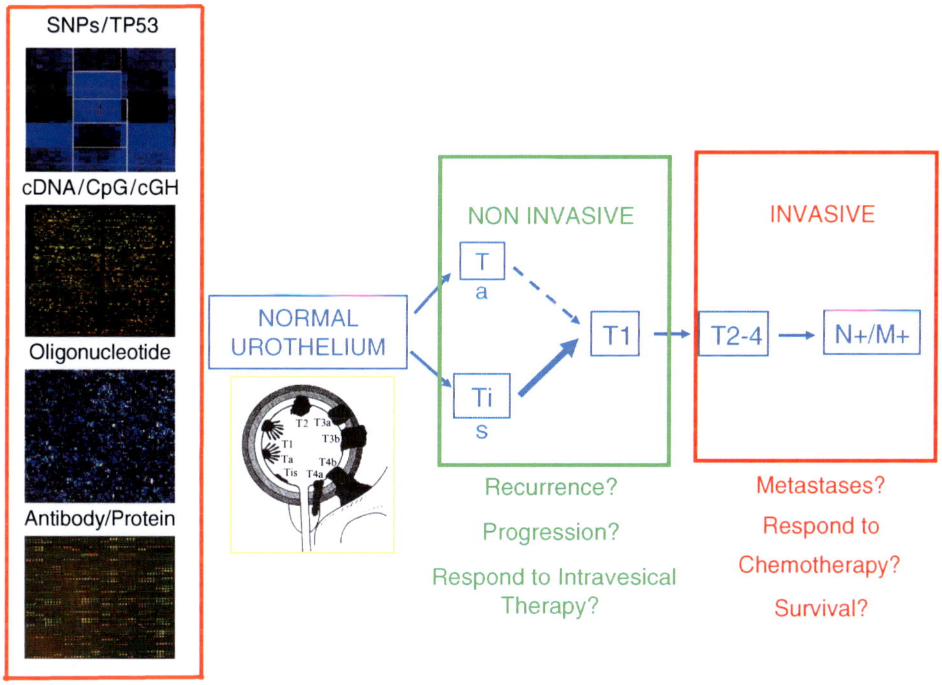

FIG. 25.1. Differential high-throughput strategies utilized for molecular profiling of bladder cancer at the DNA (CpG, CGH, SNP and TP53), RNA (oligonucleotide and cDNA) and protein (antibody and protein) level. Combined strategies of these technologies would enhance the clinical management of patients with bladder cancer to address the clinical needs of patients affected by noninvasive and muscular invasive disease

TCCSUP. Expression profiling was then analyzed at various time points, using cDNA chips. Among the many groups of genes involved in cell growth and cell cycle, a transient induction of EGR-1 was observed, relating to this event as proliferation and differentiation effects (5).

The effects of DNA methylation inhibitors, such as 5-aza-2'-deoxycytidine (5-Aza-CdR) treatment on human fibroblast cells (LD419) and a human bladder tumor cell line (T24) have also been monitored by transcript profiling. Such an approach revealed the presence of hypermethylation of the promoters of cancer-related genes (often associated with their inactivation during tumorigénesis). More genes were induced in tumorigenic cells (61 genes induced; >or = fourfold) than nontumorigenic cells (34 genes induced; >or = fourfold). Approximately 60% of induced genes did not have CpG islands within their 5' regions, suggesting that some genes activated by 5-Aza-CdR may not result from the direct inhibition of promoter methylation. Interestingly, a high percentage of genes activated in both cell types belonged to the IFN signaling pathway, confirming data from other tumor cell types (6). The clinical relevance of the study related to preclinical and clinical trials developed to use 5-Aza-CdR in attempts to reactivate silenced genes in human cancers.

Resistance to cis-diamminedichloroplatinum (II) (cisplatin) has been analyzed using two pairs of parental and cisplatin-resistant bladder cancer cell lines and cDNA microarrays. Among molecules regulating acquisition of resistance, a markedly reduced expression of inositol 1,4,5-trisphosphate (IP3) receptor type1 (IP3R1), endoplasmic reticulum membrane protein was found in cisplatin-resistant cells. The suppression of IP3R1 expression using small interfering RNA in parental cells prevented apoptosis and resulted in decreased sensitivity to cisplatin. Contrarily, overexpression of IP3R1 in resistant cells induced apoptosis and increased sensitivity to cisplatin. These results suggest that cisplatin-induced downregulation of IP3R1 expression was closely associated with the acquisition of cisplatin resistance in bladder cancer cells (7).

Another line of research has identified and monitored by means of DNA arrays, the pathways regulated after expression of critical genes involved in bladder progression. The reduced expression of the GDP dissociation inhibitor, RhoGDI2, has been shown to be associated with decreased survival of patients with advanced bladder cancer (8) and critical in lung metastasis. The effectors by which RhoGDI2 affects metastasis can be addressed by DNA microarrays to identify genes suppressed by RhoGDI2 reconstitution in lung metastatic bladder cancer cell lines. Among RNAs that also increase with the tumor stage in human bladder cancer samples, levels of endothelin-1 (ET-1), a potent vasoconstrictor, were affected by both RhoGDI2 reconstitution and tumor stage. To test the hypothesis that the endothelin axis is important in lung metastasis, lung metastatic bladder carcinoma cells were injected in mice treated with the endothelin receptor-specific antagonist, atrasentan, thereby blocking engagement of the up-regulated ET-1 ligand with its cognate receptor. Endothelin antagonism resulted in a dramatic reduction of lung metastases, similar to the effect of reexpressing RhoGDI2 in these metastatic cells. This study poses an approach of identifying therapeutic targets downstream of metastasis suppressor genes. The data also suggest that blockade of the ET-1 axis may prevent lung metastasis, a new therapeutic concept that warrants clinical evaluation (9). In order to link experimental and clinical evidence of the molecular mechanisms underlining pulmonary metastasis in bladder cancer, progressively more metastatic human bladder cancer cell lines and an in vivo bladder-cancer lung-metastasis model were developed. Such in vitro and in vivo systems were used to identify with oligonucleotide microarrays of genes of which the expression levels change according to the degree of pulmonary metastatic potential. The magnitude of gene expression changes observed during the metastatic transition correlated with the in vivo propensity for earlier lung colonization and decreased host survival. To additionally define which genes found in the experimental system were of relevance to human bladder cancer lung metastasis, gene expression profiles of 23 primary human bladder tumors of various stages and grades were evaluated and compared to the altered profiles in the model cell lines. Expression of epiregulin, urokinase-type plasminogen activator (uPA), matrix metalloproteinase (MMP)14, and tissue inhibitor of metalloproteinase (TIMP-2) were consistently and progressively up-regulated when viewed as a function of tumor stage in tissues of patients vs. the metastatic potential seen in the mouse lung model. The strong correlation of these four markers between the experimental and clinical material helped to validate this system as a useful tool for the study of lung metastasis and to define targets of therapy that may reduce the incidence of this process in such type of patients (10).

Addressing genes critical in bladder tumorigenesis includes analyses of transcript profiles after expression of the bladder tumor suppressor locus at 9q33.1 harboring the deleted gene in bladder cancer 1 (DBC1) , whose function is currently unknown. Transfection of DBC1 in a nonexpressing human bladder cancer cell line and assessing its effect on global expression patterns using cDNA microarrays revealed induced expression of 26 genes including plasminogen activator inhibitor 2, heparin-binding EGF-like growth factor precursor, small proline-rich protein 2B, metallothionein 1 isoforms, tissue-type plasminogen activator precursor and urokinase-type plasminogen activator precursor. The expression levels of these genes in 14 human bladder tumors were analyzed by real-time quantitative PCR using gene-specific primers for selected genes. Thus, this study linked the involvement of DBC1 to the urokinase-plasminogen pathway, and was validated by an independent method, in this case by RT-PCR that related genes which were clinically relevant for patients with bladder cancer (11).

An example of the *functional classification of genes* applied to bladder cancer is the study comparing the expression patterns of p53-mediated apoptosis in resistant cancer cell lines vs. sensitive ones using cDNA arrays. The ECV-304 bladder carcinoma cell line was selected for resistance to p53 by repeated infections with a p53 recombinant adenovirus Ad5CMV-p53. A number of potential p53 transcription or related targets were identified playing roles in cell cycle regulation, DNA repair, redox control, cell adhesion, apoptosis, and differentiation. Proline oxidase, a mitochondrial enzyme involved in the proline/pyrroline-5-carboxylate redox cycle, was identified and upregulated in sensitive but not in resistant cells. Further experiments showed the implication of proline oxidase and the proline/P5C pathway in p53-induced growth suppression and apoptosis (12). By addressing the role of p53 in regulating apoptosis in resistant cancer cells, this study identifies genes that represent candidate targets to evaluate therapeutic resistance in human bladder tumors.

The expression profiling of nine bladder cancer cell lines has been compared against a pool containing equal RNA quantities of each of them using cDNA arrays. Hierarchical clustering classified these tumor cells according to the histopathological characteristics of the tumors from which they were derived. Caveolin-1 and keratin 10 were differentially expressed in a squamous carcinoma cell line and certain invasive tumor cell lines when compared to cells derived from a papillary noninvasive bladder tumor. Interestingly, the expression of these genes in primary bladder tumors spotted on tissue microarrays was significantly associated with squamous differentiation, histopathological stage, and tumor grade. Additionally, when a bootstrapping resampling technique was applied on hierarchical clustering, the cells were grouped together based on their p53, RB and INK4A status. E-cadherin, zyxin and moesin were identified as genes differentially expressed in these clusters. Interestingly, the expression of these genes was significantly associated with the histopathological stage and tumor grade in bladder tumors as well (13). These results revealed that molecular profiling of clustered bladder cancer was based on histopathogenesis and biological criteria. Moreover gene profiling identified novel biomarkers of the disease that were proven to be associated with clinical and histopathological variables when validated on tumor specimens using immunohistochemistry on tissue microarrays (13).

(2) *Using clinical specimens.* Microarray studies have been used to correlate changes in the expression of specific genes and groups of genes with bladder cancer phenotypes of bladder tumors. Following the biological validation of these gene expression-phenotype correlations, the result will be a more complete list of the genes controlling cancer development and progression. Gene expression profiling of bladder cancer tissues has identified signature genes that robustly distinguish bladder cancer subclasses. Such signature genes would ideally provide a molecular basis for classification and also yield insight into the molecular events underlying the different bladder cancer clinical phenotypes.

The studies dealing with molecular classification of bladder cancer expression profiling using DNA microarrays have been increasing in the past years. The first report monitored the expression patterns of noninvasive and invasive tumor cell suspensions prepared from 36 normal and 29 bladder tumor biopsies using oligonucleotide microarrays. Pools of cells made from normal urothelium as well as pools of tumors of different stages varying from pTA grade I and II and pT2 grade III and IV bladder cancer specimens were analyzed (14). Hierarchical clustering of gene expression levels grouped bladder cancer specimens based on tumor stage and grade. By organizing genes with a similar expression patterns into clusters, several functionally related genes were identified. The most significant were obtained by examining log-fold change of expression and included genes involved in cell cycle, cell growth, immunology, cell adhesion, transcription and proteinases genes clustering into separate groups. Noninvasive papillary tumors showed increased expression of transcription factors, ribosomal and proteinase encoding genes. Invasive tumors showed increased levels of cell cycle- and immunology- related transcripts and lower cellular adhesion related mRNAs (14).

The combination of separate expression profiling studies of bladder tumors and bladder cancer cell lines has allowed the identification of KiSS-1 as a critical target in bladder cancer progression (15). Lower transcript levels of KiSS-1 were observed in bladder carcinomas as compared to noninvasive tumors and these ratios provided prognostic information. Lower expression of this gene was also observed in cells derived from advanced bladder tumors (13). The analysis of the expression patterns of KiSS-1 by in situ hybridization on tissue microarrays confirmed the loss of KiSS-1 in the progression of the disease and was associated with tumor stage, grade and overall survival. In this example, gene expression profiling identified a novel metastasis suppressor gene involved in bladder cancer progression with clinical relevance to clinical outcome stratification (15).

One of the most extensive expression profiling studies of bladder tumors reported to date has dealt with the development of a predictive classifier of Ta, T1, T2+ bladder carcinoma subclasses. The use of a support vector machine algorithm allowed prediction with 75% accuracy of these tumor subclasses in an independent set of patients. This report revealed the diagnostic and prognostic potential of bladder tumor profiling using cross-validation strategies to evaluate the clinical impact of the classifier defined using independent training and validation series of tumors. Smad6 and cyclin G2 were also identified as Ta/T1 classifier genes and their immunostaining patterns were validated on tissue microarrays by immunohistochemistry (16).

Progression into invasive disease has also been assessed in another set of gene profiles of invasive (17) and noninvasive (18) human bladder tumors from 34 patients using a commercial Clontech cDNA arrays (1185 genes). A subset of cases was contrasted with oligonucleotide Affymetrix GeneChip commercial platform (22,283 probes) and real-time reverse transcription-PCR. A subset of 41 genes validated by the oligonucleotide array classified tumor samples according to clinical outcome as noninvasive, invasive, or metastasizing. Relevant findings supported: (a) a clonal origin of noninvasive tumors, (b) highly similar gene expression patterns in different areas of invasive tumors, and (c) an invasive-like pattern observed in bladder mucosas derived from patients with locally advanced disease. In noninvasive bladder tumors, increased mRNA levels of genes encoding transcription factors, molecules involved in protein synthesis and metabolism, and some proteins involved in cell cycle progression and differentiation were observed. Transcripts for immune, extracellular matrix, adhesion, peritumoral stroma and muscle tissue components, proliferation, and cell cycle controllers were up-regulated in invasive tumors (19). Gene expression profiles of bladder tumors obtained using different platforms were consistent among themselves and also with previous reports (14).

Following the discovery of RhoGDI2 as a metastasis suppressor gene by in vivo models of bladder cancer, the expression and distribution of its encoded protein was evaluated in normal human tissues and cell lines by means of Affymetrix and tissue microarrays ($n = 51$), respectively. RhoGDI2 mRNA was inversely related to the invasive and metastatic phenotype in human bladder cancer cell lines. In patients with bladder cancer, reduced tumor RhoGDI2 transcript and protein expression was associated with worse 5-year disease-free and disease-specific survival, this latter even by multivariate analyses (20). Oligonucleotide arrays of tumor specimens along with bladder progression served to validate an in vivo model of pulmonary metastases in bladder cancer, whose investigation at the molecular level suffers from the poor availability of human metastatic tumor tissue and the absence of suitable animal models (10).

The relevance of Fibroblast growth factor receptor 3 (FGFR3) in urinary bladder carcinomas has also been addressed by means of gene profiling of 22 urinary bladder carcinomas at different stages (pTa, pT1, and pT2) and 7 nonneoplastic tissue controls together with immunohistochemistry on tissue arrays ($n = 237$). Overexpression of FGFR3 mRNA was found in pTa and pT1 stages (fold change >8) and in pT2 tumors (fold change >4). Nonneoplastic urinary bladder samples did not express FGFR3 protein. With respect to immunohistochemistry, FGFR3 was positive in 71.4% of pTa, 72% of pT1, and 49.2% of pT2 cases. In vitro studies reveal that the proliferative activity of the RT-112 cell line was inhibited with monoclonal antibodies against FGFR3. This report supported the important role of FGFR3 in transitional cell carcinoma development and as a therapeutic target (21).

The two pathways, papillary and nonpapillary, by which bladder cancer develops in the urothelial lining from intraurothelial preneoplasia have also been analyzed by means of gene expression patterns of 19 pairs of RNA samples from adjacent urothelium and tumors were analyzed using cDNA microarrays. Seven gene clusters controlling proliferation, differentiation, and programmed cell death that were common for papillary and nonpapillary cancer, were identified. In contrast, genes controlling cellular and stromal interactions were altered in the nonpapillary cancer. When validated by immunohistochemistry on tissue microarrays ($n = 251$), tumors characterized by the low expression of e-cadherin and the high expression of DNA alpha-topoisomerase II had a high propensity for distant metastasis and were associated with poor survival (17).

High-density oligonucleotide microarrays (59,619 genes and expressed sequence tags (ESTs)) have been used to identify a 45-gene signature of disease progression in a training set of 29 bladder cancer patients (13 without later disease progression and 16 with later disease progression). An independent test set (74 noninvasive tumor samples) using in house-fabricated 60-mer oligonucleotide microarrays served to monitor this progression signature, with a significant correlation between classifications and clinical outcomes ($P < 0.03$). Differentially expressed genes were involved in regulating apoptosis, cell differentiation, and cell cycle and hence may represent potential therapeutic targets. It may be possible to identify patients with a high risk of disease progression at an early stage using a molecular signature present already in the noninvasive tumors (22).

Molecular profiling of 80 bladder tumors, nine bladder cancer cell lines, and three normal bladder samples using cDNA microarrays (10,368 genes) served to identify differentially expressed genes along the course of disease progression. Unsupervised hierarchical clustering successfully separated the samples into two subgroups containing noninvasive vs. muscle-invasive tumors, supported by a 90.5% success rate by supervised techniques. Tumors could also be classified into transitional vs. squamous subtypes (89% success rate) and good vs. bad prognosis (78% success rate). The performance of stage classifiers was confirmed in silico using data from an independent tumor set. Immunohistochemistry validation on tissue microarrays was performed for cathepsin E, cyclin A2, and parathyroid hormone-related protein (18).

The changes in gene expression occurring during the neoplastic transition from normal bladder urothelium to primary Ta tumors using DNA microarrays have served to identify early events in tumorigenesis. Among the mostly changed genes between normal bladder and Ta tumors, genes related to the cytoskeleton (keratin 7 and syndecan 1), and transcription (high mobility group AT-hook 1) were identified. Altered genes in high-grade tumors were related to cell cycle (cyclin-dependent kinase 4) and transcription (jun d proto-oncogene). The presence of high keratin 7 transcript expression was validated at the protein level in the tissues by Western blotting analysis revealing three major molecular isoforms, which could also be detected in urine sediments (23).

Genetic signatures characteristic of aggressive clinical behavior in advanced bladder tumors have also been identified by transcript profiling of 52 normal urothelium, 33 noninvasive and 72 invasive tumors using oligonucleotide arrays. Unsupervised clustering classified them with 82.2% accuracy, while predictive algorithms rendered an 89%-correct rate for tumor staging using genes differentially expressed between noninvasive and invasive tumors. Accuracies of 82% and 90% were obtained for predicting overall survival when considering all patients with bladder cancer or only patients with invasive disease, respectively. A genetic profile consisting of 174 probes was identified in those patients with positive lymph nodes and poor survival. Two independent Global Test runs confirmed the robust association of this profile with lymph node metastases and overall survival simultaneously. Identification of this poor outcome profile could assist in selecting patients who may benefit from more aggressive therapeutic intervention. Target validation of synuclein by immunohistochemistry on tissue arrays (n = 294) sustained its association with tumor staging and outcome (24).

Expression profiling of 166 bladder tumor samples revealed a fivefold up-expression of human transcription factor SOX4 vs. 27 normal urothelium samples. Strong SOX4 protein expression by immunohistochemistry on a tissue array (n = 2,360) was correlated with increased patient survival. Overexpression of SOX4 in the bladder cell line HU609 strongly impaired cell viability and promoted apoptosis. Downstream target genes containing a SOX4-binding motif in the promoter sequence were characterized by means of a time-course global expression study of the overexpressed SOX4. SOX4-induced genes were involved in signal transduction (*MAP2K5*), angiogenesis (*NRP2*), and cell cycle arrest (*PIK3R3*) among others (25).

Comparison of gene profiles of small subsets of noninvasive (n = 6) and invasive (n = 6) tumors using cDNA arrays (14,551 clones) have identified genetic signatures reported in larger series. Up-regulation of 40 genes was associated with cases of noninvasive tumors, including FGFR3 or AIG1 and others involved in epithelial cell dedifferentiation and keratinization, as well as genes related to cell cycle, cell adhesion, transcription, and apoptosis. Conversely, significant up-regulation of 34 genes was associated with cases of invasive TCC, including VEGFC or MMP7 and others related to extracellular matrix degradation, immune responses, cell cycling, and angiogenesis (26).

Thus, several independent studies have analyzed tumor specimens of different stages, and identified gene signatures overlapping to a certain extent. The use of either a cDNA or oligonucleotide platforms is providing concordant results among them. The main differences may be attributed to the diverse clinic-pathological variables of the cases under study as well as each specific experimental design and the data analyses approaches undertaken. Multi-institutional analyses comparing patients from different stages, centers, and platforms on more focused arrays will in the near future define the clinical relevance of specific signatures in each of the steps along bladder cancer progression. By limiting the number of genes analyzed, it will potentially be possible to translate the specific bladder cancer gene signatures into useful tools for the diagnosis and clinical stratification of patients with bladder cancer.

(b) DNA based microarrays

In addition to transcriptome expression arrays, specific oligonucleotide microarrays have been applied to the study of DNA variation in clinical material to address tumor progression biomarkers in bladder cancer. Multiple probes of short length that differ in sequence at a single base have been designed to identify simple polymorphisms and allelic variations in DNA.

The primary applications of these types of microarrays have dealt with automated high-throughput identification of mutations in medically important genes such as TP53, a valuable predictor for bladder cancer outcome (27); and in the genotyping of single nucleotide polymorphisms (SNP) (28). Not only do SNP arrays confirm known areas of chromosomal losses, but they may also identify areas with common allelic imbalances and loss of heterozygosity loci that could harbor potential tumor suppressors in bladder cancer (28). Using a 10K SNP Affymetrix array in 37 microdissected bladder tumors, allelic imbalances and clonality were found to be strongly stage-dependent. Novel unstable chromosomal were identified at chromosomes 6q, 10p, 16q, 20p, 20q, and 22q. The tumors were separated into two distinct groups: highly stable tumors (all Ta tumors) and unstable tumors (2/3 muscle-invasive). All 11 unstable tumors had lost chromosome 17p areas and 90% chromosome 8 areas affecting Netrin-1/UNC5D/MAP2K4 genes as well as others. Allelic imbalance (AI) was present at the TP53 locus in 10 out of 11 unstable tumors, whereas six had homozygous TP53 mutations. The tumor distribution pattern reflected AI as seven out of eight patients with additional upper urinary tract tumors had genomic stable bladder tumors ($P < 0.05$). These data show the power of high-resolution SNP arrays for defining clinically relevant AIs (29). The initial chips were restricted to the polymorphic areas contained in the arrays of a few thousands of SNPs; currently high-density SNP microarrays for predefined chromosomal locations of larger regions of more than 300K and 500K SNPs have already been fabricated, making previously unknown areas quantified and informative.

Microarrays can also be used to define gene copy number changes based on cohybridization of labeled experimental and normal DNA to an array of genomic DNA. This technique is well suited to high-throughput whole genome detection of chromosomal gains and losses at high resolution, enabling rapid detection of homozygous loss that allows molecular phenotyping of tumors based on underlying abnormalities and detection of amplicons that may potentially be associated with overexpression of oncogenes. This provides a significant advantage over laborious pregenome mapping and transcript identification strategies. An additional advantage of this approach is that probes may be generated using paraffin-embedded material, greatly expanding the available specimens for analysis. This feature can allow study of genetic changes in tumor progression. The application of high-throughput CGH arrays has served to confirm transcriptome alterations at the genomic level in a similar comprehensive detailed manner. For example, the use of combined spectral karyotyping (SKY) and CGH in an invasive and metastatic variant of the T24 human bladder cell line has served to gain additional insights into the repertoire of genetic changes that may be responsible for the invasive and metastatic phenotype of these cells (8). This study identified 12p, a region of agreement among technologies harboring RhoGDI2, a candidate gene, whose expression inversely correlates with bladder tumor progression and metastasis (8–10), demonstrating the usefulness of this multimodal approach in identifying potential genetic changes that may be responsible for the invasive phenotype. Genome-wide profiles of 98 bladder tumors of diverse stages (29 pT(a), 14 pT1, 55 pT(2–4)) and grades (21 low-grade and eight high-grade noninvasive tumors) by array-based CGH (2,464 clones) showed significant increases in copy number alterations and genomic instability with increasing stage and with outcome. Array-based CGH identified quantitative and qualitative differences in DNA copy number alterations at high resolution according to the tumor stage and grade. (30).

To our knowledge, the use of high-throughput screening of bladder cancer related specimens using methylation arrays has not been reported to date. The use of such a comprehensive approach would potentially reveal novel hypermethylation targets that may be silenced and have a critical regulatory role in tumor progression (Fig. 1). The combination of SNP, CGH and CpG arrays would potentially reveal novel critical oncogenes and tumor suppressors in tumorigenesis and bladder cancer progression.

(c) Protein based arrays

Microarrays represent a convenient platform for assays involving biomolecules other than nucleic acids (31). Arrays of peptides, antibodies, proteins, and even cells have been developed (31, 32). This is further evidence of the strength and versatility of high throughput screening. These should provide means of rapidly validating at the protein level, the genes identified by expression profiling using DNA microarrays. Thus, comparative fluorescence can not only measure the relative abundance of genetic sequences, but also estimxate many antigens, once specific antibody solutions are printed on the surface of derivatized surfaces. Antibody and protein microarrays have been applied to protein profiling of cancer tissue or antibody-based detection of multiple antigens (31, 32). Toward the development of such capability, it is possible to use a practical strategy for the use of antibody microarrays for highly parallel screening of potential progression biomarkers in human serum. Very recently the use of protein profiling using antibody arrays for bladder cancer on serum specimens has been described (33). This study reports how antibody arrays can utilize the information provided by expression profiling to design targeted antibody arrays for detecting specific clinical behaviors. The highly efficient protein detection method will lead to the discovery of new and clinically useful protein biomarkers of outcome prediction for bladder cancer patients (33).

Genomic and proteomic tools can also be complimented by the use of array-based high-throughput approaches to survey tumor biopsies for a large number of individual patients. Tissue microarrays are constructed by removing cylindrical tissue samples from donor blocks and placed onto a single block with defined array coordinates (34, 35). In combination with the associated patient clinical data, this technology significantly accelerates the transition of target discovery into clinical applications (34, 35). Tissue arrays can serve to validate progression targets identified using DNA and antibody microarrays, as shown above. Tissue arrays may prove the bladder specificity at the microanatomical level, of the top discriminatory genes identified by gene profiling antibodies printed on antibody arrays by an independent method: immunohistochemistry. Moreover, they will serve to evaluate associations of targets with stage, grade and survival on independent cohorts of bladder cancer patients. In addition to validation of gene profiling analyses (Table 1), several reports have used tissue arrays also as independent studies to evaluate associations of protein expression to clinico-pathological variables. The application of tissue microarrays represents a high-throughput approach for validation of novel potential markers for bladder cancer by immunohistochemistry or fluorescence in situ hybridization in paraffin blocks. This approach allows further characterization of novel genes by in situ hybridization of ESTs and known genes when specific antibodies are not available to study their potential clinical relevance. They have served to validate the relevance of cyclin E amplification (36), 8q24 amplification on bladder tumors and metastases (37). In such studies it was possible to correlate DNA and protein profiles by immunohistochemistry for cyclin E (36), or linking 8q24 amplification to known protein expression patterns of known prognostic biomarkers in bladder cancer, such as p53 and Ki67 (37). Focus is intensified within this field to automate construction of tissue microarrays, automating readout of expression patterns and development of frozen tissue microarrays.

TABLE 25.1. Summary of markers identified by gene profiling and/or validated by tissue arrays. Reference describing the finding is shown in parenthesis.

Progression	Survival
Caveolin-1 (13)	Moesin (13)
Keratin 10 (13)	Rho GDI2 (20)
E-cadherin (13, 17)	Cyclin E (36)
Zyxin (13)	8q24 (37)
DBC 1 (11)	Clusterin (38)
FGFR3 (21)	
Keratin 7 (23)	
Smad4 (16)	
Cyclin G2 (16)	
Cathepsin E (18)	
Cyclin A2 (18)	
PTH (18)	
KiSS-1 (15)	
COX2 (39)	
Epiregulin (10)	
Urokinase plasminogen activator (10)	
Matrix metalloproteinase MMP14	
Tissue inhibitor of metalloproteinase TIMP2	
Synuclein (24)	
DNA topoisomerase II (17)	

Following the initial extensive tissue microarray studies in bladder cancer, in more than 2,000 bladder carcinomas, the prognostic utility of cyclin E in bladder cancer (36), and SOX4 (25) was revealed. The immunohistochemistry approach has also revealed associations of protein expression patterns of novel targets with tumor progression. SFRP1 loss was associated with higher tumor stage and grade and shorter overall survival. In addition, loss of sFRP1 was an independent indicator of poor survival in patients with papillary but not with muscle invasive bladder cancer (40). Higher cyclooxygenase 2 (COX2) staining was seen in muscle invasive urothelial TCC as compared to muscle invasive squamous cell carcinomas. COX2 protein expression was associated with advanced tumor stage, high-grade, solid growth pattern in invasive TCC, high Ki-67 labeling index, and positive p53 staining (39). Loss of p16 was associated with reduced progression-free in minimally invasive tumors (41), while clusterin has been revealed as an univariate survival predictive factor in muscle-invasive urothelial carcinoma (38).

3. Conclusions

Microarray technologies are certainly having a great impact in bladder cancer research. Combined experimental designs of these technologies varying from analyses in bladder cancer cell lines, tissues and body fluids are allowing identification of critical targets and signatures associated with tumorigenesis and cancer progression. The advent of high-throughput technologies has so far mainly allowed the comprehensive identification of such molecular targets specific for bladder cancer. This identification process may result not only in a better understanding of the biology associated with tumorigenesis and tumor progression, but also improve the clinical management of patients affected with bladder cancer. The challenge remains in evaluating the impact of such targets for therapeutics development and translating such information into progression and outcome biomarkers to improve early detection, clinical outcome risk stratification and monitorization of bladder cancer patients. Integrative efforts of the complementary message obtained through the diverse technologies at the DNA, RNA and protein level together with multi-institutional validation collaboration studies would result in noninvasive methods for clinical management as well as targeted and tailored therapies based on the aggressiveness of each specific bladder tumor.

References

1. Reuter VE. Bladder: Risk and prognostic factors–a pathologist' perspective. Urol Clin North Am. 26:481–492, 1999.
2. Palou J, Sanchez-Martin FM, Rosales A, et al. Intravesical bacille Calmette-Guerin in the treatment of carcinoma in situ or high-grade superficial bladder carcinoma after radiotherapy for bladder carcinoma. BJU Int. 83:429–431, 1999.
3. Bajorin DF, Dodd PM, Mazumdar M, et al. Long-term survival in metastatic transitional-cell carcinoma and prognostic factors predicting outcome of therapy. J Clin Oncol. 17:3173–3181, 1999.
4. Lotan Y, Roehrborn CG. Sensitivity and specificity of commonly available bladder tumor markers versus cytology: results of a comprehensive literature review and meta-analyses. Urology. 61:109–118, 2003.
5. Chen CC, Shieh B, Jin YT, et al. Microarray profiling of gene expression patterns in bladder tumor cells treated with genistein. J Biomed Sci. 8:214–222, 2001.
6. Liang G, Gonzales FA, Jones PA, et al. Analysis of gene induction in human fibroblasts and bladder cancer cells exposed to the methylation inhibitor 5-aza-2'-deoxycytidine. Cancer Res. 62:961–966, 2002.
7. Tsunoda T, Koga H, Yokomizo A, et al. Inositol 1,4,5--trisphosphate (IP3) receptor type1 (IP3R1) modulates the acquisition of cisplatin resistance in bladder cancer cell lines. Oncogene. 24:1396–1402, 2005.
8. Harding MA, Arden KC, Gildea JW, et al. Functional genomic comparison of lineage-related human bladder cancer cell lines with differing tumorigenic and metastatic potentials by spectral karyotyping, comparative genomic hybridization, and a novel method of positional expression profiling. Cancer Res. 62:6981–6989, 2002.
9. Titus B, Frierson HF, Jr, Conaway M, et al. Endothelin axis is a target of the lung metastasis suppressor gene RhoGDI2. Cancer Res. 65:7320–7327, 2005.
10. Nicholson BE, Frierson HF, Conaway MR, et al. Profiling the evolution of human metastatic bladder cancer. Cancer Res. 64:7813–7821, 2004.
11. Louhelainen JP, Hurst CD, Pitt E, et al. DBC1 re-expression alters the expression of multiple components of the plasminogen pathway. Oncogene. 25:2409–2419, 2006.
12. Maxwell SA, Davies GE. Differential gene expression in p53-mediated apoptosis-resistant vs. apoptosis-sensitive tumor cell lines. Proc Natl Acad Sci U S A. 97:13009–13014, 2000.
13. Sanchez-Carbayo M, Socci ND, Charytonowicz E, et al. Molecular profiling of bladder cancer using cDNA microarrays: defining histogenesis and biological phenotypes. Cancer Res. 62:6973–6980, 2002.
14. Thykjaer T, Workman C, Kruhoffer M, et al. Identification of gene expression patterns in superficial and invasive human bladder cancer. Cancer Res. 61:2492–2499, 2001.
15. Sanchez-Carbayo M, Capodieci P, Cordon- Cardo C. Tumor suppressor role of KiSS-1 in bladder cancer: Loss of KiSS-1 expression is associated with bladder cancer progression and clinical outcome. Am J Pathol. 162: 609–618, 2003.
16. Dyrskjot L, Thykjaer T, Kruhoffer M, et al. Identifying distinct classes of bladder carcinoma using microarrays. Nat Gen. 33: 90–96, 2003.
17. Kim JH, Tuziak T, Hu L, et al. Alterations in transcription clusters underlie development of bladder cancer along papillary and nonpapillary pathways. Lab Invest. 85:532–549, 2005.
18. Blaveri E, Simko JP, Korkola JE, et al. Bladder cancer outcome and subtype classification by gene expression. Clin Cancer Res. 11:4044–4055, 2005.
19. Modlich O, Prisack HB, Pitschke G, et al. Identifying superficial, muscle-invasive, and metastasizing transitional cell carcinoma of the bladder: use of cDNA array analysis of gene expression profiles. Clin Cancer Res. 10:3410–3421, 2004.
20. Theodorescu D, Sapinoso LM, Conaway MR, et al. Reduced expression of metastasis suppressor RhoGDI2 is associated with decreased survival for patients with bladder cancer. Clin Cancer Res. 10:3800–3806, 2004.
21. Gomez-Roman JJ, Saenz P, Molina M, et al. Fibroblast growth factor receptor 3 is overexpressed in urinary tract carcinomas and modulates the neoplastic cell growth. Clin Cancer Res. 11:459–465, 2005.
22. Dyrskjot L, Zieger K, Kruhoffer M, et al. A molecular signature in superficial bladder carcinoma predicts clinical outcome. Clin Cancer Res. 11:4029–4036, 2005.
23. Aaboe M, Marcussen N, Jensen KM, et al. Gene expression profiling of noninvasive primary urothelial tumours using microarrays. Br J Cancer. 93:1182–1190, 2005.

24. Sanchez-Carbayo M, Socci ND, Lozano J, et al. Defining molecular profiles of poor outcome in patients with invasive bladder cancer using oligonucleotide microarrays. J Clin Oncol. 24:778–789, 2006.
25. Aaboe M, Birkenkamp-Demtroder K, Wiuf C, et al. SOX4 expression in bladder carcinoma: clinical aspects and in vitro functional characterization. Cancer Res. 66:3434–3442, 2006.
26. Elsamman E, Fukumori T, Ewis AA, et al. Differences in gene expression between noninvasive and invasive transitional cell carcinoma of the human bladder using complementary deoxyribonucleic acid microarray: preliminary results. Urol Oncol. 24:109–115, 2006.
27. Lu M, Wikman F, Orntoft TF, et al. Impact of alterations affecting the p53 pathway in bladder cancer on clinical outcome, assessed by conventional and array-based methods. Clin Cancer Res. 8:171–179, 2002.
28. Primdahl H, Wikman FP, von der Maase H, et al. Allelic imbalances in human bladder cancer: genome-wide detection with high-density single-nucleotide polymorphism arrays. J Natl Cancer Inst. 94:216–223, 2002.
29. Koed K, Wiuf C, Christensen LL, et al. High-density single nucleotide polymorphism array defines novel stage and location-dependent allelic imbalances in human bladder tumors. Cancer Res. 65:34–45, 2005.
30. Blaveri E, Brewer JL, Roydasgupta R, et al. Bladder cancer stage and outcome by array-based comparative genomic hybridization. Clin Cancer Res. 117012–117022.
31. Pandey A, Mann M. Proteomics to study genes and genomes. Nature 405:837–846, 2000.
32. Haab BB, Dunham MJ, Brown PO. Protein microarrays for highly parallel detection and quantitation of specific proteins and antibodies in complex solutions. Genome Biol. 2:1–4, 2001
33. Sanchez-Carbayo M, Socci ND, Lozano JJ, et al. Profiling bladder cancer using targeted antibody arrays. Am J Pathol. 168:93–103, 2006.
34 Kononen J, Bubendorf L, Kallioniemi A, et al. Tissue microarrays for high-throughput molecular profiling of tumor specimens. Nat Med. 4:844–847, 1998.
35. Nocito A, Bubendorf L, Tinner EM, et al. Microarrays of bladder cancer tissue are highly representative of proliferation index and histological grade. J Pathol. 194:349–357, 2001.
36. Richter J, Wagner U, Kononen J, et al. High-throughput tissue microarray analysis of cyclin E gene amplification and overexpression in urinary bladder cancer. Am J Pathol. 157:787–794, 2000.
37. Visapaa H, Seligson D, Eeva M, et al. 8q24 amplification in transitional cell carcinoma of bladder. Appl Immunohistochem Mol Morphol. 11:33–36, 2003.
38. Kruger S, Mahnken A, Kausch I, et al. Value of clusterin immunoreactivity as a predictive factor in muscle-invasive urothelial bladder carcinoma. Urology. 67:105–109, 2006.
39. Wild PJ, Kunz-Schughart LA, Stoehr R, et al. High-throughput tissue microarray analysis of COX2 expression in urinary bladder cancer. Int J Oncol. 27:385–391, 2005.
40. Stoehr R, Wissmann C, Suzuki H, et al. Deletions of chromosome 8p and loss of sFRP1 expression are progression markers of papillary bladder cancer. Lab Invest. 84:465–478, 2004.
41. Kruger S, Mahnken A, Kausch I, Feller AC. p16 immunoreactivity is an independent predictor of tumor progression in minimally invasive urothelial bladder carcinoma. Eur Urol. 47(4):463–467, 2005.Marta Sanchez-Carbayo and Carlos Cordon-Cardo

26
Molecular Pathogenesis of Urothelial Carcinoma and the Development of Novel Therapeutic Strategies

Christopher Y. Thomas and Dan Theodorescu

Contents

Abstract The elucidation of the molecular pathogenesis of urothelial cancers (UC) has helped classify these tumors and identify candidate biomarkers and therapeutic targets. Superficial non-aggressive tumors are characterized by the expression of mutationally activated growth factor signaling molecules whereas the loss of tumor suppressor genes is a typical feature of the higher grade and more invasive tumors. Thus, assays to detect genetic anomalies or associated phenotypic markers assist in the diagnosis and management of the early stage of the disease. For more advanced diseases, the development of agents that interrupt the aberrant growth factor signals or other biochemical effects induced by specific genetic mutations may lead to novel and more effective medical therapies.

Keywords Genetics, Pathogenesis, Classification, Medical therapy

1. Introduction

Recent advances in our understanding of the genetics and molecular biology of urothelial cancers (UC) have provided new insights into the pathogenesis of the disease and also identified candidate biomarkers and therapeutic targets. These tumors appear to evolve through two major genetic pathways defined by the acquisition of specific genetic mutations and an associated clinicopathologic phenotype. A large proportion of the superficial non-aggressive tumors express mutationally activated growth factor signaling molecules whereas more aggressive tumors are typified by inactivation of tumor suppressor genes. The spectrum of genetic and biochemical alterations in UCs provides both an opportunity and challenge for the development of novel therapeutic strategies. Although the appropriate molecular targets may differ from one tumor to the next, the identification of specific

From: *Current Clinical Urology: Bladder Cancer*, Edited by: C.T. Lee and D.P. Wood,
DOI: 10.1007/978-1-59745-417-9_26, © Humana Press, a part of Springer Science+Business Media, LLC 2010

genetic and molecular markers in the tumor cells may allow tailoring of the therapy for individual patients. Efforts to improve tumor response rates include the development of agents that interrupt specific growth factor signaling or biochemical pathways, studies to determine how best to combine new targeted agents with one another and conventional therapies, and the identification and reversal of processes that mediate resistance of tumor cells to these therapies.

2. Molecular Pathogenesis of Urothelial Cancer (UC)

2.1. Genetic Mutations and the Phenotypes of Urothelial Cell Cancers

The current consensus is that urothelial cancers result from the sequential acquisition of somatic genetic mutations that confer the full malignant phenotype (1–4). The genetic aberrations found in these tumors include DNA point mutations which may result in the expression of a mutant protein with altered function; amplification of segments of the chromosome which is frequently driven by a selection for increased expression of a particular protein; and deletions of all or parts of a chromosome that usually reflects a selection for loss or down-regulation of tumor suppressor genes. The latter creates a loss of heterozygosity (LOH) for the deleted sequences or a homozygous deletion (HD) if the other copy of the chromosome has lost sequences in the same region. LOH can also produce a haploinsufficiency, i.e. the cell is left with a single copy of a given gene. In some cases, reduced expression of the gene product may be sufficient to alter normal cellular function. Gene expression can also be down regulated through epigenetic suppression, a process associated with hypermethylation of CpG-rich regions in the adjacent DNA (5, 6). As discussed below, the characterization of the various mutations and gene methylation patterns provides important clues as to the primary biochemical aberrations that drive the different tumor phenotypes and helps identify candidate biomarkers and therapeutic targets..

In general, there is a correlation between the extent and type of genetic aberration and the clinicopathologic stage and grade of the tumor. A clinically useful classification divides UCs into superficial and muscle-invasive disease as the latter requires a more aggressive therapy. By the TMN system, superficial non-invasive tumors can be subdivided into papillary carcinomas (Ta), tumors that penetrate only into the lamina propria (T1), and carcinoma in-situ (Tis; also referred to as intraepithelial or "flat tumors") (7). Muscle-invasive tumors (T2–T4) penetrate into the muscularis mucosa layer of the bladder or extend through this layer into adjacent soft tissues. UCs are also assigned a grade (G), usually from 1–3, based on the degree of cellular atypia; in general, the higher the grade the greater the risk of tumor recurrence and progression to a higher stage. All muscle-invasive tumors have features of high grade disease, whereas superficial tumors can be placed in groups based on both stage and grade, i.e. TaG1 or T1G3. However, Tis is considered a high-grade disease.

2.2. UCs Develop along Two Distinct Major Genetic Pathways

There is growing evidence that UCs develop along two major genetic pathways characterized by both clinicopathologic and genetic features (Fig. 26.1) (1, 2, 8–11). One is associated with the development of low-grade papillary and non-invasive low grade tumors (Ta; T1G1-2) that infrequently progress to a higher grade and stage. Tumors in this group have evidence of early mutational activation of growth factor signaling proteins (70–90%) along with LOH of sequences on the short (9p) and/or long (9q) arms of chromosome 9, relative genetic stability, infrequent alterations of the P53 and retinoblastoma (Rb) tumor suppressor genes, and a comparatively high expression of protein synthesis genes. In contrast, the other genetic pathway includes most of the high grade but superficially invasive tumors (T1G2-3) and in-situ (Tis) disease that not infrequently progressive to invasive disease. The genetic evolution of these tumors is typified by the early loss or inactivation of the P53 and retinoblastoma (Rb) tumor suppressor proteins, LOH of regions of chromosome 9, genetic instability, and a relative increase in the expression of cell cycle genes. This pathway can also be distinguished from the other by differences in gene expression profiles as determined by DNA microarray technology (12–17). In both pathways, tumor progression to a higher grade or stage of disease is accompanied by additional non-random chromosomal changes (18–20). The two genetic pathways may merge at the stage of high grade but non-invasive disease (T1G3) as some of these tumors contain genetic markers of both pathways, i.e. mutation of the fibroblast growth factor receptor-3 (FGFR3) and P53 genes (21).

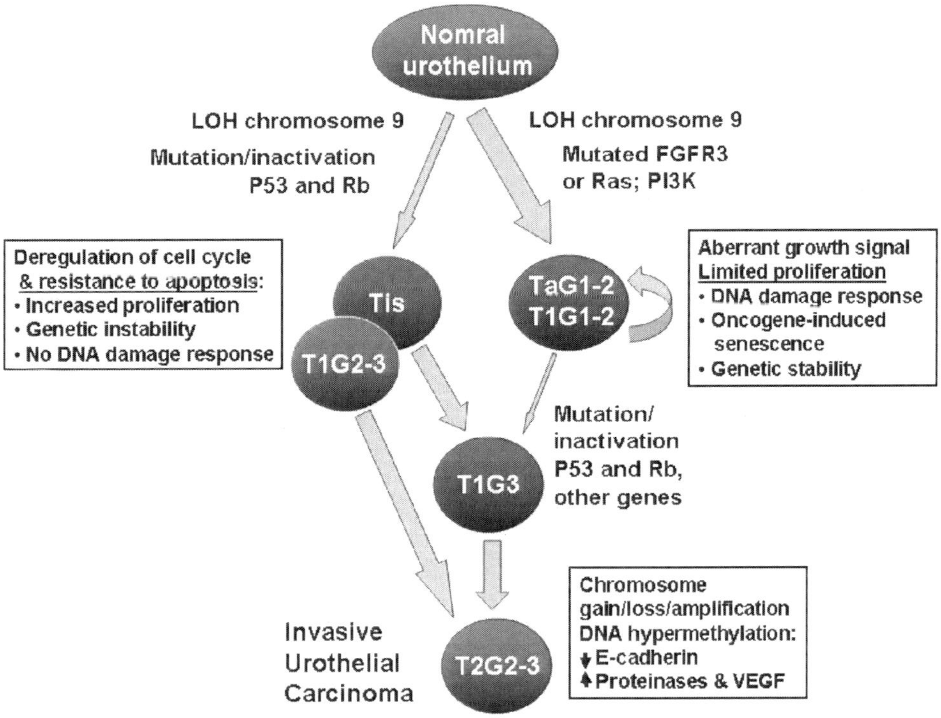

FIG. 26.1. Selected genetic and phenotypic characteristics of the two major genetic pathways in the development of the urothelial cell carcinomas. The *thickness of the arrows* represents the relative frequency of the transition. The *curved arrow* emphasizes that low grade Ta tumors tend not to progress, perhaps due to negative feedback signals generated by activated growth factor pathways. *LOH* loss of heterozygosity

2.3. Genetic Alterations Associated with the Development of UCs

2.3.1. Chromosome 9

Alterations of chromosome 9p and 9q clearly play an important role early in the development of UCs (22, 23). Depending on the techniques used and the population being surveyed, up to 90% of UCs have LOH chromosome 9, with about two-thirds having 9p deletions and 30–40% having lost 9q sequences (19, 24, 25). A detailed analyses of tumors with partial deletions of chromosome 9 have narrowed the location of the genes targeted by LOH to 9p21, 9q22, 9q32–q33 and 9q34 (2, 26–28). As noted below, LOH in the region of 9p21 likely reflects a selection for delction of the CDKN2A/ARF locus which encodes the two tumor suppressor genes, $p14^{arf1}$ and $p16^{ink4a}$, whereas the loss of the 9q34 sequences likely targets a distinct tumor suppressor gene, TSC1 (29–31). LOH of these sequences is often an indicator of complete gene activation due to a HD or point mutation of the other allele. Candidate target genes for LOH at 9q22.3 and 9q32-33 include PTCH and DBCCR1, respectively. PTCH is a known tumor suppressor gene and loss of expression is associated with the development of hereditary and spontaneous basal cell carcinomas due to activation of the sonic hedgehog (HH) signaling pathway (32, 33). However, UCs with LOH of 9q22.3 very rarely have HD or mutational inactivation of both PTCH genes which raises doubts as to the relevance of this gene to bladder tumorigenesis (34). On the other hand, loss of one allele alone may be of significance as haploinsufficiency of the PTCH gene in laboratory mice accelerates the onset of carcinogen-induced neoplastic changes in the bladder epithelium (35). The role of LOH of DBCCR1 during bladder tumorigenesis is also unclear although reduced expression may promote cell survival and proliferation (36, 37).

2.3.2. Other Chromosome Changes

As compared to low grade tumors, aggressive UCs exhibit greater genetic instability and have more numerous and diverse genetic aberrations (19, 38). For instance, chromosome changes that are more frequent in T1 and invasive tumors as compared to non-invasive Ta lesions include gains (+) or losses (-) as follows: +1q, −2q, +3p, +3q, +5p, +6p, −8p, +8q, −10q, +10p, −11p, and −11q; those more commonly seen in advanced tumors (T2–T4) are −5q, +5p, −6q, +7p, −11q, and +Xq (20, 39, 40). These and subsequent studies using single nucleotide polymorphism (SNP) arrays to evaluate chromosome changes support the hypothesis that the progression from a less aggressive to a malignant phenotype is associated with the acquisition of additional non-random gene mutations and that genetic instability is linked to the loss of P53 (19, 41–44). With a few exceptions, the target genes that drive the various chromosomal alterations are not known. Nonetheless, the elucidation of these mutations provided the rationale for the development of the UroVysion test. This assay detects cancer-related changes in chromosomes 3, 7, and 17, and/or loss of the 9p21 locus in voided urothelial cells and may be superior to standard cytology for the early detection of aggressive UCs (45).

2.4. Inactivation of the Rb and P53 Tumor Suppressors in UC

The inactivation of these two tumor suppressors is thought to facilitate progression from G1 into the S phase of the cell cycle and reduce the sensitivity of the tumor cells to apoptosis (Fig. 26.2) (46–51). The strong co-selection for inactivation of P53 and Rb during tumorigenesis is likely due to a functional interaction between the two; i.e. loss of Rb function not only stimulates cell cycle progression but also increases the sensitivity of the cells to the anti-tumor effects of P53 (51). P53 is a transcription factor that is activated in response to DNA damage and cellular stress. The resultant cellular effects that include apoptosis and cell cycle arrest are mediated to a significant degree by the induction of the pro-apoptotic Bax protein and the cyclin-dependent kinase inhibitor, p21^{waf1} (50).

In most UCs, genetic alterations are responsible for inactivation of P53. About 70% have LOH of the P53 gene which is located on chromosome 17 (17p13.1) and up to one-half of these tumors have detectable deletions or mutations within the remaining P53 gene (52–54). Erill and colleagues found that 45/76 UCs had muta-

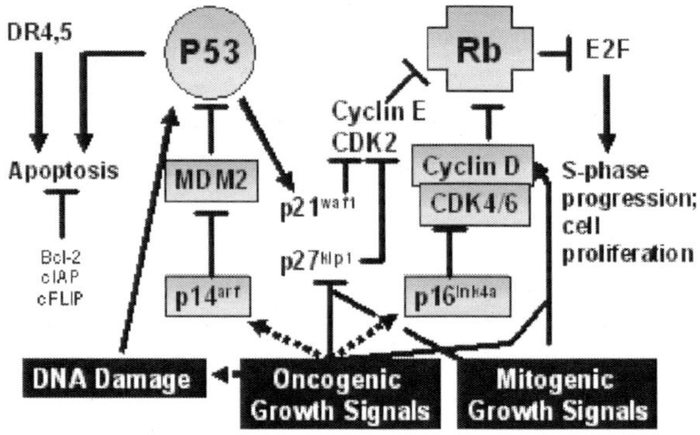

FIG. 26.2. Interactions and regulation of the p53 and Retinoblastoma (Rb) tumor suppressor pathways. The *arrows* represent positive and *bars* denote inhibitory effects. Note that oncogenic signals function may trigger responses that may limit cell proliferation and survival (*dotted arrows*). These and similar responses due to inactivation of Rb (not shown) are largely negated by concomitant loss of P53. Altered expression or function of the shaded proteins has been linked to mutations in the cognate genes. *CDK* cyclin-dependent kinase; *DR4,5* TNFR-related death receptors

tions or deletions of the P53 gene and that the presence of mutations correlated with concurrent LOH of the chromosome 17p (54). In those cases with DNA point mutations, the cells often produce mutant P53 proteins that are abnormally stable and exhibit absent or altered transcriptional activity (55). Of note, over expression of P53 in UCs as determined by immunohistochemistry correlates with mutational inactivation and is associated with a poorer prognosis, particularly when this is accompanied by abnormal or absent expression of Rb (46, 56, 57). A list of the UC-associated P53 mutations can be found in the IARC data base (58).

In other tumors, over expression of the E3 ubiquitin ligase MDM2 leads to enhanced degradation of P53. Increased activity of MDM2 may result from gene amplification or loss of the tumor suppressor p14^{arf1}, a negative regulator of MDM2, (Fig. 26.2) (59, 60). As noted above, the p14^{arf1} gene is carried in the CDKN2A/ARF locus which is a major target of the LOH on chromosome 9p21 (24, 49, 61–64). In tumors with LOH in this region, about 40% have evidence of HD of the p14^{arf1} gene.

Rb negatively regulates cycle progression primarily because of its ability to suppress E2F-dependent transcription of genes that are required entry into S phase. In UCs, the suppressor functions of Rb are abrogated primarily through genetic mutations or through hyperphosphorylation mediated by cyclin-dependent kinases (CDK). About 30% of the tumors exhibit LOH of the Rb locus located on chromosome 13q14 and about 20% of these have evidence of HD; a survey to determine how many express mutant forms of Rb has not been reported (65, 66). Inactivation of Rb by hyperphosphorylation is usually due to over expression of cyclin D or CDK4 which constitute an enzymatically active complex. Although only about 1% of UCs have evidence of CDK4 gene amplification, approximately 10% have amplification of the cyclin D1 gene (chromosome 11q13) and 30% over express the corresponding protein (60, 67–72). Reduced or absent expression of the cyclin-dependent kinase inhibitors (CDKI) such as p16^{ink4a} can also upregulate the enzymatic activity of the cyclin:CDK complexes. Remarkably, the coding sequences for p16^{ink4a} overlap with those of p14^{arf1} gene within the CDKN2A/ARF locus such that LOH of the chromosome 9p21 and a small DNA deletion in the remaining allele blocks the expression of both tumor suppressor proteins (51). In a study of tumors with LOH of 9p21, Chang et al. found HD of the p16^{ink4a} and p14^{arf1} genes in 23% and 43%, respectively, whereas 60% of the tumors had evidence of hypermethylation of the p16^{ink4a} gene which could also reduce expression (64). Some investigators have argued that haploinsufficiency of CDKN2A/ARF alone is sufficient to promote tumorigenesis (73).

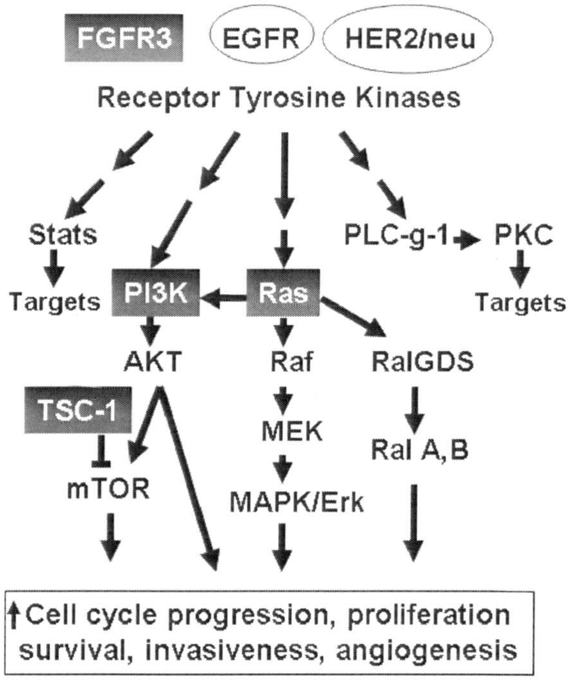

FIG. 26.3. Growth factor signaling pathways implicated in pathogenesis of bladder cancer. The darkened boxes indicate molecules that are mutationally activated (FGFR3, PI3K, Ras) or inactivated (TSC1) in a subset of the tumors. Both upstream and downstream effectors are potential therapeutic targets (see text)

2.5. Alterations in Growth Factor Signaling Pathways (Fig. 26.3)

2.5.1. *Mutational Activation of FGFR3, PI3K (PI3K-C-alpha) and Ras*

Mutational activation of the growth factor signaling proteins fibroblast growth factor receptor-3 (FGFR3), phosphatidylinositol 3-kinase alpha (PI3K), or Ras are frequent events in UCs (10, 74–81). Billerey et al. reported that the incidence of FGFR3 mutations in Ta and T1 tumors was 74% and 21%, respectively, as compared to 16% for invasive T2–T4 UCs (82). The frequency also declined with increasing the grade from 84% in G1 tumors to 0–7% in G3 and Tis cancers This and similar data from the other laboratories has led to the wide-spread impression that FGFR3 mutations are markers of low grade and stage tumors that infrequently progress to more invasive disease (10, 74, 78, 82, 83). However, for tumors of the same stage and grade, the presence or absence of FGFR3 mutations did not appear to predict the malignant potential (13).

There are four members of the fibroblast growth factor receptor (FGFR) family but the IIIB isoform of FGFR3 is most commonly associated with UCs (84–87). The majority of the mutations in this receptor consist of amino acid substitutions within the extracellular or transmembrane domain (2). Over 90% have either a cysteine in place of arginine at position 249 (S249C) or one of three other substitutions: R248C, Y375C, or G372C (75, 78). Intermolecular disulfide bonds between the cysteines in the R248C and S249C mutants result in the spontaneous formation of receptor dimers and ligand-independent activation of the receptor kinase (88–91). In other tumors, over expression of the wild-type FGFR3s has been reported which suggest that autocrine activation of these receptors may also be capable of generating oncogenic growth factor signals (92, 93).

The tumorigenic effects of FGFR3 are thought to be dependent on constitutive activation of downstream signal transduction pathways (Fig. 26.3). These include Ras, PI3K, the Stat transcriptional proteins, phospholipase-C-gamma, and their downstream effectors (94–97). Signaling by the mutant FGFRs may also influence gene expression as tumors that express these proteins are reported to have distinct gene expression profiles (11, 13). The relative contribution of the downstream effectors to FGFR3-related oncogenesis is not fully understood.

A likely target of oncogenic FGFR3 signals are the Ras proteins, which are small GTPases that act as molecular switches to regulate other signaling proteins that influence cell proliferation and survival (81). Moreover, Ras itself is a known proto-oncoprotein that itself is mutationally activated in a subset of UCs (79–81). In one study, approximately 20% of UCs that were tested contained activating mutations in the Hras, Kras2, or Nras genes (79). Interestingly, mutations of the Ras and FGFR3 genes appear to be mutually exclusive. This observation led investigators to propose that the two mutant proteins generate functionally equivalent oncogenic signals and that mutant FGFR3s promotes tumorigenesis primarily through constitutive stimulation of the wild-type Ras (Fig. 26.3) (1, 79).

Activation of RAS, either by mutation or upstream FGFR3 signaling, stimulates another set of downstream effectors. These include Raf1, which regulates the canonical Raf-MEK-mitogen-activated protein kinase/extracellular signal-regulated kinase (MAPK/Erk) pathway, as well as PI3K, and RalGDS (81). Recent studies suggests that RalGDS, a regulator of the small GTPases Ral A and B, plays a key role in bladder cancer tumorigenesis (81, 98, 99). Although signaling through Raf-MEK-MAPK may be required, indirect evidence suggests that activation of this pathway alone is not sufficient to drive Ras-related tumorigenesis. This is based on the observation that mutational activation of B-raf, which occurs frequently in melanomas that lack Ras mutations, has not been detected in bladder tumors (100). Consistent with this, FGFR3-induced transformation of NIH3T3 mouse cells is dependent on activation of MEK1 downstream of Raf, and also PI3K (81, 95, 101).

Like Ras, PI3K is a proto-oncoprotein that can be activated downstream of the FGFR3 or through mutation of PI3K itself (77, 84). PI3K is a lipid kinase whose function is critical for the maintenance of cell proliferation and survival related at least in part to secondary activation of the AKT and mTOR kinases (102, 103). Lopez-Knowles recently reported that 13% of unselected UCs contained mutations of the PIK3CA, the gene that encodes the phophatidylinositol-3-kinase-alpha isoform of PI3K (77). The point mutations predict for aminoacid substitutions (E542K, E545K, E545G, H1047L, and H1047R) which are similar or identical or similar to those found in constitutively active PI3K mutants from other human cancers (104, 105). In contrast to the situation with Ras, about one-fourth of UCs with FGFR3 mutations also contained PIK3CA gene mutations (77). This implies that the oncogenic signals produced by these two signaling molecules do not fully overlap one another despite the fact that FGFR3 signaling has the potential to activate PI3K.

PI3K signaling can also be increased by reduced or absent expression of PTEN, a tumor suppressor that deactivates the major signaling product of PI3K, phosphatidylinositol (3–5)-trisphosphate (106). In transgenic mice, homozygous deletion of PTEN in the urothelium upregulates PI3K signaling and induces the formation of papillary-like tumors (107). Although deletion or mutational inactivation of PTEN is rare in UCs, advanced stage tumors show decreased expression of PTEN and gene expression signatures indicative of PTEN-deficiency correlate with a worse clinical outcome (107–110). Taken together, these observations support the hypothesis that constitutive signaling through the PI3K pathway by one or more mechanisms promotes the early and late stages of bladder tumorigenesis (77).

2.5.2. *Mutational Activation of Signaling Proteins and the Non-Aggressive Tumor Type*

An interesting question is why mutational activation of signaling proteins is associated with low grade and non-invasive UCs rather than more aggressive tumors. The limitations of mutationally activated FGFR3s and PI3K as oncogenes are underscored by the fact that both are expressed in seborrheic keratoses, benign skin lesions that like low grade urothelial papillomas rarely if ever progress to invasive cancers (111–113). Also, individuals that inherit a mutant FGFR3 gene identical to those found in UCs develop achondroplastic dwarfism due to impaired bone growth and hypertrophic chondrocyte differentiation during development, which result in the characteristic shortening of the proximal limbs (114, 115). A favored explanation for these observations is that aberrant growth factor signals, particularly in the setting of intact tumor suppressor genes such as P53, triggers negative feedback responses that limit cell proliferation and presumably tumor progression. These responses may overlap with oncogene-induced senescence which is, associated with induction of P53 and p16^{ink4a} and cell cycle arrest. This phenomenon was first observed in non-transformed cells following the forced expression of mutationally activated Ras (116–118). Mutant FGFR3s may elicit a similar response since UCs that contain these receptors display markers of activation of the DNA damage pathway including P53 (119). In the case of Ras, studies of transgenic mouse have shown that targeted expression of moderate levels of mutant H-Ras in the urothelium produces only hyperplastic lesions, whereas concomitant inactivation of P53 leads to the development of papillary tumors, some with high-grade features (120, 121). The latter observation as well as in vitro and in vivo experiments with the fully malignant MGH-U3 and 97-7 bladder cancer cell lines that express mutated FGFR3s suggest that under certain circumstances, mutationally activated growth factor signaling proteins can contribute to the pathogenesis of the malignant as well as more benign UCs (91, 122).

2.2.3. *Other Sources of Oncogenic Growth Factor Signals*

The epidermal growth factor receptor (EGFR) and the related HER2/neu receptor have the potential to activate many of the same growth factor signaling transduction pathways as FGFR3 and have been implicated in the pathogenesis of UCs (94, 123–126). Initial reports linked expression of these receptors with tumors of higher stage and grade, but recent studies have challenged these findings (127, 128). Also, mutational activation of the EGFR that occurs in human lung and brain tumors has not been reported in bladder cancer and amplification of the HER2/neu gene is seen in only about 7% of these tumors (129–133). As reviewed below, early clinical trials of EGFR and HER2/neu inhibitors or antibodies have shown limited activity against UCs which raises doubt as to whether these receptors are appropriate therapeutic targets.

Other tyrosine receptor kinases may be relevant to the pathogenesis of UCs. Preliminary studies suggest that in some of these tumors, signaling by the platelet-derived growth factor receptor-beta (PDGFR-β) may confer resistance to the anti-proliferative effects of agents that block signaling by the EGFR family (125, 134). In addition, increased expression of the c-Met and RON receptors has been linked to the more aggressive tumor phenotype (135, 136). Over expression of the ephrin receptor EphA2 receptor is associated with higher stage UCs disease and signaling by the related EphB4 receptor may contribute to tumorigenesis (137, 138). Also, DNA sequence analysis of 518 protein kinase genes in a malignant bladder cancer revealed only three mutations, one of which predicts the expression of a mutated EphA4 (G370E) receptor (139).

The TSC1 (tuberous sclerosis-1) tumor suppressor gene appears to be the target of the LOH chromosome 9q34 in UCs as 5–33% of these tumors exhibit HD or mutational inactivation of the other allele (29–31). Reduced or absent expression of the TSC1 gene product (hamartin) may contribute to oncogenic growth factor signaling since it is an inhibitor of the serine/threonine kinase activity of mTOR, a positive regulator of cell growth that acts downstream of PI3K and AKT (102, 140–144). Germ-line mutations of TSC1 cause tuberous sclerosis, an autosomal dominant disorder that is characterized by the development of benign hamartomas and less frequently, renal cell cancers and subependymal giant cell astrocytomas (145). There is also the evidence that haploinsufficiency of TSC1 can promote tumorigenesis (142–144).

Abnormal signaling through the Wnt signaling pathway contributes to the pathogenesis of colon cancers and other human tumors (146). That this pathway is relevant to UCs is based primarily on the observation and expression that negative regulators of Wnt signaling, such as the Frizzled-related protein-1 (sFRP1), are downregulated in the tumor cells and that the cognate genes may exhibit LOH or hypermethylation (147–149, 149, 150).

2.6. Phenotypic Alterations in Urothelial Cell Cancers

UCs have been reported to produce higher levels of the angiogenic factors vascular endothelial growth factor (VEGF) and fibroblast growth factor than normal cells (151). Conversely, the tumor cells appear to have reduced expression of the angiogenesis inhibitor, thromspondin-1 (TSP-1), which may be a result of the inactivation of P53 and Rb-1 (152–154). Endothelin-1 (ET-1) is another factor that influences angiogenesis and acts through activation of the receptor tyrosine kinases, ET_A and ET_B. Signaling by these receptors alters vascular tone, stimulate mitogenesis in endothelial and other cell types, and promote angiogenesis and cell invasion (155). Expression of ET-1 is increased in UCs and levels of messenger RNA correlate with the stage of the disease (156, 157). The upregulation of ET-1 appears to be linked to reduced expression of the GDP dissociation inhibitor, RhoGDI2, which is a negative regulator of Rho GTPases (158). The latter can influence tumorigenesis through effects on gene transcription, cell structure, cell-cycle progression and cell adhesion. Recent animal experiments provide evidence that production of ET-1 by the tumor cells promotes the metastatic phenotype, perhaps by stimulating early steps in tumor angiogenesis rather than cell proliferation (157). However, the relative contribution of the different angiogenic factors to the pathogenesis of UC remains to be determined.

In addition to inactivation of P53, increased expression of the anti-apoptotic proteins (Bcl-2, survivin, cIAP, or cFLIP) or reduced levels of the pro-apoptotic protein (fragile histidine triad – FHIT) may modify the sensitivity of UC cells to apoptosis (159–165). In this regard, patients whose tumors had increased expression of Bcl-2 had a poorer outcome following treatment with radiation; however, in another study increased expression was associated with sensitivity to platinum-based chemotherapy (164–166). In view of these observations, follow-up studies are warranted to clarify the relative roles of altered expression of this and other modulators of apoptosis in determining responses to cytotoxic therapies.

Cell cycle progression in UCs may be enhanced by loss or reduced expression of the CDKI p27^{kip1}, perhaps in response to PI3K, AKT, and mTOR signaling (Fig. 26.2) (31, 167–170). Another phenotypic alteration in UCs is the sustained expression of the enzyme telomerase which occurs early in tumor development as it is required to maintain the integrity of the DNA at the chromosome tips that otherwise would erode during repetitive rounds of cell division (171). The expression of metalloproteinases such as MMP2 and MMP9 is upregulated in advanced disease and likely facilitates tissue invasion through remodeling of the basement membranes and extracellular matrix (152, 172, 173). Conversely, advanced tumors show decreased expression of E-cadherin, an adhesion molecule and tumor suppressor, most likely as a consequence of gene hypermethylation (42, 174–178). DNA hypermethylation may also down-regulate the expression of other tumor suppressors including RASSF1A (an inhibitor of Ras signaling), the death-associated protein kinase (DAPK), glutathione-S-transferase, and the VHL (von Hippel-Lindau) protein (41, 42, 179–181).

The enzyme cyclo-oxygenase-2 (COX-2) is frequently over expressed in the bladder as well as other human cancers, probably in response to the increased growth factor signaling (182–186). That COX-2 and its ability to synthesize prostaglandin PGE2 contribute to pathogenesis of the disease is supported by a number of studies of cultured cells, transplanted tumors, and transgenic mouse models (185, 187–191). However, the true role of COX-2 activity during tumorigenesis needs to be clarified.

3. Targeted and Novel Therapies for Urothelial Carcinomas

3.1. Reversal or Circumvention of P53 and Rb Inactivation

Agents that restore the tumor suppressor functions of P53 or Rb have the potential to induce responses in the majority of aggressive UCs (192, 193). One strategy is to exploit gene transfer technologies to force the expression of wild-type tumor suppressor proteins in the tumor cells. Bladder cancers lend themselves to such therapies since intravesical administration of viral vectors or other gene transfer agents allows for direct contact with the cancerous urothelium. With this in mind, Pagliaro and colleagues treated a series of UC patients with multiple intravesical infusions of the replication-defective adenoviral vector Ad5CMV-P53 which after infection of the cell, expresses wild-type P53 (194). Treatment was well tolerated and the expression of vector sequences was detectable in the target tissues. Despite this encouraging pilot study, however, clinically significant responses to this agent have yet to be reported (195). The major limitation with this and most gene therapy techniques is the inability to achieve sufficiently high rates of gene transfer to ensure expression in all or nearly all of the tumor cells. Efforts to improve upon the first generation gene therapies continue but progress has been relatively slow (196–200).

Another strategy to restore P53 function is to prevent the accelerated degradation of P53 in those tumors that overexpress MDM2 due to gene amplification or reduced or absent expression of p14^{arf1}. This has encouraged the development of MDM2 inhibitors but none have advanced to clinical trials to test activity against UCs (201). Also, activation of members of the tumor necrosis factor receptor (TNFR) family may circumvent the anti-apoptotic effects associated with loss or inactivation of P53 (202). Two members of this family, DR4 and DR5, trigger apoptosis in response to agonistic antibodies or the ligands TRAIL and FAS (203). The humanized monoclonal antibodies HGS-ETR1 and HGS-ETR2 that bind and activate these receptors have completed phase I testing and have now entered phase II trials (204). Although resistance of UCs to TRAIL-induced apoptosis has been observed in vitro, clinical trials with these stimulatory antibodies will directly determine if UCs are sensitive to TNFR-induced apoptosis in vivo (161, 205, 206). In addition, inhibitors of the anti-apoptotic protein Bcl-2 such as GX15-070 and AT-101 are under development (207–209). These inhibitors have the potential to increase tumor cell sensitivity of UCs to radiotherapy given the reported association between Bcl-2 expression and poor outcome with radiation (164, 165).

In tumors with hyperphosphorlated Rb, agents that inhibit the relevant cyclin-dependent kinases (CDK) should reduce phosphorylation and restore the tumor suppressor functions of Rb (210, 211). However, the initial clinical trials with the CDK inhibitor flavopiridol in unselected patients revealed little anti-tumor activity (211). This drug is currently being tested in combination with standard chemotherapeutic agents. Other CDK inhibitors that are under development include seliciclib (CYC202 or *R*-roscovitine), UNC01, BMS 387032, and the multi-kinase inhibitor ZK304709 (211–213).

Another approach to reduce phosphorylation of Rb is to induce the expression of the natural CDK inhibitor, $p16^{ink4a}$. In those tumors with epigenetic suppression of the $p16^{ink4a}$ gene, agents that inhibit DNA methylases or histone deacetylases (HDAC) can restore gene transcription. For example, treatment of the T24 bladder cancer cell line with the methylase inhibitors 5-azacytidine or zebularine alters gene expression and induces expression of $p16^{inka}$ (214, 215). Exposure of the same cell line to the HDAC inhibitor suberoylanilide hydroxamic acid (SAHA) also reduces cell proliferation along with upregulation of another CDKI, $p21^{waf1}$ (216). As suggested by Cote and others, these agents may suppress the malignant phenotype through the induction of multiple repressed genes in addition to those that encode $p16^{ink4a}$ and $p21^{waf1}$ (217). Of note, two patients with bladder cancer that were treated with SAHA in the context of a phase I clinical study experienced tumor regression (218). This provides a rationale for a University of Southern California phase II trial of SAHA (vorinostat) in patients with advanced UCs as well as similar study of the HDAC inhibitor FR901228 conducted by the Southwest Oncology Group (SWOG-S0400). Other inhibitors that are in various stages of clinical development are PDX 101, LAQ824, MS-275, and CI-994 (219).

3.2. Inhibition of Oncogenic Growth Factor Signaling

3.2.1. *Targeting Pathways Activated by Mutated Signaling Proteins*

In other human cancers, antibody or small molecular inhibitors of mutationally activated or over expressed growth factor receptors have produced clinically significant responses (220–222). Thus, FGFR3, PI3K, Ras, as well as their downstream effectors would be appropriate targets in UCs (Fig. 3). Based on the distribution of the gene mutations, low-grade non-invasive bladder cancers would be expected to be most sensitive to inhibitors of the mutationally activated signaling proteins. However, suppression of FGFR3 signaling may also be effective against those muscle-invasive tumors that over express wild-type FGFR3s or mutant receptors (91–93, 122). Also Ras and PI3K are downstream effectors for a large variety of upstream growth factor signals and thus likely contribute to the pathogenesis of more aggressive UCs.

FGFR3 inhibitors that are in pre-clinical and clinical testing include the small molecule inhibitors TKI258 (CHIR-258), SU5402, PD173074, and PKC412, and a receptor antibody, PRO-001/HuCAL-Fab1 (223–226). PD173074, and TKI258 are multi-kinase inhibitors that also suppress signaling by the VEGF receptors (VEGF-R) and thus have the potential to induce responses in both indolent and aggressive tumors by blocking angiogenesis as well as FGFR3 signaling (227, 228). Certainly, standard phase II trials of these agents in UC patients are indicated. An interesting issue is how best to structure trials for patients with low grade superficial tumors that express FGFR3 mutants with regards to end-points and tolerance of toxicities when treating a "pre-cancer". One possible approach is to determine if the inhibitors reduce the recurrences or tumor progression rates in those patients who have suffered at least one prior recurrence.

The initial strategy to inhibit signaling by Ras proteins was to disrupt their association with the cell membrane by blocking post-translational farnesylation (229). However, the first generation of farnesyl transferase inhibitors (FTI) had limited clinical activity in the bladder or other cancers. A phase II trial of the FTI lonafarnib/SCH6636 in patients with advanced UC was stopped early because of lack of objective responses (230). In another study, the co-administration of lonafarnib with gemcitabine chemotherapy produced tumor regression in about one-third of treated patients. However, it is not clear that this result is superior to that achieved by the administration of gemcitabine alone (231). Another FTI, tipifarnib (R115777), was tested in a group of thirty-four patients with advanced UC and produced tumor response or stabilization in two to thirteen subjects, respectively (232). A third FTI, BMS-214662, has yet to be studied in UCs (233).

The modest clinical activity of the FTIs may be explained by the subsequent observation that these compounds suppress signaling by H-Ras but have limited effects on the other Ras family members, K-Ras and N-Ras. Prenylation of the latter two Ras proteins by geranylgeranyl prenyltransferase (GGT) can maintain their association with the membrane association and signaling properties in the presence of FTIs (229, 234). This observation has also led investigators to propose that many of the anti-tumor responses seen with the FTIs are actually due to reduced farnesylation of non-Ras proteins such as Rheb, RhoB, and centromere proteins (234, 235). To more effectively inhibit Ras signaling, compounds such as the dual prenyl transferase inhibitor AZD-3409 have been developed to block both farnesylation and prenylation by GGT (236). Hopefully, these new inhibitors will exhibit greater anti-tumor activity in UCs and other human cancers.

As reviewed above, PI3K may be activated by mutation, upstream growth factor signals, or loss of negative regulators such as PTEN. Thus, the PI3K pathway is a valid therapeutic target in most UCs. Inhibitors of PI3K signaling that are under development include BEC235, PX-866, ZSTK474, SF1126, and the fused heteroaryl and imidazopyridine-based compounds. Agents that target AKT, a major downstream effector of PI3K, include perifosine, BEZ325, API-2, PX-316, A-443654, anti-AktScFv, and the cathine alkaloid analogs (237, 238). Downstream of PI3K is the mTOR whose kinase activity is suppressed by temsirolimus, Rad001, and AP23573(239, 240). Temsirolimus (Torisel) was recently approved by the FDA for treatment of renal cell carcinomas. However, trials to determine the activity of these and other mTOR, AKT and PI3K inhibitors against bladder cancer have yet to be reported.

Other therapeutic agents target molecules act downstream of Ras. Sorafenib (Bay 43-9006) is a small molecule inhibitor of B- and c-Raf that also blocks signaling by the VEGF-Rs (241–243). This drug, which was also recently approved by the FDA for treatment of renal cell cancer, is now being evaluated for efficacy against bladder cancer in an Eastern Cooperative Oncology Group phase II trial (E1804). PD0325901 and ARRY142886 are representatives of a new generation of inhibitors that target MEK, a kinase that acts immediately downstream of Raf. These compounds appear to have more favorable pharmacokinetic and pharmacodynamic than the first generation inhibitors and should be available soon for phase II trials (244, 245).

3.2.2. Targeting EGFR and HER2/neu Signaling in UC

To date, the responses of UC patients treated with EGFR and HER2/neu inhibitors have been unimpressive. Wulfing et al. recently presented the preliminary results of a phase II study of lapatinib, a small molecule inhibitor of both the EGFR and HER2/neu kinases (246). Only one of fifty-nine previously treated patients had an objective tumor response and the median survival of all subjects was 4.5 months. In other on-going studies, UCLA investigators will determine if the EGFR kinase inhibitor erlotinib will suppress recurrences following transuretheral resection of superficial UCs. A phase II sponsored by Hoffman-LaRoche will evaluate the effect of HER2/neu antibody trastuzumab as second-line treatment in patients whose tumors over express receptor protein.

Inhibitors of the EGFR family of receptors are also being tested in combination with standard chemotherapy agents for treatment of UCs. The addition of EGFR kinase inhibitor gefitinib to cisplatin and gemcitabine chemotherapy produced modest toxicity, responses in over one-half of the patients, and a median survival of 14.4 months for the entire group (247). However, in the absence of a phase III trial, the contribution of the targeted agent to the observed response rate and duration remains uncertain. Other phase II studies are testing the combinations of docetaxel chemotherapy with gefitinib or vandetanib, the latter a small molecule inhibitor of both EGFR and VEGF-R signaling. The group at Fox Chase Cancer Center is evaluating the combination of the anti-EGFR monoclonal antibody cetuximab with paclitaxel.

The observation that co-administration trastuzumab improves the efficacy of chemotherapy in breast cancer patients led investigators to adapt this strategy for treatment of advanced UCs (248). In a phase II study of patients with bladder cancers that expressed high levels of HER2/neu, the combination of trastuzumab, paclitaxel, carboplatin, and gemcitabine, produced complete or partial responses in 54% (249). Although these results are encouraging, a follow-up phase III trial will be needed to determine the contribution of trastuzumab to the observed anti-tumor effects. Trastuzumab has also been added to the combination of gemcitabine and cisplatin in a phase II trial for patients with HER2/neu-positive cancers. The Radiation Therapy Oncology Group protocol 0524 will address the safety and efficacy of adding trastuzumab to weekly paclitaxel and concomitant radiation for treatment of localized muscle-invasive disease (250).

3.3. Targeting Angiogenesis in UCs

The addition of the monoclonal VEGF antibody bevacizumab to chemotherapy improves outcome for patients with metastatic colon cancer (251). Given this and the possible contribution of VEGF to angiogenesis in UCs, investigators at the University of South Carolina have initiated a multicenter trial of bevacizumab combined with gemcitabine and cisplatin chemotherapy as adjuvant treatment for patients with muscle-invasive UCs. A similar study at M. D. Anderson Cancer Center will test the effects of bevacizumab added to neoadjuvant methotrexate, vinblastine, doxorubicin, and cisplatin (MVAC) chemotherapy. The combination of bevacizumab and gemcitabine is being evaluated in patients with metastatic disease in a phase II study sponsored by the Hoosier Oncology Group. In addition, the small molecule inhibitors of VEGF-R kinase, sorafenib, pazopanib, and sunitinib, have all been incorporated into separate phase II bladder cancer trials. The study at Case Western University will assess the activity of sunitinib in the pre- and post-operative setting and will evaluate the effects of treatment on oncogenic growth factor signaling in the tumor cells.

As discussed above, the expression of endothelin-1 (ET-1) has been implicated in the pathogenesis UCs and appears to promote the metastatic phenotype (155, 157). Atresentan, a small molecule receptor inhibitor the ET-1 receptor kinases, profoundly reduced the number of pulmonary metastases seen in mice inoculated with a human bladder cell line (157). This observation provides a rationale for a clinical trial to determine if atresentan will prevent or delay the onset of metastatic disease in high-risk UC patients who are treated with radical cystectomy and adjuvant chemotherapy.

*Note – updates on many of the clinical trials discussed above can be found on-line at the NCI-PDQ data base: http://www.cancer.gov/clinicaltrials/search.

References

1. Wu XR. Urothelial tumorigenesis: a tale of divergent pathways. [Review] [145 refs]. Nat Rev Cancer 2005;5: 713–725.
2. Knowles MA. Molecular subtypes of bladder cancer: Jekyll and Hyde or chalk and cheese? Carcinogenesis 2006;27:361–373.
3. Mhawech-Fauceglia P, Cheney RT, and Schwaller J. Genetic alterations in urothelial bladder carcinoma: an updated review. Cancer 2006;106:1205–1216.
4. Hanahan D and Weinberg RA. The hallmarks of cancer. [Review] [94 refs]. Cell 2000;100:57–70.
5. Santini V, Kantarjian HM, and Issa JP. Changes in DNA methylation in neoplasia: pathophysiology and therapeutic implications. Ann Intern Med 2001;134:573–586.
6. Baylin SB and Ohm JE. Epigenetic gene silencing in cancer – a mechanism for early oncogenic pathway addiction? Nat Rev Cancer 2006;6:107–116.
7. Greene F, Page D, Fleming I et al. AJCC Cancer Staging Handbook (6th edn), 2002. Springer, NY.
8. Wolff EM, Liang G, and Jones PA. Mechanisms of disease: genetic and epigenetic alterations that drive bladder cancer. Nat Clin Pract Urol 2005;2:502–510.
9. Spruck CH, III, Ohneseit PF, Gonzalez-Zulueta M et al. Two molecular pathways to transitional cell carcinoma of the bladder. Cancer Res 1994;54:784–788.
10. Bakkar AA, Wallerand H, Radvanyi F et al. FGFR3 and TP53 gene mutations define two distinct pathways in urothelial cell carcinoma of the bladder. Cancer Res 2003;63:8108–8112.
11. Lindgren D, Liedberg F, Andersson A et al. Molecular characterization of early-stage bladder carcinomas by expression profiles, FGFR3 mutation status, and loss of 9q. Oncogene 2006;25:2685–2696.
12. Sanchez-Carbayo M, Socci ND, Lozano JJ et al. Gene discovery in bladder cancer progression using cDNA microarrays. Am J Pathol 2003;163:505–516.
13. Zieger K, Dyrskjot L, Wiuf C et al. Role of activating fibroblast growth factor receptor 3 mutations in the development of bladder tumors. Clin Cancer Res 2005;11:7709–7719.
14. Wild PJ, Herr A, Wissmann C et al. Gene expression profiling of progressive papillary noninvasive carcinomas of the urinary bladder. Clin Cancer Res 2005;11:4415–4429.
15. Orntoft TF, Zieger K, Dyrskjot L et al. Recent developments in molecular profiling of bladder cancer. [Review] [14 refs]. Curr Opin Urol 2006;16:377–381.
16. Sanchez-Carbayo M, Socci ND, Lozano J et al. Defining molecular profiles of poor outcome in patients with invasive bladder cancer using oligonucleotide microarrays. J Clin Oncol 2006;24:778–789.
17. Dyrskjot L, Kruhoffer M, Thykjaer T et al. Gene expression in the urinary bladder: a common carcinoma in situ gene expression signature exists disregarding histopathological classification. Cancer Res 2004;64:4040–4048.
18. Blaveri E, Brewer JL, Roydasgupta R et al. Bladder cancer stage and outcome by array-based comparative genomic hybridization. Clin Cancer Res 2005;11:7012–7022.
19. Koed K, Wiuf C, Christensen LL et al. High-density single nucleotide polymorphism array defines novel stage and location-dependent allelic imbalances in human bladder tumors. Cancer Res 2005;65:34–45.
20. Placer J, Espinet B, Salido M et al. Correlation between histologic findings and cytogenetic abnormalities in bladder carcinoma: a FISH study. Urology 2005;65:913–918.
21. Hernandez S, Lopez-Knowles E, Lloreta J et al. FGFR3 and Tp53 mutations in T1G3 transitional bladder carcinomas: independent distribution and lack of association with prognosis. Clin Cancer Res 2005;11:5444–5450.

22. Hartmann A, Schlake G, Zaak D et al. Occurrence of chromosome 9 and p53 alterations in multifocal dysplasia and carcinoma in situ of human urinary bladder. Cancer Res 2002;62(3):809–818.
23. Obermann EC, Meyer S, Hellge D et al. Fluorescence in situ hybridization detects frequent chromosome 9 deletions and aneuploidy in histologically normal urothelium of bladder cancer patients. Oncol Rep 2004;11(4):745–751.
24. Wada T, Berggren P, Steineck G et al. Bladder neoplasms–regions at chromosome 9 with putative tumour suppressor genes. Scand J Urol Nephrol 2003;37:106–111.
25. Williams SV, Sibley KD, Davies AM et al. Molecular genetic analysis of chromosome 9 candidate tumor-suppressor loci in bladder cancer cell lines.[see comment]. Genes, Chromosomes Cancer 2002;34:86–96.
26. Aboulkassim TO, Larue H, Lemieux P et al. Alteration of the PATCHED locus in superficial bladder cancer. Oncogene 2003;22:2967–2971.
27. Czerniak B, Chaturvedi V, Li L et al. Superimposed histologic and genetic mapping of chromosome 9 in progression of human urinary bladder neoplasia: implications for a genetic model of multistep urothelial carcinogenesis and early detection of urinary bladder cancer. Oncogene 1999;18:1185–1196.
28. Habuchi T, Luscombe M, Elder PA et al. Structure and methylation-based silencing of a gene (DBCCR1) within a candidate bladder cancer tumor suppressor region at 9q32-q33. Genomics 1998;48:277–288.
29. van Tilborg AA, de Vries A, and Zwarthoff EC. The chromosome 9q genes TGFBR1, TSC1, and ZNF189 are rarely mutated in bladder cancer. J Pathol 2001;194:76–80.
30. Knowles MA, Habuchi T, Kennedy W et al. Mutation spectrum of the 9q34 tuberous sclerosis gene TSC1 in transitional cell carcinoma of the bladder. Cancer Res 2003;63:7652–7656.
31. Adachi H, Igawa M, Shiina H et al. Human bladder tumors with 2-hit mutations of tumor suppressor gene TSC1 and decreased expression of p27. J Urol 2003;170:601–604.
32. Daya-Grosjean L and Couve-Privat S. Sonic hedgehog signaling in basal cell carcinomas. Cancer Lett 2005; 225:181–192.
33. Kasper M, Regl G, Frischauf AM et al. GLI transcription factors: mediators of oncogenic Hedgehog signalling. Eur J Cancer 2006;42:437–445.
34. McGarvey TW, Maruta Y, Tomaszewski JE et al. PTCH gene mutations in invasive transitional cell carcinoma of the bladder. Oncogene 1998;17:1167–1172.
35. Hamed S, Larue H, Hovington H et al. Accelerated induction of bladder cancer in patched heterozygous mutant mice. Cancer Res 2004;64:1938–1942.
36. Wright KO, Messing EM, and Reeder JE. DBCCR1 mediates death in cultured bladder tumor cells. Oncogene 2004;23:82–90.
37. Nishiyama H, Gill JH, Pitt E et al. Negative regulation of G(1)/S transition by the candidate bladder tumour suppressor gene DBCCR1. Oncogene 2001;20:2956–2964.
38. Blaveri E, Simko JP, Korkola JE et al. Bladder cancer outcome and subtype classification by gene expression. Clin Cancer Res 2005;11:4044–4055.
39. Simon R, Burger H, Brinkschmidt C et al. Chromosomal aberrations associated with invasion in papillary superficial bladder cancer. J Pathol 1998;185:345–351.
40. Richter J, Beffa L, Wagner U et al. Patterns of chromosomal imbalances in advanced urinary bladder cancer detected by comparative genomic hybridization. Am J Pathol 1998;153:1615–1621.
41. Catto JWF, Azzouzi AR, Rehman I et al. Promoter hypermethylation is associated with tumor location, stage, and subsequent progression in transitional cell carcinoma. J Clin Oncol 2005;23:2903–2910.
42. Maruyama R, Toyooka S, Toyooka KO et al. Aberrant promoter methylation profile of bladder cancer and its relationship to clinicopathological features. Cancer Res 2001;61(24):8659–8663.
43. Oeggerli M, Tomovska S, Schraml P et al. E2F3 amplification and overexpression is associated with invasive tumor growth and rapid tumor cell proliferation in urinary bladder cancer. Oncogene 2004;23:5616–5623.
44. Richter J, Wagner U, Kononen J et al. High-throughput tissue microarray analysis of cyclin E gene amplification and overexpression in urinary bladder cancer. Am J Pathol 2000;157:787–794.
45. Sarosdy MF, Kahn PR, Ziffer MD et al. Use of a multitarget fluorescence in situ hybridization assay to diagnose bladder cancer in patients with hematuria. J Urol 2006;176:44–47.
46. Esrig D, Elmajian D, Groshen S et al. Accumulation of nuclear p53 and tumor progression in bladder cancer. N Engl J Med 1994;331:1259–1264.
47. Sarkis AS, Dalbagni G, Cordon-Cardo C et al. Nuclear overexpression of p53 protein in transitional cell bladder carcinoma: a marker for disease progression. J Natl Cancer Inst 1993;85(1):53–59.
48. Markl ID and Jones PA. Presence and location of TP53 mutation determines pattern of CDKN2A/ARF pathway inactivation in bladder cancer. Cancer Res 1998;58: 5348–5353.
49. Le Frere-Belda MA, Gil Diez de MS, Daher A et al. Profiles of the 2 INK4a gene products, p16 and p14ARF, in human reference urothelium and bladder carcinomas, according to pRb and p53 protein status. Hum Pathol 2004;35:817–824.
50. Sengupta S and Harris CC. p53: traffic cop at the crossroads of DNA repair and recombination. Nat Rev Mol Cell Biol 2005;6:44–55.
51. Sherr CJ. Principles of tumor suppression. Cell 2004;116:235–246.
52. Lorenzo-Romero JG, Salinas-Sanchez AS, Gimenez-Bachs JM et al. Prognostic implications of p53 gene mutations in bladder tumors. J Urol 2003;169:492–499.
53. Schroeder JC, Conway K, Li Y et al. p53 mutations in bladder cancer: evidence for exogenous versus endogenous risk factors. Cancer Res 2003;63:7530–7538.
54. Erill N, Colomer A, Verdu M et al. Genetic and immunophenotype analyses of TP53 in bladder cancer: TP53 alterations are associated with tumor progression. Diagn Mol Pathol 2004;13:217–223.
55. Levine AJ, Hu W, and Feng Z. The P53 pathway: what questions remain to be explored? Cell Death Differ 2006;13:1027–1036.
56. Chatterjee SJ, Datar R, Youssefzadeh D et al. Combined effects of p53, p21, and pRb expression in the progression of bladder transitional cell carcinoma. J Clin Oncol 2004;22:1007–1013.

57. Shariat SF, Tokunaga H, Zhou J et al. p53, p21, pRB, and p16 expression predict clinical outcome in cystectomy with bladder cancer.[see comment]. J Clin Oncol 2004;22:1014–1024.
58. Petijean A, Mathe E, Kato S et al. Impact of mutant p53 functional properties on TP53 mutation patterns and tumor phenotype: lessons from recent developments in the IARC TP53 database. Hum Mutation 2007;28:622–629.
59. Lianes P, Orlow I, Zhang ZF et al. Altered patterns of MDM2 and TP53 expression in human bladder cancer. [see comment]. J Natl Cancer Inst 1994;86:1325–1330.
60. Simon R, Struckmann K, Schraml P et al. Amplification pattern of 12q13-q15 genes (MDM2, CDK4, GLI) in urinary bladder cancer. Oncogene 2002;21:2476–2483.
61. Baud E, Catilina P, Bignon YJ et al. p16 involvement in primary bladder tumors: analysis of deletions and mutations. Int J Oncol 1999;14:441–445.
62. Orlow I, Lacombe L, Hannon GJ et al. Deletion of the p16 and p15 genes in human bladder tumors.[see comment]. J Natl Cancer Inst 1995;87:1524–1529.
63. Berggren P, Kumar R, Sakano S et al. Detecting homozygous deletions in the CDKN2A(p16(INK4a))/ARF(p14(ARF)) gene in urinary bladder cancer using real-time quantitative PCR. Clin Cancer Res 2003;9:235–242.
64. Chang LL, Yeh WT, Yang SY et al. Genetic alterations of p16INK4a and p14ARF genes in human bladder cancer. J Urol 2003;170:595–600.
65. Cairns P, Proctor AJ, and Knowles MA. Loss of heterozygosity at the RB locus is frequent and correlates with muscle invasion in bladder carcinoma. Oncogene 1991;6:2305–2309.
66. Sparano A, Quesnelle KM, Kumar MS et al. Genome-wide profiling of oral squamous cell carcinoma by array-based comparative genomic hybridization. Laryngoscope 2006;116:735–741.
67. Zaharieva BM, Simon R, Diener PA et al. High-throughput tissue microarray analysis of 11q13 gene amplification (CCND1, FGF3, FGF4, EMS1) in urinary bladder cancer. J Pathol 2003;201:603–608.
68. Suwa Y, Takano Y, Iki M et al. Cyclin D1 protein overexpression is related to tumor differentiation, but not to tumor progression or proliferative activity, in transitional cell carcinoma of the bladder. J Urol 1998;160:897–900.
69. Tut VM, Braithwaite KL, Angus B et al. Cyclin D1 expression in transitional cell carcinoma of the bladder: correlation with p53, waf1, pRb and Ki67. Br J Cancer 2001;84:270–275.
70. Lee CC, Yamamoto S, Morimura K et al. Significance of cyclin D1 overexpression in transitional cell carcinomas of the urinary bladder and its correlation with histopathologic features. Cancer 1997;79:780–789.
71. Watters AD, Latif Z, Forsyth A et al. Genetic aberrations of c-myc and CCND1 in the development of invasive bladder cancer. Br J Cancer 2002;87:654–658.
72. Veltman JA, Fridlyand J, Pejavar S et al. Array-based comparative genomic hybridization for genome-wide screening of DNA copy number in bladder tumors. Cancer Res 2003;63:2872–2880.
73. Chapman EJ, Harnden P, Chambers P et al. Comprehensive analysis of CDKN2A status in microdissected urothelial cell carcinoma reveals potential haploinsufficiency, a high frequency of homozygous co-deletion and associations with clinical phenotype. Clin Cancer Res 2005;11:5740–5747.
74. van Rhijn BW, van der Kwast TH, Vis AN et al. FGFR3 and P53 characterize alternative genetic pathways in the pathogenesis of urothelial cell carcinoma. Cancer Res 2004;64:1911–1914.
75. Billerey C, Chopin D, Aubriot-Lorton MH et al. Frequent FGFR3 mutations in papillary non-invasive bladder (pTa) tumors. Am J Pathol 2001;158:1955–1959.
76. van Rhijn BW, Vis AN, van der Kwast TH et al. Molecular grading of urothelial cell carcinoma with fibroblast growth factor receptor 3 and MIB-1 is superior to pathologic grade for the prediction of clinical outcome. J Clin Oncol 2003;21:1912–1921.
77. Lopez-Knowles E, Hernandez S, Malats N et al. PIK3CA mutations are an early genetic alteration associated with FGFR3 mutations in superficial papillary bladder tumors. Cancer Res 2006;66:7401–7404.
78. Hernandez S, Lopez-Knowles E, Lloreta J et al. Prospective study of FGFR3 mutations as a prognostic factor in non-muscle invasive urothelial bladder carcinomas. J Clin Oncol 2006;24:3664–3671.
79. Jebar AH, Hurst CD, Tomlinson DC et al. FGFR3 and Ras gene mutations are mutually exclusive genetic events in urothelial cell carcinoma. Oncogene 2005;24:5218–5225.
80. Uchida T, Wada C, Ishida H et al. Infrequent involvement of mutations on neurofibromatosis type 1, H-ras, K-ras and N-ras in urothelial tumors. Urol Int 1995;55:63–67.
81. Oxford G and Theodorescu D. The role of Ras superfamily proteins in bladder cancer progression. J Urol 2003;170:1987–1993.
82. Billerey C, Chopin D, Aubriot-Lorton MH et al. Frequent FGFR3 mutations in papillary non-invasive bladder (pTa) tumors. Am J Pathol 2001;158:1955–1959.
83. van Rhijn BW, Lurkin I, Radvanyi F et al. The fibroblast growth factor receptor 3 (FGFR3) mutation is a strong indicator of superficial bladder cancer with low recurrence rate. Cancer Res 2001;61:1265–1268.
84. Eswarakumar VP, Lax I, and Schlessinger J. Cellular signaling by fibroblast growth factor receptors. [Review] [112 refs]. Cytokine Growth Factor Rev 2005;16:139–149.
85. L'Hote CG and Knowles MA. Cell responses to FGFR3 signalling: growth, differentiation and apoptosis. [Review] [139 refs]. Exp Cell Res 2005;304:417–431.
86. Dailey L, Ambrosetti D, Mansukhani A et al. Mechanisms underlying differential responses to FGF signaling. Cytokine Growth Factor Rev 2005;16:233–247.
87. Tomlinson DC, L'Hote CG, Kennedy W et al. Alternative splicing of fibroblast growth factor receptor 3 produces a secreted isoform that inhibits fibroblast growth factor-induced proliferation and is repressed in urothelial carcinoma cell lines. Cancer Res 2005;65:10441–10449.
88. Naski MC, Wang Q, Xu J et al. Graded activation of fibroblast growth factor receptor 3 by mutations causing achondroplasia and thanatophoric dysplasia. Nat Genet 1996;13:233–237.
89. Li Y, Mangasarian K, Mansukhani A et al. Activation of FGF receptors by mutations in the transmembrane domain. Oncogene 1997;14:1397–1406.
90. Monsonego-Ornan E, Adar R, Feferman T et al. The transmembrane mutation G380R in fibroblast growth factor

receptor 3 uncouples ligand-mediated receptor activation from down-regulation. Mol Cell Biol 2000;20:516–522.
91. Tomlinson DC, Hurst CD, and Knowles MA. Knockdown by shRNA identifies S249C mutant FGFR3 as a potential therapeutic target in bladder cancer. Oncogene 2007;26:5889–5999.
92. Tomlinson D, Baldo O, Harnden P et al. FGFR3 protein expression and its relationship to mutation status and prognostic variables in bladder cancer. J Pathol 2007;213:91–98.
93. Gomez-Roman JJ, Saenz P, Molina M et al. Fibroblast growth factor receptor 3 is overexpressed in urinary tract carcinomas and modulates the neoplastic cell growth. Clin Cancer Res 2005;11:459–465.
94. Schlessinger J. Common and distinct elements in cellular signaling via EGF and FGF receptors. Science 2004;306:1506–1507.
95. Agazie YM, Movilla N, Ischenko I et al. The phosphotyrosine phosphatase SHP2 is a critical mediator of transformation induced by the oncogenic fibroblast growth factor receptor 3. Oncogene 2003;22:6909–6918.
96. Kanai M, Goke M, Tsunekawa S et al. Signal transduction pathway of human fibroblast growth factor receptor 3. Identification of a novel 66-kDa phosphoprotein. J Biol Chem 1997;272:6621–6628.
97. Hart KC, Robertson SC, Kanemitsu MY et al. Transformation and Stat activation by derivatives of FGFR1, FGFR3, and FGFR4. Oncogene 2000;19:3309–3320.
98. Swiatkowski S, Seifert HH, Steinhoff C et al. Activities of MAP-kinase pathways in normal uroepithelial cells and urothelial carcinoma cell lines. Exp Cell Res 2003;282(1):48–57.
99. Smith SC, Oxford G, Baras AS et al. Expression of ral GTPases, their effectors, and activators in human bladder cancer. Clin Cancer Res 2007;13:3803–3813.
100. Stoehr R, Brinkmann A, Filbeck T et al. No evidence for mutation of B-RAF in urothelial carcinomas of the bladder and upper urinary tract. Oncol Rep 2004;11:137–141.
101. Hart KC, Robertson SC, and Donoghue DJ. Identification of tyrosine residues in constitutively activated fibroblast growth factor receptor 3 involved in mitogenesis, Stat activation, and phosphatidylinositol 3-kinase activation. Mol Biol Cell 2001;12:931–942.
102. Hay N. The Akt-mTOR tango and its relevance to cancer. [Review] [41 refs]. Cancer Cell 2005;8(3):179–83.
103. Shaw RJ and Cantley LC. Ras, PI(3)K and mTOR signalling controls tumour cell growth. Nature 2006;441:424–430.
104. Karakas B, Bachman KE, and Park BH. Mutation of the PIK3CA oncogene in human cancers. Br J Cancer 2006;94:455–459.
105. Samuels Y, Wang Z, Bardelli A et al. High frequency of mutations of the PIK3CA gene in human cancers. Science 2004;304:554.
106. Hawkins PT, Anderson KE, Davidson K et al. Signalling through Class I PI3Ks in mammalian cells. Biochem Soc Trans 2006;34:647–662.
107. Tsuruta H, Kishimoto H, Sasaki T et al. Hyperplasia and carcinomas in Pten-deficient mice and reduced PTEN protein in human bladder cancer patients. Cancer Res 2006;66:8389–8396.
108. Cairns P, Evron E, Okami K et al. Point mutation and homozygous deletion of PTEN/MMAC1 in primary bladder cancers. Oncogene 1998;16:3215–3218.
109. Aveyard JS, Skilleter A, Habuchi T et al. Somatic mutation of PTEN in bladder carcinoma. Br J Cancer 1999;80:904–908.
110. Saal LH, Johansson P, Holm K et al. Poor prognosis in carcinoma is associated with a gene expression signature of aberrant PTEN tumor suppressor pathway activity. Proc Natl Acad Sci USA 2007;104:7564–7569.
111. Logie A, Dunois-Larde C, Rosty C et al. Activating mutations of the tyrosine kinase receptor FGFR3 are associated with benign skin tumors in mice and humans. Hum Mol Genet 2005;14:1153–1160.
112. van Rhijn BW, Montironi R, Zwarthoff EC et al. Frequent FGFR3 mutations in urothelial papilloma. J Pathol 2002;198:245–251.
113. Hafner C, Lopez-Knowles E, Luis NM et al. Oncogenic PIK3CA mutations occur in epidermal nevi and seborrheic keratoses with a characteristic mutation pattern. PNAS 2007;104:13450–13454.
114. Vajo Z, Francomano CA, and Wilkin DJ. The molecular and genetic basis of fibroblast growth factor receptor 3 disorders: the achondroplasia family of skeletal dysplasias, Muenke craniosynostosis, and Crouzon syndrome with acanthosis nigricans. Endocr Rev 2000;21:23–39.
115. Murakami S, Balmes G, McKinney S et al. Constitutive activation of MEK1 in chondrocytes causes Stat1-independent achondroplasia-like dwarfism and rescues the Fgfr3-deficient mouse phenotype. Genes Dev 2004;18:290–305.
116. Serrano M, Lin AW, McCurrach ME et al. Oncogenic ras provokes premature cell senescence associated with accumulation of p53 and p16INK4a. Cell 1997;88:593–602.
117. Braig M and Schmitt CA. Oncogene-induced senescence: putting the brakes on tumor development. Cancer Res 2006;66:2881–2884.
118. Gorgoulis VG, Vassiliou LV, Karakaidos P et al. Activation of the DNA damage checkpoint and genomic instability in human precancerous lesions. Nature 2005;434:907–913.
119. Bartkova J, Horejsi Z, Koed K et al. DNA damage response as a candidate anti-cancer barrier in early human tumorigenesis. Nature 2005;434:864–870.
120. Gao J, Huang HY, Pak J et al. p53 deficiency provokes urothelial proliferation and synergizes with activated Ha-ras in promoting urothelial tumorigenesis. Oncogene 2004;23:687–696.
121. Zhang ZT, Pak J, Huang HY et al. Role of Ha-ras activation in superficial papillary pathway of urothelial tumor formation. Oncogene 2001;20:1973–1980.
122. Bernard-Pierrot I, Brams A, Dunois-Larde C et al. Oncogenic properties of the mutated forms of fibroblast growth factor receptor 3b. Carcinogenesis 2006;27: 740–747.
123. Mellon K, Wright C, Kelly P et al. Long-term outcome related to epidermal growth factor receptor status in bladder cancer. J Urol 1995;153:919–925.
124. Villares GJ, Zigler M, Blehm K et al. Targeting EGFR in bladder cancer. World J Urol 2007;25(6):573–579.
125. Black PC, Agarwal PK, and Dinney CP. Targeted therapies in bladder cancer-an update. Urol Oncol 2007;25:433–438.

126. Cheng J, Huang H, Zhang ZT et al. Overexpression of epidermal growth factor receptor in urothelium elicits urothelial hyperplasia and promotes bladder tumor growth. Cancer Res 2002;62:4157–4163.
127. Rajjayabun PH, Keegan PE, Lunec J et al. erbB receptor expression patterns in human bladder cancer. Urology 2005;66:196–200.
128. Rotterud R, Nesland JM, Berner A et al. Expression of the epidermal growth factor receptor family in normal and malignant urothelium. BJU Int 2005;95:1344–1350.
129. Frederick L, Wang XY, Eley G et al. Diversity and frequency of epidermal growth factor receptor mutations in human glioblastomas. Cancer Res 2000;60:1383–1387.
130. Riely GJ, Politi KA, Miller VA et al. Update on epidermal growth factor receptor mutations in non-small cell lung cancer. Clin Cancer Res 2006;12:7232–7241.
131. Coogan CL, Estrada CR, Kapur S et al. HER-2/neu protein overexpression and gene amplification in human transitional cell carcinoma of the bladder. Urology 2004;63:786–790.
132. Latif Z, Watters AD, Dunn I et al. HER2/neu gene amplification and protein overexpression in G3 pT2 transitional cell carcinoma of the bladder: a role for anti-HER2 therapy? Eur J Cancer 2004;40:56–63.
133. Kruger S, Weitsch G, Buttner H et al. Overexpression of c-erbB-2 oncoprotein in muscle-invasive bladder carcinoma: relationship with gene amplification, clinicopathological parameters and prognostic outcome. Int J Oncol 2002;21:981–987.
134. Kassouf W, Dinney CP, Brown G et al. Uncoupling between epidermal growth factor receptor and downstream signals defines resistance to the antiproliferative effect of Gefitinib in bladder cancer cells. Cancer Res 2005;65:10524–10535.
135. Cheng HL, Liu HS, Lin YJ et al. Co-expression of RON and MET is a prognostic indicator for patients with transitional-cell carcinoma of the bladder. Br J Cancer 2005;92:1906–1914.
136. Cheng HL, Trink B, Tzai TS et al. Overexpression of c-met as a prognostic indicator for transitional cell carcinoma of the urinary bladder: a comparison with p53 nuclear accumulation. J Clin Oncol 2002;20:1544–1550.
137. Xia G, Kumar SR, Stein JP et al. EphB4 receptor tyrosine kinase is expressed in bladder cancer and provides signals for cell survival. Oncogene 2006;25:769–780.
138. Abraham S, Knapp DW, Cheng L et al. Expression of EphA2 and Ephrin A-1 in carcinoma of the urinary bladder. Clin Cancer Res 2006;12:353–360.
139. Greenman C, Stephens P, Smith R et al. Patterns of somatic mutation in human cancer genomes. Nature 2007;446:153–158.
140. Astrinidis A and Henske EP. Tuberous sclerosis complex: linking growth and energy signaling pathways with human disease. Oncogene 2005;24:7475–7481.
141. Kwiatkowski DJ and Manning BD. Tuberous sclerosis: a GAP at the crossroads of multiple signaling pathways. Hum Mol Genet 2005;14 Spec No. 2:R251–R258.
142. Niida Y, Stemmer-Rachamimov AO, Logrip M et al. Survey of somatic mutations in tuberous sclerosis complex (TSC) hamartomas suggests different genetic mechanisms for pathogenesis of TSC lesions. Am J Hum Genet 2001;69:493–503.
143. Edwards J, Duncan P, Going JJ et al. Identification of loci associated with putative recurrence genes in transitional cell carcinoma of the urinary bladder. J Pathol 2002;196: 380–385.
144. Hirao S, Hirao T, Marsit CJ et al. Loss of heterozygosity on chromosome 9q and p53 alterations in human bladder cancer. Cancer 2005;104:1918–1923.
145. Kandt RS. Tuberous sclerosis complex and neurofibromatosis type 1: the two most common neurocutaneous diseases. Neurol Clin 2003;21:983–1004.
146. Polakis P. The many ways of Wnt in cancer. Curr Opin Genet Dev 2007;17:45–51.
147. Marsit CJ, Karagas MR, Andrew A et al. Epigenetic inactivation of SFRP genes and TP53 alteration act jointly as markers of invasive bladder cancer. Cancer Res 2005;65: 7081–7085.
148. Urakami S, Shiina H, Enokida H et al. Epigenetic inactivation of Wnt inhibitory factor-1 plays an important role in bladder cancer through aberrant canonical Wnt/beta-catenin signaling pathway. Clin Cancer Res 2006;12:383–391.
149. Stoehr R, Wissmann C, Suzuki H et al. Deletions of chromosome 8p and loss of sFRP1 expression are progression markers of papillary bladder cancer. Lab Invest 2004;84:465–478.
150. Hooper JE and Scott MP. Communicating with Hedgehogs. Nat Rev Mol Cell Biol 2005;6:306–317.
151. Black PC and Dinney CP. Bladder cancer angiogenesis and metastasis-translation from murine model to clinical trial. Cancer Metastasis Rev 2007;26(3–4):623–634.
152. Gontero P, Banisadr S, Frea B et al. Metastasis markers in bladder cancer: a review of the literature and clinical considerations. Eur Urol 2004;46:296–311.
153. Charlesworth PJ and Harris AL. Mechanisms of disease: angiogenesis in urologic malignancies. Nat Clin Pract Urol 2006;3:157–169.
154. Ren B, Yee KO, Lawler J et al. Regulation of tumor angiogenesis by thrombospondin-1. [Review] [145 refs]. Biochimica et Biophysica Acta 2006;1765:178–188.
155. Masaki T. Historical review: Endothelin. Trends Pharmacol Sci 2004;25:219–224.
156. Wulfing C, Eltze E, Yamini J et al. Expression of the endothelin axis in bladder cancer: relationship to clinicopathologic parameters and long-term survival. Eur Urol 2005;47:593–600.
157. Titus B, Frierson HF, Jr., Conaway M et al. Endothelin axis is a target of the lung metastasis suppressor gene RhoGDI2. Cancer Res 2005;65:7320–7327.
158. Theodorescu D, Sapinoso LM, Conaway MR et al. Reduced expression of metastasis suppressor RhoGDI2 is associated with decreased survival for patients with bladder cancer. Clin Cancer Res 2004;10:3800–3806.
159. Swana HS, Grossman D, Anthony JN et al. Tumor content of the antiapoptosis molecule survivin and recurrence of bladder cancer. New Engl J Med 1999;341:452–453.
160. Jonsson G, Paulie S, Grandien A et al. cIAP-2 block apoptotic events in bladder cancer cells. Anticancer Res 2003;23:3311–3316.

161. Jonsson G, Paulie S, Grandien A et al. High level of cFLIP correlates with resistance to death receptor-induced apoptosis in bladder carcinoma cells. Anticancer Res 2003;23:1213–1218.
162. Duggan BJ, Maxwell P, Kelly JD et al. The effect of antisense Bcl-2 oligonucleotides on Bcl-2 protein expression and apoptosis in human bladder transitional cell carcinoma. J Urol 2001;166:1098–1105.
163. Matsumoto H, Wada T, Fukunaga K et al. Bax to Bcl-2 ratio and Ki-67 index are useful predictors of neoadjuvant chemoradiation therapy in bladder cancer. Jpn J Clin Oncol 2004;34:124–130.
164. Ong F, Moonen LM, Gallee MP et al. Prognostic factors in transitional cell cancer of the bladder: an emerging role for Bcl-2 and p53. Radiotherapy & Oncology 2001;61: 169–175.
165. Pollack A, Wu CS, Czerniak B et al. Abnormal bcl-2 and pRb expression are independent correlates of radiation response in muscle-invasive bladder cancer. Clin Cancer Res 1997;3:1823–1829.
166. Cooke PW, James ND, Ganesan R et al. Bcl-2 expression identifies patients with advanced bladder cancer treated by radiotherapy who benefit from neoadjuvant chemotherapy. [see comment]. BJU Int 2000;85:829–835.
167. Del Pizzo JJ, Borkowski A, Jacobs SC et al. Loss of cell cycle regulators p27(Kip1) and cyclin E in transitional cell carcinoma of the bladder correlates with tumor grade and patient survival. Am J Pathol 1999;155:1129–1136.
168. Korkolopoulou P, Christodoulou P, Konstantinidou AE et al. Cell cycle regulators in bladder cancer: a multivariate survival study with emphasis on p27Kip1. Hum Pathol 2000;31(6):751–60.
169. Liang J, Zubovitz J, Petrocelli T et al. PKB/Akt phosphorylates p27, impairs nuclear import of p27 and opposes p27-mediated G1 arrest. Nat Med 2002;8:1153–1160.
170. Medema RH, Kops GJ, Bos JL et al. AFX-like Forkhead transcription factors mediate cell-cycle regulation by Ras and PKB through p27kip1. Nature 2000;404:782–787.
171. Orlando C, Gelmini S, Selli C et al. Telomerase in urological malignancy. [Review] [159 refs]. J Urol 2001;166:666–673.
172. Papathoma AS, Petraki C, Grigorakis A et al. Prognostic significance of matrix metalloproteinases 2 and 9 in bladder cancer. Anticancer Res 2000;20:2009–2013.
173. Kanayama H. Matrix metalloproteinases and bladder cancer. J Med Invest 2001;48:31–43.
174. Mhawech-Fauceglia P, Fischer G, Beck A et al. Raf1, Aurora-A/STK15 and E-cadherin biomarkers expression in patients with pTa/pT1 urothelial bladder carcinoma; a retrospective TMA study of 246 patients with long-term follow-up. Eur J Surg Oncol 2006;32:439–444.
175. Fromont G, Roupret M, Amira N et al. Tissue microarray analysis of the prognostic value of E-cadherin, Ki67, p53, p27, survivin and MSH2 expression in upper urinary tract transitional cell carcinoma. Eur Urol 2005;48:764–770.
176. Mahnken A, Kausch I, Feller AC et al. E-cadherin immunoreactivity correlates with recurrence and progression of minimally invasive transitional cell carcinomas of the urinary bladder. Oncol Rep 2005;14:1065–1070.
177. Ribeiro-Filho LA, Franks J, Sasaki M et al. CpG hypermethylation of promoter region and inactivation of E-cadherin gene in human bladder cancer. Mol Carcinog 2002;34:187–198.
178. Bornman DM, Mathew S, Alsruhe J et al. Methylation of the E-cadherin gene in bladder neoplasia and in normal urothelial epithelium from elderly individuals. Am J Pathol 2001;159:831–835.
179. Friedrich MG, Chandrasoma S, Siegmund KD et al. Prognostic relevance of methylation markers in patients with non-muscle invasive bladder carcinoma. Eur J Cancer 2005;41(17):2769–2778.
180. Dulaimi E, Uzzo RG, Greenberg RE et al. Detection of bladder cancer in urine by a tumor suppressor gene hypermethylation panel. Clin Cancer Res 2004;10:1887–1893.
181. Tada Y, Wada M, Taguchi K et al. The association of death-associated protein kinase hypermethylation with early recurrence in superficial bladder cancers. Cancer Res 2002;62:4048–4053.
182. Shirahama T and Shirahama T. Cyclooxygenase-2 expression is up-regulated in transitional cell carcinoma and its preneoplastic lesions in the human urinary bladder. Clin Cancer Res 2000;6:2424–2430.
183. Wild PJ, Kunz-Schughart LA, Stoehr R et al. High-throughput tissue microarray analysis of COX2 expression in urinary bladder cancer. Int J Oncol 2005;27:385–391.
184. Komhoff M, Guan Y, Shappell HW et al. Enhanced expression of cyclooxygenase-2 in high grade human transitional cell bladder carcinomas. Am J Pathol 2000;157:29–35.
185. Dannenberg AJ and Subbaramaiah K. Targeting cyclooxygenase-2 in human neoplasia: rationale and promise. Cancer Cell 2003;4:431–436.
186. Koehne CH and Dubois RN. COX-2 inhibition and colorectal cancer. Semin Oncol 2004;31:12–21.
187. Klein RD, Van Pelt CS, Sabichi AL et al. Transitional cell hyperplasia and carcinomas in urinary bladders of transgenic mice with keratin 5 promoter-driven cyclooxygenase-2 overexpression. Cancer Res 2005;65:1808–1813.
188. Mohammed SI, Dhawan D, Abraham S et al. Cyclooxygenase inhibitors in urinary bladder cancer: in vitro and in vivo effects. Mol Cancer Ther 2006;5:329–336.
189. Smakman N, Schaap N, Snijckers CM et al. NS-398, a selective cyclooxygenase-2 inhibitor, reduces experimental bladder carcinoma outgrowth by inhibiting tumor cell proliferation. Urology 2005;66:434–440.
190. Grubbs CJ, Lubet RA, Koki AT et al. Celecoxib Inhibits N-Butyl-N-(4-hydroxybutyl)-nitrosamine-induced urinary bladder cancers in male B6D2F1 Mice and female fischer-344 rats. Cancer Res 2000;60:5599–5602.
191. Sabichi AL and Lippman SM. COX-2 inhibitors and other nonsteroidal anti-inflammatory drugs in genitourinary cancer. Semin Oncol 2004;31:36–44.
192. McNeish IA, Bell SJ, and Lemoine NR. Gene therapy progress and prospects: cancer gene therapy using tumour suppressor genes. Gene Ther 2004;11:497–503.
193. Wang S and El-Deiry WS. The p53 pathway: targets for the development of novel cancer therapeutics. Cancer Treat Res 2004;119:175–187.
194. Pagliaro LC, Keyhani A, Williams D et al. Repeated intravesical instillations of an adenoviral vector in patients with locally advanced bladder cancer: a phase I study of p53 gene therapy. J Clin Oncol 2003;21:2247–2253.

195. Connell PP, Weichselbaum RR, Connell PP et al. Gene therapy: the challenges of translating laboratory research into clinical practice. [comment]. J Clin Oncol 2003;21:2230–2231.
196. El Zawahry A, Lu P, White SJ et al. In vitro efficacy of AdTRAIL gene therapy of bladder cancer is enhanced by trichostatin A-mediated restoration of CAR expression and downregulation of cFLIP and Bcl-XL. Cancer Gene Ther 2006;13:281–289.
197. Kikuchi E, Menendez S, Ozu C et al. Highly efficient gene delivery for bladder cancers by intravesically administered replication-competent retroviral vectors. Clin Cancer Res 2007;13:4511–4518.
198. McKeown SR, Ward C, and Robson T. Gene-directed enzyme prodrug therapy: a current assessment. Curr Opin Mol Ther 2004;6:421–435.
199. Inoue M, Tomizawa K, Matsushita M et al. p53 protein transduction therapy: successful targeting and inhibition of the growth of the bladder cancer cells. Eur Urol 2006;49:161–168.
200. Ruifa H, Liwei L, Binxin L et al. Additional gene therapy with rAAV-wt-p53 enhanced the efficacy of cisplatin in human bladder cancer cells. Urol Int 2006;77:355–361.
201. Tovar C, Rosinski J, Filipovic Z et al. From the cover: small-molecule MDM2 antagonists reveal aberrant p53 signaling in cancer: implications for therapy. PNAS 2006;103:1888–1893.
202. O'Kane HF, Watson CJ, Johnston SR et al. Targeting death receptors in bladder, prostate and renal cancer. J Urol 2006;175:432–438.
203. Sheikh MS and Huang Y. Death receptors as targets of cancer therapeutics. Curr Cancer Drug Targets 2004;4:97–104.
204. Pukac L, Kanakaraj P, Humphreys R et al. HGS-ETR1, a fully human TRAIL-receptor 1 monoclonal antibody, induces cell death in multiple tumour types in vitro and in vivo. Br J Cancer 2005;92:1430–1441.
205. Korkolopoulou P, Goudopoulou A, Voutsinas G et al. c-FLIP expression in bladder urothelial carcinomas: its role in resistance to Fas-mediated apoptosis and clinicopathologic correlations. Urology 2004;63:1198–1204.
206. Maas S, Warskulat U, Steinhoff C et al. Decreased Fas expression in advanced-stage bladder cancer is not related to p53 status. Urology 2004;63:392–397.
207. Wang JL, Liu D, Zhang ZJ et al. Structure-based discovery of an organic compound that binds Bcl-2 protein and induces apoptosis of tumor cells. PNAS 2000;97:7124–7129.
208. James D, Castro J, Loria O et al. AT-101, a small molecule Bcl-2 antagonist, in treatment naïve CLL patients (pts) with high risk features; Preliminary results from an ongoing phase I trial. J Clin Oncol 2006;24:abstract 6605.
209. Li J, Viallet J, and Haura EB. A small molecule pan-Bcl-2 family inhibitor, GX15-070, induces apoptosis and enhances cisplatin-induced apoptosis in non-small cell lung cancer cells. Cancer Chemother Pharmacol 2008;61:525–534.
210. Shapiro GI. Cyclin-dependent kinase pathways as targets for cancer treatment. J Clin Oncol 2006;24:1770–1783.
211. Benson C, Kaye S, Workman P et al. Clinical anticancer drug development: targeting the cyclin-dependent kinases. [Review] [54 refs]. Br J Cancer 2005;92:7–12.
212. Misra RN, Xiao HY, Kim KS et al. N-(cycloalkylamino) acyl-2-aminothiazole inhibitors of cyclin-dependent kinase 2. N-[5-[[[5-(1,1-dimethylethyl)-2-oxazolyl]methyl]thio]-2-thiazolyl]-4- piperidinecarboxamide (BMS-387032), a highly efficacious and selective antitumor agent. J Med Chem 2004;47:1719–1728.
213. Ahmed S, Molife R, Shaw H et al. Phase I dose-escalation study of ZK 304709, an oral multi-target tumor growth inhibitor (MTGI), administered for 14 days of a 28-day cycle. Proc Am Soc Clin Oncol 2006;24:abstract 2076.
214. Cheng JC, Weisenberger DJ, Gonzales FA et al. Continuous zebularine treatment effectively sustains demethylation in human bladder cancer cells. Mol Cell Biol 2004;24:1270–1278.
215. Liang G, Gonzales FA, Jones PA et al. Analysis of gene induction in human fibroblasts and bladder cancer cells exposed to the methylation inhibitor 5-aza-2′-deoxycytidine. Cancer Res 2002;62:961–966.
216. Richon VM, Sandhoff TW, Rifkind RA et al. Histone deacetylase inhibitor selectively induces p21WAF1 expression and gene-associated histone acetylation. Proc Natl Acad Sci USA 2000;97:10014–10019.
217. Cote RJ, Laird PW, and Datar RH. Promoter hypermethylation: a new therapeutic target emerges in urothelial cancer. J Clin Oncol 2005;23:2879–2881.
218. Kelly WK, Richon VM, O'Connor O et al. Phase I clinical trial of histone deacetylase inhibitor: suberoylanilide hydroxamic acid administered intravenously. Clin Cancer Res 2003;9:3578–3588.
219. Monneret C. Histone deacetylase inhibitors. Eur J Med Chem 2005;40:1–13.
220. Lynch TJ, Bell DW, Sordella R et al. Activating mutations in the epidermal growth factor receptor underlying responsiveness of non-small-cell lung cancer to gefitinib. N Engl J Med 2004;350:2129–2139.
221. Sanborn RE and Blanke CD. Gastrointestinal stromal tumors and the evolution of targeted therapy. Clin Adv Hematol Oncol 2005;3:647–657.
222. Deininger MW and Druker BJ. Specific targeted therapy of chronic myelogenous leukemia with imatinib. Pharmacol Rev 2003;55:401–423.
223. Rauchenberger R, Borges E, Thomassen-Wolf E et al. Human combinatorial Fab library yielding specific and functional antibodies against the human fibroblast growth factor receptor 3. J Biol Chem 2003;278: 38194–38205.
224. Trudel S, Stewart AK, Rom E et al. The inhibitory anti-FGFR3 antibody, PRO-001, is cytotoxic to t(4;14) multiple myeloma cells. Blood 2006;107:4039–4046.
225. Chen J, Lee BH, Williams IR et al. FGFR3 as a therapeutic target of the small molecule inhibitor PKC412 in hematopoietic malignancies. Oncogene 2005;24:8259–8267.
226. Monnerat C, Henriksson R, Le Chevalier T et al. Phase I study of PKC412 (N-benzoyl-staurosporine), a novel oral protein kinase C inhibitor, combined with gemcitabine and cisplatin in patients with non-small-cell lung cancer. Ann Oncol 2004;15:316–323.
227. Lee SH, Lopes de Menezes D, Vora J et al. In vivo target modulation and biological activity of CHIR-258, a multitargeted growth factor receptor kinase inhibitor, in colon cancer models. Clin Cancer Res 2005;11:3633–3641.

228. Dimitroff CJ, Klohs W, Sharma A et al. Anti-angiogenic activity of selected receptor tyrosine kinase inhibitors, PD166285 and PD173074: implications for combination treatment with photodynamic therapy. Invest New Drugs 1999;17:121–135.
229. Sebti SM. Protein farnesylation: implications for normal physiology, malignant transformation, and cancer therapy. Cancer Cell 2005;7:297–300.
230. Winquist E, Moore MJ, Chi KN et al. A multinomial Phase II study of lonafarnib (SCH 66336) in patients with refractory urothelial cancer. Urol Oncol 2005;23:143–149.
231. Theodore C, Geoffrois L, Vermorken JB et al. Multicentre EORTC study 16997: feasibility and phase II trial of farnesyl transferase inhibitor & gemcitabine combination in salvage treatment of advanced urothelial tract cancers. Eur J Cancer 2005;41:1150–1157.
232. Rosenberg JE, von der MH, Seigne JD et al. A phase II trial of R115777, an oral farnesyl transferase inhibitor, in patients with advanced urothelial tract transitional cell carcinoma. Cancer 2005;103:2035–2041.
233. Cortes J, Faderl S, Estey E et al. Phase I study of BMS-214662, a farnesyl transferase inhibitor in patients with acute leukemias and high-risk myelodysplastic syndromes. J Clin Oncol 2005;23:2805–2812.
234. Basso AD, Kirschmeier P, and Bishop WR. Lipid posttranslational modifications. Farnesyl transferase inhibitors. J Lipid Res 2006;47:15–31.
235. Pan J and Yeung SCJ. Recent advances in understanding the antineoplastic mechanisms of farnesyltransferase inhibitors. Cancer Res 2005;65:9109–9112.
236. Appels NMGM, Beijnen JH, and Schellens JHM. Development of farnesyl transferase inhibitors: a review. Oncologist 2005;10:565–578.
237. Granville C, Memmott RM, Gills JJ et al. Handicapping the race to develop inhibitors of the phosphoinositide 3-Kinase/Akt/mammalian target of rapamycin pathway. Clin Cancer Res 2006;12:679–689.
238. Powis G, Ihle N, and Kirkpatrick DL. Practicalities of drugging the Phosphatidylinositol-3-Kinase/Akt cell survival signaling pathway. Clin Cancer Res 2006;12:2964–2966.
239. Mita M, Rowinsky E, Godston M et al. Phase I, pharmacokinetic and pharmacodynamic study of an mTOR inhibitor administered IV daily x 5 every other week in patients with refractory or advanced malignancies. Proc Am Soc Clin Oncol 2004;24:abstract 3076.
240. Tabernero J, Rojo F, Burris H et al. A phase I study with tumor molecular pharmacodynamic (MPD) evaluation of dose and schedule of the oral mTOR-inhibitor everolimus (RAD001) in patients (pts) with advanced solid tumors. Proc Am Soc Clin Oncol 2005;23:abstract 3007.
241. Wilhelm SM, Carter C, Tang L et al. BAY 43-9006 exhibits broad spectrum oral antitumor activity and targets the RAF/MEK/ERK pathway and receptor tyrosine kinases involved in tumor progression and angiogenesis. Cancer Res 2004;64:7099–7109.
242. Lyons JF, Wilhelm S, Hibner B et al. Discovery of a novel Raf kinase inhibitor. Endocr Relat Cancer 2001;8:219–225.
243. Strumberg D. Preclinical and clinical development of the oral multikinase inhibitor sorafenib in cancer treatment. Drugs Today (Barc) 2005;41:773–784.
244. Rinehart J, Adjei AA, Lorusso PM et al. Multicenter phase II study of the oral MEK inhibitor, CI-1040, in patients with advanced non-small-cell lung, breast, colon, and pancreatic cancer. [see comment]. J Clin Oncol 2004;22:4456–4462.
245. Kohno M, Pouyssegur J, Kohno M et al. Targeting the ERK signaling pathway in cancer therapy. [Review] [73 refs]. Ann Med 2006;38:200–211.
246. Wulfing C, Machiels J, Richel M et al. A single arm, multicenter, open label, phase II study of lapatinib as second-line treatment of patients with advanced/metastatic transitional cell carcinoma of the urothelial tract. Proc Am Soc Clin Oncol 2005;23:abstract 4594.
247. Philips G, Sanford S, Halabi D et al. Phase II study of cisplatin, gemcitabine, and gefitinib for advanced urothelial carcinoma: Analysis of the second cohort of CALGB 90102. Proc Am Soc Clin Oncol 2006;24:abstract 4578.
248. Slamon DJ, Leyland-Jones B, Shak S et al. Use of chemotherapy plus a monoclonal antibody against HER2 for metastatic breast cancer that overexpresses HER2. N Engl J Med 2001;344:783–792.
249. Hussain M, Petrylak DP, Dunn R et al. Trastuzumab, paclitaxel, carboplatin, and gemcitabine in advanced her2-positive urothelial carcinoma: results of a multi-center phase II NCI trial. Proc Am Soc Clin Oncol 2005;23:abstract 4507.
250. Vieillefond A, Beuzeboc P, Mignot L et al. HER2 status in urothelial bladder cancer (UC): screening of patients eligible for a phase II randomized study of gemcitabine plus platinum salt with or without trastuzumab. Proc Am Soc Clin Oncol 2005;23:abstract 4700.
251. Hurwitz H, Fehrenbacher L, Novotny W et al. Bevacizumab plus irinotecan, fluorouracil, and leucovorin for metastatic colorectal cancer. N Engl J Med 2004;350:2335–2342.

27
Tools for Study: National Databanking

Randall E. Millikan, Stuart O. Zimmerman, and Shida Jin

Contents

Abstract Some considerations bearing on the creation of a national databank for urotheilal cancer are discussed, including some potential applications of such a resource. A brief discussion of database design issues and caBIG™ serve to highlight the importance of teamwork and semantic interoperability. Finally, some specific data elements are put forward as a starting framework for the design of such a national repository.

Keywords Database, caBIG, Nomogram, Urothelial cancer

1. Introduction

To an extent that is truly humbling, this volume has documented the many facets of urothelial cancer that remain unsettled, and sometimes, controversial. In order to make progress, there is a broad consensus that we need data from which evidence-based practice can emerge for the benefit of patients with cancer. Indeed, large-scale collection and sharing of clinical data (a "National Databank") would seem to be a notion as unimpugnable as motherhood. Unfortunately however, structured information characterizing clinical medicine is hard to come by. Those who have tried to organize clinical "databases" have typically had an experience reminiscent of the proverbial Little Red Hen–everyone likes the smell and taste of freshly baked bread (or freshly collated data), but there are few as enthusiastic about the planting, watering, weeding, tending, harvesting, threshing, kneading, and baking required to produce it.

Nonetheless, it is almost certainly true that a large repository of high quality, structured clinical data related to the diagnosis, management and outcome of patients with urothelial cancer would be of enormous importance, and would accelerate both the pace of

From: *Current Clinical Urology: Bladder Cancer*, Edited by: C.T. Lee and D.P. Wood,
DOI: 10.1007/978-1-59745-417-9_27, © Humana Press, a part of Springer Science+Business Media, LLC 2010

new discovery and its clinical application. Some fairly obvious applications of such a resource include the support required to:

1. *Refine diagnostic criteria for, and define the natural history of, uncommon variants of bladder cancer.* For example, currently we have some centers finding micropapillary histology in up to 5–10% of cases, but most report this histology in less than 1%. While a portion of this discrepancy may reflect referral bias, it seems likely that the lack of clear diagnostic criteria also contributes. The true prognostic and therapeutic implications of a subtype will be difficult to define until we know who has that subtype! By definition, no single center has enough experience to establish such criteria for a rare disease, making this a particularly attractive area for cooperative data sharing.
2. *Establish clinical data elements that are needed to support inter-institutional translational studies.* Sharing biospecimen resources across institutions has proven to be extremely difficult. Part of this difficulty is that in order to be meaningful, the clinical annotation attached to a biospecimen must be standardized. It is surprisingly difficult to establish what the "core data elements" should be, and even harder to make sure that those elements have a consistent definition and usage across institutions.
3. *Refine staging systems and prognostic models.* It is obvious that we need to start incorporating more biological information into our prognostic models, since "Stage" is no longer a purely anatomic concept. For example, there is good evidence that the following clinical features (among others) are associated with a poor prognosis: hydronephrosis at presentation, muscle-invasion in the area of the bladder neck, variant histologies (such as small cell, sarcomatoid, focal lympho-epithelioma-like, and micropapillary), a long interval from diagnosis to cystectomy and an inadequate node dissection. None of these features are currently accounted for in the standard assessment of stage, even though some of these are powerful predictors of outcome in small series. Without question, future attempts to refine the staging system by incorporating clinical features such as these, as well as emerging genotypic and phenotypic markers, would greatly benefit from a national databank. This is not to say that prospective, rigorous validation will not be required, as it obviously will be. The point is only that at present, it is hard even to prioritize such investigations, and difficult to build a case for funding such trials when we have so little hard data available.
4. *Provide historical data to refine targets for statistical power calculations and accrual.* All trial designs start with some assumptions related to the question "What magnitude of a trial effect would be of interest?" Having a large dataset to serve as a more objective basis for defining the expectation of outcome with standard therapy would be a great benefit. In addition, such a resource would contribute considerable efficiency by making it possible to have confidence on the feasibility of proposed trials and their accrual goals.

While these and other benefits of a national databank are fairly easy to imagine, the particular tactical approach to creating such a resource is less clear. It is also apparent that the benefits we can envision for bladder cancer research are by no means confined to this context. In fact, the need to support these important tasks for all cancer researches is at the heart of the National Cancer Institute's initiative to provide both infrastructure and software tools for facilitating cooperative cancer research. This program, known as the cancer Biomedical Informatics Grid™ (caBIG™) is a very large effort, now involving hundreds of people in academia and industry. It is useful to keep in mind that the problems we seek to solve in the context of bladder cancer are just one facet of a much more general problem for which a more general solution is desirable. This chapter will provide a brief overview of some particular challenges that arise in constructing a databank, followed by a short description of the caBIG initiative, and finally some consideration of what data elements might be included in a national databank. It is of course awkward to provide a chapter on something that does not yet exist, and thus this is a necessarily hypothetical treatment.

2. Challenges

A few of the more prominent challenges for building a proper databank are outlined below. Only the more philosophical (as opposed to technical) aspects are discussed, since these are of greatest interest to clinicians and investigators. This discussion is intended only to give the broadest outline of the problem, as any meaningful treatment would require an entire chapter for each issue. Nonetheless, these vignettes are offered in the hope of establishing some basis for appreciating the magnitude of the task, and especially, the need to form partnerships between investigators and experts in informatics and information technology.

2.1. Medical Information is Always Observer Dependent

There is no such thing as truly "objective" clinical data. Consider the innocent question "Does the patient have a heart murmur?" The answer depends on whether you ask the medical student, resident, attending or cardiology consultant. Again, "What medication is the patient taking?" turns out to be a very difficult question to answer, since it depends on the skill of the provider to elicit the full extent of the list from the patient. Even a very "objective" question such as "How many lymph nodes were in the surgical specimen?" is not so objective–it depends on how hard the pathologist looks, and what the conventions are for describing confluent or matted nodes. As a final example, consider the question "Was there lympho-vascular invasion?" Well, should we insist on seeing endothelial-lined spaces, or is the overall architecture enough? and again, How hard must one look, and how prominent does the phenotype have to be–does one high-powered-field among all sections examined count?

It is immediately apparent that one of the interesting side effects of initiating a databanking effort is the need (opportunity!) to standardize the definition and understanding of clinical terms. Even so, all clinical data retain some trace of observer dependence. (This is one reason why there are many case-series reports that are limited to a small group of providers and pathologists who can at least use words in a way that is understandable by the members of the team.) A well-designed databank should have some provision for capturing who is vouching for the veracity of each data element, what role that individual plays, and for annotating the database with the results of auditors and others who provide "review" of the data.

2.2. Data Elements are Difficult to Define Properly

When clinicians are asked to define data elements for a "database", it seems that they are naturally inclined to put forward needlessly categorical or derivable data elements. Most people tend to think in terms of what data will appear on a spreadsheet report or in a data table for publication, and not necessarily in terms of how the data are best represented in relational database schema. (If you do not know what "relational database schema" are, please keep in mind that your information technology colleagues do not know what an Indiana pouch is; a large part of successful database development consists of mutual vocabulary expansion!) Consider a very simple but real example: "age at diagnosis" is a data element that we can all relate to, and it seems obvious that having this in the database would be appropriate. In fact however, it is far better for the database to contain the date of birth and the date of diagnosis. If it does, then age at diagnosis is easily derived and reported, even though it does not reside in the database as such. Moreover, if the database contains the date of birth, the date of diagnosis *and* the age at diagnosis, then internal inconsistencies can arise because essentially the same information is contained in two places in the database. In the parlance of informatics, having the same bit of information in the database more than once is called denormalization, and usually, it is a very bad thing for data integrity. It is not a trivial undertaking to design a large database that is normalized, but this is an essential feature for a robust repository that will be useful over time.

A related problem is the collection of information that has been made categorical or ordinal, throwing away granularity that may in fact be important in the fullness of time. Usually this happens in the context of a specific perceived use for the data, instead of a more detached perspective cognizant of long-term flexibility. For example, a particular cut point for tumor size might be established by a "standard" staging system and thus we get data elements like "Tumor >5 cm". This may look like a respectable data element on the surface, but in fact a database filled with these sorts of data elements can be quite frustrating over time. What happens when a reanalysis of a more complete data set suggests that the proper cut off is 4 cm? Those with only categorical or ordinal data will not be able to play; while those with the insight to have recorded "Size of Primary" will be able to accommodate any arbitrary categorization.

Physicians have a predilection for grading disease categories on a four-point ordinal scale; e.g. none, mild, moderate, severe; Stage I to IV, adverse events of grade 1–4, etc. This tendency to record derived data elements such as this is a major cause for different databases not being able to "talk to each other." This problem is virtually impossible to fix once established; but fortunately, it is rather easy to avoid in the first place. Thus, a very important general rule: put as much granularity in the database as is practical, and put the rules for making categories in the business logic, not embedded in the structure of the database per se.

It should be clear from these simple examples that when building a databank it is a good idea to get some professional help from someone experienced with database architecture, and not just make your list of "data elements" the columns in the database tables.

2.3. We Do not all Speak the Same Language

It is quite difficult to standardize medical terminology. For example, we have already seen that objective and reproducible criteria for histopathologic classification and grading are hard to come by. By definition, all standard systems for listing, naming, and classifying things are several years behind the thought leaders in any field. Thus the task of having academic pathologists (who make a living on the cutting edge of cancer classification and subdivision) use a standard vocabulary to do their work could be stifling and counterproductive. Likewise, research on perioperative outcomes may require defining and collecting data elements that are not part of routine operative reports or clinical care notes. Thus there are good reasons that "nonstandard" terminology needs to be used and supported by information systems. Nonetheless, it is almost impossible to achieve interoperability between information systems without attention to the problem of establishing a shared semantic meaning for terminology.

Of course, the nice thing about standards is that there are so many to choose from; which really is another way of saying that it will never work to make everyone use the same vocabulary. Although it is good to strive for universal definitions, it is necessary to realize that many different terminologies will need to coexist, and a robust information system should be able to "translate" as needed.

2.4. Patient Protection and Oversight

The need to handle protected health information (PHI), which is already challenging in the single institution setting, is obviously much more difficult in the multicenter setting of a shared databank. Moreover, the complexity introduced by multiple Institutional Review Boards overseeing research conducted in a multiinstitution setting can be quite challenging. Sometimes these difficulties have led to tissue studies no longer linkable to clinical data, a rather extreme impact on the whole point of translational research! A national databank obviously will require methods for stripping patient identifiers from shared narrative material, but should preserve the ability (for persons with the appropriate IRB oversight) to get back to the clinical data, and the information system should preserve the possibility of adding follow-up information over time. Simple "slice of time" datasets are likely to be obfuscating at best, and can often support conclusions at odds with those that arise from more mature follow up. Thus, it would seem to be necessary for a national databank to be committed to longitudinal data collection and not merely one-time characterizations.

2.5. Intellectual Property

Simply put, what are we going to do to make sure that if a surgeon shares 20 years of outcome data about a particular procedure in a national databank, some second-year fellow at another institution will not be able to sift that data and write a paper about it? This problem has no simple solution, aside perhaps from a few public hangings to set the proper tone. In fact however, there are many things that can be done to safeguard intellectual property and proper academic recognition. For example, a national databank would require a sophisticated system for granting access to data, and would need to support "feasibility queries" for an informed assessment of research prospects, without actually providing real data until the proper research oversight is in place. No matter how sophisticated the information system however, it seems clear that some altruism and trust must drive sharing for the benefit of collective progress against cancer.

3. Cancer Biomedical Informatics Grid™ (caBIG™)

Both the enormous potential benefits, and the substantial challenges, of developing the means for investigators to share clinical and translational data about patients with cancer have been recognized as high priority concerns by the National Cancer Institute. In response, caBIG™ was created as a three-year pilot project to create computing infrastructure and software tools (https://cabig.nci.nih.gov/overview). The program was initiated in the fall of 2003 and is officially described in the following way:

The cancer Biomedical Informatics Grid™, or caBIG™, is a voluntary network or grid connecting individuals and institutions to enable the sharing of data and tools, creating a world-wide web of cancer research. The goal is to speed delivery of innovative approaches for the prevention and treatment of cancer. The infrastructure and tools created by caBIG™ also have broad utility outside the cancer community. caBIG™ is being developed under the leadership of the National Cancer Institute's Center for Bioinformatics.

The importance of such an infrastructure, and the power of creating a truly interoperable cancer research community, can hardly be overstated. As of this writing, much progress has been made in defining common data elements via the cancer data standards repository (caDSR) which will serve as key infrastructure for the entire effort. Version 1.1 releases of applications related to tissue banking have appeared, and the effort to make them interoperable and mature enough to support clinical investigations is making good progress. Clinical data elements of the sort required for a national bladder databank are not yet available within the caBIG paradigm, but this is expected to be remedied in parallel with progress on the HL7 Reference Information Model.

An important current initiative is the attempt to use the nascent grid infrastructure to support a multisite collaboration among the prostate SPOREs. This project, known as the Inter-SPORE Prostate Biomarker Study, will provide proof-of-principle for many caBIG components. Its objectives are to share prostate tissues for biomarker analysis, requiring the ability to post tissue bank information on the grid, physically share biomaterials, post translational (e.g. biomarker staining) results on the grid, and allow participants to query across the institutions using the grid technologies. The emerging caBIG applications will be used as a way of interacting with the grid.

4. Data elements

If we are to have a national databank, whether it is built in concert with caBIG tools or not, we will need to decide on what data elements should be collected. Clearly, the answer depends in part on what questions would be asked of such a repository. Although flexibility to address questions other than those in mind at the time a databank is created is a laudable goal and an aspect of good design, the lessons of history strongly suggest that having some specific questions in mind will be an indispensable guide to getting such an effort successfully launched. Thus, before it is built, there will need to be some concensus on what the priority questions are likely to be.

Nonetheless, some discussion of specific data elements seems appropriate here. It is instructive in this regard to consider the nomogram, recently published by International Bladder Cancer Nomogram Consortium, for predicting the risk of recurrence within 5 years following radical cystectomy (1). This was a very significant effort, spanning 2.5 years and involving 13 institutions, to pool data on 9,064 patients. The 14 data elements solicited for each patient are listed in Table 27.1. Note that date of birth was not included (in violation of the principle espoused above) since date of birth is a "patient identifier," and it was felt that the pooled dataset should not contain PHI (illustrating the profound effect that considerations of patient protection appropriately have). Other noteworthy features of the data includetelescoping of histology to just three values, the characterization of nodal status as simply involved or not and the lumping of T4a disease (invasion of the prostate or vagina) with T4b (invasion of pelvic sidewall, pubis, or abdominal wall). For the final nomogram, patients receiving preoperative or postoperative systemic therapy, or definitive pelvic radiation were excluded, leaving 8,522 patients in the analysis. This provided a final model with a concordance index (CI identical to the area under the curve of a receiver-operator curve) of 0.75. This compared favorably wih the performance of standard TNM values, which gave a CI of 0.68, or the use of standard stage groupings, which gave a CI of only 0.62. Although a CI of 0.75 is fairly good for a clinical prognostic index, it is clear that more detailed data elements would be required

TABLE 27.1. Data elements solicited for use by the international bladder cancer nomogram consortium.

Gender
Age at cystectomy
Preoperative radiotherapy (Y/N)
Preoperative systemic chemotherapy (Y/N)
Date of diagnosis
Date of cystectomy
Histology (TCC, adenocarcinoma, squamous carcinoma)
Grade (high/low)
pT-Stage ('97 system)
pN-Stage ('97 system)
Number of nodes in surgical specimen
Number of involved nodes in surgical specimen
Recurrence status; date recurrence if applicable
Vital status; date of death if deceased

if the goal of a national databank were to establish a more powerful predictor of recurrence after cystectomy. In addition, a more contemporary dataset would need to include some information about perioperative chemotherapy since this is far more common now than just a few years ago. For example, 18% of the patients in the analysis had node-positive disease, and it would be unlikely that patients with such a high risk of recurrence would not be offered chemotherapy in current practice.

The more data elements that would be solicited for a national databank, the greater the risk that the effort to collect the information will not be rewarded with proportional gain. As with so many things, complexity is associated with diminishing returns in a databanking project. Nonetheless, more detailed annotation may be required for many questions of interest. The College of American Pathologists (CAP) have produced very detailed protocols for commonly encountered cancer procedures. These are essentially concerned with pathologic staging and data elements that are available at the time of definitive resection. These protocols can be downloaded at http://www.cap.org/apps/docs/cancer_protocols/protocols_index.html, and they are rapidly becoming widely accepted standards. They have been placed in the Federal Register, and they are expected to be incorporated in the infrastructure of caBIG very soon. A dataset based on the CAP data elements, along with the enumerated values, is shown in Table 27.2. Here we have expanded from 14 data elements in the International Consortium dataset, to 23 elements, with a significant expansion of the available enumerated values. For example, for histology the CAP protocol provides 11 values, as opposed to only three in the set of elements used to create the nomogram. As noted previously, the CAP protocols are focused on pathologic staging, and thus this set of data elements might be especially well suited for addressing questions related to surgical technique or postoperative outcomes. By contrast, these elements would be much less relevant if the questions to be addressed were concerned with outcomes in the setting of systemic therapy for metastatic disease.

Although it is hazardous to put forward a suggestion about specific data elements in the absence of a consensus on what the most important questions are, a possible set of elements that could fairly comprehensively support a national databank for bladder cancer is shown in Table 27.3. Here the number of discrete elements has ballooned to just over 40, and many of these can be multivalued. Those listed in

TABLE 27.2. CAP data elements, with enumerated values, for cystectomy.

Procedure (pick one)
Partial cystectomy
Total cystectomy
Radical cystectomy
Radical cystoprostatectomy
Anterior exenteration
Other
Location of primary tumor (all that apply)
Trigone
Right lateral wall
Left lateral wall
Anterior
Posterior
Dome
Other
Dimensions of primary tumor
Largest dimension
Others (up to 3 total)
Histologic type
TCC
TCC with squamous differentiation
TCC with glandular differentiation
TCC with variant histology (specify)
Squamous cell, typical
Squamous cell, variant histology (specify)
Adenocarcinoma, typical
Adenocarcinoma, variant histology (specify)
Small cell carcinoma
Undifferentiated carcinoma (specify)
Mixed cell type (specify)
Other (specify)
Carcinoma, type cannot be determined
Grade
for TCC (pick one)
High
Low
For adenocarcinoma and squamous carcinoma (pick one)
Grade 1
Grade 2
Grade3
Gross tumor configuration (pick one)
Papillary
Solid
Flat
Ulcerated
Indeterminate
Associated lesions (all that apply)
Papilloma, normal
Papilloma, inverted
Papilloma, low malignant potential
Other pathologic findings (all that apply)
c.i.s.
Inflammation / regenerative changes
Therapy-related changes

(continued)

TABLE 27.2. (continued)

Cystitis cystica glandularis
Keratinizing squamous metaplasia
Intestinal metaplasia
Other
Nodal involvement
pNx – pN3 (pick one)
Number of nodes examined
Number involved
Extent of invasion
pTx – pT4 (pick one)
Margin status
Cannot be assessed
Margins uninvolved
Distance from invasive carcinoma
Distance from c.i.s.
Margins involved
Involved by invasive cancer
Site(s) (specify)
Involved by c.i.s.
Other
Lymphovascular invasion (pick one)
Absent
Present
Indeterminate
Direct extension of invasive tumor (all that apply)
None
Perivesical fat
Rectum
Prostatic stroma
Seminal vesicles(s) (specify side)
Vagina
Uterus and adnexae
Pelvic sidewall
Ureter(s) (specify side)
Other

italics would point to lists of valid values that in turn would reflect standard terminologies that could be readily related to data elements defined in the context of CAP, caBIG™, etc.

5. Conclusion

There is a lot of information about bladder cancer sitting in databases around the world, and almost certainly, there would be important conclusions that would improve patient care if the information could be aggregated and queried. Perhaps more importantly, facilitation of cooperative translational studies, particularly for less common clinical problems, should significantly accelerate the pace of discovery and the application of those new discoveries to therapeutic interventions. The possibility of leveraging what is emerging from the caBIG™ effort is particularly exciting. If the trail-blazing efforts of the Inter-SPORE Prostate Biomarker Study to leverage the caBIG™ infrastructure are successful, this will provide a

Table 27.3. Proposed data elements for a national databank for bladder cancer.

I. Patient characterization
DOB
Place of birth (city and country)
Self-described ethnicity
Self-described racial heritage (could have 2 values in keeping with census policy)
Smoking exposure characterized as:
Age (or date) of onset
Age (or date) of quitting
Heaviest pack-per-day use
Total exposure (estimated pack-years)
Occupation(s), with associated dates or number of years in each (could be multi-valued)
Highest educational level
Smoking status of parents (as smoke-exposed years)
Smoking status of workplace (as smoke-exposed years)
Toxic exposures
II. Disease characterization
Histologies present (could be multi-valued)
Type of sample
Date first symptom
Date first tissue diagnosis
Local extent of disease at diagnosis (could be multi-valued)
Signs and symptoms at presentation (could be multi-valued)
Sites involved (could be multi-valued)
Baseline creatinine at diagnosis
Creatinine postcystectomy
Disease state at diagnosis
III. Treatment characterization
Procedure(s) and date (could be multi-valued)
Findings (could be multi-valued)
Radiotherapy (could be multi-valued)
Technique
Start date
Total dose
Site (could be multi-valued)
Chemotherapy drugs and cycle start dates (could be multi-valued)
IV. Outcome characterization
Local recurrence: Cytology vs. cystoscopy vs. diagnostic imaging
Distant recurrence site(s) (could be multi-valued)
Disease state at serial follow-up, with date (could be multi-valued)
Date of death
Cause of death
V. Translational studies
Phenotypic characterization (could be multi-valued)
Molecular characterization (could be multi-valued)

path for many to follow as a practical approach to establishing a national (or international) databank. At the very least, the forces coalescing around the creation of national standards for electronic medical records, the necessity of teamwork to pool experience for rare diseases, and the increasingly global nature of biomedical research, ensure that we will certainly have a national (or even international) databank for bladder cancer within the next decade. Sooner would be better.

Reference

1. International Bladder Cancer Nomogram Consortium. Postoperative nomogram predicting risk of recurrence after radical cystectomy for bladder cancer. J Clin Oncol 24:3967–3972, 2006.

28
Vaccine Development

Nicholas Karanikolas and Jonathan Coleman

Contents

Abstract Intravesical immunotherapy has been proven to be an effective approach for the management of carcinoma in situ and a proportion of high-grade, non-muscle invasive bladder cancers. The use of intravesical Bacillus Calmette-Guerin (BCG) has been extensively studied in this setting, allowing insight into the therapeutic cascade of immune response following BCG exposure. A number of virus-based strategies have been investigated that target tumor-specific epitopes in the hope of developing more effective and durable forms of treatment. Herein, we review the mechanistic action of vaccine therapies and report on the rationale and progress of vaccine-based strategies for the treatment of localized bladder cancer.

Keywords Bladder cancer, Vaccine therapy, Bacillus calmette guerin, Immunotherapy, Intravesical

1. Introduction

Approximately 70% of bladder cancers can be broadly classified as superficial; this comprises both noninvasive and invasive variants into the lamina propria. Superficial bladder cancers constitute a heterogeneous group of cancers with variable recurrence and progression rates. Initial treatment for all such cancers, however, is focused on bladder preservation; employing fundamental tenets of treatment that include complete transurethral resection followed by intravesical instillation of immunotherapeutic or chemotherapeutic agents for curative intent. The proven track record of intravesical vaccine strategies has set the benchmark for successful treatment by inhibiting recurrence of superficial cancers and delaying progression to muscle-invasive disease (1).

Immunotherapeutic strategies produce antitumor effects by either passive or active immunity. Most of the current work in bladder cancer immunotherapy is focused on active immunity; the recruitment and imprinting of the host immune system to recognize and effectively destroy tumor cells (1). Efforts to use passive immunity (i.e. IFN) have yielded only modest results against bladder cancer either alone or in combination with other agents (2).

Intravesical instillation of immunotherapeutic and chemotherapeutic agents is the treatment of choice as a superior route for the use of local therapies in the prevention of superficial bladder cancer progression and

From: *Current Clinical Urology: Bladder Cancer*, Edited by: C.T. Lee and D.P. Wood,
DOI: 10.1007/978-1-59745-417-9_28,

recurrence following complete transurethral resection, particularly for high-grade tumors. Still, a substantial subset of patients do not respond to intravesical therapies. The use of BCG, a notable triumph in the approach of localized immunotherapy, has an associated 50% of risk progression to muscle-invasive disease and further metastases occurring in up to one-third of these patients (3). Treatment for BCG refractory cases is dictated by a number of factors including histology and time interval of recurrence. Late recurrence with noninvasive disease may be amenable to repeat or additional intravesical regimens. While long-term data on the success of repeat treatment may be lacking, the indication that a meaningful proportion of these patients can respond to further intravesical vaccine treatments with or without IFN is encouraging (4–6).

The significant toxicity and modest response rates often associated with BCG treatment have fostered a growing interest in novel bladder cancer treatments. Efforts in improving immune-dependent treatments have centered on boosting antitumor immune response by using cytokine gene transfer techniques or enhancing systemic response to tumor-specific epitopes. This form of active immunity mimics the response observed with BCG therapy though intended to increase specificity and prolonged duration. The second one employs the delivery of specific gene products known to be aberrantly expressed in high-grade tumors, or directed gene therapy.

2. BCG Immunotherapy and the Immune Response

The association between tuberculosis (TB) and cancer dates back to the nineteenth century with Coley's observation that patients who were infected with TB had a lower incidence of cancer. BCG was introduced in 1921 for use as a tuberculosis vaccine and its first use as a cancer vaccine was established in Sweden during the 1930's as described by Holmgren. Beginning in the 1950's, clinical studies utilized BCG as a vaccine in the treatment of a number of various malignancies including leukemia, melanoma, colon and lung cancers. More contemporary clinical trials, however, failed to confirm earlier reports of limited success in these diseases and BCG was abandoned in favor of more modern chemotherapy and radiotherapy.

The work of Coe and Feldman demonstrated that bladder was capable of mounting a strong immune response, forming the experimental prerequisite for using BCG intravesically (7). In 1976, intravesical BCG was first employed by Morales and colleagues on a small group of patients with bladder cancer (8). Widespread acceptance for the use of BCG for superficial bladder cancer did not occur until the 1980's when the Southwest Oncology Group published results of prospective randomized treatment demonstrating decreased recurrence in patients who had been given BCG following transurethral resection (9).

In the wake of the success with this approach, several trials have compared BCG with various alternative forms of intravesical chemotherapy. When used in appropriately selected patients, BCG has been proven to be more effective than any other form of intravesical chemotherapeutic agent. BCG has shown effectiveness against small residual tumors and a 70–75% complete response for carcinoma in situ. Sustained responses to BCG with remission rates averaging 70% over 5 years have also been reported.

BCG usage is associated with significant adverse toxicities limiting the ability for many patients to complete a full course of therapy. Such treatment inconsistencies have complicated the design and interpretation of treatment response on study regimens. Most patients experience local symptoms of cystitis and some mild systemic symptoms, but severe symptoms occur in up to 5% of patients including treatment-associated mortality being reported 10. Additionally, there are difficulties in accurately assessing the response or durability of initial BCG responders since urine cytologies are frequently unreliable and biopsies may not be predictive of ultimate response.

2.1. Immune Response

For intravesical immunotherapy approaches to be effective, it is important that an appropriate and sustained antitumor response be obtained. Defining this type of response has been problematic although studies with BCG have been helpful in understanding the complex cascade of local immunological events that can lead to successful treatment. The postulated mode of action using intravesical BCG involves binding of the BCG organism to the urothelium of both cancer and normal cells. The binding is mediated by fibronectin and subsequent endocytosis resulting in the induction of several immunologically active chemokines and cytokines (Table 28.1). Resulting induction of

TABLE 28.1. Detectable urinary cytokines following 6-week BCG and purported mechanism of action.

Cytokine	Function	Peak levels
IL-18	Activates helper T and NK Cells	
IL-12	Activates helper T and NK Cells	
IL-8	Recruitment of neutrophils	
IL-6	Promotes BCG adherence	Week 6
IL-2	Cytotoxic T-cell differentiation, activation	Week 5 and 6
IL-1 (α/β)	Promotes adhesion, leukocyte transmigration	
TNFα	Induce MHC class II, apoptosis	Week 3–6
IFN-γ	Cell surface antigen expression	Week 4
G-CSF	Motility and invasion	
GM-CSF	Monocyte differentiation	Week 5 and 6

Interleukin-8 is a likely promoter of leukocyte aggregation. The release of proinflammatory cytokines such as tumor necrosis factor alpha (TNFa) and Interleukin 6 (IL-6) as well as upregulation of adhesion-molecule expression (intracellular adhesion molecule 1) has been found to facilitate effector cell–tumor cell interactions. These cytokines may themselves promote an antiproliferative affect; however, it is largely believed that they set the groundwork for subsequent cell-mediated reactions. Cytokines may cause tumor cells to display molecules that serve as sites of leukocyte attachment and activation (10). The expression of cytokines in response to BCG treatment is not uniform in all the patients prompting the search for a pattern of inflammatory response that may be predictive of treatment success. The expression of Interleukin 2 (IL-2) appears to be helpful in discriminating between those who may respond to BCG treatment, at least in the short-term analysis.

Prolonged treatment is associated with bladder wall infiltration by T lymphocytes, macrophages and neutrophils, as well as further induction of intercellular adhesion molecule 1, MHC class I and II molecules (11). It is believed that this leukocyte infiltrate secretes numerous cytokines, including IL-2 and interferon gamma (IFNγ), that are the hallmark of activated T cells and natural killer cells. Maximal levels of cytokine secretion, cellular influx, intercellular adhesion molecule 1 and MHC expression and clinical response are attained by the fifth and sixth instillation.

T lymphocytes are believed to play a central role in the antitumor response. Studies by Ratliff and colleagues had shown that both CD4 and CD8 T lymphocytes are required for effective response. CD4 T cells contribute to cytokine secretion that results in maturation of cytotoxic T lymphocytes or BCG-activated killer cells. These natural killer cells are unique in that they are able to discern between normal and tumor cells. Additionally, CD4 T cells also exert bystander antitumor effects through ligand interactions of fatty acid synthetase and CD40. CD40 ligand interactions play a crucial role in the activation of cytotoxic T lymphocytes and CD40-expressing tumor cells could substitute for antigen-presenting cells. In contrast, CD8 T cells presumably have an affect either by induction of necrosis or by apoptosis.

The type of immune response may largely be determined by the nature of the T cell generated. TH1 response is associated with IL-2, IL-12 and IFN-γ and favor the development of a cellular immune response. TH2 response is characterized by the synthesis of cytokines such as Il-4, IL-5 and IL-6, which favor the generation of a humoral immune response. It could be extrapolated that success with BCG treatment may result from preferential induction of TH1, as has been substantiated by studies with urine samples demonstrating activation of TH1-associated cytokines in treated patients. Problems exist, however, with measuring urinary levels of TH1 and TH2 cytokines because of their intrinsic instability in this medium.

After completion of BCG treatment, the activity of the immune system gradually subsides. There is a decrease in the amount of infiltrating leukocytes, MHC expression on epithelium and cytokine levels. This argument has formed the basis for maintenance instillation regimens, although studies with several maintenance regimens, with and without combination immunotherapy, show inconsistent or variable benefit.

3. Vaccine Strategies

There are several intrinsic limitations to cancer vaccine derivation that involve both host and vector factors; the identification of appropriate target antigens, the distribution of antigens in tumors and the effective immunization strategies that can induce a tumoricidal immune response (12). The choice of appropriate transgene product becomes integral to the formulation of an effective vaccine therapy for bladder cancer. However, alterations of tumor suppressor genes located on chromosome 9, such as p53 and pRb, are common events in bladder cancer and believed to be associated with progression (13). An increasing body of literature supports a cooperative effect of p53, p21 and pRB in cancer progression (14, 15). It has been questioned as to whether correcting a single genetic alteration is sufficient to address the heterogenous and complex interaction of oncogenic pathways activated by cancer cells, or if approaches to deliver tumor-specific suicide and immunomodulatory transgenes are more suitable (16).

Cell-surface antigens that are either overexpressed or specific to tumor cells have been sought to facilitate vaccine strategies. Coxsackie adenovirus receptor (CAR) is one of the more promising and most studied such targets. To identify variations in CAR expression in urothelial derived cells, Sabichi et al. characterized ten separate urothelial cancer cell lines. While CAR expression was identified in nine of the ten cell lines studied, significant variability in the amount of expression was found which poorly correlated with the degree of adenoviral-mediated gene transduction (17). Additionally, they identified a large degree of variation with respect to expression of p53, p16 and pRB. Studies such as these in human derived bladder cell lines serve to highlight the significant heterogeneity and complexity of genetic alterations associated with bladder tumors, even in the select tumor lines and subclones that can be established in cell culture. While these models serve as useful tools for the study of bladder cancer, they also highlight the complexity associated with creating vaccine therapies based on highly specific markers.

A different approach to generating generalized immune-mediated responses may be obtained with transduction of bladder cells with immune-modulating factors. Clinical studies using MB-49 cell line, a well-characterized transitional cell carcinoma derived from a mouse bladder tumor, had shown that transduction with CD154, a second signal costimulatory molecule that induces a T lymphocyte antitumor response, resulted in a potent antitumor response (18). Loskog et al. evaluated the tumorgenicity of the MB-49 cell line transduced with a variety of immune-modulating adenoviral vectors including CD154, CD80, IL-2 and combinations of CD154 and IL-2 (18). Dose-dependent protection against subsequent tumor challenges were noted after vaccination with CD154 modified tumor cells. They noted that the mice which received four vaccinations were completely protected whereas fewer vaccinations yielded intermediate results. These investigators have suggested a role for CD154 as immunomodulatory therapy in the treatment of bladder cancer.

Ephrin receptor type A2 (EphA2) is a receptor tyrosine kinase that has been reported to regulate growth and survival of several tumor cells. There is evidence demonstrating overexpression of these proteins in advanced stage of urothelial cancer. Eph receptors encompass the largest family of receptor tyrosine kinase known to have an effect on cell behaviors in both normal tissue and in states of disease. Events such as embryonic vascular development, cell migration and neovascularization have been linked to activity mediated by EphA2–ligand binding (19). EphA2 was originally isolated from cervical cancer lines and increased expression has since been shown to correlate with metastases and decreased survival. Overexpression of EphA2 has been reported to induce malignant transformation from nontransformed cell lines (20). In human urothelial cancer, overexpression of EphA2 has been identified and associated with advanced stage disease. Abraham et al. had shown that urothelial carcinoma growth can be inhibited by therapies that target EphA2–ligand binding (19). Delivery of Ephrin A-1fc utilizing an adenoviral vector decreased proliferation of bladder cancer cells. Their studies have shown the potential benefit of utilizing EphA2 agonists to treat urinary bladder cancer.

Cancer-testis antigens (CTA) are found in various types of cancers and expressed in normal adult germ cells (12). Several CTAs have been studied as target antigens in vaccine clinical trials. Included within this class are the MAGE, GAGE, BAGE and NY-ESO-1family of genes. Sharma et al. had evaluated the expression of CTAs in urothelial carcinoma and identified that expression was evident in a large portion of high-grade cancers (12). Additionally, they found that expression of specific CTAs may be independently predictive of survival. Their findings supported the potential for CTAs to be used in vaccine development and as potential prognostic markers.

The human MUC-1 mucin is a transmembrane glycoprotein that is expressed by both normal and malignant epithelium (2). Variable degrees of glycosylation are associated with the malignant phenotype exposing tumor-specific epitopes on the peptide core. These epitopes are recognized by the immune system and results in both MHC-restricted and -unrestricted recognition of target cells containing the exposed MUC-1 core protein (2). High levels of MUC-1 expression have been correlated with high-grade bladder cancers and implicated in the aggressive phenotype of micropapillary variants of urothelial carcinoma (21, 22). Phase I vaccine trials have revealed their safety and tolerability in patients with metastatic or locally advanced prostate and breast cancer (2, 23). This makes MUC-1 a desirable candidate for future vaccine trials, but at present vaccine trials with MUC-1 have not been conducted.

Transfection of tumor cells with immunomodulating agents, including IL-2 and GM-CSF, resulted in the enhanced tumor antigen recognition and an increase in antigen-specific immune response (14, 24, 25). In vitro studies using retroviral vectors to transfect the mouse MBT-2 bladder tumor cell line, which grossly and histologically resembles human transitional cell carcinoma, had shown successful integration and expression of these cytokines (26, 27). Retroviral vector transfections, however, were time-consuming and often resulted in low expressions of the gene product (28). An alternative transduction mechanism utilizing a cationic liposome was proposed by Larchian et al. (29). Liposome-mediated transfections allowed a higher concentration of plasmid to be introduced facilitating a high, though transient, concentration of gene product. In vivo studies utilizing a murine model with MBT-2 cells, orthotopically implanted in the mouse bladder, revealed a survival advantage for those liposome-mediated transfections as compared to the retroviral system. Additionally, multi-agent cytokine gene-modified tumor vaccines were beneficial as opposed to single-agent vaccines (29).

4. Vectors

The efficiency of gene transfer and cell-targeted therapy is contingent upon the ability of the recombinant viral vector to bind, enter and deliver the transfectant to the host cell. The variable expression of surface receptors by malignant urothelium and the attenuated nature of the viral vectors are major obstacles to vaccine development. Siemens et al. compared gene transfer efficiencies of attenuated vaccinia virus (NYVAC), canarypox virus (ALVAC) and replication-deficient adenovirus (30). They found significant variability in the transfecting efficiencies of these separate vectors in the cellular models used. Importantly, these findings appear to be related to differences in cell surface binding and the virus–cell interaction, highlighting the need for further work in identifying suitable targets and defining the level of efficiency necessary for effective vaccine strategies.

4.1. Adenovirus

The adenovirus particle is not surrounded by a lipid envelope; it enters the cytoplasm by disrupting the endosome and not through membrane fusion events (31). The virus enters the cells by receptor-mediated endocytosis that requires its attachment to cell-surface receptors. Interaction with the coxsackievirus group B cell surface receptor (CVADR) has been identified for adenovirus serotypes of subgroups A, C, D, E and F to attach to the cell surface (31). Additionally, the virus interacts with the vitronectin receptors, integrins $\alpha_v\beta_3$ and $\alpha_v\beta_5$. Loskog and colleagues demonstrated that bladder cancer cell lines express CVADR (31). Superficial tumors were broadly CVADR-positive as were tumor cells close to blood vessels. Invasive tumors, however, were weakly positive for CVADR. The cell lines with lower CVADR expression required twice the amount of vector for effective transduction. Tumor cells were weakly positive for integrin $\alpha_v\beta_3$ and nearly half expressed $\alpha_v\beta_5$. Evaluation of the stromal components of normal bladder also demonstrated expression in normal urothelium and in subepithelial tissues as well that could affect transfection efficiency, specificity and clinical effects of therapy. These preliminary data may suggest a role for this approach in patients with superficial low-grade tumors which are typically less effectively treated with more conventional intravesical immunotherapies such as BCG.

An open-label phase I dose-escalation study compared vector distribution of an intratumoral vs. intravesical instilled replication-deficient adenoviral vector containing wild-type p53 (SCH 58500) in patients with localized bladder cancer undergoing cystectomy (32). Analysis of tissue sections revealed high transduction efficacy and vector penetration into malignant and normal urothelium in patients who received intravesical treatments, but not in patients who underwent intratumoral injections (32). This study was not designed to address survival benefits to treatment but the authors had shown that adenoviral-mediated p53 gene transduction can be performed safely and with minimal side effects.

Pagliaro and colleagues performed a phase I dose-escalation study of a replication-defective adenoviral vector Ad5CMV-p53 (33). Intravesical instillations of the vector were performed on patients who were not candidates for cystectomy. Thirteen patients comprised the study cohort and they were randomized to a variable instillation schedule and viral particle dosing. Dose-limiting toxicity was not appreciated in any patient group.

Seven patients underwent RT-PCR of biopsy specimens to confirm effective gene transfer. They confirmed that bladder cancer cells were successfully transfected but no detectable changes in the immunostaining pattern of the transfected cells were appreciated. The authors attributed this to the glycosaminoglycan (gag) layer of the bladder mucosa that may serve as a natural barrier to adenoviral penetration. Additionally, low levels of coxsackie receptor and adenovirus receptor on the surface urothelium may be a major deterrent to effective transduction (34, 35). One patient in the study cohort was noted to have a clinical benefit from the treatment but the authors attributed this to a nonspecific inflammatory response, similar to BCG, rather than a p53-mediated antitumor effect.

5. Vaccinia Virus

Vaccinia virus belongs to the Poxviridae family of viruses. It was the first widely used vaccine, utilized for small-pox immunizations. Mastrangelo et al. performed intratumoral injections of vaccinia-GM-CSF in patients with malignant melanoma refractory to prior therapies (34, 36, 37). All patients had dermal lesions and some had visceral involvement. The lesions demonstrated a dense concentration of CD4 and CD8 T lymphocytes positive for CD3 and CD45 R0 activation indicating an intense local response. Also, they did not observe the regression of lesions in the primary injection field. RT-PCR confirmed the high level of expression of virally encoded GM-CSF and thymidine kinase mRNA. The same researchers then performed a phase I study on nonrecombinant vaccinia vector in patients with advanced urothelial carcinoma. Patients received three intravesical doses over 2 weeks and all patients underwent cystectomy 1 day after the third dose. Immunohistochemical staining of vaccinia-treated bladders revealed significant recruitment of activated T lymphocytes and dendritic cells indicating enhanced antitumor activity.

A phase I study evaluating the safety and complication profile of live intravesical vaccinia instillations were conducted by Gomella and colleagues (3). The study cohort consisted of four subjects with invasive bladder cancer who were candidates for cystectomy. The subjects were immunized prior to treatment with the small-pox vaccine. Intravesical instillations up to 100×10^6 colony-forming units were performed. Histological analyses of cystectomy specimens revealed mucosal and submucosal infiltration with lymphocytes, eosinophils and plasma cells in the areas of normal and malignant urothelium. Both tumor and normal urothelium showed evidence of viral infection with enlarged vacuolated cells and cytoplasmic inclusions. Immunohistochemical staining revealed a marked CD3+ T lymphocyte infiltration that expressed the CD45RO marker. Dendritic cell recruitment was also appreciated, indicating the ability for antigen presenting cell recruitment with intravesical vaccinia. The study supported the use of vaccinia as a vector for intravesical gene therapy and the authors are presently conducting a phase II trial using native vaccinia in patients with BCG-refractory bladder cancer (3).

Yang et al. performed intratumoral injections of vaccinia and granulocyte colony stimulating factor (GM-CSF) in a murine model to determine whether a tumor specific systemic immune response would result (38). They performed either intratumoral or contra lateral flank vaccinations of MB49-bearing female B6 mice. A systemic response was appreciated with intratumoral injections of the combination vaccinia and GM-CSF but not with vaccinia injection alone or when contra-lateral flank vaccinations were performed (38). They hypothesized that the increased tumor antigen at the tumor site facilitated the observed systemic immune response. Their findings supported intratumoral vaccinations as a means of immunotherapy for established tumors. Interestingly, despite the enhanced systemic response to the tumor, the tumors themselves did not regress. They postulated that the tumor kill to growth rate was insufficient to facilitate the appropriate antitumor response. Additionally, the tumor-specific T cells may be insufficient or inactive at the tumor site because of immunosuppressive factors.

6. Conclusion

The development of an effective bladder cancer vaccine will depend largely on the identification of specific tumor epitopes, vector selection and transgenic product utilized. A large number of specific tumor proteins are being evaluated as potential treatment targets; some with promising potential. Effective gene transduction into malignant and normal urothelium has been documented using varicella and adenoviral vectors, cytokine gene transfer as well as the development of an active immune response to intratumoral and intravesical vaccinations. Additionally, phase I studies have shown that intravesical instillations of attenuated and live viral vector are well tolerated with a low complication and toxicity profile and good transduction into normal and malignant urothelium.

Further development and clinical studies of this promising approach may provide an effective second-line therapy for patients who fail conventional treatment.

References

1. Shah, J.B. and J.M. McKiernan, *Novel therapeutics in the treatment of bladder cancer*. Curr Opin Urol, 2004. **14**(5): 287–293.
2. Pantuck, A.J., et al., *Phase I trial of antigen-specific gene therapy using a recombinant vaccinia virus encoding MUC-1 and IL-2 in MUC-1-positive patients with advanced prostate cancer*. J Immunother, 2004. **27**(3): 240–253.
3. Gomella, L.G., et al., *Phase I study of intravesical vaccinia virus as a vector for gene therapy of bladder cancer*. J Urol, 2001. **166**(4): 1291–1295.
4. Lam, J.S., et al., *Bacillus Calmete-Guerin plus interferon-alpha2B intravesical therapy maintains an extended treatment plan for superficial bladder cancer with minimal toxicity*. Urol Oncol, 2003. **21**(5): 354–360.
5. O'Donnell, M.A., *Combined bacillus Calmette-Guerin and interferon use in superficial bladder cancer*. Expert Rev Anticancer Ther, 2003. **3**(6): 809–821.
6. Punnen, S.P., J.L. Chin, and M.A. Jewett, *Management of bacillus Calmette-Guerin (BCG) refractory superficial bladder cancer: results with intravesical BCG and Interferon combination therapy*. Can J Urol, 2003. **10**(2): 1790–1795.
7. Coe, J.E. and J.D. Feldman, *Extracutaneous delayed hypersensitivity, particularly in the guinea-pig bladder. Immunology*, 1966. **10**(2): 127–136.
8. Morales, A., D. Eidinger, and A.W. Bruce, *Intracavitary Bacillus Calmette-Guerin in the treatment of superficial bladder tumors*. J Urol, 1976. **116**(2): 180–183.
9. Lamm, D.L., et al., *Bacillus Calmette-Guerin immunotherapy of superficial bladder cancer*. J Urol, 1980. **124**(1): 38–40.
10. Alexandroff, A.B., et al., *BCG immunotherapy of bladder cancer: 20 years on*. Lancet, 1999. **353**(9165): 1689–1694.
11. Prescott, S., et al., *Intravesical Evans strain BCG therapy: quantitative immunohistochemical analysis of the immune response within the bladder wall*. J Urol, 1992. **147**(6): 1636–1642.
12. Sharma, P., et al., *Cancer-testis antigens: expression and correlation with survival in human urothelial carcinoma*. Clin Cancer Res, 2006. **12**(18): 5442–5447.
13. Chatterjee, S.J., et al., *Combined effects of p53, p21, and pRb expression in the progression of bladder transitional cell carcinoma*. J Clin Oncol, 2004. **22**(6): 1007–1013.
14. Fearon, E.R., et al., *Interleukin-2 production by tumor cells bypasses T helper function in the generation of an antitumor response*. Cell, 1990. **60**(3): 397–403.
15. Cote, R.J., et al., *Elevated and absent pRb expression is associated with bladder cancer progression and has cooperative effects with p53*. Cancer Res, 1998. **58**(6): 1090–1094.
16. Casado, E., et al., *Doomed trials for promising adenoviruses: a rationale for success*. J Clin Oncol, 2004. **22**(6): 1162-3; author reply 1163–1164.
17. Sabichi, A., et al., *Characterization of a panel of cell lines derived from urothelial neoplasms: genetic alterations, growth in vivo and the relationship of adenoviral mediated gene transfer to coxsackie adenovirus receptor expression*. J Urol, 2006. **175**(3 Pt 1): 1133–1137.
18. Loskog, A., et al., *Potent antitumor effects of CD154 transduced tumor cells in experimental bladder cancer*. J Urol, 2001. **166**(3): 1093–1097.
19. Abraham, S., et al., *Expression of EphA2 and Ephrin A-1 in carcinoma of the urinary bladder*. Clin Cancer Res, 2006. **12**(2): 353–360.
20. Zelinski, D.P., et al., *EphA2 overexpression causes tumorigenesis of mammary epithelial cells*. Cancer Res, 2001. **61**(5): 2301–2306.
21. Cardillo, M.R., et al., *Epidermal growth factor receptor, MUC-1 and MUC-2 in bladder cancer*. J Exp Clin Cancer Res, 2000. **19**(2): 225–233.
22. Nassar, H., et al., *Pathogenesis of invasive micropapillary carcinoma: role of MUC1 glycoprotein*. Mod Pathol, 2004. **17**(9): 1045–1050.
23. Scholl, S.M., et al., *Recombinant vaccinia virus encoding human MUC1 and IL2 as immunotherapy in patients with breast cancer*. J Immunother, 2000. **23**(5): 570–580.
24. Gilboa, E., et al., *Immunotherapy of cancer using cytokine gene-modified tumor vaccines*. Semin Cancer Biol, 1994. **5**(6): 409–417.
25. Gansbacher, B., et al., *Interleukin 2 gene transfer into tumor cells abrogates tumorigenicity and induces protective immunity*. J Exp Med, 1990. **172**(4): 1217–1224.
26. Saito, S., et al., *Immunotherapy of bladder cancer with cytokine gene-modified tumor vaccines*. Cancer Res, 1994. **54**(13): 3516–3520.
27. Connor, J., et al., *Regression of bladder tumors in mice treated with interleukin 2 gene-modified tumor cells*. J Exp Med, 1993. **177**(4): 1127–1134.
28. Jaffee, E.M., et al., *High efficiency gene transfer into primary human tumor explants without cell selection*. Cancer Res, 1993. **53**(10 Suppl): 2221–2226.
29. Larchian, W.A., et al., *Effectiveness of combined interleukin 2 and B7.1 vaccination strategy is dependent on the sequence and order: a liposome-mediated gene therapy treatment for bladder cancer*. Clin Cancer Res, 2000. **6**(7): 2913–2920.
30. Siemens, D.R., et al., *Comparison of viral vectors: gene transfer efficiency and tissue specificity in a bladder cancer model*. J Urol, 2003. **170**(3): 979–984.
31. Loskog, A., et al., *Human urinary bladder carcinomas express adenovirus attachment and internalization receptors*. Gene Ther, 2002. 9(9): 547–553.
32. Kuball, J., et al., *Successful adenovirus-mediated wild-type p53 gene transfer in patients with bladder cancer by intravesical vector instillation*. J Clin Oncol, 2002. **20**(4): 957–965.
33. Pagliaro, L.C., et al., *Repeated intravesical instillations of an adenoviral vector in patients with locally advanced bladder cancer: a phase I study of p53 gene therapy*. J Clin Oncol, 2003. **21**(12): 2247–2253.
34. Mastrangelo, M.J., et al., *Intratumoral recombinant GM-CSF-encoding virus as gene therapy in patients with cutaneous melanoma*. Cancer Gene Ther, 1999. **6**(5): 409–422.
35. Okegawa, T., et al., *The mechanism of the growth-inhibitory effect of coxsackie and adenovirus receptor (CAR) on human bladder cancer: a functional analysis of car protein structure*. Cancer Res, 2001. **61**(17): 6592–6600.

36. Mastrangelo, M.J. and E.C. Lattime, *Virotherapy clinical trials for regional disease: in situ immune modulation using recombinant poxvirus vectors*. Cancer Gene Ther, 2002. **9**(12): 1013–1021.
37. Mastrangelo, M.J., et al., *Poxvirus vectors: orphaned and underappreciated*. J Clin Invest, 2000. **105**(8): 1031–1034.
38. Yang, A.S., C.E. Monken, and E.C. Lattime, *Intratumoral vaccination with vaccinia-expressed tumor antigen and granulocyte macrophage colony-stimulating factor overcomes immunological ignorance to tumor antigen*. Cancer Res, 2003. **63**(20): 6956–6961.

29
Advances in Gene Therapy for Bladder Cancer

Niels-Erik B. Jacobsen and Thomas A. Gardner

Contents

Abstract Bladder cancer continues to be a lethal disease despite advances in surgical, chemotherapy and radiotherapy techniques. As the understanding of the molecular mechanisms of bladder cancer development, progression, and metastases increases, new opportunities for therapeutic advances arise. The advances in vector development and production also provide additional opportunities for therapeutic advances for all diseases including cancer. This chapter reviews the past, present and future gene therapy approaches and will serve as a valuable resource for anyone who wishes to understand the role of gene therapy in the future management of bladder cancer. In particular the molecular alterations, cytoreductive, corrective and immunomodulation approaches are reviewed.

Keywords Bladder cancer, Gene therapy, Vector, Oncogene, Tumor suppressor gene, Oncolytic, Immunomodulation, Vaccine

1. Introduction

Bladder cancer is the fourth and ninth most common cancer in men and women, respectively, and accounts for approximately 13,000 deaths in the United States in 2006 (1). Transitional cell carcinoma (TCC), which accounts for more than 90% of all cases of bladder cancer, presents in two forms. Seventy percent of cases consist of a low grade superficial papillary variant that carries with it a 50–70% recurrence rate and a 10% risk of progression to muscle invasion. High grade TCC, on the other hand, has a much higher malignant potential wherein 15–50% of cases present with or progress to muscle invasive disease. Overall, 25% of patients harbor muscle invasive bladder cancer at the time of initial diagnosis and an additional 10–15% of patients with superficial disease develop invasion during follow-up.

Although the risk of recurrence of superficial TCC after endoscopic resection can be reduced through

From: *Current Clinical Urology: Bladder Cancer*, Edited by: C.T. Lee and D.P. Wood,
DOI: 10.1007/978-1-59745-417-9_29,

the use of adjuvant intravesical chemotherapy or immunotherapy, 33–66% of patients will develop a recurrence within five years (2). Furthermore, high-grade superficial TCC refractory to intravesical BCG portends a high risk of progression to muscle invasion, metastases and subsequent mortality if definitive surgical therapy is delayed. The prognosis for patients presenting with muscle invasive TCC remains equally guarded since up to 50% have micrometastatic disease at the time of cystectomy. While numerous trials evaluating multi-agent chemotherapy regimens have demonstrated high response rates in the neoadjuvant, adjuvant and palliative settings, the 5-year survival rate for patients with locally advanced or metastatic disease remains low (13–15%) as does the median survival (14–15 months) (3, 4). Such sobering results argue strongly for the development of novel treatment strategies for both superficial and invasive TCC.

During the past two decades great strides have been made in our understanding of the molecular and genetic events responsible for the initiation and progression of bladder cancer. With such insight has come the realization that therapies targeted against specific genetic aberrations may halt or reverse the neoplastic process. Although clinical trials evaluating gene therapy for bladder cancer remain in their infancy, the results of numerous in vitro and in vivo studies support this treatment concept. This paper serves to review the current knowledge base, highlight active research protocols, and outline future directions in the field of gene therapy as it relates to bladder cancer.

2. Molecular Genetics and Bladder Cancer Biology

Basic research has identified a vast array of genetic abnormalities associated with the initiation, promotion and progression of urothelial carcinoma. Such variety helps to explain the heterogeneous clinical behavior of bladder cancer. In fact, low grade superficial TCC and high-grade invasive TCC appear to represent two distinct disease processes each with their own unique genetic profile. Genetic changes integral to the development of the neoplastic state include the over-expression of oncogenes and the under-expression or inactivation of tumor suppressor genes, both of which lead to uncontrolled cellular proliferation. Additional mutations in the urothelial genotype allow TCC to escape normal immune surveillance mechanisms through a reduction in tumor antigenicity or through active suppression of the host immune response. Recognizing the importance these genetic events, researchers have begun to translate this knowledge into the development of viable gene therapy techniques.

Gene therapy for the treatment of cancer can be divided into three broad categories: corrective, cytotoxic and immunomodulatory (5, 6). The goal of corrective gene therapy is to repair a critical genetic mutation by either inactivating an over-expressed oncogene or by replacing a non-functional tumor suppressor gene (TSG). Cytotoxic gene therapy aims to kill tumor cells through the induction of suicide genes, or through the transfection of replication-competent oncolytic viruses. Finally, immunomodulatory gene therapy seeks to stimulate a tumor-specific host immune response through the induction of cytokines, the transfection of genetically enhanced cytotoxic lymphocytes, or through the use of autologous tumor vaccines.

3. Vector Delivery

An important determinant of the therapeutic efficacy of any gene therapy technique is the efficiency of transgene delivery. The ideal delivery system maximizes target specificity, vector uptake, and transgene expression while minimizing local and systemic toxicity. Improving transgene delivery has been the focus of numerous studies in recent years with special attention given to vector construction, delivery route, and vector uptake by tumor cells.

Vectors serve as the delivery vehicles for gene transport into target cells. Viruses, specifically retrovirus and adenovirus, represent the original vectors used in early gene therapy studies. Case reports of vector-induced pediatric leukemia with retrovirus and vector-specific immunity and sensitization-induced inflammatory toxicity with adenovirus have spurred intense research into the development of modified viral vectors as well as non-viral delivery systems (7–10). The risk of insertional mutagenesis with retrovirus is rare and may be further reduced with improvements in vector design (11). Likewise, the immunogenicity of adenoviruses can be reduced through vector modification as demonstrated by helper-dependent adenoviruses which are completely devoid of viral genes and, as a result, weakly immunogenic (12). Non-viral vector systems, which include both physical (microinjection, jet injection, electroporation) and chemical (liposomes) subtypes, provide efficient genetic transduction and carry no risk of insertional mutagenesis or immunogenicity as can occur with viral vectors (13, 14). Regardless of the above, viral vectors represent the simplest and most effective means for genetic transduction and, as a result, remain the most commonly used delivery systems for gene therapy today.

A second issue of importance concerns the route for vector delivery. Options for vector delivery in the case of localized bladder cancer include direct intralesional injection and intravesical instillation, while locally-advanced or metastatic cases require systemic therapy. Gene therapy for most other solid tumors (ex. prostate) is delivered via intratumoral injection, however, the bladder, by virtue of its accessibility and capability to maintain prolonged dwell times, is ideally suited for intravesical instillation. In fact, phase one clinical data demonstrates that transgene expression after intravesical instillation of a recombinant adenoviral vector encoding wild-type p53 cDNA is superior to that achieved with intratumoral injection (15). Intravesical instillation is not without its limitations, however. The protectant glycosaminoglycan (GAG) lining of the urothelium represents a significant barrier to efficient vector transduction. This has necessitated the development and incorporation of numerous permeability agents such as the non-ionic detergent Big CHAP and the polyamide compound Syn3. Both of these agents have been shown to improve transgene delivery and transduction with minimal side-effects (15–17).

Once in contact with bladder urothelium, viral vectors must gain entrance into the target cells before transgene expression can take place. The primary mechanism by which this occurs is receptor-mediated endocytosis. Coxsackie adenovirus receptor (CAR) has been identified as an important determinant of adenoviral infectivity (18). Unfortunately, CAR expression is not uniform and has been shown to be low, or even nonexistent, in high grade bladder cancer (19, 20). This has obvious implications for the efficiency and specificity of gene therapy techniques which make use of an adenoviral vector. One method to overcome this limitation involves the co-administration of CAR cDNA which improves adenoviral transfection through an up-regulation of receptor density in target cell membranes (21). Treatment with the histone deacetylase inhibitor FR901228 has also been shown to increase CAR expression and adenoviral p53-mediated cytotoxicity (22). Alternate strategies include the utilization of epidermal growth factor receptor (EGFR), which appears to be more commonly expressed by human bladder cancer. By tagging replication-competent adenoviral vectors with antibodies to EGFR, transfection efficiency is improved as is the tumor response rate (23). Most adenoviral vectors currently in use are based on the Ad type 5 (Ad5) fiber which uses CAR as the initial receptor. Modified Ad vectors which carry the fiber shaft domain of both Ad5 and Ad35 (Ad5/35) overcome this limitation and demonstrate improved transfection efficiency based on expanded tropism for such receptors as the CD46 membrane cofactor protein (24). Instillation volume, pressure, and viral concentration have also been identified as important determinants of transfection efficiency in viral vector delivery systems (25, 26).

Three phase I trials have demonstrated that intravesical vector delivery is safe, feasible and biologically efficacious in the clinical setting (15, 27, 28). It is readily apparent, however, that intravesical instillation cannot achieve the systemic levels required to eradicate distant metastatic disease. This can only occur through systemic administration which, in turn, necessitates a delivery system of high specificity for target cells. Tumor specificity may be achieved through either selective transfection or site-restricted expression. As already discussed, transfection specificity may be improved by increasing target receptor density or by constructing vectors with receptor-specific antibodies. Site-restrictive expression, on the other hand, involves the use of tissue-specific promoters that ensure selective transgene expression within target cells regardless of the transfection specificity. The cyclooxygenase-2 (Cox-2) and uroplakinII (UPII) promoters represent two such promoters with potential application in gene therapy (29, 30).

4. Corrective Strategies

4.1. Oncogene Suppression

Proto-oncogenes encode for various proteins involved in the normal regulation of cellular growth and differentiation. Oncogenes represent mutated proto-oncogenes which, when over-expressed, act in a positive fashion to promote tumorigenesis. The goal of corrective gene therapy in this regard is to inhibit aberrant oncogene expression. This can be achieved at the DNA, RNA or protein level by one of four suppressive strategies including anti-sense oligonucleotides (AS), ribozymes (RZ), dominant negative mutants (DNM) and RNA interference (RNAi).

Anti-sense oligonucleotides are short segments of DNA or RNA which bind to and prevent the transcription or translation of complementary oncogenes. Ribozymes are small RNA strands which posses catalytic activity towards specific sequences of oncogene mRNA. Together, AS and RZ represent the two most commonly employed strategies in oncogene suppression. Dominant negative mutants are mutated oncogenes that encode for defective protein products. These non-functional proteins, when produced in great excess, suppress the neoplastic process through the sequestration of targets critical to tumor-specific oncogene function. RNA interference is a recently discovered gene silencing strategy in which small segments of double stranded RNA, termed short inhibitory RNA (siRNA), suppress the expression of genes with partial sequence homology through the degradation of target mRNA. The advantage of RNAi is that it can be used to target a large number of genes involving multiple aberrant cellular pathways as typically occurs in cancer. Such technology obviously holds great promise in the field of cancer therapy.

Over the past decade, suppressive gene therapy targeting a range of oncogenes and gene products have demonstrated efficacy towards TCC of the bladder in vitro and in vivo (31–37). Although there is no published clinical data as of yet, the findings of certain pre-clinical bladder cancer studies deserve mention. The H-ras oncogene, a member of the Ras G protein family, is mutated or over-expressed in 39–58% of bladder cancers and portends a two-fold increased risk of tumor recurrence following standard therapy (38). The transduction of a ribozyme targeting H-ras has been shown to cause significant tumor regression in a murine bladder cancer model (31). The tumor response was dose-dependent and optimal results were achieved using multiple doses set at lower viral titres. C-myc, an oncogene over-expressed in 58% of bladder cancers, represents an important determinant of cell-cycle progression and may also play a role in the development of resistance to chemotherapy (39). In vitro, anti-myc-AS has demonstrated significant cytotoxic activity against human bladder cancer cells (34). Interestingly, the combined administration of cisplatin or carboplatin with anti-myc-AS resulted in synergistic tumor cell kill. Anti-myc-AS appeared to enhance tumor chemosensitivity by increasing the intracellular concentration of cisplatin or carboplatin. Similarly, anti-mdr-1 AS/RZ directed towards the multi-drug resistance gene-1 (mdr-1), has been shown to improve response rates to chemotherapeutic agents (40).

The over-expression of polo-like kinase-1 (PLK-1), an oncogene with important regulatory control over cell-cycle progression, is associated with high-grade, muscle-invasive bladder cancer and is predictive of a poor prognosis among human subjects (41). The intravesical administration of liposomes containing a combination of four siRNAs specific to PLK-1 has been shown to result in significant tumor regression in an orthotopic bladder cancer model. In vitro, PLK-1 siRNAs inhibited the expression of endogenous PLK-1 causing a reduction in tumor cell proliferation and an increase in apoptotic activity. Similarly, siRNAs (SVV284 and SVV094) targeting survivin, an oncogene with anti-apoptotic activity, inhibited the growth of TCC in vitro through the induction of cell-cycle arrest and apoptosis (42). A follow-up study found that pre-treatment with the anti-survivin siRNA SVV284, followed by chemotherapy, improved tumor cell kill in a synergistic fashion indicating potential use for this agent as a chemosensitizing agent (43). Multi-target siRNA therapy appears to be more efficacious than single-target therapy. The transfection of multiple siRNAs targeting VEGF (vascular endothelial growth factor), hTERT (human telomerase reverse transcriptase) and survivin, in vitro, resulted in superior tumor control relative to siRNAs targeting individual genes (44). This makes intuitive sense since the initiation, promotion and progression of most common cancers, including bladder cancer, involves multiple genetic events affecting a number of distinct cellular pathways.

In summary, numerous in vitro and in vivo studies have shown that corrective strategies targeting aberrant oncogene expression provide significant anti-tumor effect in bladder cancer models. While corrective strategies have not yet been evaluated in phase I clinical trials, the results of pre-clinical studies performed thus far certainly set the foundation to do so. Future trials may further examine the apparent synergism between suppressive gene therapy and cytotoxic chemotherapy, and its potential role in the multimodal treatment of advanced bladder cancer.

4.2. Induction of Tumor Suppressor Genes

Tumor suppressor genes (TSG) serve to control cellular proliferation through the regulation of cell-cycle progression, DNA repair, transcriptional activity, and apoptosis. Mutation of critical TSGs has been shown to lead to malignant transformation by abrogating strict proliferative control. Through the transfection of wild-type TSGs into malignant cells, the goal of corrective gene therapy is to re-institute normal control mechanisms and, in turn, induce tumor regression.

The TSG that has garnered the most attention in the oncologic literature, including that of bladder cancer, is p53. Through the regulation of cell-cycle progression, angiogenesis, and apoptosis, wild-type p53 serves to prevent the development of neoplastic growth. The association of p53 mutation with bladder cancer has been well-documented with an incidence ranging from 10 to 70% (45, 46). Laboratory studies have shown that transfection of bladder cancer with vectors encoding wild-type p53 leads to tumor regression (47–49). The exact mechanism of action is a matter of debate. Some studies suggest the dominant effect is one of cell cycle arrest while others point to the stimulation of apoptosis as more important (50, 51). In actuality, the tumor regression observed with p53 corrective gene therapy is likely to occur via multiple pathways commensurate with the numerous functions that this TSG performs. With preliminary work having established the feasibility of gene therapy directed towards p53, subsequent efforts have focused on expanding its therapeutic potential and testing its clinical efficacy.

One such study sought to improve the specificity of p53 transgene expression for tumor cells through the combined use of an hTRT promoter (human telomerase reverse transcriptase promoter) and a Cre/loxP site-specific recombination system. Since bladder cancer cells are typically telomerase-positive and Cre-negative, this dual targeting system ensures that the expression of vector-specific p53 only occurs in telomerase-positive cells. Although most benign cells are telomerase-negative, the few that are positive are protected through Cre expression which allows the deletion of the transfected p53 (52).

Similar to the c-myc oncogene, over-expression of the mutated p53 correlates with bladder cancer resistance to cytotoxic chemotherapy (53). The transduction of recombinant wild-type p53 has been shown to improve tumor chemosensitivity independent from its direct growth inhibitory effects. Pre-treatment with Ad5CMV-p53, in vitro, improved the chemosensitivity of TCC towards cisplatin in a dose-dependent manner, reducing the median IC_{50} (half maximal inhibitory concentration) by more than 50% (54). In vivo, this combination synergistically inhibited tumor cell growth and reduced the incidence of metastases in an orthotopic murine bladder cancer model. Dual gene therapy regimens which combine the transfection of wild-type p53 with suppressive techniques targeting the oncogenes erbB2 or clusterin have also demonstrated synergistic activity against bladder cancer (55, 56). The addition of cisplatin to these same dual gene therapy regimens appears to provide even further improvement in local and distant tumor control. Apart from improved therapeutic efficacy, an obvious advantage of dual gene therapy or combined gene/chemotherapy is the capacity for dose reduction which, in turn, will improve vector- or chemotherapy-related toxicity profiles.

Of the three published clinical trials evaluating gene therapy in bladder cancer, two involve p53. The first trial compared the results of a single intratumoral injection of rAd-p53 to that of a single intravesical instillation of rAd-p53 in eleven patients with muscle-invasive bladder cancer scheduled for cystectomy three days after treatment. Whereas vector-specific p53 expression was identified in seven out of eight patients after intravesical instillation, no transgene expression could be found in the cystectomy specimens of the three patients treated by intratumoral injection. Furthermore, intravesical instillation of rAd-p53, in conjunction with the transduction-enhancing agent Big CHAP, provided uniform vector penetration throughout the urothelium including submucosal tumor. Both transgene expression and biologic activity, as determined by RT-PCR (reverse transcriptase polymerase chain reaction) for p53 and p21, respectively, correlated with the dose. Side-effects consisted of mild tos moderate dysuria or abdominal pain, both of which resolved immediately upon the cessation of intravesical instillation. Although this study cannot confirm the clinical efficacy of p53 gene therapy in bladder cancer, it does establish the safety, feasibility and transfection efficiency of intravesical rAd-p53 instillation in the clinical setting (15).

A more recent phase I trial, using an adenoviral vector encoding the cytomegalovirus (CMV) promoter and wild-type p53 gene (Ad5CMV-p53), evaluated the role of intravesical dose-escalation. Thirteen patients with locally-advanced or BCG-refractory bladder cancer, who were not candidates for cystectomy, received intravesical instillations of Ad5CMV-p53 at dosages ranging from 10^{10} to 10^{12} virions. Analysis of post-treatment biopsy specimens by RT-PCR found vector-specific p53 expression in two of seven patients, both of which had received the highest viral particle dose (10^{12}). Further immunohistochemical analysis demonstrated that none of the eleven patients had identifiable changes in p53 or p21 levels. Side-effects were generally minor, consisting of mild bladder spasms in three patients and asymptomatic bladder ulcerations in one patient. Importantly, no patient experienced dose-limiting toxicity. All patients with positive cytology at study entry retained positive cytology at one month and eleven of thirteen patients developed disease progression at a median time of two months. These results corroborate the safety and feasibility of intravesical Ad5CMV-p53 gene therapy, however the sub-optimal transfection efficiency and biologic activity highlight the need for improvements in gene transfer and expression (28).

The retinoblastoma TSG (Rb), which exerts control over cell-cycle progression, is mutated in up to 30% of bladder tumors and appears to be associated with high grade disease (45). With this in mind, recent studies have sought to determine the therapeutic potential of Rb-directed gene therapy. One such study evaluated both full-length Rb110 and N-terminal truncated Rb94 gene transduction in a murine model and found that both forms induced tumor regression, however, Rb94 was more effective (57). The superiority of Rb94 has since been confirmed in a second study which also found that induction of telomere erosion and caspase-dependent apoptosis appear to be the major pathways by which Rb94 exerts its cytotoxic effect (58).

In addition to p53 and Rb, corrective strategies targeting such TSGs as p21, p16, and gelsolin have demonstrated anti-tumor effect in preclinical bladder cancer models (59–62). While published clinical data is only available for p53, Rb has recently been the focus of a phase I dose-escalation trial. Patients with superficial or muscle invasive disease refractory to at least one course of standard therapy will receive a single intravesical dose of a replication-defective adenoviral construct encoding the Rb gene (ACNRb). This trial, which is now closed, hopes to shed light on the safety, efficiency and efficacy of Rb gene transfer. Until the results of this trial are known, the current status of TSG gene therapy can only be drawn from our experience with p53 (15, 28). First and foremost, it appears that corrective gene therapy targeting TSGs is both safe and feasible for the treatment of localized bladder cancer. Unfortunately, this knowledge must be tempered with the realization that inadequate transfection efficiency and suboptimal biologic activity have translated into poor clinical efficacy thus far. Future clinical trials evaluating TSG corrective strategies must therefore focus on improving vector delivery systems and subsequent transgene biologic activity before a full determination of the clinical efficacy of such a strategy can be made. Certainly, the successes of preclinical studies provide the impetus to do so.

5. Cytotoxic Strategies

The selective killing of tumor cells by cytotoxic gene therapy can be accomplished through two approaches, suicide gene transduction or replication-competent oncolytic viral transfection. Suicide genes encode for products with direct cytotoxicity towards tumor cells, or for enzymatic products which convert inactive pro-drugs into tumor-toxic substances. One strategy of great promise combines delivery of the suicide gene herpes simplex virus thymidine kinase (HSV-TK) with the systemic delivery of ganciclovir (GCV), a purine nucleoside analog. Since mammalian thymidine kinase (TK) cannot metabolize GCV, only transfected tumor cells which express HSV-TK are able to phosphorylate GCV into the monophosphate form. Mammalian TK can then convert GCV monophosphate into GCV triphosphate which leads to tumor cell death through competitive inhibition of DNA synthesis. Based on the successful pre-clinical results of this cytotoxic strategy towards other malignancies, including those of brain and prostate, HSV-TK/GCV has also been tested against bladder cancer (63). The first study to do so evaluated a replication-defective adenoviral construct containing HSV-TK linked to the rous sarcoma virus (RSV) promoter (Ad/RSV-TK). In vitro, this construct provided efficient genetic transduction and a tumor cell kill rate in excess of 95% upon the administration of GCV. In vivo, Ad/RSV-TK plus GCV led to a four-fold reduction in tumor growth and improved long-term host survival, without significant toxicity, relative to control animals (64). Effective tumor cell kill appears to be maintained with either intravesical instillation or intratumoral injection of HSV-TK (65, 66). Recent efforts have focused upon improving the oncologic efficacy of HSV-TK/GCV through a combination therapy or modification of the genetic construct. Substitution of the RSV promoter with the cytomegalovirus (CMV) promoter has been found to improve the tumoricidal potency of HSV-TK three to four-fold. However, this improvement in tumor cell kill was accomplished at the expense of higher dose-related hepatotoxicity with the CMV promoter construct (67). Although combination strategies have proven successful for other gene therapy techniques, the same cannot be said for HSV-TK/GCV. One such endeavour involved a dual gene construct encoding both HSV-TK and IL-2. While each agent lead to growth inhibition, sequential cytotoxic and cytokine gene therapy was not superior to HSV-TK/GCV alone (68). Similarly, the addition of doxorubicin, cisplatin, mitomycin C, or methotrexate to HSV-TK/GCV, individually, had no apparent benefit unless both agents were given at high dosages. Even with high-dose combination therapy, however, the incremental improvement in tumor cell kill amounts to only 10–20% (69).

The second approach to cytotoxic gene therapy involves replication-competent oncolytic viruses. These are genetically engineered, tumor-targeting viruses whose intracellular replication is directly toxic to tumor cells. The modified adenovirus, ONYX-015, which replicates preferentially in p53-mutated cells has demonstrated consistent safety and efficacy in phase I and II trials against tumors at other sites including hepatocellular carcinoma and metastatic sarcomas (70, 71). Although bladder cancer, with a high incidence of p53 mutation, would appear to be well-suited to this form of gene therapy, ONXY-015 has yet to be tested against urothelial carcinoma. More attention has been given to G207, a modified herpes simplex virus which preferentially targets rapidly dividing cells. Following transfection, tumor cell death occurs through viral-mediated cell lysis. In vivo, G207 appears to provide safe and effective local tumor control through both intravesical instillation and intratumoral injection. Of even greater significance, tumor regression has been demonstrated at distant metastatic sites after intravenous administration of G207. The importance of this finding cannot be understated because effective gene therapy options for metastatic bladder cancer are lacking (72). A third oncolytic virus with apparent efficacy against bladder cancer is NV1020, a mutant form of HSV-1 with a 700 base pair deletion in the thymidine kinase locus. Comparison of NV1020 and G207, both in vitro and in vivo, found that NV1020 provides superior tumor cell kill while maintaining a favourable toxicity profile (73). The adenovirus Ad-BSP-E1a has recently been added to the growing list of oncolytic viruses with potential use in bladder cancer. This conditionally replicating virus contains the gene E1a/b, a key regulator for viral replication, linked to a truncated bone sialoprotein (BSP) promoter. Instillation of Ad-BSP-E1a in an orthotopic murine bladder cancer model resulted in tumor growth inhibition and apoptosis based on the constitutive expression of BSP by TCC (74).

As with suicide gene therapy, the therapeutic potential of oncolytic viruses in combination with chemotherapy has also been investigated. NV1066, a modified herpes simplex type-1 virus lacking the genes ICP0 and ICP4, was administered in combination with intravesical mitomycin C. In vitro, NV1066 enhanced the cytotoxicity of mitomycin C which permitted a significant dose reduction of both agents while maintaining 90% cell kill (75). Although such a dose reduction is likely to improve the safety profile of oncolytic viruses, other efforts have focused on improving target specificity. One such method involves the manipulation of receptor-mediated viral transfection. As outlined earlier, receptor profiling studies have shown that CAR expression is not ubiquitous in bladder cancer, particularly among high-grade variants (19, 20). Epidermal growth factor receptor, on the other hand, appears to be more prevalent. Through the use of flow cytometry, EGF-R expression has been identified in seven out of seven human bladder cancer cell lines analyzed in one study. This same study found that the cytotoxicity of an oncolytic adenovirus could be improved by tagging virions with single chain Fv fragment antibodies specific for EGFR (23).

No phase I trials of cytotoxic gene therapy for bladder cancer have been performed to date. However, the safety and short-term efficacy of this treatment strategy in prostate cancer has been established in numerous clinical studies. The earliest study, a dose escalation trial, involved the intraprostatic injection of Ad/HSV-TK followed by systemic delivery of GCV into eighteen patients with biopsy-proven local recurrence after definitive radiotherapy. Three patients demonstrated a 50% or greater reduction in serum prostate specific antigen (PSA) lasting between 6 and 52 weeks. Side-effects were generally mild, with reversible grade 3 hepatotoxicity and grade 4 thrombocytopenia developing in only one patient at the highest dose level. Although vector-specific DNA remained detectable in urine up to one month post-treatment, cultures of both blood and urine were negative for adenoviral growth (76). In a similar study design, a cytosine deaminase/HSV-TK dual suicide gene construct led to a significant reduction in serum PSA in 3 of 16 patients, two of whom remained disease-free at one year. No dose-limiting toxicities were encountered and 94% of the adverse events were of mild to moderate severity (77). Suicide gene therapy has recently been tested in combination with definitive radiotherapy against moderate to high-risk localized prostate cancer. Recognizing that ionizing radiation improves the transfection and transduction efficiency of gene therapy and gene therapy interferes with the repair of radiation-induced DNA damage, it is hypothesized that such a combination may act against malignant cells in a synergistic manner (78). Phase I and II trials of single or dual suicide gene constructs, in combination with three-dimensional conformal or intensity-modulated radiotherapy for patients with localized prostate cancer, demonstrate acceptable toxicity and encouraging short term oncologic results. One such study found that the time interval to the serum PSA nadir correlated indirectly with the duration of pro-drug (5-fluorocytosine and valganciclovir) administration and may occur much earlier in patients receiving combination therapy relative to those receiving radiotherapy alone (79, 80).

In summary, numerous preclinical bladder cancer studies have demonstrated that cytotoxic gene therapy provides safe and effective local tumor control through the induction of suicide genes or viral-mediated tumor cell lysis. Also, the systemic delivery of replication competent oncolytic viruses such as G207, unlike other gene therapy techniques, has been shown to result in significant reduction of metastatic deposits. While the clinical safety of cytotoxic gene therapy may be extrapolated from the prostate cancer experience, the efficacy of this strategy against bladder cannot be determined until proper phase I and II trials are conducted. At the moment, a phase I trial of Ad/HSV-TK plus ganciclovir is actively accruing patients with locally advanced or treatment-refractory superficial bladder cancer (81). Patients will be observed for toxic side effects and will undergo transurethral resection or radical cystectomy two weeks after completing treatment in order to quantify the efficiency and efficacy of this suicide gene strategy. Future endeavours may focus on the use of cytotoxic gene therapy in the primary or neoadjuvant setting for local or locoregional control, respectively. Attention should also be directed towards combination strategies with radiotherapy, as well as determining the role of oncolytic viruses in the management of metastatic disease.

6. Immunomodulatory Gene Therapy

Similar to other malignancies, the initiation and propagation of bladder TCC often proceeds unchecked by the host immune system. Transitional cell carcinoma actively evades immunosurveillance or impairs effector cell function through numerous mechanisms, the most common of which include the altered presentation of tumor-specific antigens and the secretion of immunosuppressive cytokines (82). The goal of immunomodulatory gene therapy is to selectively stimulate the host immune system against tumor cells through the induction of genes encoding tumor-specific antigens or immune stimulatory cytokines. The transfection of target cells with vectors encoding such genes can take place in situ or ex vivo. Tumor cells which are genetically-modified ex vivo and subsequently returned to the host in order to stimulate the immune system constitute a "tumor vaccine."

Immunohistochemical studies demonstrate that the majority of bladder cancer cell lines are weak or non-immunogenic as a result of aberrant antigen presentation (83). Gene therapy techniques which induce antigen presentation in a tumor-specific manner have proven successful for other types of tumors and have recently also been applied to bladder cancer. One of the first studies to do so transfected murine bladder cancer cells with the cDNA of MPT59, an antigen isolated from mycobacteria. Transduction of the MPT59 antigen elicited a tumor-specific cytotoxic T cell response which led to complete regression of the transfected tumor. The establishment of protective immunity was also apparent since vaccinated animals were able to reject subsequent orthotopic tumor challenges (84). These results have since been duplicated using a variety of antigens including CD154, CD40L as well as a multicomponent antigen complex specific to mycobacterium bovis bacillus Calmette-Guerin (BCG) (85–87). When applied to a heterotopic murine bladder cancer model, the combination of four subcomponent BCG DNA vaccines (poly-rBCG) stimulated an intense T helper type 1 (Th1) cytokine response which significantly inhibited tumor growth and improved host survival. Indeed, a common finding among tumor vaccination studies is the stimulation of a Th1 immune response following antigen presentation. Based on data extrapolated from other tumor types, it does appear that the Th1 response is the primary mechanism by which the immune system eradicates tumor cells (88).

A second approach to immunomodulatory gene therapy involves the transduction of genes encoding potent immune stimulating cytokines. Prior experience has shown that the systemic delivery of certain cytokines, most notably interleukin-2 (IL-2), can result in the development of toxic side-effects including the capillary leak syndrome (89). The selective transduction of cytokine genes into malignant cells is advantageous in that it provides a high local concentration of cytokine without the potential toxicity associated with systemic delivery. Cytokines with established efficacy in preclinical gene therapy studies include IL-2, IL-12, IL-21, interferon-alpha (IFNα) and INFγ (26, 90, 91). The primary mechanism by which the transduction of such cytokines inhibits tumor cell growth is through the activation of a Th1 CD8 immune response; however, additional mechanisms clearly play an important role. Interferon-α2b has recently been shown to inhibit angiogenesis through the down-regulation of VEGF (92). Interleukin-2, which has received the most attention in cytokine gene therapy, has demonstrated significant anti-tumor effect in at least four separate in vivo bladder cancer models (93–96). Using various IL-2 transfection methods, each of these studies observed significant regression of the primary tumor, as well as the prevention of malignant re-growth, indicating the development of tumor-specific immunologic memory. The efficacy of IL-2 and INFγ have been compared in an orthotopic animal model in which tumor cells were transfected by a retroviral vector ex vivo and then re-administered systemically. While the expression of both cytokines established an immunologic memory against future tumor growth, only IL-2 resulted in significant regression of established tumor deposits. Furthermore, there did not appear to be any added benefit to combination therapy (93). A second study of similar design compared the results of five separately transfected cytokines and found that only IL-2 and granulocyte-macrophage colony stimulating factor (GM-CSF) effectively controlled primary tumors while IL-1α, IL-1β and IFNγ were ineffective (96). Of interest, two other studies evaluating the efficacy of IFNγ vaccination through in vivo transfection demonstrated a complete response rate of up to 50% as well as improved overall survival (97, 98). Although numerous methodological differences may explain the conflicting results of these IFNγ studies, it remains to be determined if in vivo transfection is more efficacious than ex vivo. At the present time, no cytokine has been subject to such a comparison in a bladder cancer model. The results of two other studies do, however, advocate for in vivo liposome-mediated transduction. Citing a 40% complete response rate and strong immunologic memory with intravesical instillation of liposomes containing the IL-2 gene, the first study points out that in situ liposome delivery obviates the need for tissue procurement, a necessity with ex vivo transduction (95). The second study, an objective comparison of retroviral and liposome IL-2 vectors in a murine model, demonstrated superior tumor regression and host survival in the liposome arm (99).

Immunomodulatory studies performed in other tumor types, such as lung cancer and sarcoma, have demonstrated the importance of co-stimulation. Whereas tumor vaccination based on the transduction of a single immunogenic molecule consistently prevents the growth of new tumors, regression of an established tumor is often incomplete. Co-stimulation involves the transduction of multiple antigens or cytokines and has been shown to improve the primary tumor response in both lung cancer and sarcoma (100, 101). Evidence also exists for the use of dual immunogene therapy in bladder cancer. One study comparing the efficacy of a combination rBCG/IL-2 vaccine to either vaccine alone found a stronger Th1 immune response, superior tumor reduction and improved host survival with dual vaccination (85). Likewise, the transduction and vaccination of IL-2 together with the co-stimulatory molecule B7.1 demonstrated clear superiority to IL-2 alone in terms of primary tumor regression, complete response rate, immunity to subsequent tumor re-challenge, and host survival (99).

As is the case for most gene therapy strategies, there is little clinical data available regarding the safety and efficacy of immunomodulatory gene therapy in bladder cancer. Recently, the preliminary results of a phase I dose-escalation trial of CG0070 in patients with BCG-refractory superficial bladder cancer have been presented (102). CG0070, a replication competent adenovirus modified to express GM-CSF, replicates preferentially in cells with defective Rb function as found in TCC. Based on preclinical evidence of selective cytotoxicity and immunostimulation, CG0070 was delivered intravesically to six patients with Ta, T1, or CIS bladder cancer refractory to BCG. Treatment-related side effects were generally mild and consisted of dysuria, urgency and malaise. No grade three or four adverse events were noted. At this time, data concerning treatment efficacy is only available for three patients. Cystoscopy performed 8 days after treatment demonstrated tumor regression in all cases, and a complete response was noted in one patient at 12 weeks. This would appear to provide initial evidence of anti-tumor activity with CG0070 in a relatively treatment-resistant subgroup of bladder cancer patients. A second phase I trial is actively accruing patients with invasive bladder cancer awaiting cystectomy to undergo intravesical therapy with fowlpox-GM-CSF and/or fowlpox-TRICOM which encodes three separate co-stimulatory molecules

(B7.1, ICAM-I and LFA-3) (103). The purpose of this study is to determine the maximum tolerated dose and safety profile of these two regimens alone or in combination as well as to clarify the importance of co-stimulation with regard to the generation of a local and systemic immunologic response. A third clinical trial, which is not yet open, plans to evaluate the safety and tolerability of recombinant INF-α2b gene transfer via an intravesically-delivered adenoviral vector (104). Additional questions which deserve future clinical study include the relative potency of available cytokines and transfection methods, as well as the relative value of dual immunogene therapy. Perhaps most important is the issue of protective immunity. Should clinical trials duplicate the tumor-specific immunologic memory observed in some pre-clinical gene therapy studies, the implications for bladder cancer with a recurrence rate approaching 70% would be significant.

7. Summary

The propensity of bladder cancer to recur or progress in the face of standard treatment begs strongly for the development of new and improved therapeutic modalities. Gene therapy clearly represents one such modality. Inspired by the recognition of aberrant genetic events involved in the initiation, promotion and progression of the neoplastic process, numerous genetic strategies have been developed and evaluated. Corrective, cytotoxic and immunomodulatory strategies directed against a wide variety of genetic targets have all demonstrated efficacy against bladder cancer in vitro and in vivo. Furthermore, numerous gene therapy techniques appear to work in a synergistic manner with conventional chemotherapeutic agents. Immunogene therapy offers the additional prospect of long term protective immunity against the formation of recurrent bladder tumors.

While only a few phase I trials examining the role of gene therapy in bladder cancer have reached completion, it does appear that intravesical gene therapy is both safe and feasible. However, the sub-optimal transfection efficiency and minimal biologic activity demonstrated in recent trials represent significant obstacles that must be addressed. Likewise, target specificity, through the manipulation of receptor-mediated transfection or site-restricted expression, must be optimized in order to improve the efficacy and safety profile of local and systemic gene therapy. Only then can we hope to translate the successes of preclinical gene therapy studies into a clinical reality.

References

1. Jemal A, Siegel R, Ward E, Murray T, Xu J et al. Cancer statistics, 2005. CA Cancer J Clin 2006; 56(2):106–30.
2. Shelley MD, Wilt TJ, Court J, Coles B, Kynaston H, Mason MD. Intravesical bacillus Calmette-Guerin is superior to mitomycin C in reducing tumour recurrence in high-risk superficial bladder cancer: a meta-analysis of randomized trials. BJU Int 2004; 93(4):485–90.
3. Sternberg CN. Current perspectives in muscle invasive bladder cancer. Eur J Cancer 2002; 38(4):460–7.
4. von der Masse H, Sengelov L, Roberts JT, Ricci S, Dogliotti L, Oliver T, Moore MJ, Zimmermann A, Arning M. Long-term survival results of a randomized trial comparing gemcitabine plus cisplatin, with methotrexate, vinblastine, doxorubicin, plus cisplatin in patients with bladder cancer. J Clin Oncol 2005; 23(21):4602–8.
5. Ardelt P, Bohle A. Molecular aspects of bladder cancer IV: gene therapy of bladder cancer. Eur Urol 2002; 41(4):372–80.
6. Irie A. Advances in gene therapy for bladder cancer. Curr Gene Ther 2003; 3(1):1–11.
7. Check E. Harmful potential of viral vectors fuels doubts over gene therapy. Nature 2003; 423:573–574.
8. Crystal RG. Transfer of genes to humans: early lessons and obstacles to success. Science 1995; 270:404.
9. Yang Y, Nunes F, Berencsi K et al. Cellular immunity to viral antigens limits E1-deleted adenoviruses for gene therapy. Proc Natl Acad Sci USA 1994; 91:4407.
10. Assessment of adenoviral vector safety and toxicity: report of the National Institutes of Health Recombinant DNA Advisory Committee. Hum Gene Ther 2002;13(1):3–13.
11. Tomanin R, Scarpa M. Why do we need new gene therapy viral vectors? Characteristics, limitations and future perspectives of viral vector transduction. Curr Gene Ther 2004; 4(4):357–72.
12. Palmer DJ, Ng P. Helper-dependent adenoviral vectors for gene therapy. Hum Gene Ther 2005; 16(1):1–16.
13. Harimoto K, Sugimura K, Lee CR, Kuratsukuri K, Kishimoto T. In vivo gene transfer methods in the bladder without viral vectors. Br J Urol 1998; 81(6):870–4.
14. Haviernik P, Bunting KD. Safety concerns related to hematopoietic stem cell gene transfer using retroviral vectors. Curr Gene Ther 2004; 4(3):263–76.
15. Kuball J, Wen SF, Leissner J, Atkins D, Meinhardt P et al. Successful adenovirus-mediated wild-type p53 gene transfer in patients with bladder cancer by intravesical vector instillation. J Clin Oncol 2002; 20(4):957–65.

16. Connor RJ, Engler H, Machemer T, Philopena JM, Horn MT et al. Identification of polyamides that enhance adenovirus-mediated gene expression in the urothelium. Gene Ther 2001; 8(1):41–8.
17. Yamashita M, Rosser CJ, Zhou JH, Zhang XQ, Connor RJ et al. Syn3 provides high levels of intravesical adenoviral-mediated gene transfer for gene therapy of genetically altered urothelium and superficial bladder cancer. Cancer Gene Ther 2002; 9(8):687–91.
18. Loskog A, Hedlund T, Wester K, de al Torre M, Philipson L et al. Human urinary bladder carcinomas express adenovirus attachment and internalization receptors. Gene Ther 2002; 9(9):547–53.
19. Li Y, Pong RC, Bergelson JM, Hall MC, Sagalowsky AI, Tseng CP, Wang Z et al. Loss of adenoviral receptor expression in human bladder cancer cells: a potential impact on the efficacy of gene therapy. Cancer Res 1999; 59(2):325–30.
20. Sachs MD, Rauen KA, Ramamurthy M, Dodson JL, De Marzo AM et al. Integrin alpha(v) and coxsackie adenovirus receptor expression in clinical bladder cancer. Urology 2002; 60(3):531–6.
21. Okegawa T, Pong RC, Li Y, Bergelson JM, Sagalowsky AI, Hsieh JT. The mechanism of the growth-inhibitory effect of coxsackie and adenovirus receptor (CAR) on human bladder cancer: a functional analysis of car protein structure. Cancer Res 2001; 61(17):6592–600.
22. Okegawa T, Nutahara K, Pong RC, Higashihara E, Hsieh JT. Enhanced transgene expression in urothelial cancer gene therapy with histone deacetylase inhibitor. J Urol 2005; 174(2):747–52.
23. van der Poel HG, Molenaar B, van Beusechem VW, Haisma HJ, Rodriguez R et al. Epidermal growth factor receptor targeting of replication competent adenovirus enhances cytotoxicity in bladder cancer. J Urol 2002; 168(1):266–72.
24. Mizuguchi H, Hayakawa T. Adenovirus vectors containing chimeric type 5 and type 35 fiber proteins exhibit altered and expanded tropism and increase the size limit of foreign genes. Gene 2002; 285(1–2):69–77.
25. Siemens DR, Austin JC, See WA, Tartaglia J, Ratliff TL. Evaluation of gene transfer efficiency by viral vectors to murine bladder epithelium. J Urol 2001; 165(2):667–71.
26. Tao Z, Connor RJ, Ashoori F, Dinney CP, Munsell M et al. Efficacy of a single intravesical treatment with Ad-IFN/Syn 3 is dependent on dose and urine IFN concentration obtained: implications for clinical investigation. Cancer Gene Ther 2006; 13(2):125–30.
27. Gomella LG, Mastrangelo MJ, McCue PA, Maguire HC Jr, Mulholland SG et al. Phase i study of intravesical vaccinia virus as a vector for gene therapy of bladder cancer. J Urol 2001; 166(4):1291–5.
28. Pagliaro LC, Keyhani A, Williams D, Woods D, Liu B et al. Repeated intravesical instillations of an adenoviral vector in patients with locally advanced bladder cancer: a phase I study of p53 gene therapy. J Clin Oncol 2003; 21(12):2247–53.
29. Shirakawa T, Hamada K, Zhang Z, Okada H, Tagawa M et al. A cox-2 promoter-based replication-selective adenoviral vector to target the cox-2-expressing human bladder cancer cells. Clin Cancer Res 2004; 10(13):4342–8.
30. Zhu HJ, Zhang ZQ, Zeng XF, Wei SS, Zhang ZW, Guo YL. Cloning and analysis of human UroplakinII promoter and its application for gene therapy in bladder cancer. Cancer Gene Ther 2004; 11(4):263–72.
31. Irie A, Anderegg B, Kashani-Sabet M, Ohkawa T, Suzuki T et al. Therapeutic efficacy of an adenovirus-mediated anti-H-ras ribozyme in experimental bladder cancer. Antisense Nucleic Acid Drug Dev 1999; 9(4):341–9.
32. Watanabe T, Shinohara N, Sazawa A, Takimoto M, Hashimoto A et al. Adenovirus-mediated gene therapy for bladder cancer in an orthotopic model using a dominant negative H-ras mutant. Int J Cancer 2001; 92(5):712–7.
33. Irie A, Kashani-Sabet M, Scanlon KJ, Uchida T, Baba S. Hammerhead ribozymes as therapeutic agents for bladder cancer. Mol Urol 2000; 4(2):61–6.
34. Mizutani Y, Fukumoto M, Bonavida B, Yoshida O. Enhancement of sensitivity of urinary bladder tumor cells to cisplatin by c-myc antisense oligonucleotide. Cancer; 74(9):2546–54.
35. Bilim V, Kashara T, Noboru H, Takahashi K, Tomita Y. Caspase involved synergistic cytotoxicity of bcl-2 antisense oligonucleotides and adriamycin on transitional cell cancer cells. Cancer Lett 2000; 155(2):191–8.
36. Zhang Z, Zeng G, Zhang Z. Impact of extracellular gene of VEGF receptor KDR on growth of human bladder carcinoma in nude rats. Zhonghua Yi Xue Za Zhi 2001; 81(11):684–6.
37. Inoue K, Perrotte P, Wood CG, Slaton JW, Sweeney P et al. Gene therapy of human bladder cancer with adenovirus-mediated antisense basic fibroblast growth factor. Clin Cancer Res 2000; 6(11):4422–31.
38. Oxford G, Theodorescu D. The role of Ras superfamily proteins in bladder cancer progression. J Urol 2003; 170(5):1987–93
39. Schmitz-Drager BJ, Schulz WA, Jurgens B, Gerharz CD, van Roeyen CR et al. C-myc in bladder cancer. Clinical findings and analysis of mechanism. Urol Res; 25(Suppl 1):S45–9.
40. Scanlon KJ, Ishida H, Kashani-Sabet M. Ribozyme-mediated reversal of the multidrug-resistant phenotype. Proc Natl Acad Sci USA 1994; 91(23):11123–7.
41. Nogawa M, Yuasa Ti, Kimura S, Tanaka M, Kuroda J et al. Intravesical administration of small interfering RNA targeting PLK-1 successfully prevents the growth of bladder cancer. J Clin Invest 2005; 115(4):978–85.

42. Ning S, Fuessel S, Kotzsch M, Kraemer K, Kappler M et al. siRNA-mediated down-regulation of survivin inhibits bladder cancer cell growth. Int J Oncol 2004; 25(4):1065–71.
43. Fuessel S, Herrmann J, Ning S, Kotzsch M, Kraemer K et al. Chemosensitization of bladder cancer cells by survivin-directed antisense oligodeoxynucleotides and siRNA. Cancer Lett 2006; 232(2):243–54.
44. Burmeister Y, Kraemer K, Fuessel S, Kotzsch M, Meye A et al. Multitarget gene inhibition by synthetic nucleic acids in bladder cancer cells. J Urol 2006; 175(Supp 4):202.
45. Knowles MA. The genetics of transitional cell carcinoma: progress and potential clinical application. BJU Int 1999; 84(4):412–27.
46. Reznikoff CA, Belair CD, Yeager TR, Savelieva E, Blelloch RH et al. A molecular genetic model of human bladder cancer pathogenesis. Semin Oncol 1996; 23(5):571–84.
47. Wada Y, Gotoh A, Chirakawa T, Hamada K, Kamidono S. Gene therapy for bladder cancer using adenoviral vector. Mol Urol 2001; 5(2):47–52.
48. Irie A, Uchida T, Ishida H, Matsumoto K, Iwamura M, Baba S. p53 mutation in bladder cancer patients in Japan and inhibition of growth by in vitro adenovirus-mediated wild-type p53 transduction in bladder cancer cells. Mol Urol 2001; 5(2):53–8.
49. Fodor I, Timiryasova T, Denes B, Yoshida J, Ruckle H, Lilly M. Vaccinia virus mediated p53 gene therapy for bladder cancer in an orthotopic murine model. J Urol 2005; 173(2):604–9.
50. Yang C, Cirielli C, Capogrossi MC, Passaniti A. Adenovirus-mediated wild-type p53 expression induces apoptosis and suppresses tumorigenesis of prostatic tumor cells. Cancer Res 1995; 55(19):4210–3.
51. Sugrue MM, Shin DY, Lee SW, Aaronson SA. Wild-type p53 triggers a rapid senescence program in human tumor cells lacking functional p53. Proc Natl Acad Sci USA 1997; 94(18):9648–53.
52. Pan CX, Koeneman KS. A novel tumor-specific gene therapy for bladder cancer. Med Hypotheses 1999; 53(2):130–5.
53. Miyake H, Hara I, Gohji K, Yamanaka K, Arakawa S, Kamidono S. Enhancement of chemosensitivity in human bladder cancer cells by adenoviral-mediated p53 gene transfer. Anticancer Res 1998; 18(4C): 3087–92.
54. Miyake H, Hara I, Hara S, Arakawa S, Kamidono S. Synergistic chemosensitization and inhibition of tumor growth and metastasis by adenovirus-mediated P53 gene transfer in human bladder cancer model. Urology 2000; 56(2):332–6.
55. Irie A, Matsumoto K, Anderegg B, Kuruma H, Kashani-Sabet M et al. Growth inhibition efficacy of an adenovirus expressing dual therapeutic genes, wild-type p53, and anti-erbB2 ribozyme, against human bladder cancer cells. Cancer Gene Ther 2006; 13(3):298–305.
56. Miyake H, Yamanaka K, Muramaki M, Hara I, Gleave ME. Therapeutic efficacy of adenoviral-mediated p53 gene transfer is synergistically enhanced by combined use of antisense oligodeoxynucleotide targeting clusterin gene in a human bladder cancer model. Neoplasia 2005; 7(2):171–9.
57. Xu HJ, Zhou Y, Seigne J, Perng GS, Mixon M et al. Enhanced tumor suppressor gene therapy via replication-deficient adenovirus vectors expressing an N-terminal truncated retinoblastoma protein. Cancer Res 1996; 56(10):2245–9.
58. Zhang X, Multani AS, Zhou JH, Shay JW, McConkey D et al. Adenoviral-mediated retinoblastoma 94 produces rapid telomere erosion, chromosomal crisis, and caspase-dependent apoptosis in bladder cancer and immortalized human urothelial cells but not in normal urothelial cells. Cancer Res 2003; 63(4):760–5.
59. Sazawa A, Watanabe T, Tanaka M, Haga K, Fujita H et al. Adenovirus mediated gelsolin gene therapy for orthotopic human bladder cancer in nude mice. J Urol 2002; 168(3):1182–7.
60. Sudarshan S, Holman DH, Hyer ML, Voelkel-Johnson C, Dong JY et al. In vitro efficacy of Fas ligand gene therapy for the treatment of bladder cancer. Cancer Gene Ther 2005; 12(1):12–8.
61. Hall MC, Li Y, Pong RC, Ely B, Sagalowsky AI, Hsieh JT. The growth inhibitory effect of p21 adenovirus on human bladder cancer cells. J Urol 2000; 163(3): 1033–8.
62. Lee CT, Seol JY, Park KH, Yoo CG, Kim YW et al. Differential effects of adenovirus-p16 on bladder cancer cell lines can be overcome by the addition of butyrate. Clin Cancer Res 2001; 7(1):210–4.
63. Culver KW, Van Gilder J, Link CJ, Carlstrom T, Buroker T et al. Gene therapy for the treatment of malignant brain tumors with in vivo tumor transduction with the herpes simplex thymidine kinase gene/ganciclovir system. Hum Gene Ther 1994; 5(3):343–79.
64. Sutton MA, Berkman SA, Chen SH, Block A, Dang TD et al. Adenovirus-mediated suicide gene therapy for experimental bladder cancer. Urology 1997; 49(2): 173–80.
65. Cheon J, Moon du G, Cho HY, Park HS, Kim JJ et al. Adenovirus-mediated suicide-gene therapy in an orthotopic murine bladder tumor model. Int J Urol 2002; 9(5):261–7.
66. Akasaka S, Suzuki H, Igarashi T, Akimoto M, Shimada T. Suicide gene therapy for chemically induced rat bladder tumor entailing instillation of adenoviral vectors. Jpn J Cancer Res 2001; 92(5):568–75.
67. Freund CT, Tong XW, Block A, Contant CF, Kieback DG et al. Adenovirus-mediated suicide gene therapy for bladder cancer: comparison of the cytomegalovirus- and

Rous sarcoma virus-promoter. Anticancer Res 2000; 20(5A):2811–6.
68. Freund CT, Sutton MA, Dang T, Contant CF, Rowley D et al. Adenovirus-mediated combination suicide and cytokine gene therapy for bladder cancer. Anticancer Res 2000; 20(3A):1359–65.
69. Freund CT, Tong XW, Rowley D, Engehausen D, Frolov A et al. Combination of adenovirus-mediated thymidine kinase gene therapy with cytotoxic chemotherapy in bladder cancer in vitro. Urol Oncol 2003; 21(3): 197–205.
70. Galanis E, Okuno SH, Nascimento AG, Lewis BD, Lee RA et al. Phase I-II trial of ONYX-015 in combination with MAP chemotherapy in patients with advanced sarcomas. Gene Ther 2005; 12(5):437–45.
71. Makower D, Rozenblit A, Kaufman H, Edelman M, Lane ME et al. Phase II clinical trial of intralesional administration of the oncolytic adenovirus ONYX-015 in patients with hepatobiliary tumors with correlative p53 studies. Clin Cancer Res 2003; 9(2):693–702.
72. Oyama M, Ohigashi T, Hoshi M, Nakashima J, Tachibana M et al. Intravesical and intravenous therapy of human bladder cancer by the herpes vector G207. Hum Gene Ther 2000; 11(12):1683–93.
73. Cozzi PJ, Malhotra S, McAuliffe P, Kooby DA, Federoff HJ et al. Intravesical oncolytic viral therapy using attenuated, replication-competent herpes simplex viruses G207 and Nv1020 is effective in the treatment of bladder cancer in an orthotopic syngeneic model. FASEB J 2001; 15(7):1306–8.
74. Melquist JJ, Kacka M, Li Y, Malaeb BS, Elmore J et al. Conditionally replicating adenovirus-mediated gene therapy in bladder cancer: an orthotopic in vivo model. Urol Oncol 2006; 24(4):362–71.
75. Mullerad M, Bochner BH, Adusumilli PS, Bhargava A, Kikuchi E et al. Herpes simplex virus based gene therapy enhances the efficacy of mitomycin C for the treatment of human bladder transitional cell carcinoma. J Urol 2005; 174(2):741–6.
76. Herman JR, Adler HL, Aguilar-Cordova E, Rojas-Martinez A, Woo S et al. In situ gene therapy for adenocarcinoma of the prostate: a phase I clinical trial. Hum Gene Ther 1999; 10(7):1239–49.
77. Freytag SO, Khil M, Stricker H, Peabody J, Menon M et al. Phase I study of replication-competent adenovirus-mediated double suicide gene therapy for the treatment of locally recurrent prostate cancer. Cancer Res 2002; 62(17):4968–76.
78. Teh BS, Aguilar-Cordova E, Vlachaki MT, Aguilar L, Mai WY et al. Combining radiotherapy with gene therapy (from the bench to the bedside): a novel treatment strategy for prostate cancer. Oncologist 2002; 7(5):458–66.
79. Freytag SO, Stricker H, Pegg J, Paielli D, Pradhan DG et al. Phase I study of replication-competent adenovirus-mediated double-suicide gene therapy in combination with conventional-dose three-dimensional conformal radiation therapy for the treatment of newly diagnosed, intermediate- to high-risk prostate cancer. Cancer Res 2003; 63(21):7497–506.
80. Teh BS, Ayala G, Aguilar L, Mai WY, Timme TL et al. Phase I-II trial evaluating combined intensity-modulated radiotherapy and in situ gene therapy with or without hormonal therapy in treatment of prostate cancer-interim report on PSA response and biopsy data. Int J Radiat Oncol Biol Phys 2004; 58(5): 1520–9.
81. Lerner, SP. Phase I Trial of Adenoviral Mediated Suicide Gene Therapy with HSV-tk Followed by Intravenous Administration of Ganciclovir in Patients with Locally Advanced and Refractory Superficial Bladder Cancer. Protocol # 0110-500. GeMCRIS July 2006. http://www.gemcris.od.nih.gov.
82. Radoja S, Frey AB. Cancer-induced defective cytotoxic T lymphocyte effector function: another mechanism how antigenic tumors escape immune-mediated killing. Mol Med 2000; 6(6):465–79.
83. Nouri AM, Hussain RF, Oliver RT. The frequency of major histocompatibility complex antigen abnormalities in urological tumours and their correction by gene transfection or cytokine stimulation. Cancer Gene Ther 1994; 1(2):119–23.
84. Kuromatsu I, Matsuo K, Takamura S, Kim G, Takebe Y et al. Induction of effective antitumor immune responses in a mouse bladder tumor model by using DNA of an alpha antigen from mycobacteria. Cancer Gene Ther 2001; 8(7):483–90.
85. Lee CF, Chang SY, Hsieh DS, Yu DS. Treatment of bladder carcinomas using recombinant BCG DNA vaccines and electroporative gene immunotherapy. Cancer Gene Ther 2004; 11(3):194–207.
86. Loskog A, Bjorkland A, Brown MP, Korsgren O, Malmstrom PU, Totterman TH. Potent antitumor effects of CD154 transduced tumor cells in experimental bladder cancer. J Urol 2001; 166(3):1093–7.
87. Loskog AS, Fransson ME, Totterman TT. AdCD40L gene therapy counteracts T regulatory cells and cures aggressive tumors in an orthotopic bladder cancer model. Clin Cancer Res 2005; 11(24):8816–21.
88. Nishimura T, Iwakabe K, Sekimoto M, Ohmi Y, Yahata T et al. Distinct role of antigen-specific T helper type 1 (Th1) and Th2 cells in tumor eradication in vivo. J Exp Med 1999; 190(5):617–27.
89. Lindemann A, Hoffken K, Schmidt RE, Diehl V, Kloke O et al. phase-II study of low-dose cyclophosphamide and recombinant human interleukin-2 in metastatic renal cell carcinoma and malignant melanoma. Cancer Immunol Immunother 1989; 28(4):275–81.
90. Horinaga M, Harsch KM, Fukuyama R, Heston W, Larchian W. Intravesical interleukin-12 gene therapy

in an orthotopic bladder cancer model. Urology 2005; 66(2):461–6.
91. Hara I, Furukawa J, Yamanaka K, Yamada Y, Fujisawa M. Usefulness of cancer vaccine therapy using bladder cancer cell line introduced with interleukin-21 gene. J Urol 2006; 175(Supp 4):201.
92. Adam L, Kassouf W, McConkey D, Munsell M, Benedict W et al. Adenoviral-mediated IFN-alpha2b expression suppresses proangiogenic factors in bladder cancer. J Urol 2006; 175(Supp 4):270.
93. Connor J, Bannerji R, Saito S, Heston W, Fair W et al. Regression of bladder tumors in mice treated with interleukin 2 gene-modified tumor cells. J Exp Med 1993; 177(4):1127–34.
94. Milella M, Jacobelli J, Cavallo F, Guarini A, Velotti F et al. Interleukin-2 gene transfer into human transitional cell carcinoma of the urinary bladder. Br J Cancer 1999; 79(5–6):770–9.
95. Horiguchi Y, Larchian WA, Kaplinsky R, Fair WR, Heston WD. Intravesical liposome-mediated interleukin-2 gene therapy in orthotopic murine bladder cancer model. Gene Ther 2000; 7(10):844–51.
96. Saito S, Bannerji R, Gansbacher B, Rosenthal FM, Romanenko P et al. Immunotherapy of bladder cancer with cytokine gene-modified tumor vaccines. Cancer Res 1994; 54(13):3516–20.
97. Hashimura T, Ueda T, Hiura M, Yoshida O, Kawabata K et al. Gene therapy by in vivo interferon-gamma gene transfer to murine bladder tumor. Hinyokika Kiyo 1997; 43(11):809–13.
98. Shiau AL, Lin CY, Tzai TS, Wu CL. Postoperative immuno-gene therapy of murine bladder tumor by in vivo administration of retroviruses expressing mouse interferon-gamma. Cancer Gene Ther 2001; 8(1):73–81.
99. Larchian WA, Horiguchi Y, Nair SK, Fair WR, Heston WD et al. Effectiveness of combined interleukin 2 and B7.1 vaccination strategy is dependent on the sequence and order: a liposome-mediated gene therapy treatment for bladder cancer. Clin Cancer Res 2000; 6(7): 2913–20.
100. Fujii H, Inobe M, Kimura F, Murata J, Murakami M et al. Vaccination of tumor cells transfected with the B7-1 (CD80) gene induces the anti-metastatic effect and tumor immunity in mice. Int J Cancer 1996; 66(2):219–24.
101. Baskar S, Glimcher L, Nabavi N, Jones RT, Ostrand-Rosenberg S. Major histocompatibility complex class II + B7-1+ tumor cells are potent vaccines for stimulating tumor rejection in tumor-bearing mice. J Exp Med 1995; 181(2):619–29.
102. Lamm D, Stephensom J, Tsai H, Nemunaitis J, Goldstein M et al. A phase I dose-escalation trial of intravesical CG0070 for superficial transitional cell carcinoma (TCC) of the bladder after bacillus calmette-guerin (BCG) failure. J Urol 2006; 175(Supp 4):272.
103. Weiss, RJ. Phase I Study of Intravesical Recombinant Fowlpox-Gm-CSF (rF-GM-CSF) and/or Recombinant Fowlpox-Tricom (rF-TRICOM) in Patients with Bladder Carcinoma Scheduled for Cystectomy. 0304-581. GeMCRIS July 2006. http://www.gemcris.od.nih.gov.
104. Dinney, CP. A Phase I Study of the Safety and Tolerability of Intravesical Administration of SCH 721015 (rAd-IFN) in Patients with Transitional Cell Carcinoma of the Bladder. Protocol # 0501-688. GeMCRIS July 2006. http://www.gemcris.od.nih.gov.

Index

L

M

N

O